Bo Tice.

AN ATLAS OF

Normal Radiographic Anatomy

By

ISADORE MESCHAN, M.A., M.D.

Professor and Director, Department of Radiology, Bowman
Gray School of Medicine of Wake Forest College,
Winston-Salem, North Carolina; Consultant, Walter Reed Army
Medical Center, Washington, D.C.; Formerly
Professor and Head of the Department of Radiology,
University of Arkansas School of Medicine

With the assistance of

R. M. F. FARRER-MESCHAN,
M.B., B.S. (Melbourne, Australia), M.D.

Research Associate, Department of Radiology,
Bowman Gray School of Medicine of Wake Forest College,
Winston-Salem, North Carolina

SECOND EDITION – 1446 Illustrations on 412 Figures

W. B. SAUNDERS COMPANY

Philadelphia and London

W. B. Saunders Company: West Washington Square
Philadelphia, Pa. 19105

12 Dyott Street
London, WC1A 1DB

An Atlas of Normal Radiographic Anatomy.   SBN   0–7216–6270–6

Print No.   15   14   13   12   11

TO
OUR PARENTS

PREFACE TO THE SECOND EDITION

RADIOGRAPHIC ANATOMY has now achieved a definite place in most medical and para-medical curricula and progress in the past eight years has been so great as to necessitate this new edition.

Anatomists are gaining an increasing awareness of the value of the x-ray beam as a dissecting tool, and as a valuable technique for supplementing conventional dissection exercises with demonstrations of in vivo anatomic study. Practically every discipline in clinical medicine is also making increasing use of this diagnostic medium.

Once again it has not been our purpose to present an encyclopedic reference, but rather a practical, useful text for medical students, general practictioners, residents, especially in radiology, and x-ray technicians.

The areas of major revision or addition are as follows:

A chapter on radiation protection has been added in view of the increasing necessity for consideration of this facet by anyone who would utilize x-radiation for any purpose.

The chapter dealing with bone growth and development has been completely rewritten in the light of more dynamic concepts of this area. Also, more comprehensive bone growth tables have been included.

The radiographic reproductions and their tracings have been replaced by new illustrations where some loss of detail has been encountered in the engravure process. Log Etronic prints have been utilized in many areas—particularly in the skull.

The chapter on the radiographic study of the brain has been considerably modified. The selective study of the posterior fossa by pneumoencephalography has been introduced; and greater emphasis has been placed on arteriography and venography of the brain.

Additions have been made to the chapter on the spine. The increasing importance of cervical myelography has necessitated greater emphasis in this area.

The special studies of the heart and major blood vessels probably represent the area of greatest development in radiographic anatomy. These studies have kept pace with newer surgical efforts in the area of attempted correction of cardiovascular abnormalities. Advances in cardiovascular radiographic anatomy (and physiology) are basic to this progress and have been included here.

Advances in gastrointestinal radiographic anatomy have been included, such as: (1) the new concepts of the swallowing function gained from cineradiography, and the esophago-gastric junction; (2) measurements of the stomach and

v

its relationship to the spine and retrogastric structures with special emphasis on the importance of the left lateral erect stomach film study; and (3) the improved double contrast colloidal barium and air colon study.

It has been possible to visualize the biliary passages in greater detail; and with improved media for this purpose, the radiographic anatomy of this area has been revised.

New illustrations have been introduced wherever possible to demonstrate confusing appearances and variations of normal.

Medical textbook writing and revision are severe task masters. The authors are grateful to many people who have made the project less arduous. We are especially indebted to Mr. George Lynch, who, as artist, student of anatomy and Director of the Department of Medical Illustration of the Bowman Gray School of Medicine has given us incomparable aid and guidance. Photographers, Tom Webster and Jack Dent, have done their utmost to give us true photographic prints of the transilluminated roentgen image. Mrs. Rolene Ward, Chief X-Ray Technician at the North Carolina Baptist Hospital, has helped greatly in obtaining improved radiographs whenever they were deemed necessary. Mrs. Joan Cave deserves special mention for typing the revised manuscript and index.

Frequent critical comments by our associates and students have helped us greatly in formulating our concept of what should or should not be included or clarified. A special note of gratitude in this regard is directed to our associates, Dr. James F. Martin and Dr. Damon D. Blake.

Once again we also express our deep appreciation to the publishers who have always encouraged and helped us unstintingly in our endeavor to present this subject in the best possible way.

THE AUTHORS

PREFACE TO THE FIRST EDITION

DIAGNOSTIC radiology has progressed with tremendous strides and now occupies a most important position in clinical medicine. Whereas only a few years ago the practice of diagnostic radiology was confined to a relatively few highly trained specialists, it is now recognized that some knowledge of the fundamentals of radiology is a requirement for any medical practice.

The organization of the teaching of radiology in medical schools is therefore undergoing considerable change. Only a few years ago it was deemed adequate for a well-balanced medical curriculum to include only a single didactic course in radiology of perhaps fifteen one-hour lectures. By popular demand and by necessity this has been changed, for the following reasons:

1. Teachers of morbid anatomy are attempting to correlate the anatomy of the dead more closely with that of the living. Radiographic anatomy furnishes an excellent opportunity for such correlation.

2. Teachers of radiology have realized that before the student or resident can learn pathologic concepts in radiology, a basic knowledge of the *normal* must be obtained

3. Teachers of clinical medicine have felt a lack of basic training in radiology which requires a knowledge of the normal, before the abnormal can be understood.

4. General practitioners, who have long comprised the backbone of medical practice, have needed a ready guide and reference for their everyday problems, and for more intelligent consultation with the specialist in radiology.

This present book was undertaken in an effort to fulfill some of the needs for these four diverse and yet related groups of individuals. It has been our purpose to make convenient for the student a single compendium of normal radiographic anatomy which will include: (1) basic morbid anatomy as it is applicable to radiography; (2) the manner in which the routine projections employed in radiography are obtained; (3) a concept of the film so obtained; (4) the anatomic parts best visualized on these views; (5) changes with growth and development; and (6) some of the more common variations of normal.

Any one of these objectives could in itself occupy an entire text. It has been our purpose to achieve clarity with an emphasis only on fundamentals.

The authors are particularly indebted to a number of individuals without whose assistance this work would have been impossible. Many of the original sketches and tracings were made by a medical student, Mr. Gil Brogdon; these sketches were then completed by our artist, Mr. Ruben Hawkins.

The entire text has been critically reviewed by several physicians. Dr. Jeff Banks, Professor of Gross Anatomy at the University of Arkansas School of Medicine, criticized the text from the anatomic standpoint, and has been most encouraging and helpful in its every phase. Dr. E. S. Kerekes, Assistant Professor of Radiology, and Dr. Joseph D. Calhoun, Clinical Instructor in Radiology, assisted materially from the radiologic aspects. The authors, however, accept full responsibility for the contents of this text.

To our photographer, Mr. Herbert Lyle, and our secretaries, Mrs. Guyla Berry and Mrs. Gil Brogdon, we make record of our sincere gratitude.

Mrs. Helen Matthews, R.T., and Mr. Earl Pearson, Jr., R.T., performed the arduous task of seeking out the radiographs reproduced herein.

It is virtually impossible to acknowledge fully all the sources of information for a textbook of this type. Some of these are discrete references and others are teachings passed down to us by our preceptors. Some of these are modified from technical manuals which have been published by the General Electric X-Ray Corporation, Eastman Kodak Company, Keleket, and the like. To all of these we are deeply indebted.

Our Miss Mona Brooks has frequently been called upon to act in the capacity of both mother and father for our children during the preparation of this text. To her we owe a very great debt of gratitude.

To our publishers, we owe many thanks for their encouragement and forbearance, and the sincerity of their endeavor.

THE AUTHORS

CONTENTS

CHAPTER 1

Fundamental Background
for Radiologic Anatomy

HISTORICAL BACKGROUND*

IN COMPARISON with other sciences, the science of radiology is relatively young. The development of this new science was made possible by the discovery of x-rays by Wilhelm Konrad Röntgen on November 8, 1895. This discovery was the culmination of efforts of many scientists over a period of three hundred years, and has been the basis of further research in medical, dental, biologic, chemical and industrial fields. In addition, Röntgen's investigations introduced many of the experiments which led to the discovery of natural radioactivity and radium by the Curies one year later, and, more recently, to the discovery of artificial radioactivity.

NATURE OF X-RAYS

Spectrum of Electromagnetic Radiations. X-rays resemble visible light rays very closely but have the distinguishing feature that their wave lengths are very short—only about 1/10,000 the wave length of visible light. It is this characteristic that permits x-rays to penetrate materials which otherwise would absorb or reflect light. X-rays form a part of the spectrum of electromagnetic radiations, where the long electric and radio waves are found at the one end; the infrared, visible and ultraviolet light waves in the middle; and the x-rays, gamma rays and cosmic rays at the short wave length end (Fig. 1–1). These wave lengths are

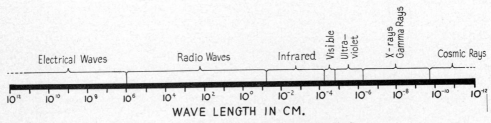

FIG. 1–1. Spectrum of electromagnetic radiations.

* For greater detail see: Otto Glasser, Editor: The Science of Radiology. Springfield, Illinois Charles C Thomas, 1933.

1

VERY RADIOLUCENT	MODERATELY RADIOLUCENT	INTERMEDIATE	MODERATELY RADIOPAQUE	VERY RADIOPAQUE
Gas	Fatty Tissue	Connective Tissue Muscle Tissue Blood Cartilage Epithelium Cholesterol Stones Uric Acid Stones	Bone Calcium Salts	Heavy Metals

FIG. 1–2. Classification of tissues and other substances with medical application in accordance with five general categories of radiopacity and radiolucency.

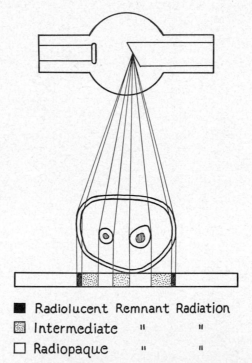

■ Radiolucent Remnant Radiation
▨ Intermediate   "   "
☐ Radiopaque   "   "

FIG. 1–3. Diagrammatic illustration of how remnant radiation will vary in intensity and radiopacity when x-rays pass through the tissues of the forearm, shown in cross section.

measured in terms of Ångstrom units, where 1 Å is defined as 10^{-8} cm. or 1/100,000,000 cm. The useful range of wave lengths for medical radiography is approximately 0.50 to 0.125 Ångstrom unit.

Propagation of X-rays. It is probable that radiant energy, such as light waves of all kinds, is propagated by means of both waves and corpuscles, with one or the other form predominating, depending upon the energy level of the propagation.

Radiolucency and Radiopacity. X-rays do not penetrate all matter with similar ease. Some substances such as fats and gases are more readily penetrated than others such as heavy metals, bone or calcium salts. *Radiolucency* refers to matter which is penetrated by x-rays with relative ease, whereas *radiopacity* is descriptive of matter in which x-rays are absorbed in great measure. Anatomic tissues can be arranged in a scale from the most radiolucent graduating to the most radiopaque (Fig. 1–2), and this difference in opacity when reproduced on photosensitive film makes possible the science of radiography. The x-rays which finally penetrate the anatomic part and produce the x-ray image are spoken of as the "remnant x-rays" (Fig. 1–3).

THE PRODUCTION OF X-RAYS

General Principle. In order to produce x-rays one must obtain electrons, and allow these electrons to strike a target with sufficient energy. This is a complex physical process in which most of the electron energy is converted to heat, and a very minute amount (less than 1 per cent) is converted to x-rays

X-ray Tube. The device in which x-rays are produced is the x-ray tube (Fig. 1–4). This consists of the following essential componant parts:

1. An evacuated glass bulb.
2. A negative electrode called the cathode.
3. A positive electrode called the anode.
4. A spiral incandescent filament of tungsten wire, which when heated emits electrons.
5. A means of dissipation of the heat produced when the electrons are made to strike their target, the anode.

Surrounding the filament is a focusing cup (Fig. 1–5) which focuses the electron stream upon the so-called focal spot on the anode. Upon impact with this focal spot, the electrons give rise to a stream of x-rays which are emitted over a 180 degrees hemispherical angle surrounding the focal spot. A lead-shielded window (Fig. 1–6) is provided, along with a lead tube casing, so that only a small fraction of these x-rays passes through the portal of the tube.

The actual target is a small rectangular plate of tungsten fused into the beveled end of a large copper bar, causing an angulation of the target of about 20 degrees. This angulation affects the size of the focal spot. The copper bar acts to dissipate the heat from the target.

Filament Circuit. In addition, a means of regulating the number of electrons must be provided, and also a means of regulating the energy with which the electrons strike their target so that the number of x-rays and the heat can be controlled.

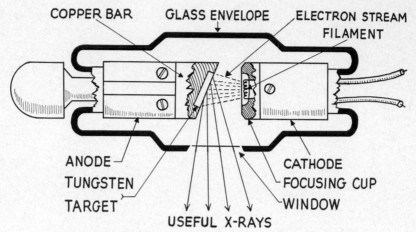

FIG. 1–4.   Diagram of standard stationary anode x-ray tube.

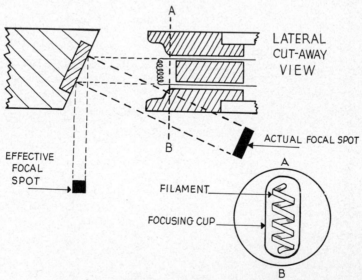

FIG. 1–5.   Diagram of focusing cup and filament.

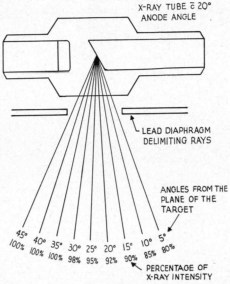

FIG. 1-6. Diagram to illustrate stream of x-rays emitted from target through a delimiting lead diaphragm.

The higher the temperature of the filament, the greater is the number of electrons emitted. The number of electrons emitted can be controlled by means of controlling the temperature of the filament by means of a separate filament circuit (Fig. 1-7). The filament is heated by about 4 to 8 amperes of current from a low-voltage step-down transformer.

It must be assumed that the student is already familiar with these basic electrical terms.

The Major Circuit. To provide the energy behind the electron, another circuit is obtained (Fig. 1-7) which allows a tremendous voltage or "electrical pressure" difference to exist between the cathode, of which the tungsten filament is an integral part, and the anode, which is the target for the electrons. This voltage is measured in terms of thousands of volts (35,000 to 150,000) on most medical diagnostic x-ray machines, and may be regulated at will by various interposed regulatory mechanisms such as the autotransformer.

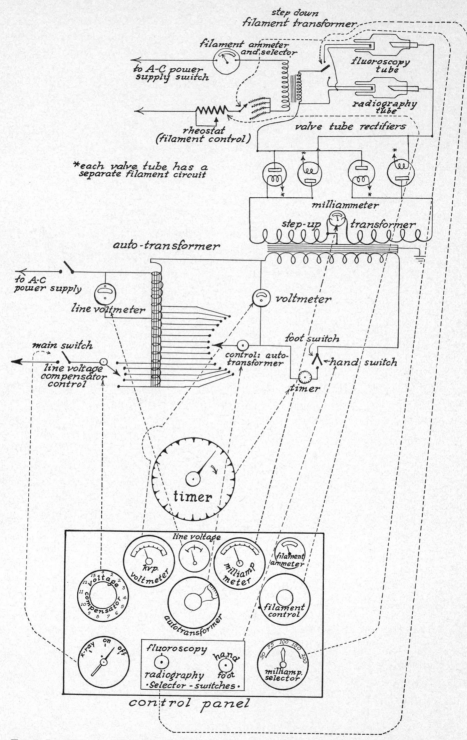

Fig. 1–7. Diagram illustrating the basic control panel for a universal type x-ray machine, with demonstration of how each item on the panel fits into the basic wiring diagram of a simple x-ray machine.

THE MANNER IN WHICH A BASIC X-RAY MACHINE OPERATES

The Basic Control Panel of an X-ray Machine. There is some variation in control panels of different x-ray machines but there is usually a basic design which can be recognized in all types, if the many automatic features in present day machines are disregarded.

The essential elements of a control panel are shown in Figure 1–7; in the line drawing above the panel, the position of each control is indicated in a schematic diagram. The controls consist of:

1. A main switch to connect the x-ray circuit with the main power supply. This may have a supplemental connection to close the entire x-ray circuit after initially closing only the primary circuit.

2. A line voltage meter to indicate when the line voltage is at proper level.

3. A line voltage compensator to adjust the line voltage if necessary.

4. An autotransformer control to select the proper kilovoltage to be applied for a particular examination.

5. A voltmeter on the primary side of the step-up transformer calibrated to indicate the kilovoltage being obtained on the secondary side of the transformer in the x-ray tube circuit. This indirect engineering expedient of indicating the kilovoltage in the secondary circuit is necessary because of the difficulty of inserting a suitable high tension voltmeter in a shock-proof manner on the high tension side of the circuit, although this could be done.

6. A timer circuit, which automatically cuts off the exposure at the preset time.

7. A selector switch which usually permits one to select either the hand switch or the foot switch and either radiography or fluoroscopy. Occasionally, the additional selection of spot-film radiography combined with fluoroscopy is permitted, but to have included this would have made the diagram too complex.

8. A milliampere selector which automatically indicates the desired milliamperage and which is wired in with an ammeter on the primary side of the filament circuit so that adjustment can be made if necessary by means of the filament control. With age changes in the x-ray tube, slight adjustment may be necessary to obtain the desired milliamperage. In some x-ray machines, this adjustment is automatically obtained. Also, changes in kilovoltage setting require automatic regulation with each change of milliamperage in automatic or monitor controls. In many machines, the filament ammeter does not appear on the control panel, but its equivalent is concealed.

It is possible to trace the action of the operator and the circuit in the following manner:

1. When the operator turns the x-ray switch on, the current passes into the filament circuit and heats the filament, giving rise to an abundance of electrons around the tube filament.

2. Assuming that no further adjustment in line voltage is necessary, the autotransformer is set, the timer is set, the selector switches connected appropriately to either foot switch or hand switch, fluoroscopy or radiography, and the hand or foot switch is turned on.

3. Current passes through the autotransformer and through the primary side of the step-up transformer; then the induced oppositely directed current passes through the secondary side of the step-up transformer, through the rectifier circuit and then to the x-ray tube.

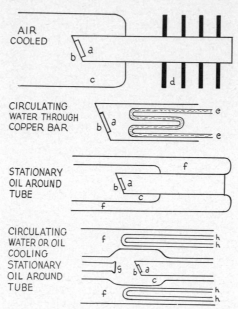

FIG. 1-8. Diagram of various types of target-cooling systems. *a*, Copper bar; *b*, tungsten target; *c*, glass envelope—vacuum within; *d*, metal radial fins; *e*, water coils; *f*, oil around tube; *g*, filament; *h*, coils for circulating water or oil within stationary oil.

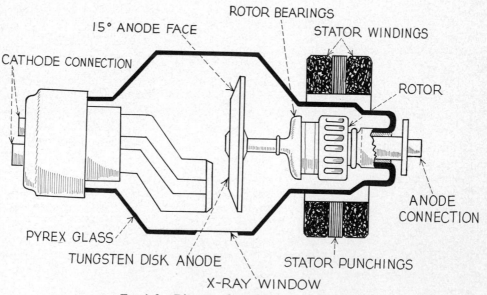

FIG. 1-9. Diagram of rotating anode x-ray tube.

4. A high potential difference is thus applied between the tube filament and the target, forcing the electrons derived from the already heated filament to strike the target; thus x-rays are produced.

Various Methods of Cooling Anode. There are various means of cooling the anode stem (Fig. 1–8):

1. Radial fins outside the glass bulb in continuity with the copper bar (air-cooling).
2. Circulating water within or around the copper bar (water-cooling).
3. Circulating oil around or within the copper bar (oil-cooling).
4. Various combinations of circulating or stationary oil, and circulating water, to cool the oil.

The Rotating Anode. A much more efficient anode is provided if the anode is made to rotate (Fig. 1–9) while the electrons strike the target, so that the electrons never strike a single rectangular area, but rather the rim of a wheel which is angled at about 15 degrees. In this type of "rotating anode" tube the effective focal spot can be very small, and yet the actual target is the rim of a wheel, and hence does not heat up as readily as it would in a "stationary anode" type tube.

Advantages and Limitations of Small Focal Spot. As in all instances of light emission, the smaller the light source in size, the sharper is the image produced; just so in radiography, the smaller the focal spot, the sharper is the radiographic image. However, the smaller the focal spot, the lower the amount of energy that can be applied without producing damage to the target, so that heat dissipation and mechanical design of the x-ray tube are of fundamental importance in radiography.

Rectification. The design of the x-ray circuit is also of importance—particularly the mode of rectification—but this is beyond the scope of the present text, and can be obtained from many other books devoted to this subject.

FUNDAMENTAL PROPERTIES OF X-RAYS

Ionization. The primary effect of x-rays when they strike matter is the ionization of particles. This ionization produces various phenomena which are observable, depending upon the matter which is struck. Many of these phenomena are utilized in radiography and the ionization of air by x-rays has been used in their quantitative measurement.

Fluorescence. When x-rays strike certain substances called "phosphors" (such as barium platinocyanide, zinc sulfide or calcium tungstate), they cause them to fluoresce (Fig. 1–10). In other words, the x-rays are converted to light waves of longer wave length in the visible and ultraviolet light range.

Photographic Effect. When x-rays strike a photographic silver-salt emulsion, they produce the same type of photosensitization which is produced by visible light. All the steps in this photochemical process are not fully understood, but this effect of x-rays is fundamental. The photosensitized silver salt is partially precipitated, depending upon the degree of photosensitization; when the film is developed and fixed by a special chemical process a photographic image is obtained. This characteristic makes possible the recording of internal structures of many objects of interest to man in medicine, biology and industry.

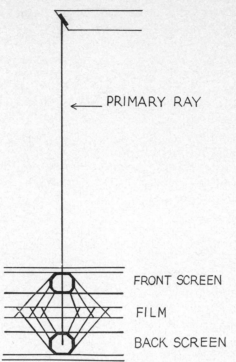

FIG. 1–10.   Diagram illustrating fluorescence from intensifying screen.

The latter two properties, the fluorescent and photosensitization effects of x-rays, are the two most important characteristics of x-rays with regard to radiography. These will be discussed in greater detail below.

Chemical Effects.   Certain chemical changes are also produced by x-rays by altering atomic structure. Ordinary salt, for example, turns yellow from liberation of chlorine.

Heat Production.   There is also a small amount of heat which is produced when x-rays strike matter. This is an infinitesimally small quantity and is very difficult to measure.

Biologic Effects.   There are certain very important biologic changes produced by x-rays which are utilized constantly in x-ray therapy. These alterations in both normal and abnormal tissues fall outside the scope of this text.

ACCESSORIES NECESSARY FOR THE RECORDING OF THE X-RAY IMAGE

X-ray Film.   X-ray film is composed of photosensitive emulsion of silver bromide especially adapted for that use, and a blue-tinted, transparent, cellulose acetate support or base. The emulsion is coated on both sides about 0.001 inch thick, thereby producing a greater photographic effect than would be possible with a single emulsion film. The silver bromide crystals are affected variably depending upon the intensity of the light striking them, and metallic silver is precipitated. X-ray "developing solution" is then applied which changes the affected crystals into black metallic silver. The silver bromide crystals which have not been affected by the x-rays or developer are removed by treatment with another solution known as "fixer," and thus a permanent image is obtained. Two types of x-ray film are now employed in medical radiography: (1) *screen* *film* which is especially sensitive to the fluorescent light of intensifying screens (to be discussed below) and not so sensitive to the direct action of x-rays; and (2) *direct exposure* film which is highly sensitive to the direct action of x-rays and not so to screens.

Since x-ray film is very sensitive and easily damaged, one must be constantly on the alert to detect artefacts that may have been produced by the handling of the film, in the developing or fixing process, by dust particles on the screens, or by static electricity.

Intensifying Screens (Fig. 1–11).   An intensifying screen is a special cardboard containing a thin layer of a fine phosphor emulsion with a suitable binder. Calcium tungstate is the compound that is most frequently employed for this purpose. When the x-rays strike the crystals of this compound, there

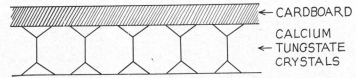

← CARDBOARD

CALCIUM
← TUNGSTATE
CRYSTALS

FIG. 1–11.   Diagrammatic presentation of intensifying screen in cross section.

is an instantaneous conversion of the x-rays to ultraviolet and visible light, called "fluorescence." These screens increase the effect of the irradiation on the sensitive emulsion of the film, and thus reduce the x-ray exposure necessary. When intensifying screens are employed, the film is placed between the active faces of two screens. The image is, therefore, a combination of an image obtained by x-rays and fluorescence. There is some loss of detail as the result of diffusion, and screens are rated in accordance with the size of the crystals employed in their structure. Small crystals in the screen are less efficient fluorescent agents ("slower"), but attain maximum sharpness in definition. One disadvantage of screens, however, is that dust particles, stains, scratches or cracks, or any faulty contact of the screen with the film, produces artefacts in the film image.

Ordinarily, when an x-ray beam strikes x-ray film, less than 1 per cent of the radiant energy is absorbed by the emulsion, and as a result more than 99 per cent fails to perform any useful radiographic work. This degree of efficiency is markedly improved with the aid of the intensifying screens.

The Fluoroscopic Screen.   The fluoroscopic screen is a specially constructed intensifying screen which converts most of the x-rays to visible light rather than ultraviolet, as is the case with the radiographic screen. It offers the advantage of immediate visualization of an x-ray image, but this image is not nearly so clearly delineated as is the photographic image on x-ray film. It is ordinarily covered with lead glass so that the penetrating x-rays which are not absorbed by the intensifying screen are absorbed by the lead, and do not strike the observer.

By placing an x-ray tube under the radiographic table, the patient on the table, and a fluoroscopic screen over the patient in direct line with the x-rays (Fig. 1–12), the physician may under suitable conditions study many anatomic parts in motion or while they function and thus gain additional information of a physiologic nature as an adjunct to the anatomic study. The fluoroscope is an extremely useful instrument when used judiciously, but in the hands of the unwary or the careless it can become virtually an instrument of destruction.

DIAGRAM OF A FLUOROSCOPE

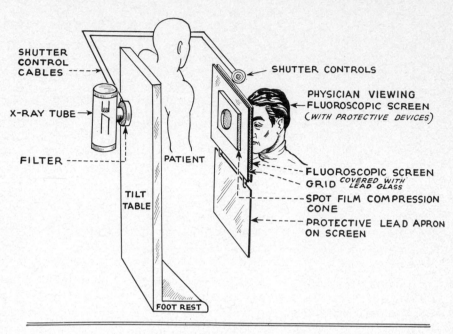

SHUTTER
CONTROL
CABLES

SHUTTER CONTROLS

X-RAY TUBE

PHYSICIAN VIEWING
FLUOROSCOPIC SCREEN
(*WITH PROTECTIVE DEVICES*)

FILTER

PATIENT

FLUOROSCOPIC SCREEN
GRID *COVERED WITH LEAD GLASS*

TILT
TABLE

SPOT FILM COMPRESSION
CONE

PROTECTIVE LEAD APRON
ON SCREEN

FOOT REST

FIG. 1–12.   Diagram of a fluoroscope.

Shutter Mechanism.   Immediately in front of the x-ray tube under the table is a lead shutter mechanism which may be opened and closed in both the vertical and horizontal directions. The opening and closure are controlled by cables connected to knobs beside the fluoroscopic screen or by electrical switches similarly connected. The lead is of sufficient thickness to prevent any primary radiation from escaping in a forward direction and is so constructed that secondary emanations are also largely absorbed. The field of vision of the fluoroscopic screen is thus delimited by these controls beside the screen. The field should always be no larger than is absolutely necessary for vision of the part in question, and one should always be able to see the margins of the shutters on the screen for safety. The smaller the field, the better the detail—an added inducement for maintaining this status.

Filtration.   Additional filters should always be added in front of the fluoroscopic tube to the extent of even 4 mm. of aluminum if possible. Only the more highly penetrating rays are effective in fluoroscopy in any case, and the addition of such filters removes a higher percentage of the less penetrating rays than of the more penetrating. The patient's skin has a much higher tolerance for the more penetrating rays, and thus the fluoroscopic time so far as the patient's skin is concerned is increased. This will be more fully discussed in the succeeding section on protection.

Distance of Tube Target to Table Top.   In former years tables were constructed so that only a 12-inch distance was possible between the tube target and table top; newer tables have provided an 18- to 30-inch distance. This greater distance is desirable for further protecting the patient's skin as well as for obtaining better detail on the fluoroscopic screen. As we pointed out previously, the greater the target-to-film (or, in this case, screen) distance, the greater is the detail. The added protection will be discussed below.

Use of Stationary Grid. A stationary grid wafer may be interposed between the patient and the screen in an appropriate slot. This improves the contrast, particularly in the more opaque areas, but it requires an increase of 8 to 10 kilovolts peak to compensate for the energy absorption by the grid. A focused grid is most desirable in this regard, remembering that the grid radius must be known, and the tube side must be properly placed.

Spot-Film Radiography. An increasing amount of radiography is being done with the fluoroscopic tube, especially in gastrointestinal examinations, but also in the examination of other areas, such as the spine, chest and heart. The use of the fluoroscope permits the physician to position the patient accurately prior to obtaining the radiograph and to obtain the radiograph instantaneously. In view of the close tube-target-to-screen distances, a relatively small focal spot is desirable in this regard (no greater than 2.5 to 3.0 mm.) to promote better detail. Actually, a rotating anode is most desirable in this respect, but unfortunately, it is most costly. It is usually desirable to use a maximum kilovoltage setting (around 85 KvP) and an average of about 50 milliampere-seconds for adult spot-film radiography. A compression cone between the screen and the patient is also desirable since it allows both a reduction of the amount of tissue to be penetrated and a better relief picture of mucosal pattern. Some modern equipment has provided for the introduction of a photoelectric cell, and thus the time of exposure is automatically regulated by a special "phototiming" circuit. Also, a moving grid may be interposed.

Amplification of the Fluoroscopic Image. There are at least three different methods employing either complex mirror systems or electronic amplification. Although these methods will undoubtedly come into greater use in the near future, it is doubtful that they will be within the economic range of the general practitioner; hence, they are beyond the scope of the present volume. Such amplification is a decided advantage from the standpoints of both greater accuracy and less x-ray exposure for the patient and physician. It will also prove to be a great teaching aid since the fluoroscopic image may by this means be televised and viewed by large groups or photographed with a movie camera (cineradiography).

Eye Accommodation Preceding Fluoroscopy. At least 20 minutes are required for the proper accommodation of the eyes, by either remaining in a dark room or wearing appropriate goggles. Failure to observe this rule will result in inadequate accommodation and will tempt the operator to increase the milliamperage, kilovoltage or time of fluoroscopy and possibly expose himself and the patient to dangerous amounts of radiation.

Physical Factors. Ordinarily 3 to 5 milliamperes are adequate for all types of fluoroscopy, and under no circumstances should one exceed 8 milliamperes. It is common practice to use 85 kilovolts peak for abdominal fluoroscopy, 70 kilovolts for chest and 60 kilovolts for the extremities. In fluoroscoping children, 60 kilovolts need never be exceeded, and, of course, a small field is imperative for children since a much greater proportion of the entire body of a child is covered by the radiation.

Use of X-ray Protective Devices. X-ray protective devices such as lead-lined gloves, lead rubber or lead glass fiber aprons, and small lead rubber shields dangling beneath the fluoroscopic screen are imperative. The operator should never permit his unprotected hands, wrists, arms or other parts to be exposed to the x-ray beam. Palpation with the hand or other manipulation under the fluoroscope for setting fractures, foreign body localization, or other such procedures should be avoided. Intermittent and serial radiography is much to be preferred to such dangerous exposure.

Head Type Fluoroscopic Screen. This device should be condemned and never used. It is virtually impossible to avoid exposure to the primary x-ray beam when this instrument is used and it is very tempting to avoid adequate accommodation when using it, thus further imperiling oneself by increasing the physical dangers to obtain good fluoroscopic vision. If an operating fluoroscope is necessary, it is far better to move the operation to an x-ray table where frequent radiography should be employed by preference, and short term fluoroscopy only as an expedient.

Photoroentgenograms are now also achieving increasing importance. In this device, a photograph of the fluoroscopic image is obtained by means of a specially constructed camera. The usual film sizes employed for this purpose are: 4 x 5 inches, 70 mm. and 35 mm. Photoroentgenography offers an economical method for radiographic survey of large populations. The main disadvantages of this method are: (1) loss of accuracy in detail, and (2) increased radiation exposure to the patient. With newer developments, however, this method offers great promise for the future, particularly along the lines of electronic image amplification and television.

Cassette (Figs. 1–13a and **b**). An x-ray cassette is a permanent light-proof container for two intensifying screens, which permit the easy introduction of the x-ray film between them. From the tube side outward, a cassette has the following layers: an outer light-proof but relatively radiolucent layer of bakelite, aluminum or some similar substance; an upper intensifying screen, which has a thinner layer of phosphor emulsion than the lower intensifying screen; the lower intensifying screen, so placed that the two screen phosphor layers make contact with the film when it is introduced between them; a lead foil back to absorb any x-rays which penetrate the outer screen; and a metal spring back which allows good contact between the screens and film. A layer of felt is usually interposed between the outer screen and cassette back.

Cardboard Film Holder. This is a light-proof cardboard folder into which the film can be placed. Ordinarily this is accomplished by means of heavy black paper folded properly inside two cardboards. The back cardboard (away from the x-ray tube) ordinarily contains some lead foil for absorption of the x-rays which have penetrated the upper cardboard and film, to prevent the scattering effect from the table top. Adequately light-protected and individually wrapped nonscreen films are available commercially (without the lead backing) which avoid the necessity for darkroom loading, and prevent confusion from storage of both nonscreen and screen film in the darkroom. Although the efficiency of the production of the x-ray image is not so great here as in the case of intensifying screens, there is no loss of detail from fluorescent diffusion of light, and in the thinner parts of the body it is advantageous to use this method of radiography. Also, when it is necessary to look for extremely minute foreign bodies as in the case of the eye, this method of radiography offers greater accuracy. Similar film holders are made of plastic.

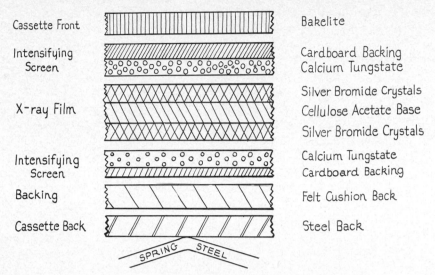

Cassette Front		Bakelite
Intensifying Screen		Cardboard Backing Calcium Tungstate
X-ray Film		Silver Bromide Crystals Cellulose Acetate Base Silver Bromide Crystals
Intensifying Screen		Calcium Tungstate Cardboard Backing
Backing		Felt Cushion Back
Cassette Back		Steel Back

SPRING STEEL

FIG. 1–13. **a,** Diagrammatic cross section of x-ray cassette.

THE CASSETTE AND ITS CARE

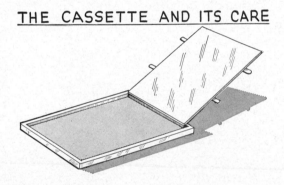

1. AVOID INJURY OR DROPPING.
2. AVOID CHEMICAL CONTACT WITH SCREENS.
3. HANDLE ON DRY BENCH.
4. AVOID STORAGE OF ITEMS ABOVE LOADING BENCH.
5. DO NOT LEAVE CASSETTE OPEN.
6. INSPECT FREQUENTLY TO DETECT WEARING OF FELT OR BENDING OF HINGES.
7. TEST SCREEN FILM CONTACT WITH FLAT WIRE MESH.

FIG. 1–13. **b,** The cassette and its care.

Stationary and Moving Grid (Fig. 1–14).   When an x-ray beam strikes any matter some of the x-rays are absorbed, some are deflected and partially absorbed, and some pass directly through. There is a considerable percentage which is scattered in all directions by the atoms of the object struck. This is known as "secondary radiation," and although the wave length of such radiation is longer than that of the primary beam, nevertheless it is photographically effective, and overcasts the x-ray image with a loss of image detail. It is desirable in radiography to reduce this secondary radiation to a minimum. This is particularly true in the radiography of the larger anatomic parts.

The grid is a device for eliminating much of this scattered radiation. It is composed of a series of very thin strips of lead held in position by intervening

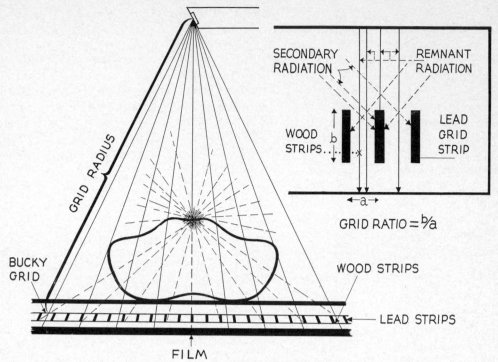

FIG. 1–14.   Diagram of a Potter-Bucky diaphragm and how it is used.

strips of wood or bakelite. It is interposed between the part to be radiographed and the film. The lead strips are obliquely placed so that the plane of each is parallel with the radial projections from the focal spot. Thus, a special grid must be employed for each major change in grid to tube-target distance and this is called the "grid radius." The wood-filled slots between the lead strips are usually about six to 16 times as deep as they are wide, and this ratio of the height to the width of the wood slots is the "grid ratio." The strips of lead have the function of absorbing the scattered rays as they come from the body part before they can strike the film, so that the image is formed by the primary parallel radiation that has penetrated the body part (so-called "remnant radiation"). The greater the grid ratio, the more efficient is the grid in absorbing scattered radiation.

If the grid is stationary, the lead lines will be reproduced on the radiograph, and are objectionable unless the lead strips are extremely fine; but if the grid is placed in motion by a spring or motor device while the exposure is being made, the grid lines are not seen, and the efficiency of the grid is improved. This moving grid is also called the "Potter-Bucky diaphragm."

In the Camp grid cassette, a stationary grid of special design has been incorporated directly in the cover of the cassette. Although such cassettes are expensive, they delimit scattered radiation very efficiently, and the grid lines (due to the lead strips) are visible only on the closest inspection. Great care must be exercised in the handling of these wafer grids, since the slightest bending of the grid will distort the relationship of the lead strips to the primary beam and diminish the efficiency of the grid.

It is important to recognize that a focused grid (i.e., a grid with oblique lead strips to conform to a known grid radius) has a "tube side" and a "film side." These must not be reversed or a virtually blank radiograph will be obtained.

If the lead strips are all perpendicular to the grid surface (an unfocused grid) either side may be used as the tube side.

A focused grid must be carefully centered with respect to the x-ray tube. Otherwise, there will be more absorption of radiation on one side of the grid than on the other and an uneven radiograph will result.

The grid method of eliminating the major portion of secondary radiation requires considerably more exposure; therefore the intensifying screens are usually employed along with the grid. In addition, the device increases the distance of the part to be radiographed from the film, and thereby increases distortion of the image unless a long tube target-skin distance is employed, and a small focal spot.

Cones and Aperture Diaphragms (Fig. 1–15). Cones and aperture diaphragms are applied to the tube window to delimit the x-ray beam and thus reduce the secondary radiation. Cones have the additional advantage of reducing the stray radiation toward the operator, and thus they furnish a protective mechanism as well.

X-RAY CONING DEVICES

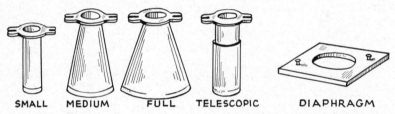

SMALL   MEDIUM   FULL   TELESCOPIC   DIAPHRAGM

FIG. 1–15. **a,** Various accessories used to delimit secondary irradiation. An adjustable cone for various field sizes with a light localizer and centering device is also available commercially (not illustrated).

FIG. 1–15. **b,** Diagram illustrating effect of cone in delimiting scattered radiation.

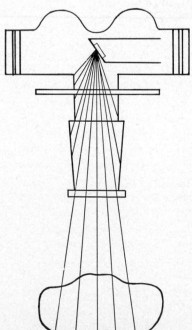

SPECIAL ACCESSORIES IN THE PRODUCTION OF SPECIAL TYPES OF X-RAY IMAGES

Body-Section Radiography. The body-section radiograph is known by various names, depending on slightly different operating principles (laminagraph, stratograph, tomograph, etc.). The main factor in each of these, however, is the rotation of the x-ray tube and the x-ray film about a fixed axis, so that all images are blurred except that at the chosen axis. By this means, a certain section of the body is brought into focus while other interfering parts are diffused and a clearer image at the chosen level is obtained. This is a useful adjunct, particularly in the visualization of certain lung structures, brain structures, larynx, nasopharynx and the like.

X-ray Kymograph. The single-slit kymograph is a device for recording the sequential movement of adjoining points on a given organ such as the heart. It consists of a single slit cut in a lead sheet which permits the recording of only a narrow segment of the organ at one time. It moves vertically at a pre-set desired speed while the exposure is made so that there is a sequential record on the film of the movement of adjoining parts of the organ in question. The multiple-slit kymograph records several areas simultaneously, and is the type most frequently used. The photoelectric kymograph is a device with a similar purpose, but a beam of light is focused on a given point, and variations in its intensity are recorded by means of a photoelectric cell on photographic paper. This is a far more accurate method of recording the movements of a given organ or structure.

Stereoradiography. A single radiographic image is a two-dimensional representation and does not possess perspective. To some extent, our mind's eye can be trained to overcome this deficiency when we project our knowledge of gross anatomy into the x-ray image and visualize the structure in three dimensions. This projection process is not a true visualization in space, but is most helpful in roentgenographic interpretation. To obtain radiographs that can give a true stereoscopic effect, two slightly different views are obtained—first as though the one eye were looking at the part, and then as though the other eye were seeing it. This is done by making two radiographs from two separate tube positions, the amount of tube shift bearing a definite ratio to the normal interpupillary distance. These two radiographs are then placed in a stereoscope or viewed with special prismatic lenses so that each eye will see the separate image. The brain fuses the two images into one in which the various parts stand out in striking relief in their true perspective and correct spatial relationship.

Stereoscopy is of definite value in visualizing a structure in three dimensions and seeing its spatial relationship. Stereoscopic films also have value since when viewed separately, we can see the part in question from two different perspectives, and a structure obscured by an overlying part may be seen more clearly. *However, it is important to realize that stereoscopy will not reveal anything which is not readily seen on one or the other of the two films,* and it will not permit seeing more of an object than the two eyes could see if they were looking at it.

Contrast Media. The differential radiopacity and radiolucency of many of the organs of the body is very similar, and it would be difficult to diagnose many structural aberrations and abnormalities, were it not possible to introduce substances within these organs to accentuate this contrast. It is desirable that the substance so introduced should be physiologically inert, or harmless. There have been many substances devised for this purpose. They fall into two main categories: those that are radiopaque, and those that are radiolucent.

The common radiopaque compounds are as follows:

1. *Barium sulfate* is particularly useful in studies of the gastrointestinal tract. It is inert and is not absorbed, nor does it alter the normal physiologic function of the gastrointestinal tract.

2. *Bismuth subcarbonate* may be used in lieu of barium sulfate, but does not produce as good contrast.

3. *Tetraiodophenolphthalein* is an organic iodide which was formerly widely used for visualization of the gallbladder, since it was selectively concentrated by the normal gallbladder which then became visualized.

4. *Priodax, Telepaque, Teridax, Monophen, Orabilex* and similar substances for gallbladder visualization have replaced the above because of less nausea, vomiting and diarrhea than are produced by the phenolphthalein derivative. In excessive doses, Priodax may also cause a diarrhea.

Cholografin (Biligrafin) by intravenous administration may visualize the main biliary ducts and gallbladder.

5. *Inorganic iodides* (e.g., sodium iodide) are still occasionally used in the retrograde visualization of the urinary tract, but less irritating organic iodides have largely replaced these.

6. *Organic iodides* are selectively concentrated by the normal kidney. There are many of these water-soluble compounds both in this country and abroad, such as Hypaque, Renografin, Diodrast, Neo-iopax, Uropac, Abrodil, and so on. These are injected intravenously, and are quite irritating if they leak into the subcutaneous tissues. However, in our experience Diodrast can be used intramuscularly and is not so irritating locally as is Neo-iopax. The latter, however, has fewer undesirable side effects such as nausea and vomiting. These organic iodides in double strength are also used in angiography (the visualization of blood vessels), in angiocardiography (the visualization of the chambers of the heart), and in the visualization of fistulous tracts. They may also be used in visualization of hepatic and biliary radicles by T-tube or operative cholangiography (see appropriate sections in text).

7. *Iodized oils* such as Visciodol, Lipiodol, Iodochloral and other iodized, bromated or chlorinated oils are particularly of value in the visualization of the bronchial tree; the uterine cavity and oviducts; the biliary and hepatic duct system when injected directly into these structures either at the time of operation or thereafter through a T-tube in the common duct; the subarachnoid space of the spinal column; fistulous tracts; the paranasal sinuses; and other duct systems, such as the salivary ducts.

Absorbable organic iodides suspended in oil such as Dionosil are advantageous for visualization of the bronchial tree since they disappear in about four days. We have found aqueous Dionosil quite irritating and less tolerable.

Other absorbable organic iodides such as Skiodan Acacia and Salpix are useful in hysterosalpingography.

8. *Pantopaque* is particularly of value in the visualization of the subarachnoid space of the spinal column. It has the advantage over Lipiodol in having a lesser viscosity which permits its withdrawal through a lumbar puncture needle after the diagnostic study is completed.

9. *Thorotrast, Umbrathor and other thorium compounds* have been and are still being used for visualization of body cavities, vascular systems and the reticuloendothelial system but have the disadvantage of being radioactive. Some disparaging reports have appeared regarding their use, for example the development of sarcomas. Hence, these compounds are not in great favor and are not in general use.

The common radiolucent substances used are mostly *gases*, although it is conceivable that fatty substances could be employed. Air, oxygen, nitrogen, helium and carbon dioxide have all been used for visualization of the body cavities. These are most commonly employed in visualization of the ventricular system of the brain (pneumoencephalograms and ventriculograms), and in the demonstration of some of the joint spaces such as the knee joint. Air is also used as a contrast medium in the pleural, peritoneal and pericardial spaces.

Carbon dioxide is achieving particular importance since it is resorbed extremely rapidly, and it is well tolerated even when injected into the blood stream.

THE FUNDAMENTAL GEOMETRY OF X-RAY IMAGE FORMATION AND INTERPRETATION

X-rays obey the common laws of light. The manner in which any object placed in the path of the x-ray beam is projected depends on: (1) the size of the light source (focal spot), i.e., whether pin-point or a larger surface; (2) the alignment of the object with respect to the light source (focal spot) and the screen or film; (3) the distance of the object from the light source; (4) the distance of the object from the screen or film; and (5) the plane of the object with respect to the screen or film.

When an image is projected from a pin-point light source, the borders of the image are sharp, but if the light source is a larger surface, as in the case of the focal spot of an x-ray tube, the image is ill-defined at its periphery owing to penumbra formation (Fig. 1–16). Measures must be taken to reduce the penumbra as much as possible. To accomplish this the focal spot must be as small as possible, and the object-to-film distance as short as possible. The object-to-focal-spot distance should be as long as possible (Fig. 1–17). Also, the film should be perpendicular to the central ray arising from the focal spot.

When the object is not centrally placed with respect to the central ray its image will be distorted, and this distortion may be considerable (Fig. 1–18). Sometimes this distortion is unavoidable if one is to visualize a part, and in some of the radiographic positions, this distortion brings a part into view which otherwise would be hidden (Fig. 1–19). Thus, the phenomenon of projection may be utilized to good advantage.

The farther an object is from the light source and the closer it is to the film, the less will be the magnification (Fig. 1–17). The magnification of an object as much as 15 cm. from the film when a relatively usual focal spot-film distance is employed (such as 36 inches) is approximately 20 per cent. Such magnification must be considered in interpreting the size of the heart, the pelvis or any other structure which is to be measured.

These various phenomena of magnification, projection, distortion and penumbra formation must be constantly borne in mind in viewing radiographic images.

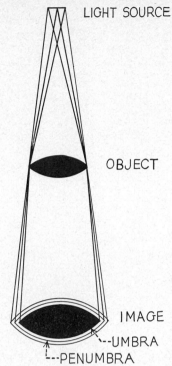

FIG. 1–16. Diagram of penumbra formation from surface light source.

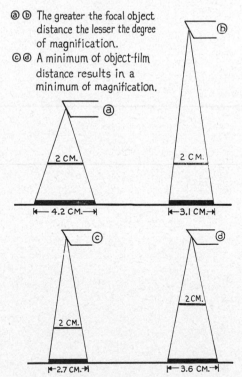

ⓐ ⓑ The greater the focal object distance the lesser the degree of magnification.

ⓒ ⓓ A minimum of object-film distance results in a minimum of magnification.

FIG. 1–17. Diagram illustrating effect of focal-object distance and object-film distance on magnification.

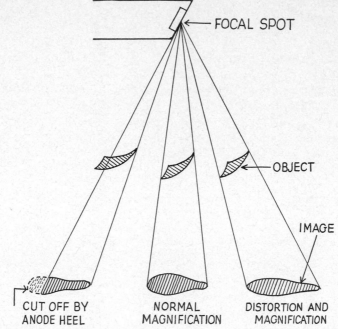

FIG. 1–18.   Diagram illustrating effect of position of object with respect to central ray on distortion, magnification, and anode-heel effect.

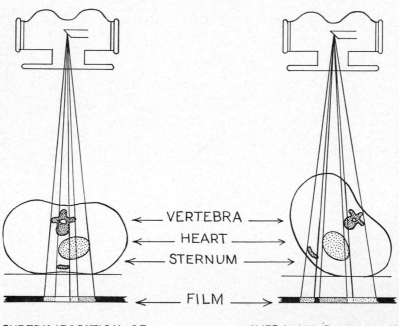

FIG. 1–19.   Diagram illustrating utilization of projection to overcome superimposition of anatomic parts.

THE NECESSITY FOR DIFFERENT VIEWS OR PROJECTIONS OF AN ANATOMIC PART

The obvious method of examining a part is to look at it from several different aspects. This allows a proper perspective of the entire structure. Similarly, when examining an anatomic part, it is radiographed from a minimum of two different views, and a three-dimensional concept is thus obtained.

This method of obtaining several views of a given anatomic part has the additional advantage of separating overlying or overlapping structures—of separating the gallbladder, for example, from interfering gas shadows, the stomach from the spine, and so on.

STEPS IN THE PRODUCTION OF A RADIOGRAPH

There are many steps in the production and final interpretation of a radiograph (Fig. 1–20), and it is well to have some concept of all of them. Given the problem of the radiography of an anatomic part, the following steps are pursued:

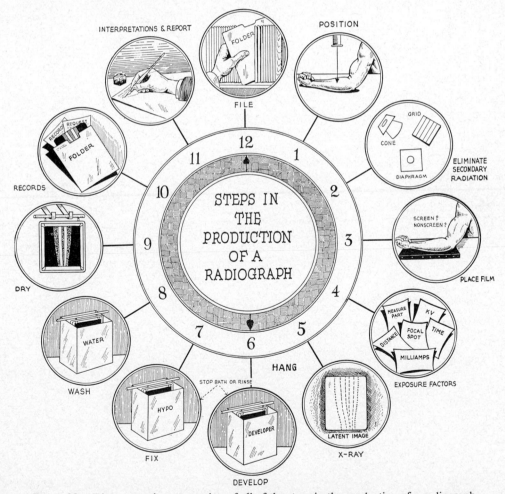

Fig. 1–20. Diagrammatic presentation of all of the steps in the production of a radiograph.

1. The patient is placed in a position with respect to the central ray of the x-ray tube in full accordance with our knowledge of the gross anatomy.
2. The most suitable method to eliminate secondary radiation is chosen, whether it be a diaphragm, cone, grid, or all three. In some types of movable grids, a grid movement time must be chosen depending upon the exposure time, and the moving mechanism must be cocked.
3. The proper type of film and the film holder or cassette are placed in position with respect to the central ray, either directly under the anatomic part, or under the grid in a special carriage.
4. Optimum exposure factors are chosen: (*a*) milliamperage; (*b*) kilovoltage; (*c*) time; (*d*) distance; and (*e*) focal spot after the anatomic part has been measured as to its relative size.
5. A latent image is obtained on the film by the x-rays.
6. The cassette or film holder is taken to the darkroom where the film is carefully removed, placed on a film hanger of appropriate size, and allowed to remain in the developing solution for a definite time depending upon the temperature and degree of exhaustion of the developer.
7. The film is removed from the developer and inserted into a s op-bath or it is quickly rinsed and transferred to a fixing solution for approximately ten minutes.
8. The film is then allowed to "fix" in hypo solution for at least twice the developing time, and then transferred to the 'wash" for at least one-half hour.
9. The film is then dried.
10. The finished radiograph is then attached to the original film consultation request, and other pertinent records of the patient in the office, and the entire folder on the patient is brought to the radiologist (physician) for interpretation in the light of all information on the patient.
11. The radiologist writes or dictates his consultation report.
12. The radiologist's report is filed in duplicate in his office, and the original copy is sent to the physician who originally requested the consultation. The patient's films are returned to the central office of the radiologist for filing also.

REFERENCES

Glasser, Otto: *The Science of Radiology.* Charles C Thomas, Springfield, Illinois, 1933.
Glasser, Otto, Quimby, Edith, Taylor, Lauriston, and Weatherwax, J.: *Physical Foundations of Radiology.* Paul B. Hoeber, New York, 1952.

CHAPTER 2

Protection from
Roentgen Irradiation

Definition of Physical Terms. QUALITY OF IRRADIATION. In the previous chapter we have stated that x-rays are produced when the electron beam strikes the anode or target in the evacuated glass tube. The quantity of rays produced is proportional to the milliamperage of the current. The quality is dependent in great part on the kilovoltage. The rays are of heterogeneous quality in a broad spectrum, but in general terms two types of irradiation may be identified:

1. The rays of relatively long wave length which are known as "soft" rays and which have a marked relative effect upon the skin and superficial tissues. This is the type of irradiation used in diagnostic roentgenology and in superficial (dermatologic) x-ray therapy.

2. The rays of short wave length which are responsible for the penetration of the tissues at a depth and whose dosage is calculated as "percentage depth dose" in relation to the dose on the skin. *Filters* are strips of varying thickness of one or more metals which are placed beneath the window of the x-ray tube and serve to diminish the soft radiations which are damaging to patient or physician. The type of filter used is dependent upon the kilovoltage and the penetration desired. In diagnostic roentgenology, 35 to 120 KvP and 2 to 4 mm. of aluminum added filtration are recommended.

THE ROENTGEN. The internationally accepted unit for quantity of radiation is the roentgen. The roentgen is defined as the "quantity of x- or gamma radiation such that the associated corpuscular emission per 0.001293 grams of air produces, in air, ions carrying 1 e.s.u. of quantity of electricity of either sign." This definition in terms of everyday radiologic practice is best understood if compared with the average dosage required to produce "skin erythema"—approximately 300 roentgens for intermediate voltage radiation. Skin erythema represents the first stage of clinically recognizable response to x-ray exposure on the skin. More severe effects are obtained with progressively larger doses, to the point of necrosis with acute exposure or skin carcinoma with intermittent protracted exposure. The hazards of exposure to x-rays are great for the technician, physician or patient unless properly controlled. First, the general effects of irradiation must be understood. Thereafter, consideration must be given to protection of the patient, the physician and the technician.

THE GENERAL EFFECTS OF IRRADIATION

In 1950, the International Commission on Radiological Protection listed the effects of x-rays to be observed as follows:[7]

1. Superficial injuries.
2. General effects on the body, particularly the blood-forming organs; e.g., production of anemia and leukemia.
3. Induction of malignant tumors.
4. Other deleterious effects, including cataracts, obesity, impaired fertility, and reduction of the life span.
5. Genetic effects.

Superficial Injuries may either be immediate as with severe sunburn or manifest only after a prolonged period of time, with thin scaly skin, telangiectasia, striation and brittleness of nails, keratoses, and finally carcinoma. The maximum permissible dose for the skin is not known, but in persons subject to daily radiation over a period of years it is thought to be less than 1 roentgen per day; in patients subject to radiation over a relatively short period of time (85 KvP, 5 Ma., total filtration 2 mm. aluminum) it is thought to be about 250 roentgens over any one region of the body, this dose not to be repeated for at least four weeks.[16]

One hundred and thirty-five physicians were seen at the Mayo Clinic between 1919 and 1935 for advice about or treatment of roentgen-ray injuries. Ninety-one had contracted their injuries during reduction of fractures with the fluoroscope; 78 of these admitted use of no protection at all and 11 began using lead protection gloves only after the injury became apparent. Only 8 had had any formal roentgen training and all had failed to follow recommended measures of protection until they had been injured.[2]

Effects on the Blood and Hematopoietic Tissues. Various effects on the blood of man and experimental animals have been noted with extremely small doses of x-ray radiation administered daily over relatively long periods of time. Leukopenia and relative lymphopenia in man and lymphocytosis in animals have been noted with as little as 0.02 to 0.05 roentgen per day.[16] March reports 14 deaths from leukemia among a total of 299 deaths among radiologists—an incidence nine times as frequent among radiologists as among other physicians.[11] Henshaw and Hawkins have shown that the incidence of leukemia in all physicians is almost twice as great as that in the population as a whole.[6] From experiments on animals it appears that leukemia is induced by chronic irradiation mainly in animals in which the disease develops spontaneously. The maximum permissible dose in this regard is actually not known.

Induction of Malignant Tumors. Frequent low-grade exposure to x-rays over several years has long been known to result in highly malignant skin carcinomata. Animal experiments suggest as little as 0.11 r per day (eight hours) causes some deleterious and irreversible changes associated with the development of malignancies. Therefore, these factors must be taken into account in forming a concept of the maximum permissible dose.[16]

Other Deleterious Effects. Within the range of permissible doses to the skin for x-rays and gamma rays, and probably for beta rays, there is likely to be no change in the cornea or lens. It is not uncommon, however, for iridocyclitis to develop when the eye cannot be shielded from intense irradiation such as is given for malignant neoplasm in the vicinity of the eye. Lenticular cataract may be produced by 800 to 1000 roentgens.

Experimental data on animals indicate that small daily doses in the order even of 0.1 r per day may produce significant reduction in the life span of these animals. The reduction was definite with daily exposure in excess of 0.5 r.

With regard to fertility in humans, little can be said except that it requires in excess of 625 roentgens delivered to both ovaries within a few days to produce permanent amenorrhea. To produce complete aspermia in men, an even higher dose is required. However, the data in experimental animals would seem to indicate that effects on the ovaries of mice are observed with 1.1 r per day over long periods of time and on the testicles in dogs and mice with 0.5 r to 1.0 r per day.

Genetic Effects.   Genetic radiation effects may be due either to gene mutations or to chromosomal aberrations. Geneticists indicate that any amount of radiation is deleterious. It is almost impossible to be certain how to translate the work of the geneticist on experimental animals to use in man. "A warning is needed, however, lest exposures for [x-ray] diagnosis and for surveys cause more genetic change in the population at large than a lifetime of work with ionizing radiation."[16]

Summary.   In recent years the National Committee on Radiation Protection and Measurements as well as the International Commission on Radiological Protection have made certain recommendations in relation to radiation protection, which have been reproduced in various handbooks published by the National Bureau of Standards.[5]

These recommendations may be summarized as follows:

1. The revised recommendations are not based on any positive evidence of damage at the earlier higher levels of radiation but are rather in accordance with trends of scientific opinion to reduce radiation exposure to an absolute minimum.

2. The entire population has been divided into two groups, a small one consisting of those who work with radiation or radioactive substances under the supervision of a radiation safety officer, and second, a very large group consisting of everyone else. The exposure in controlled areas to individuals occupationally exposed to radiation is such that the hazard will be no greater than might be anticipated in any industry.

The exposure to the rest of the population is dictated on the basis of the desire to diminish radiation so that there will not exist any significant genetic hazard to the population as a whole.

3. The unit of the present recommendations is the *REM*. This is the quantity of any ionizing radiation which has the same biological effectiveness as one RAD of x-rays in the usual energy range. Various radiations have various relative biological effectiveness differing according to specific ionization. The dose in REMS is equal to the dose in RADS multiplied by the relative biological effectiveness for the radiation in question. The RAD has been defined as: "100 ergs of energy absorbed from radiation per gram of tissue." This is a unit of "absorbed dose" differing from the roentgen which is a unit based upon ionization of air by radiation. Suffice it that with radiation in the million volt range, the roentgen and the RAD are almost interchangeable. However, with the lower energy radiations such as are used in diagnostic roentgenology, there is a very considerable difference in that a roentgen absorbed in air, in soft tissues such as fat, and in bone, gives rise to a widely differing number of ergs per gram. Thus the ergs per gram for one roentgen in air are 84; for fat 84; but for bone 245.

4. The maximum permissible accumulated dose to the whole body in REMS at any age is equal to five times the number of years beyond 18, provided no annual increment exceeds 15 REMS. Occupational exposure may not start before age 18. This implies an average weekly dose of 0.1 REM if the exposure is a regular part of the occupation. However there are provisions for fluctuations as long as the annual total is kept at about 5 REMS. A permissible weekly whole body dose of 0.3 REM may be maintained for an appreciable period, provided in another period the dose is sufficient to keep the total for the year within the set limit. Thus the total accumulation in 13 consecutive weeks must not exceed 3 REMS. Such a period of high exposure must be compensated for by an adequate period of low exposure.

The hands and forearms are often exposed to more radiation than any other part of the body. Since they do not constitute a critical region involving either gonads or vital organs, it is permissible for them to receive a maximum weekly dose of 1.5 REMS on the skin.

The maximum permissible dose to the gonads for the population of the United States as a whole shall not exceed an average of 14 REMS per individual over the period from conception to age 30 and one-third that for each decade thereafter during the reproductive period.

5. Radiation levels for radioisotopes deposited within the body must conform to the same general principles as for external radiation. Thus whole body radiation to individuals in controlled areas should be limited to 0.3 REM for the first week after administration of a short-lived isotope. For a long-lived isotope this may be too high a dose level, and the 3 REMS in 13 weeks must not be exceeded.

6. When it is a question of isotope therapy or of diagnostic procedures from which the patient is expected to receive some advantage, it is evident that these limits cannot be imposed any more than they can on diagnostic or therapeutic applications of x-rays. Here the matter of benefit to be obtained from the radiation must be weighed against the possible harm and the patient's physician must make the final decision.

7. For individuals outside controlled areas, dose levels should in general be not more than 1/10 those inside.

This has been further supplemented by the Atomic Energy Commission and read into the Federal Register (January 29, 1957) as follows (Table 2–1):

It will be noted from the above, that two different categories of individuals are recognized: (1) those who by choice of occupation must of necessity be exposed to radiation. These individuals must not receive more exposure than that recommended by the International Commission of Radiation Protection. (2) All other individuals must not exceed approximately one-third that exposure.

In line with these statements are those of the Summary Report to the Public from the National Academy of Sciences (1956)[17] which are summarized as follows:

1. Records should be kept for every individual, showing his total accumulated lifetime exposure to radiation.

2. The medical use of x-rays should be reduced as much as is consistent with medical necessity.

Table 2–1. Permissible Weekly Dose of Radiation

CONDITIONS OF EXPOSURE		DOSE IN CRITICAL ORGANS (mrem)			
Parts of body	Radiation	Skin, at basal layer of epidermis	Blood-forming organs	Gonads	Lens of eye
Whole body	Any radiation with half-value-layer greater than 1 mm. of soft tissue.	[1]600	[1]300	[1]300	[1]300
Whole body	Any radiation with half-value-layer less than 1 mm. of soft tissue.	1500	300	300	300
Hands and forearms or feet and ankles or head and neck	Any radiation	[2]1500	—	—	—

[1] For exposure of the whole body to X or gamma rays up to 3 mev, this condition may be assumed to be met if the "air dose" does not exceed 300 mr. provided the dose to the gonads does not exceed 300 mrem. "Air dose" means that the dose is measured by an appropriate instrument in air in the region of highest dosage rate to be occupied by an individual, without the presence of the human body or other absorbing and scattering material.

[2] Exposure of these limited portions of the body under these conditions does not alter the total weekly dose of 300 mrem permitted to the blood-forming organs in the main portion of the body, to the gonads, or to the lens of the eye.

3. The average exposure of the population's reproductive cells to radiation above the natural background should be limited to 10 roentgens from conception to age 30.

4. The 10 roentgen limit should be reconsidered periodically with a view to keeping the reproductive cell exposure at the lowest practicable level.

5. Individual persons should not receive a total accumulated dose to the reproductive cells of more than 50 roentgens up to age 30 years, and not more than 50 roentgens additional up to age 40. (About half of all children in the United States are born to parents under 30, nine-tenths to parents under 40.)

From this mass of recommendations and accumulated data, what course shall we as physicians follow? From the practical point of view, we must always weigh what we do for our patients in the light of the benefit to be derived by the patient. This is true for all phases of medicine whether they be therapeutic, surgical, medical or radiologic. Hence, if the care of the patient *requires* radiation exposure, we must not deny him of its benefits. The promiscuous, unwarranted use of radiation, however, is to be condemned.

With these basic observations in mind, we can proceed to practical considerations.[5]

PROTECTION OF THE PATIENT IN X-RAY DIAGNOSIS[5, 8]

Exposure of the patient in x-ray diagnosis may be considered from the standpoint of protection against the acute effects and the chronic effects of overexposure, each being dealt with in relation to fluoroscopy on the one hand and radiography on the other. The acute effects are epilation and erythema; the chronic effects may be reflected in the blood-forming organs, may cause induction of malignant tumors, cataracts, impaired fertility, reduction of the life span, and produce genetic changes.

The methods of diminishing x-ray exposure of the patient may be outlined as follows:

THE USE OF MAXIMUM FILTRATION IN THE PRIMARY BEAM.   The inherent filtration of the tube structure is ordinarily equivalent to 0.5 mm. of aluminum. The addition of 2.0 to 4.0 mm. of aluminum is highly desirable. In the usually employed voltage range (40 KvP to 120 KvP), 1 mm. of aluminum will reduce the dose to the skin about 60 per cent; 2 mm. of aluminum about 80 per cent at 50 KvP and 60 per cent at 130 KvP; and 3 mm. of aluminum about 80 to 85 per cent.

It is also interesting that added filtration of this order has very little effect on the resulting roentgenograms. The effective radiation is that which is transmitted through the part being radiographed and hence is the more penetrating, "hard" type previously mentioned. The addition of a filter increases the transmission by a large factor, at the same time reducing the percentage of soft radiations. The quality of the resulting radiograph is not materially altered by the additional filtration, and the increase in the exposure time necessary is relatively small.

It is concluded that it is advisable to use 2 mm. of aluminum filter for voltages of 50 to 70 KvP and 3 mm. of aluminum for voltage above 70 KvP. If voltages above 100 KvP are employed, use ¼ mm. of copper added filtration.

THE USE OF HIGHER VOLTAGES WHENEVER POSSIBLE WITHOUT SIGNIFICANTLY ALTERING THE QUALITY OF THE RADIOGRAPH.   This expedient also increases the penetration of the beam, thereby relatively diminishing the total quanta of rays which must strike the skin of the patient to produce a satisfactory radiograph.

This, of course, is of particular importance in pregnancy examinations.

INCREASED TARGET-TO-SKIN DISTANCE AS MUCH AS IS PRACTICABLE.   On the basis of the inverse square law, this increases the intensity of the remnant radiation (producing the radiographic or fluoroscopic image) for a given entry dose. In fluoroscopy a minimum target-skin distance of 18 inches should be used. In radiography, a minimum target-film distance of 36 inches is recommended.

THE USE OF AS SMALL A FIELD OF RADIATION AS IS NECESSARY TO ACHIEVE THE DESIRED DIAGNOSTIC RESULT.   This may be achieved with cones in radiography and an adjustable diaphragm in fluoroscopy.

DIMINISHING FLUOROSCOPIC EXPOSURE AS MUCH AS POSSIBLE.   Thus, using a 18-inch target-to-table-top distance, 80 KvP, and 4 Ma., with 3 mm. of aluminum filtration added, fluoroscopy adds 5 to 8 roentgens per minute to the skin of the irradiated area. Five minutes of fluoroscopy to one area must be considered maximum.

CALCULATION OF DOSAGE TO PATIENTS IN DIAGNOSTIC EXAMINATIONS. Various tables and nomograms have been provided which permit ready calculation of dose delivered. Table 2–2 is representative.

Needless to say, these are representative values and will vary with the techniques employed. It is advised that each radiologist become familiar with the dosages obtained by his techniques.

Although maximum tolerance doses are established for workers with radiation at 0.3 roentgen per week, the maximum permissible dose to patients is not established.

As a guide, however, in determining the safe patient exposure factors for fluoroscopy and radiography, the accompanying tables of maximum permissible exposure values in milliampere-seconds are included. Milliampere-seconds are

Table 2–2. Skin Dose per Film and Central Body Dose per Total Examination at the Center of the Beam[12, 13, 15]

EXAMINATION	SKIN DOSE (ROENTGENS/ FILM)	DOSE IN ROENTGENS TO CENTER OF ORGAN (17 cm. cone 3.0 mm. Al filter 90 Kv) AFTER COMPLETE ROUTINE EXAMINA-TION (Several Films)	TESTIS[9]	OVARY[9]
Teeth (Whole mouth)	33			
Skull or Sinuses	4	0.4		
Chest, P.A.	0.16		P.A. .005	.010
Lateral	0.42	0.1		
Body-section	0.36			
Abdomen				
KUB film	2.2	0.26	.003	.040
Obstetric, AP	2.6	1.0 to 4.2		
Lat.	12.4			
Gallbladder	2.6	1.0		
Pelvis, AP	4.7	0.2	.020	.080
I.V.P.	2.5	1.0		
Spines, Cervical, AP	1.5	0.6		
Lat.	1.1	0.6		
Dorsal, AP	4.7	0.7		
Lat.	10.5	0.6		
Lumbar, AP	5.2	1.3	.005	.100
Lat.	12.4		.025	1.0/0.5
Shoulder, AP	1.3	0.6		
Extremities	0.44	0.6	.006	.001 (knee)
Stomach fluoroscopy	75 to 100	3.0		

36-inch T.F.D. except chest which is 72-inch T.F.D.; 2 mm. Al filter.

Table 2–3. Maximum Permissible Exposure Values in Milliampere-Seconds for All Parts of the Body Except the Head (At 85 KvP)

TARGET-SKIN DISTANCE (INCHES)	FILTER (mm. Al) External......None Inherent.......0.5 Total..........0.5	FILTER (mm. Al) External.......0.5 Inherent.......0.5 Total..........1.0	FILTER (mm. Al) External.......1.0 Inherent.......0.5 Total..........1.5
10	265	510	810
12	380	730	1090
14	520	1000	1500
16	680	1300	1950
18	870	1650	2500
20	1060	2050	3000
22	1280	2450	3640
24	1530	2900	4360
30	2400	4500	6800
36	3460	6500	9800
42	4700	8850	13300
48	6150	11600	17400

Table 2–4.   Maximum Permissible Exposure Values in Milliampere-Seconds for the Head
(At 85 KvP)

TARGET-SKIN DISTANCE (INCHES)	FILTER (mm. Al) External.....None Inherent.......0.5 Total.........0.5	FILTER (mm. Al) External.......0.5 Inherent.......0.5 Total.........1.0	FILTER (mm. Al) External.......1.0 Inherent.......0.5 Total.........1.5
10	200	380	610
12	290	550	875
14	390	750	1190
16	510	970	1560
18	650	1240	1980
20	800	1530	2450
22	960	1840	2970
24	1150	2150	3540
30	1790	3360	5540
36	2585	4840	7950
42	3600	6560	10850
48	4600	8550	14100

Table 2–5.   Changes in Tables 2–3 and 2–4 When Kilovoltage Is Altered

KVP	CHANGE IN MAXIMUM PERMISSIBLE EXPOSURE VALUES
100	Reduce by 25%
90	Reduce by 8%
85	No change
80	Increase by 10%
70	Increase by 35%
60	Increase by 80%

the product of milliamperes and total actual exposure time in seconds. The kilovoltage presented is 85 KvP. When higher voltage is used, a reduced value must be applied as indicated in Table 2–5, and likewise when lesser voltages are used, the change in permissible exposure value is increased as shown. Table 2–3 applies to all parts of the body except the head. Table 2–4 applies only to the head and represents a reduction of approximately 25 per cent. The values of these tables are based on: (1) the average output of a typical installation, (2) the average figure of 275 roentgens for a "threshold erythema," and (3) a factor of 50 per cent which is necessary to cover unpredictable variations in either of the first two factors. These tables are meant to cover a four year period at least.[4]

We do not actually know the limitation to impose on diagnostic procedures, except to avoid untoward reaction or visible reactions of any kind. Radiation hazards to the embryo and fetus are particularly important to bear in mind.[13] The developing embryos of a great variety of animals, including several mammals, are highly susceptible to the induction of malformations by radiation. These malformations occur in a well-defined critical period for each genus. There is no reason to doubt that this also applies to human embryos. In man this would correspond with the second to the sixth week of gestation for the majority of characters, when doses of less than 25 roentgens may be detrimental. Beyond this period, the effects are less obvious or possibly delayed with such doses. *Certainly, if pregnancy is known, radiation should be avoided in the first trimester of pregnancy at all costs and as much as possible in pregnancy thereafter.*

PROTECTION OF THE PHYSICIAN IN X-RAY DIAGNOSIS

As pointed out previously, most local injuries sustained by the physician are of the hands. Such injuries can be avoided by certain protective measures:

1. The physician should at all times wear protective lead gloves of at least 0.5 mm. lead equivalent, as well as a lead-lined apron or its equivalent. Roentgenoscopic screens with lead-rubber drapes also diminish radiation exposure.

2. The physician's unprotected hands, wrists, arms or other parts should never be exposed to the x-ray beam.

3. Eye accommodation preceding fluoroscopy should be at least 20 minutes.

4. Suitable kilovoltage and milliamperage settings at fluoroscopy should be adopted, as follows:

Abdomen	80 KvP	3–4 Ma.
Chest	70 KvP	3.0 Ma.
Thick extremities	60 KvP	3.0 Ma.
Thin extremities	50 KvP	3.0 Ma.
Children	50–55 KvP	3.0 Ma.

5. General Principles of Fluoroscope Use:

(a) Shutters must be closed down to no more than 30 to 40 square centimeters.

(b) The fluoroscope should be used intermittently, and should be avoided when the patient is not intercepting the beam.

(c) The examination should be concluded as quickly as possible, usually within five minutes. It is well to have a special timing device in the circuit to turn off the machine automatically when this time is exceeded.

(d) When fractures are being set or foreign bodies located, alternating radiography with intermittent manipulation should be used, if possible, rather than fluoroscopy.

(e) Head fluoroscopy should never be used.

Metabolic changes are perhaps incurred by physicians even though sufficient protection is worn. The high incidence of leukemia in radiologists, and even among non-radiologists, has already been alluded to; it is possible that when certain susceptible individuals receive even the minimal exposure allowed for in the above methods, they ultimately develop leukemia.[3]

Figure 2–1 shows the approximate number of milliroentgens received by physicians in 43 fluoroscopic examinations (80 KvP, 3 to 5 Ma.) in various parts of their bodies when no protection was used.[1] Even when aprons and conventional lead-lined gloves are used, it is thought that about 35 gastr intestinal fluoroscopic examinations weekly or their equivalent are probably maximum for the average physician in an average installation.[10] The maximum, of course, will vary with different physicians and the technique they employ. Actually, it would be well for every individual to study his technique very closely, even to the point of taking measurements over various exposed parts of his body to see how he may diminish his exposure with adequate attention to these regions. Archer's[1] lead glass fabric may have further value in that it can be purchased so that it covers the body completely; when it is so purchased, the manufacturers make a survey of the individual's technique and exposure and protect him accordingly by constructing a gown especially for his use. Such a service is quite expensive but in terms of life, death, and disease it is certainly

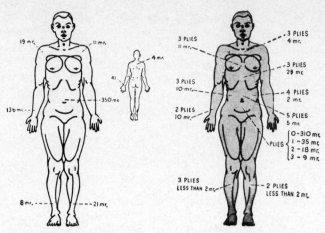

Fig. 2–1. Drawing showing radiation in milliroentgens received by operator when no protection was used during 43 fluoroscopic examinations (left) and radiation received through various thicknesses of lead glass fabric during 43 fluoroscopic examinations (right). (From Archer, Cooper, and Kroll: Protection against x-ray and beta radiation. J.A.M.A. vol. *148:* 1952.)

well worth serious consideration. "If reduction in life span is proportional to the dose received, it may be inferred that radiologists using present safeguards do not need to fear any significant future reduction in their life span due to irradiation."[3]

PROTECTION AGAINST ELECTRICAL HAZARD. In addition to the radiation hazard, an electrical hazard may also be present. The voltages used to energize x-ray tubes are highly dangerous. The best assurance of safety is the enclosure of all high voltage parts in a shock-proof container. Most x-ray machines now being made for diagnostic use are of shock-proof design, but where the design is such that high voltage conductors are exposed, operators should keep at a liberal distance from them and should guard against spark-gap formation. A space of at least one foot should always be allowed between such a conductor and any body part.

X-ray apparatus should not be installed or operated in dangerous locations. When used in a room with anesthetic gases, the machine and all switches should be explosion proof, or all electrical contacts should be 5 feet or more above floor level. Provision should be made to protect all exposed cables from mechanical damage, and these should be periodically inspected for defects or abrasions.

Table 2–6. Methods to Insure Adequate Protection

FOR PATIENT	FOR PHYSICIAN
1. Avoid examination in the first trimester of pregnancy.	1. Wear lead impregnated gloves and apron.
2. Work with a minimum of 2 to 3 mm. of aluminum filter over aperture of tube.	2. Never expose unprotected areas to x-ray beam.
3. Use as high a kilovoltage as possible.	3. Always use repeated x-ray film examination rather than fluoroscopic unit in the setting of fractures.
4. Increase target-skin distance as much as possible.	4. Avoid head fluoroscopy.
5. Use narrow shutter for fluoroscopy screen and use unit intermittently with limitation of time.	5. Accommodate eyes for 20 minutes prior to fluoroscopy.

All of the exposed non-current-carrying parts of the apparatus should be permanently grounded in acceptable fashion with good ground leads.

It is well to bear in mind first aid practices such as artificial respiration and emergency treatment for burns, in the event the need for these should arise.

Although the high tension does not extend to the dark room, the hazard of electrical shock in the darkroom is great. Lighting fixtures form the greatest potential hazard in this regard and must be carefully installed with every attention to proper insulation and grounding.

REFERENCES

1. Archer, V. W., Cooper, G., Kroll, J. G., and Cunningham, D. A.: Protection against X-ray and Beta Ray Radiation. J.A.M.A., *148:* 106–108, 1952.
2. Bacon, J. F., and Leddy, E. T.: Protection in Roentgenoscopy. M. Clin. North America, *29:* 1036–1041, 1945.
3. Braestrup, C. B.: Past and Present Radiation Exposure to Radiologists from the Point of View of Life Expectancy. Am. J. Roentgenol., *78:* 988–992, 1957.
4. General Electric X-Ray Corporation: What You Should Know About X-Ray Protection.
5. Handbook No. 42, Safe Handling of Radioactive Isotopes.
   Handbook No. 52, Maximum Permissible Amounts of Radioisotopes in the Human Body and Maximum Permissible Concentrations in Air and Water.
   Handbook No. 54, Protection Against Radiations from Radium, Co 60, and Cesium-137.
   Handbook No. 59, Permissible Dose from External Sources of Ionizing Radiation.
   Handbook No. 65, Safe Handling of Bodies Containing Radioactive Isotopes.
   Addendum which has been published in Radiology, *71:* 263–266, 1958.
6. Henshaw, P. S., and Hawkins, J. W.: Incidence of Leukemia in Physicians. J. National Cancer Inst., *4:* 339–346, 1944.
7. International Recommendations on Radiological Protection. Revised by the International Commission on Radiological Protection at the Sixth International Congress of Radiology, London, July 1950. Radiology, *6:* 421–439, 1951.
8. Laughlin, J. S., Meurk, M. L., Pullman, I., and Sherman, R. S.: Bone, Skin, and Gonadal Doses in Routine Diagnostic Procedures. Am. J. Roentgenol., *78:* 962–982, 1957.
9. Lincoln, T. A., and Gupton, E. D.: Radiation Dose to Gonads from Diagnostic X-ray Exposure. J.A.M.A., *166:* 233–239, 1958.
10. Macht, S. H., and Kutz, E. R.: Detection of Faulty Roentgenoscopic Technique by Direct Radiation Measurement. Am. J. Roentgenol., *68:* 809–814, 1952.
11. March, H. C.: Leukemia in Radiologists. Radiology, *43:* 275–278, 1944.
12. Ritter, V. W., Warren, S. R., Jr., and Pendergrass, E. P.: Roentgen Doses During Diagnostic Procedures. Radiology, *59:* 238–250, 1952.
13. Russell, L. B., and Russell, W. L.: Radiation Hazards to the Embryo and Fetus. Radiology, *58:* 369–376, 1952.
14. Sorrentino, J., and Yalow, R.: A Nomogram for Dose Determinations in Diagnostic Roentgenology. Radiology, *55:* 748–753, 1950.
15. Stanford, R. W., and Vance, J.: The Quantity of Radiation Received by Reproductive Organs or Patients during Routine Diagnostic X-ray Examinations. Brit. J. Radiology, *28:* 266–273, 1955.
16. Stone, R. S.: The Concept of a Maximum Permissible Exposure. Radiology, *58:* 639, 1952.
17. The Biological Effects of Atomic Radiation: A Summary Report to the Public from the National Academy of Sciences—National Research Council, 1956.

CHAPTER 3

The Development
of Bone

OSTEOBLASTS, the cells which are responsible for the deposition of bone, are normally differentiated from mesenchyme in two different environments:

In the first, exemplified by the skull, they form within fibroblastic and collagenous membranes—and bone formed in such an environment is called *intramembranous ossification*.

In the second type of ossification (*endochondral*), osteoblasts develop in a cartilaginous environment. Their source is thought to be perichondrial cells, or fibrous connective tissue cells, and the means by which these penetrate the cartilage cells is described below.

INTRAMEMBRANOUS OSSIFICATION

Intramembranous ossification begins when certain mesenchymal cells differentiate into osteoblasts. These appear in clusters called *centers of ossification*.

Osteoblasts secrete or form the intercellular organic matrix of bone called *osteoid*, and ultimately this matrix surrounds the osteoblast in a chamber called a *lacuna*, which is then said to contain the *osteocyte*, or bone cell.

Simultaneously, phosphatase is secreted which causes calcification of the osteoid.

Near the margin of the bony anlage the osteoblasts proliferate, producing growth by spider-like processes or "spicules." These spicules join one another in a lattice-work called *bony trabeculae*. When the lattice spaces predominate, the bone is called *cancellous*. When the trabeculae are compactly arranged and the lattice spaces are sparse, the bone is called *compact* (Fig. 3–2).

The lattice spaces in both cases contain the main blood supply and marrow tissues.

ENDOCHONDRAL OSSIFICATION (Fig. 3–1)

Most of the skeleton forms as a result of endochondral ossification.

In the various sites where bones are to form, the mesenchyme of that area begins to differentiate into cartilage with a surrounding membrane called the *perichondrium*.

Cartilage grows by one of two methods:

1. *Interstitial* growth, in which the cartilage cells themselves retain their capacity to divide. This capacity is retained by young cartilage cells only. These

cells are responsible for the addition of intercellular substance, which enables the cartilage to expand from within.

2. *Appositional* growth is defined as the adding of new cartilage to a pre-existing surface, and is due to differentiation of the deep perichondrial cells into chondroblasts and later to chondrocytes.

The cartilaginous anlage increases in length by interstitial growth. This growth is greater near the ends than the mid-section. The chondrocytes go through a definite cycle of maturation which is characteristic wherever cartilage is undergoing transformation into bone. The areas of such transformation are: (1) The primary center of ossification in the center of the shaft; (2) in linear fashion in the epiphyseal plate and (3) in the subarticular region of the growing end, where the epiphysis is formed.

This cycle develops as follows:

1. Cartilaginous interstitial growth.

2. Swelling, vacuolation and maturation of these cells, with the secretion of phosphatase.

3. Intercellular calcification of cartilaginous matrix.

4. Death of the cartilage cells and fragmentation of the calcified intercellular substance.

5. Invasion of the disintegrating calcific zone by blood vessels and osteogenic cells.

6. Elaboration of bony matrix around the calcific foci remaining, forming trabeculae of bone.

With the progressive development of the vascular system, the perichondrium is invaded by blood vessels. The cells which were chondroblasts and chondrocytes within the perichondrium become osteoblasts, and a thin layer or shell of bone is laid down around the cartilaginous anlage. The perichondrium has thus become the periosteum (Fig. 3–1, *B*).

Thereafter, osteogenic cells together with capillaries grow from the inner layer of the periosteum into the breaking down mid-section of the cartilage. These vessels provide the osteoblastic source for the primary center of ossification and epiphyseal plate, the latter by extension along the shaft. Ossification gradually extends toward the ends of the anlage (Fig. 3–1, *C*). Periosteum also continues to add bone to the sides of the anlage, and as this becomes more compact, the central area becomes more cancellous, ultimately forming the marrow cavity (Fig. 3–1, *C*).

However, ossification stops short of replacing all the cartilage near the end of the anlage. The cartilage cells on the shaft side of the articular cartilage go through the maturation cycle which is responsible for the ossification of the shaft. Ossification also stops short of "a plate" between the epiphyseal and diaphyseal centers of ossification (*epiphyseal disk or plate*).

In the epiphyseal disk, there are two processes occurring constantly:

1. Proliferation of cartilage cells which tend to thicken it and make it grow, and,

2. Calcification, death and replacement of cartilage on its diaphyseal side which tends to thin it out.

This allows the bone to grow, and is identical with the maturation cycle described above.

Any interference with any of these processes is quickly reflected in an aberration of bone growth.

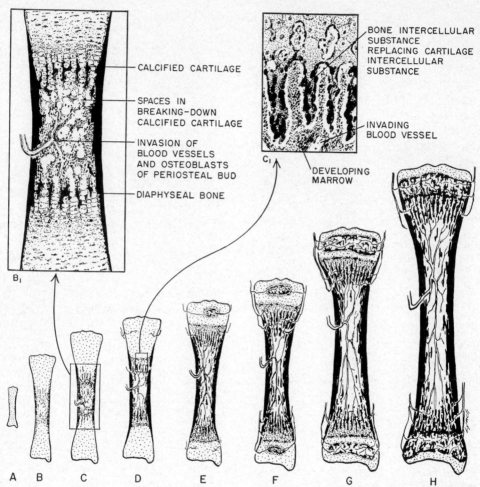

CALCIFIED CARTILAGE

SPACES IN
BREAKING-DOWN
CALCIFIED CARTILAGE

INVASION OF
BLOOD VESSELS
AND OSTEOBLASTS
OF PERIOSTEAL BUD

DIAPHYSEAL BONE

B₁

BONE INTERCELLULAR
SUBSTANCE
REPLACING CARTILAGE
INTERCELLULAR
SUBSTANCE

INVADING
BLOOD VESSEL

C₁

DEVELOPING
MARROW

A   B   C   D   E   F   G   H

FIG. 3–1. Diagram to illustrate the growth and ossification of a typical long bone: *A*, Primary cartilaginous anlage. *B*, Primary center of ossification in shaft with early conversion of perichondrium to periosteum. *C*, Further progression of the perichondrial ossification and extension of the partially calcified cartilage upward toward the metaphysis. *D*, Continued absorption of the inner compact bony wall and new bone deposition beneath the periosteum. Note the bone intercellular substance replacing the cartilage intercellular substance and the invasion of the blood vessels from the region of the marrow. *E, F* and *G*, Commencement and continued ossification of the epiphyses. Note the demarcation between the metaphysis and epiphyseal plate, *H*, The ossification of the epiphyseal plate and cessation of growth. Note the covering of articular cartilage which remains unossified.

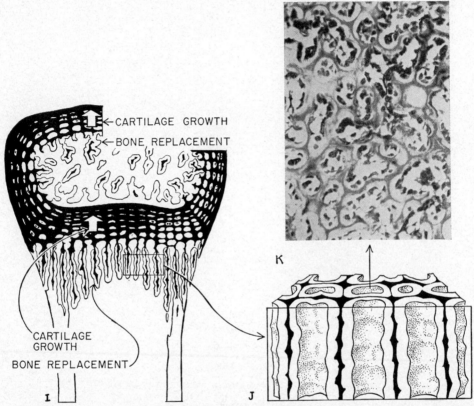

CARTILAGE GROWTH
BONE REPLACEMENT
CARTILAGE
GROWTH
BONE REPLACEMENT
I
J
K

Fig. 3–1. *I*, Diagram which illustrates in longitudinal section an end of a growing long bone. The trabeculae appear stalactite-like in such a preparation. However, if they could be seen in three dimensions, as is illustrated in *J*, it would be seen that close to the plate the structures that appear as trabeculae in a longitudinal section are slices that have been cut through walls that surround spaces; they are slices cut through walls of tunnels. Photomicrograph *K* represents what is seen in a cross-section cut through the metaphysis of a growing long bone of a rabbit, close to the epiphyseal disk. In it the trabeculae of bone have cartilaginous cores and they surround spaces. These spaces under the periphery of the disk become filled in to form haversian systems and such compact bone as is present in the flared extremities of bone is built by spaces such as these becoming filled in. (Modified from Ham: *Histology*, J. B. Lippincott Co., 3rd Ed. 1957.)

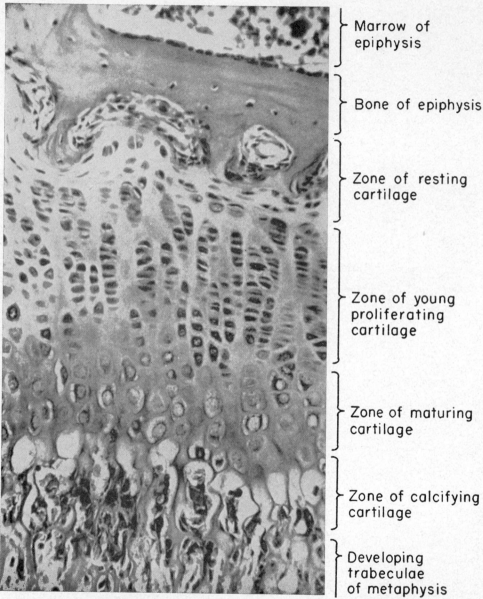

Marrow of epiphysis

Bone of epiphysis

Zone of resting cartilage

Zone of young proliferating cartilage

Zone of maturing cartilage

Zone of calcifying cartilage

Developing trabeculae of metaphysis

Fig. 3–1. *L*, High-power photomicrograph of a longitudinal section cut through the upper end of the tibia of a guinea pig. This picture illustrates the different zones of cells in the epiphyseal plate. (Modified from Ham: *Histology.*)

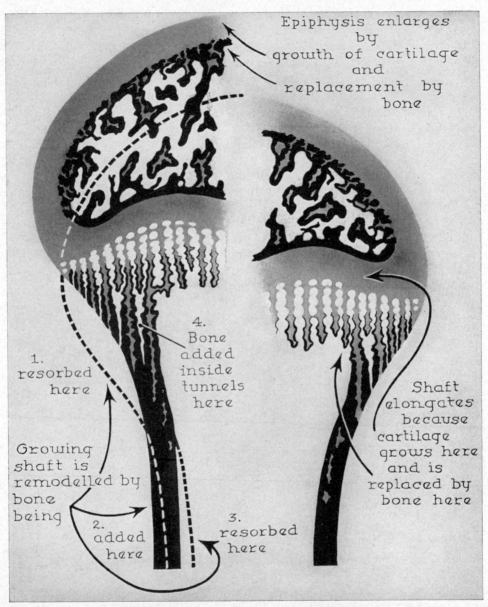

Epiphysis enlarges
by
growth of cartilage
and
replacement by
bone

4.
Bone
added
inside
tunnels
here

1.
resorbed
here

Growing
shaft is
remodelled by
bone
being

2.
added
here

3.
resorbed
here

Shaft
elongates
because
cartilage
grows here
and is
replaced by
bone here

FIG. 3–1. *M*, Diagram showing the manner in which bone is deposited and resorbed to account for the remodeling that takes place at the ends of growing long bones that have flared extremities. (From Ham: J. Bone and Joint Surg., vol. 34A, 1952.)

Thus, the epiphyseal disk is composed of four different zones passing from the diaphysis to the epiphysis (Fig. 3–1, *L*):

1. Zone of calcified cartilage.
2. Zone of maturing cartilage.
3. Zone of proliferating young cartilage.
4. Zone of "resting" cartilage which binds the plate to the bone of the epiphysis.

The zones of maturing and proliferating cartilage are arranged in columns, and any deviation from regularity is an indication of an abnormal process at work.

The zone of calcified cartilage is thin and intermingles with the bone of the diaphysis arranged in longitudinally disposed trabeculae. This zone of calcified cartilage is seen in the x-ray as the provisional zone of calcification (Fig. 3–3). As rapidly as bone is added to the epiphyseal plate side of the metaphysis, it is resorbed by osteoblasts on the marrow side.

The growth in diameter of the shaft of the bone as well as the normal flaring is accomplished by continuous resorption at the outer periphery of the epiphyseal plate, and adding to the shaft below this level (Fig. 3–1, *M*). The shaft of the bone grows in width by apposition of new bone under the periosteum while at the same time bone is dissolved away from the inside of the shaft.

These added layers of bone are called "circumferential lamellae" and tend to surround the entire shaft (Fig. 3–4). Some of these are converted to haversian systems as more and more lamellae are added. The persistent blood supply to these lamellae and haversian systems from the periosteum are contained within canals called Volkmann's canals.

The bone marrow contained in the medullary spaces contains connective tissue, fat, blood vessels, nerve fibers, all of the hematogenic elements of the blood and osteogenic elements as well. Yellow marrow consists mainly of fat and thus differs from the red marrow.

The periosteum of bone is not normally detected in the radiograph because it is not calcified and offers no contrast to overlying structures. When it is seen, it is an indication of abnormality.

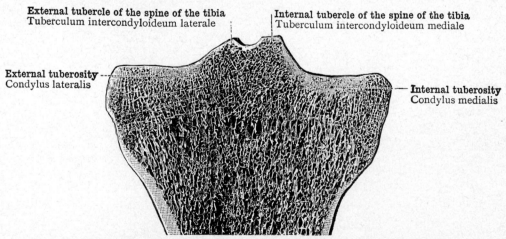

External tubercle of the spine of the tibia
Tuberculum intercondyloideum laterale

Internal tubercle of the spine of the tibia
Tuberculum intercondyloideum mediale

External tuberosity
Condylus lateralis

Internal tuberosity
Condylus medialis

FIG. 3–2.   Macroscopic longitudinal section through a typical long bone (tibia) to show cancellous and compact bone. (From C. Toldt, *An Atlas of Human Anatomy*, Macmillan Co., New York, 1926.)

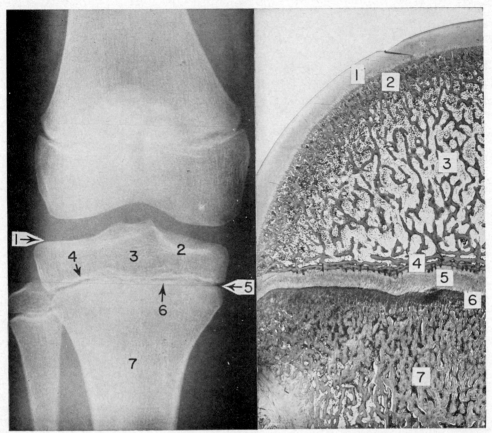

FIG. 3–3. (From Pyle and Hoerr: *Radiographic Atlas of Skeletal Development of the Knee*, Charles C Thomas, 1955.)

RADIOLOGICAL TERMS:

1. Articular cartilage does not show in a film.
2. White outline of subarticular margin of epiphysis.
3. Epiphysis.
4. Increased density of terminal plate; inner bone margin of epiphysis.
5. Epiphyseal line; strip of lesser density; epiphyseal plate; diaphyseal-epiphyseal gap. Radiographically, these terms exclude the recently calcified cartilage, which appears as part of the metaphysis.
6. Metaphysis; includes both calcified cartilage and newly-formed bone. (Zone of provisional calcification.)
7. Diaphysis or shaft.

HISTOLOGICAL TERMS:

1. Articular cartilage.
2. Compact bone of subarticular margin.
3. Epiphysis, spongy bone.
4. Terminal plate.
5. Epiphyseal disk; growth cartilage. Histologically, these terms include the calcified cartilage.
6. Metaphysis; includes only newly formed bone of primary ossification.
7. Spongy bone of diaphysis.

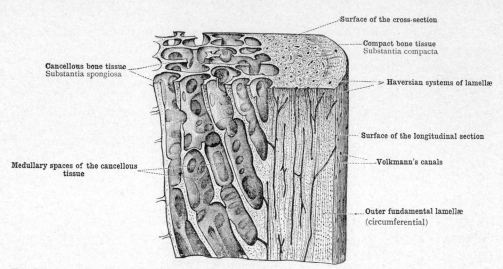

FIG. 3–4.   **a,** Diagram to illustrate the structure of bone. (From C. Toldt, *An Atlas of Human Anatomy.* Macmillan Co., New York, 1926).

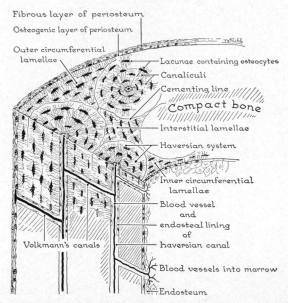

FIG. 3–4.   **b,** A three-dimensional diagram showing the appearance of both a cross and a longitudinal section of the various components that enter into the structure of the cortex of the shaft of a long bone. The diagram shows the different kinds of lamellae that are present and the relation between the blood vessels of the periosteum, Volkmann's canals, haversian canals and the marrow cavity. (From Ham: *Histology*, 3rd edition, J. B. Lippincott Co.)

THE BLOOD SUPPLY OF A LONG BONE (Figs. 3–5, 3–6)

There are three sets of vessels supplying a long bone:

1. *The nutrient artery* (or arteries), derived from the original periosteal bud to the primary ossification center.

2. *The metaphyseal and epiphyseal vessels,* entering these regions directly. Epiphyseal vessels are of two types: (a) In epiphyses completely surrounded by articular cartilage (like the head of the femur), the epiphyseal vessel enters between the articular and epiphyseal plate cartilages. (b) In other epiphyses, the vessel may enter the epiphyses directly.

After growth in length ceases, the cartilage of the epiphyseal plate is resorbed and replaced by bony trabeculae (Fig. 3–1, *H*). Anastomoses between the epiphyseal and metaphyseal vessels thus occur and these are called metaphyseal-epiphyseal vessels.

3. *The periosteal vessels* contribute to the arterioles in the haversian systems and Volkmann's canals.

The blood supply of the *bone marrow* is very rich. The nutrient or medullary artery penetrates obliquely through the nutrient foramen where it divides into an ascending and descending branch and supplies an abundance of small arteries to all portions of the medullary portion of the bone.

The terminal arteries end in broad capillaries which simulate sinusoids. Certain of the terminal arteries anastomose with those of the cancellous epiphyses and with the arteries which enter the haversian system of the compact bone from the periosteum, which have already been described. Afferent veins return the blood as companion veins to the arterial system described above.

The nerves accompany the blood vessels throughout.

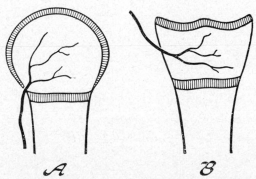

A　　　　　*B*

Fig. 3–5. Drawings to show the two types of epiphyseal blood supply. When separation of the epiphyseal plate occurs in *A*, the blood vessels are torn and the bone of the epiphysis dies. (Preparation by G. Dale and W. R. Harris.) (From Ham: *Histology.* 3rd edition, J. B. Lippincott Co.)

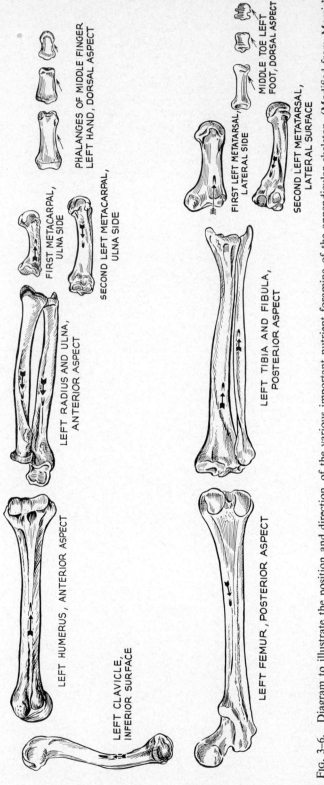

PHALANGES OF MIDDLE FINGER
LEFT HAND, DORSAL ASPECT

MIDDLE TOE LEFT
FOOT, DORSAL ASPECT

FIRST LEFT METATARSAL,
LATERAL SIDE

SECOND LEFT METATARSAL,
LATERAL SURFACE

FIRST METACARPAL,
ULNA SIDE

SECOND LEFT METACARPAL,
ULNA SIDE

LEFT RADIUS AND ULNA,
ANTERIOR ASPECT

LEFT TIBIA AND FIBULA,
POSTERIOR ASPECT

LEFT HUMERUS, ANTERIOR ASPECT

LEFT FEMUR, POSTERIOR ASPECT

LEFT CLAVICLE,
INFERIOR SURFACE

FIG. 3-6.   Diagram to illustrate the position and direction of the various important nutrient foramina of the appendicular skeleton. (Modified from Morris' *Human Anatomy*.)

WOLFF'S LAW

Wolff's law postulates that the internal architecture and external structure of bone are related to its function and change with altered function. The arrangement of trabeculae in the upper end of the femure is an example of this principle

"BONE AGE" VERSUS "CHRONOLOGIC AGE"

The ossification of epiphyses is frequently quite irregular in its general outline, which produces confusing appearances on the radiograph. It is always helpful whenever possible to obtain comparison views with the normal opposite side in the same individual so that such confusing appearances can properly be related to a physiologic process in the individual.

The ossification of bone follows a rather well-defined pattern. After study of many hundreds of individuals, certain growth charts have been constructed whereby the so-called "bone age" can be stated up to the early twenties. "Bone age" can therefore be compared with the actual calendar or chronologic age to determine whether or not a growth deterring or accelerating process has been in operation.

Although most epiphyseal centers of ossification appear after birth, there are several notable exceptions: The center of the distal end of the femur appears during the ninth month of intra-uterine life; the center for the proximal end of the tibia and the center for the head of the humerus often appear toward the end of the intra-uterine period also. Most of the other centers of long bones appear during infancy and childhood with the exception of the clavicle. This has an epiphysis at its medial end only and this does not appear until the eighteenth or twentieth year. It is one of the last to unite.

In any given long bone the epiphysis which appears first is usually the last to fuse. The fibula, femur and tibia are frequently exceptions to this rule.

The nutrient canal of a long bone is directed away from the epiphysis which fuses last (Fig. 3–6).

Some epiphyseal centers do not appear until puberty or thereafter, such as those of the innominate bone, scapula, ribs and vertebrae.

The following techniques are used in establishing a normal bone age.

The Determination of Bone Age from Birth to Five Years of Age. In this early period one may use either the methods recommended by Sontag, Snell, and Anderson[5] or those of Elgenmark[1] of counting the ossification centers visible on roentgenograms of half of the skeleton and correlating these with bone age. As an alternate method in this early period one may use the standards of Francis as indicated in Figure 3–7, Figure 3–8, Table 3–1 and Table 3–2.

The methods avoid reliance upon any single small group of ossification centers during an age period when variation in their time of appearance is great.

Only if the technique of skeletal survey of several areas is impractical for any given case should the estimation of any bone age in infancy be made from a single roentgenogram of either the hand or the foot. Nevertheless, these latter prove to be very useful standards and are reproduced here for reference, together with alternate charts.

Table 3–1.   Time Order of Appearance of Ossification Centers from 5 to 15 Years: Male, White.

Age	Center
5 years 2 months	Hum. med. epicondyle
5 years 6 months	Ulna, dist.
6 years 2 months	Epiphysis of calcaneus
8 years 0 months	Epiphysis of talus
8 years 4 months	Trochlea of humerus
8 years 8 months	Olecranon
9 years 4 months	Lesser troch. femur
9 years 10 months	Pisiform
10 years 4 months	Sesamoids of flex. hall. brevis
10 years 5 months	Hum. lat. epicondyle
10 years 10 months	Tib. tubercle
11 years 0 months	5 metat. prox.
11 years 8 months	Sesamoid of flex. poll. brevis
13 years 3 months	Tubercle, rib 1
13 years 4 months	Ant. inf. iliac spine; Trans. proc. T 1
13 years 5 months	Acromion; iliac crest
13 years 10 months	Coracoid angle
15 years 0 months	Ischial tuber.*
15 years plus	Med. clav.

* Provisional.

Table 3–2.   Time Order of Appearance of Ossification Centers from 6 to 15 Years: Female, White.

Age	Center
6 years 8 months	Olecranon
6 years 10 months	Epiphysis of talus
7 years 1 month	Pisiform
7 years 2 months	Trochlea of humerus
7 years 7 months	Lesser troch. femur
8 years 2 months	Sesamoids of flex. hall. brevis
8 years 3 months	Hum. lat. epicondyle
8 years 7 months	5 metat. prox.
9 years 0 months	Tib. tubercle
9 years 3 months	Ant. inf. iliac spine*
9 years 4 months	Sesamoid of flex. poll. brevis
10 years 10 months	Tubercle, rib 1
11 years 3 months	Coracoid angle
11 years 4 months	Trans. proc. T 1; Acromion
12 years 0 months	Iliac crest
13 years 2 months	Ischial tuber.*
14 years 6 months	Med. clav.

* Provisional.

DATES OF APPEARANCE OF CENTERS OF OSSIFICATION
BIRTH TO 5 YRS. OF AGE - WHITE MALES

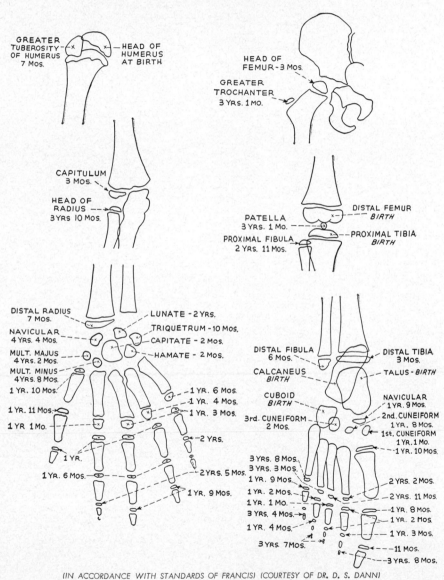

(IN ACCORDANCE WITH STANDARDS OF FRANCIS) (COURTESY OF DR. D. S. DANN)

FIG. 3–7. Dates of appearance of centers of ossification. Birth to five years of age—white males.

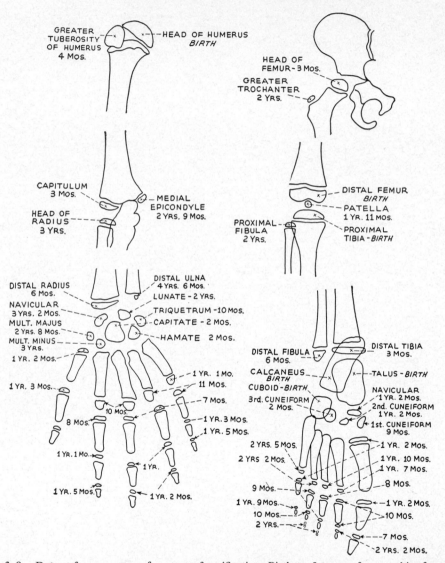

Fig. 3–8.   Dates of appearance of centers of ossification. Birth to 5 years of age—white females.

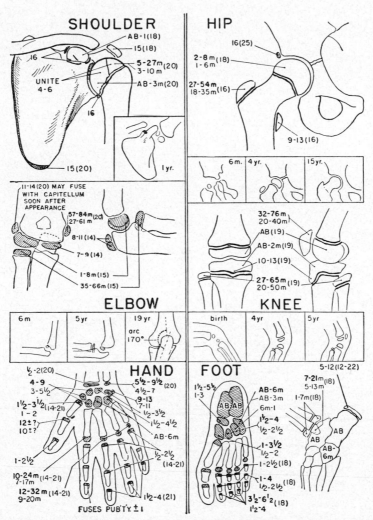

FIG. 3–9.   The figures indicate the range from the 10th to the 90th percentile in appearance time of centers of ossification, obtained from the studies on bone growth available in 1950. Statistically significant studies of the time of appearance of ossification centers have been made of relatively few portions of the skeleton after the sixth year of life. Figure followed by "m" mean months, otherwise all numbers indicate years. Where two sets of numbers are given for one center of ossification, the upper heavier figures refer to males and the lower lighter figures refer to females. A single set of figures applies to both sexes. "AB" indicates that the ossification center is visible at birth. Figures in parentheses give approximate time of fusion. (From Girdany, B. R., and Golden, R.: Am. J. Roentgenol. vol. 68, 1952.)

Table 3-3

OSSIFICATION OF UPPER EXTREMITY and SHOULDER GIRDLE

	SCAPULA	CLAVICLE	HUMERUS	ULNA	RADIUS	CARPUS	METACARPUS	PHALANGES
BIRTH			HEAD A					
1 yr	CORACOID PROCESS A		CAPITULUM and LATERAL PART OF TROCHLEA A			CAPITATUM — A, HAMATUM		
2 yrs					DISTAL END A	TRIQUETRUM ♀		BASES ♀ A
3 yrs			GREATER TUBERCLE A			TRIQUETRUM ♂	BASE OF FIRST A, HEADS OF ALL REST A	BASES ♂ A
4 yrs				HEAD EXTENDING INTO STYLOID A		LUNATUM ♀, NAVICULAR ♀, LUNATUM ♂		
5 yrs			LESSER TUBERCLE A		HEAD ♀ A	MULTANGULAR MAJUS ♀, NAVICULAR ♂, MULTANGULAR MAJUS ♂		
6 yrs			MEDIAL EPICONDYLE ♀ A, TUBERCLES UNITE WITH HEAD			MULTANGULAR MINUS ♀		
7 yrs					HEAD ♂ A	MULTANGULAR MINUS ♂		
8 yrs			MEDIAL EPICONDYLE ♂ A	DISTAL END A				
9 yrs								
10 yrs	SUBCORACOID (UPPER 1/3 OF GLENOID) A					PISIFORM ♂ AND ♀		
11 yrs			MEDIAL PART OF TROCHLEA A	TOP OF OLECRANON A				
12 yrs	MARGINS OF GLENOID A, INFERIOR ANGLE A, VERTEBRAL BORDER A, TWO FOR ACROMION A		LAT. EPICONDYLE A		TUBEROSITY A			
13 yrs								
14 yrs			CAPITULUM, TROCHLEA LAT. and MED. EPICONDYLE	TOP OF OLECRANON ♀ F	HEAD ♀ F, TUBEROSITY F			
15 yrs	CORACOID AND SUBCORACOID F		LATERAL EPICONDYLE UNITES WITH ARTICULAR SURFACES					
16 yrs		MEDIAL END A					ALL FUSE ♀	ALL FUSE ♀
17 yrs								
18 yrs			ALL PROXIMAL EPIPHYSES ♀ F	TOP OF OLECRANON ♂ F	HEAD ♂ F			
19 yrs			ALL DISTAL EPIPHYSES F	DISTAL END ♀ F	DISTAL END ♀ F		FUSE ♂	ALL FUSE ♂
20 yrs	TWO FOR ACROMION F, VERTEBRAL BORDER F, MARGINS OF GLENOID F, INFERIOR ANGLE F							
21 yrs			ALL PROXIMAL EPIPHYSES ♂ F	DISTAL END ♂ F	DISTAL END ♂ F			
22 yrs or more		MEDIAL END F (25)						

Table 3-4

OSSIFICATION OF LOWER EXTREMITY AND PELVIS

	HIP BONE	FEMUR	PATELLA	TIBIA	FIBULA	TARSUS	METATARSUS	PHALANGES
BIRTH		DISTAL EPIPHYSIS A				CALCANEOUS, TALUS, CUBOID A		
1 yr.		HEAD A		PROXIMAL END A	DISTAL END A	THIRD CUNEIFORM A		BASE OF PROXIMAL PHALANGES ♀ A
2 yrs.				DISTAL END A			BASE OF FIRST / HEAD OF OTHERS ♀ A	BASE OF PROXIMAL PHALANGES ♂ A
3 yrs.		GREATER TROCHANTER ♀ A			PROXIMAL END A	NAVICULAR, SECOND CUNEIFORM, FIRST CUNEIFORM A	BASE OF FIRST / HEAD OF OTHERS ♂ A	
4 yrs.		GREATER TROCHANTER ♂ A	APPEARS					
5 yrs.								
6 yrs.								BASE OF DISTAL PHALANGES A
7 yrs.								
8 yrs.	CONJOINED RAMI F			MEDIAL MALLEOLUS BEGINS TO OSSIFY		SECONDARY CALCANEAL ♀ A		
9 yrs.								
10 yrs.		LESSER TROCHANTER A		OSSIFICATION OF TIBIAL TUBERCLE BEGINS		SECONDARY CALCANEAL ♂ A		
11 yrs.								
12 yrs.			COMPLETED					
13 yrs.								
14 yrs.	ILIAC CREST A, ANT. INF. SPINE A, ISCHIAL TUBEROSITY A, PUBIC SYMPHYSIS (SECONDARY) A					ALL TARSALS COMPLETED EXCEPT SECONDARY CALCANEAL ♀ F		
15 yrs.								
16 yrs.		ALL SECONDARY EPIPHYSES F ♀		BOTH F ♀				
17 yrs.	TRI-RADIATE F	ALL SECONDARY EPIPHYSES F ♂						
18 yrs.				BOTH F ♂	DISTAL EPIPHYSIS F *	SECONDARY CALCANEAL ♂ F		
19 yrs.							ALL FUSE *	ALL FUSE *
20 yrs.								
21 yrs.	ALL SECONDARY EPIPHYSES F (EXCEPT TRI-RADIATE)							
22 yrs. or more					PROXIMAL EPIPHYSIS F *			

* FEMALE EPIPHYSES FUSE SOMEWHAT EARLIER THAN THOSE OF MALE

Bone Age Determination Between Ages Six and Fifteen Years. Tables 3–1, 3–2, 3–3 and 3–4 give the time order of appearance of ossification centers in male and female white children in the various age groups indicated. In the latter two tables, the letter A indicates appearance and the letter F indicates time of fusion. The appropriate symbols also indicate male and female.

Changes in the Wrist and Hand Which Occur with the Growth of the Individual (Fig. 3–10). The wrist and hand furnish excellent opportunity to determine the bone age of a child between birth and 10 years of age. Not only is the time of appearance of the epiphyses of importance in this regard, but also their configuration. This has been very carefully depicted in standards set up after study of large groups of children. The most widely used standards are those of Todd,[6] traced in Figure 3–10.

The carpus is ordinarily cartilaginous at birth, but the centers of ossification for the capitate and hamate carpal bones soon make their appearance—usually by the sixth month. Thereafter, usually no new centers appear until 2 years of age in the female and 2 to 3 in the male, when the triquetrum makes its appearance. The lunate, navicular, greater multangular, lesser multangular and pisiform appear thereafter at approximately yearly intervals.

The epiphyses of the metacarpals usually make their appearance at approximately 2 years of age in the female and 3 in the male. They fuse between 17 and 19 years of age.

At birth the phalanges are usually fairly well formed, and the primary centers of ossification are central with the exception of the ungual phalanges where the primary centers are more distal.

The epiphyses are found at the bases of the phalanges and they appear at about 2 years of age in the female and slightly later in the male. Their growth and development parallel that of the metacarpals closely. Several standard charts are illustrative of the mode of application of bone age studies. (See Tables 3–3 and 3–4.)

The distal epiphysis of the radius ordinarily appears at about 9 months of age, and is quite well developed when the distal epiphysis of the ulna appears radiographically at about 4 years. The styloid process of the ulna becomes ossified at about 8 years in the female and 9 years in the male. The distal radial and ulnar epiphyses fuse at about 19 years in the female, and about one to two years later in the male.

The Utilization of the Knee in Assay of Growth and Development.[4] Pyle and Hoerr have developed a set of radiographic standards of reference in relation to the maturation of the knee, similar to those of Todd's for the hand (Fig. 3–10), and subsequently further studied by Greulich and Pyle.[3] This was accomplished by developing what they called "intermediate skeletal maturity indicators" from the beginning of ossification of the growing end of the bone to the time of fusion of the epiphysis. These maturity indicators at birth are the ossified portions of the epiphyses around the knee, and the indentation of the adjoining metaphysis of the femur. At 6 months, the characteristic thinness of the growth cartilage of the femur is the indicator; at 9 months (male) the indicator is the thinness of the growth cartilage of the tibia. As the knee grows, further indicators are: the shaping of the epiphyses and the adjoining metaphyses; the width of the epiphyseal plates; the width of the joint space; the vertical heights of the condyles in relation to one another; the shaping of the joint surfaces; and finally, the fusion of the epiphyses with the metaphyses. An effort is made in the accompanying tracings of these standards (Fig. 3–11) to reproduce these changes as accurately as possible in accordance with the standards as published by these authors, but, needless to say, it is difficult in these tracings to do complete justice to the original radiographs in relation to the various maturation indicators.

The authors caution that a skeletal age of the whole knee of 20 per cent more or less than the actual chronologic age of the child should not in itself be evidence of abnormality.

Indeed, it is not wise to rely on any single area of the skeleton to assess bone age but rather several areas must be assessed, and the bone age interpreted as a whole.

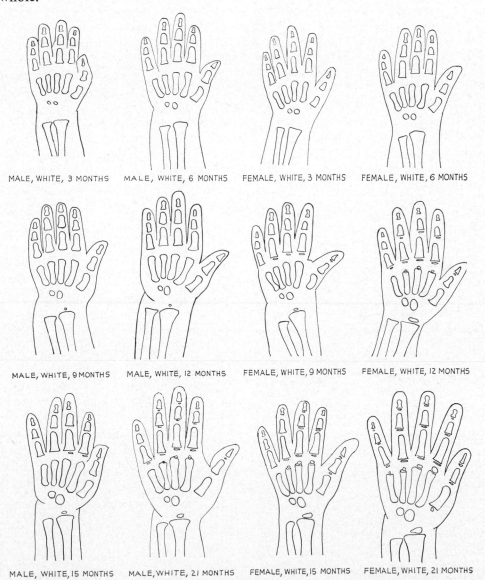

MALE, WHITE, 3 MONTHS   MALE, WHITE, 6 MONTHS   FEMALE, WHITE, 3 MONTHS   FEMALE, WHITE, 6 MONTHS

MALE, WHITE, 9 MONTHS   MALE, WHITE, 12 MONTHS   FEMALE, WHITE, 9 MONTHS   FEMALE, WHITE, 12 MONTHS

MALE, WHITE, 15 MONTHS   MALE, WHITE, 21 MONTHS   FEMALE, WHITE, 15 MONTHS   FEMALE, WHITE, 21 MONTHS

FIG. 3–10.   Osseous changes in the wrist and hand which occur with age in the male and female. These tracings may be used as standards for bone age determination by comparison with the actual radiograph. (Modified from T. W. Todd: *Atlas of Skeletal Maturation* [*Hand*]. C. V. Mosby Co., St. Louis, 1937.) Figure continued on following pages.

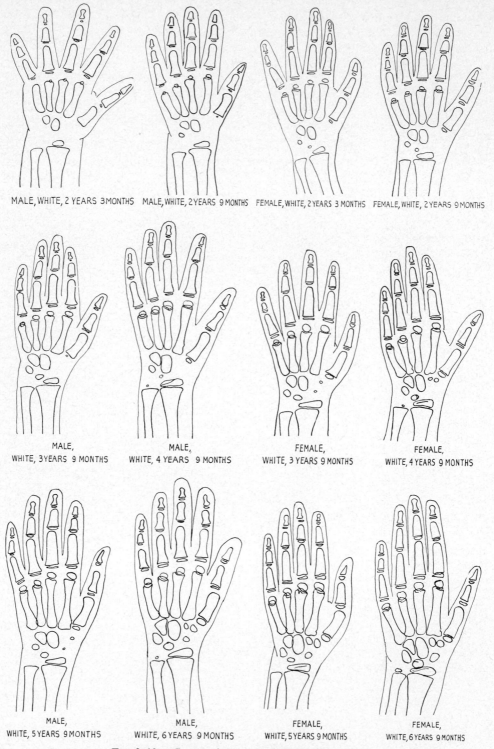

MALE, WHITE, 2 YEARS 3 MONTHS   MALE, WHITE, 2 YEARS 9 MONTHS   FEMALE, WHITE, 2 YEARS 3 MONTHS   FEMALE, WHITE, 2 YEARS 9 MONTHS

MALE,
WHITE, 3 YEARS 9 MONTHS

MALE,
WHITE, 4 YEARS 9 MONTHS

FEMALE,
WHITE, 3 YEARS 9 MONTHS

FEMALE,
WHITE, 4 YEARS 9 MONTHS

MALE,
WHITE, 5 YEARS 9 MONTHS

MALE,
WHITE, 6 YEARS 9 MONTHS

FEMALE,
WHITE, 5 YEARS 9 MONTHS

FEMALE,
WHITE, 6 YEARS 9 MONTHS

FIG. 3–10. *Continued.* See preceding page for legend.

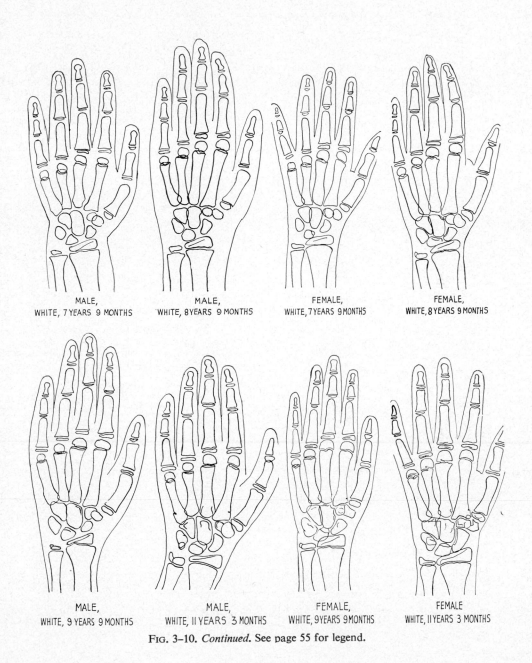

MALE,
WHITE, 7 YEARS 9 MONTHS

MALE,
WHITE, 8 YEARS 9 MONTHS

FEMALE,
WHITE, 7 YEARS 9 MONTHS

FEMALE,
WHITE, 8 YEARS 9 MONTHS

MALE,
WHITE, 9 YEARS 9 MONTHS

MALE,
WHITE, 11 YEARS 3 MONTHS

FEMALE,
WHITE, 9 YEARS 9 MONTHS

FEMALE
WHITE, 11 YEARS 3 MONTHS

FIG. 3–10. *Continued.* See page 55 for legend.

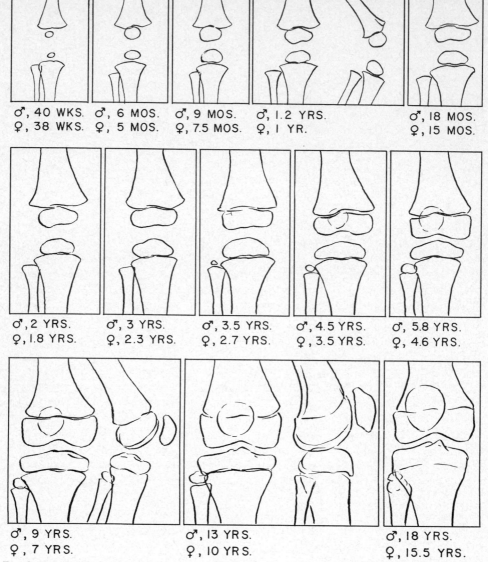

♂, 40 WKS.   ♂, 6 MOS.   ♂, 9 MOS.   ♂, 1.2 YRS.   ♂, 18 MOS.
♀, 38 WKS.   ♀, 5 MOS.   ♀, 7.5 MOS. ♀, 1 YR.   ♀, 15 MOS.

♂, 2 YRS.   ♂, 3 YRS.   ♂, 3.5 YRS.   ♂, 4.5 YRS.   ♂, 5.8 YRS.
♀, 1.8 YRS. ♀, 2.3 YRS. ♀, 2.7 YRS.   ♀, 3.5 YRS.   ♀, 4.6 YRS.

♂, 9 YRS.   ♂, 13 YRS.   ♂, 18 YRS.
♀, 7 YRS.   ♀, 10 YRS.   ♀, 15.5 YRS.

FIG. 3–11.   Osseous changes in the knee with age in the male and female (after Pyle and Hoerr).

SUGGESTED ROUTINE FOR BONE AGE DETERMINATIONS

From birth to age 5, it is suggested that the following regions be radiographed (AP refers to antero-posterior):

1. An AP view of the shoulder.
2. An AP view of the elbow.
3. An AP view of the hand and wrist.
4. An AP view of the hip.
5. An AP view of the knee.
6. An AP view including the ankle and foot.

From age 6 to 11 years the following are recommended:

1. AP views of the elbow.
2. AP views of the wrist and hand.

3. AP view of the foot.

4. Lateral view of the knee.

For individuals 12 years to 15 years of age the following are recommended:

1. AP views of both hands and wrists.

2. AP views of both feet.

3. AP views of both elbows.

4. An AP view of the shoulder.

5. An AP view of at least one half of the pelvis including the ilium and hip region as well as one half of the sacrum.

Beyond the age of 15 years one is primarily interested in studying the closure of the epiphyses, and it is well under these circumstances to obtain AP views of the shoulders, elbows, hands and wrists, hips, knees and ankles.

In spite of all of the foregoing tabular and pictorial data, the comment is justified that statistically significant studies of the time of appearance of the ossification centers have been made of relatively few portions of the skeleton after the sixth year of life. Actually, the time of fusion of the epiphyses, with the exception of those of the hands, has not been adequately investigated.

One should not negate the value of the x-ray examination of the various epiphyseal standards, since definite bone retardation implies some constitutional imbalance and this in turn should stimulate further investigation of the patient.

CARTILAGE

Hyaline cartilage forms the articular surfaces of joints, the costochondral junctions, the nasal cartilage, the bronchial rings, and parts of the trachea and larynx. Articular cartilage has the following layer-like structure as one proceeds from the epiphysis adjoining the joint surface proper: a zone of calcified cartilage nearest the bone; a zone of transition, consisting of longitudinal columns of large chondrocytes, and a gliding zone, which is the true articular zone and in which the cells tend to be flat and elongated and lie in the plane of the articular surface. The perichondrium is a continuation of the periosteum laterally but does not extend over the gliding zone proper. The actual thickness of articular cartilage is from 0.2 to 0.5 mm. in small joints, 2 to 3 mm. in larger joints, and as much as 4 mm. in the knee joint. The actual joint space on the radiograph in children is considerably wider since there is included a greater portion of cartilaginous epiphysis as well. The osseous articular surfaces are smooth and the limiting contour lines of the joints sharp in the adult, but they may be irregular and blurred in the child.

Fibrocartilage is found normally in such locations as the intervertebral disks, symphysis pubis, sternoclavicular joints and articular menisci, and it represents a modified fibrous tissue.

Elastic cartilage is hyaline cartilage to which have been added elastic fibers. It is found in the ligamentum nuchae, ligamentum flavae, the external auditory canal and the external ear.

Hyaline and elastic cartilage may undergo calcification and degeneration following trauma and during senility.

JOINTS (Figs. 3–12, 3–13)

There are three main types of joints: the movable (diarthroses), the slightly movable (amphiarthroses) and the immovable (synarthroses).

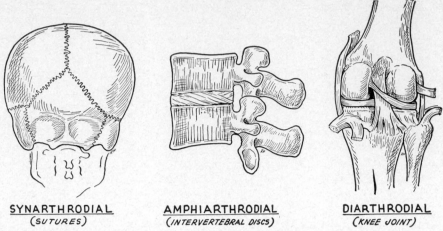

| SYNARTHRODIAL | AMPHIARTHRODIAL | DIARTHRODIAL |
| (SUTURES) | (INTERVERTEBRAL DISCS) | (KNEE JOINT) |

FIG. 3–12.   Classification of joints.

SCHEMATIC DIAGRAMS SHOWING FOUR STAGES IN THE DEVELOPMENT OF A JOINT

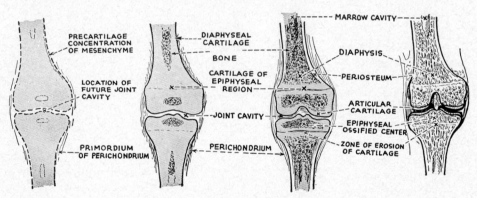

FIG. 3–13.

The *diarthroses* (movable joints) are invested by a joint capsule which consists of two layers: an outer fibroelastic layer continuous with the periosteum and an inner cellular layer, the synovial membrane. The synovial membrane is lined by an incomplete layer of mesenchymal cells which lie upon variable thicknesses of fibrous, adipose or areolar tissue. The loose areolar tissue may form villi, which are highly vascular and which have considerable regenerative powers when destroyed by disease or trauma. Synovial fluid is secreted by the cells lining the synovial membrane and acts as a lubricant by virtue of its mucin content. In hypertrophic arthritis there is increased mucin formation, and in rheumatoid arthritis there is decreased mucin. The following synovial joints contain fibrocartilaginous menisci: temporomandibular, radiocarpal, sternocostal, sternoclavicular, acromioclavicular, knee and glenohumeral.

The *amphiarthroses* (intervertebral disks) are composed of three parts: the nucleus pulposus, which forms the center of the disk; the annulus fibrosus, which is the fibrocartilaginous substance around the nucleus; and thin hyaline cartilaginous plates which form the upper and lower surfaces of the disk adjacent to the vertebral bodies. The nucleus pulposus absorbs and transmits pressure from one vertebral body to the other and moves about within the annulus fibrosus. Schmorl found that in 38 per cent of autopsied spines there was a protrusion of the nucleus pulposus into the adjoining vertebral bodies (hence called "Schmorl's nodes") and that occasionally such protrusion occurred toward the spinal canal. The disk may be destroyed by pyogenic infection, chronic non-specific infection, or tuberculosis, but there is considerable resistance to invasion by malignant neoplasm, although the latter may occur also.

The synarthroses (immovable joints) are represented by the sutures in the skull.

GENERAL PRINCIPLES OF IMPORTANCE IN THE RADIOGRAPHIC ANATOMY OF THE SKELETAL SYSTEM

1. In clinical radiography our emphasis is regional rather than sharply confined to a single anatomic structure. An area is investigated as a whole and it is not unusual, for example, to detect abnormality in the apex of the lung when viewing a shoulder for pain in that region.

2. The radiographic method for study of a region will vary with the clinical problem at hand. This will become readily apparent when it is evident that there are numerous views to be obtained with regard to each anatomic region and only those applicable to the case at hand are utilized. It is, therefore, most important to adapt the radiographic anatomic study to each individual problem.

3. The epiphyseal development varies somewhat from one individual to another, and in the anatomic study of epiphyses it is most important to compare both sides wherever possible. This is also true for the study of other symmetrical parts of the body such as the two sides of the skull or face. Thus the normal side of a given individual becomes one base line for comparison with the potentially abnormal structure.

4. In the study of the extremities we always include at least one joint in the radiograph, or one of the joints on either end of that bone, if possible. The main purpose of this is to demonstrate clearly the alignment of the bone with respect to the joints which it serves.

5. Certain distortions are sometimes inevitable and the observer must become familiar with the normal appearance of such distortion; e.g., when the head of the radius is injured, it is impossible for the patient to extend his elbow fully and a film of the unextended elbow results in considerable distortion (Chap. 4, Figs. 4–23, 4–24).

REFERENCES

1. Elgenmark, O.: Normal Development of Ossific Centers During Infancy and Childhood: Clinical Roentgenologic and Statistical Studies. Acta Paediat. (Supp. 1), *33:* 1–79, 1946.
2. Girdany, B. R., and Golden, R.: Centers of Ossification of the Skeleton. Am. J. Roentgenol., *68:* 922–924, 1952.
3. Greulich, W. W., and Pyle, S. I.: Radiographic Atlas of Skeletal Development of the Hand and Wrist. Stanford University Press, 1950.
4. Pyle, S. I., and Hoerr, N. I.: Radiographic Atlas of Skeletal Development of the Knee. Charles C Thomas, Springfield, Ill., 1955.
5. Sontag, L. W., Snell, D., and Anderson, M.: Rate of Appearance of Ossification Centers from Birth to the Age of Five Years. Am. J. Dis. Child., *58:* 949–956, 1939.
6. Todd, T. W.: Atlas of Skeletal Maturation (Hand). C. V. Mosby Co., St. Louis, 1937.

CHAPTER 4

The Upper Extremity

THE PRIMARY INTEREST, when reviewing the radiographic anatomy of the extremities, lies in the bony structures, since for the most part muscles are blended into a homogeneous mass. Joint capsular shadows can be distinguished, the fatty subcutaneous layer identified in soft films, and vascular channels visualized by special contrast media, but the bones by virtue of their radiopacity offer greatest scope to the diagnostic powers of the radiologist. The vascular channels visualized by special contrast studies are considered separately in Chapter 12.

The main function of the upper extremity is that of a prehensile organ. To perform at maximum efficiency, definite anatomic relationships between the various parts are maintained. In the event of the fracture of the bone or dislocation at a joint, its normal axis of operation should be restored, and from that standpoint the position of the fragments in relation to the normal must be understood. A system of lining has been developed to indicate normal position and alignment, and these will be described in greater detail in subsequent paragraphs.

THE SHOULDER

Related Gross Anatomy. The shoulder girdle consists of the clavicles and scapulas. These structures articulate with one another at the acromioclavicular joint and furnish a suspension type of support for the arm by means of the glenohumeral joint. They are firmly attached to the axial skeleton by the muscles of the vertebral column and the anterolateral thoracic wall.

The clavicle, when viewed from above, presents a double curvature (Fig. 4–1). The medial two thirds of the bone is convex forward and has the form of a triangular prism. The middle of the shaft is considerably smoother than either

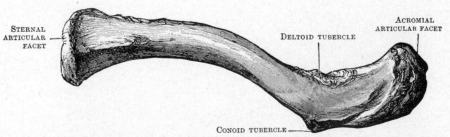

FIG. 4–1. Clavicle viewed from above. (From Cunningham's *Text-Book of Anatomy*, Edited by Arthur Robinson, published by Oxford University Press.)

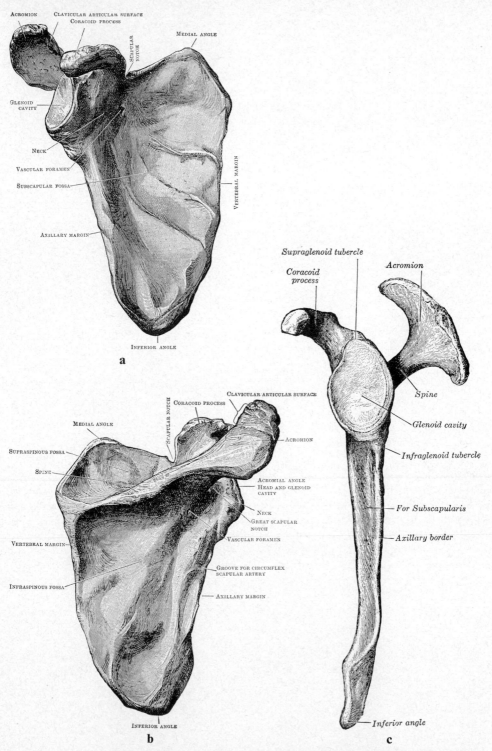

FIG. 4–2.   VIEWS OF THE SCAPULA: **a**, anterior; **b**, posterior; **c**, lateral. (**a** and **b**, From Cunningham's *Text-Book of Anatomy*, Edited by Arthur Robinson, Published by Oxford University Press. **c**, From Gray, *Anatomy of the Human Body*, Edited by C. W. Goss, Courtesy of Lea & Febiger.)

of the ends. The posterior border on the medial two thirds is variably indented and roughened by the "costal tuberosity" for the attachment of the costoclavicular ligament.

The lateral third of the clavicle with an anterior concavity tends to be flattened supero-inferiorly. On its inferior surface is a rough elevation, "the conoid tubercle," which overhangs the coracoid process of the scapula. This may be quite as prominent as the coracoid process in some individuals.

The scapula (Fig. 4–2) is a large flat bone on the dorsal aspect of the thorax between the second and the seventh ribs. The body of the scapula is a triangle from which the coracoid process extends anteriorly, and the spine extends posteriorly. The posterior part of the upper surface of the coracoid process is roughened for the attachment of the coraco-clavicular ligament. On occasion a small joint may be present between the two bones (Fig. 4–3). The spine continues laterally to form the acromion process which articulates with the clavicle. The anterior surface, or subscapular fossa, is marked by several oblique lines or ridges from which the subscapularis muscle takes origin (in part). The posterior surface is divided by the spine into supraspinatus and infraspinatus fossae. The lateral boundary of the infraspinatus fossa is formed by an oblique ridge of bone which runs from the glenoid cavity downward and backward to the inferior angle of the scapula. This ridge is crossed by an arterial groove and several smaller ridges. These various grooves and ridges are of importance from the standpoint of differentiation from fractures.

The various anatomic parts of radiographic significance are the coracoid process, glenoid process, neck, acromion process, spine, inferior angle, axillary border, vertebral border and supraspinatus fossa.

Radiographic Variation of the Shoulder in Children (Fig. 4–4). In the scapula at birth, the acromion, the coracoid process, the glenoid cavity, the inferior angle and the vertebral border are still cartilaginous, and hence are not visualized radiographically. The secondary center of ossification for the coracoid process proper appears about the first year, and fuses with the main body of the scapula around puberty. There is a subcoracoid center of ossification for the lateral part of the coracoid process and upper third of the glenoid cavity which appears about 10 years of age and fuses at puberty. The other secondary

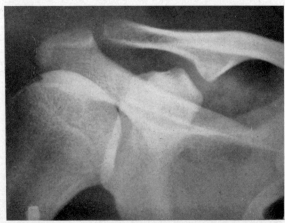

FIG. 4–3.   Roentgenogram showing coraco-clavicular joint. (From Moore, R. D., and Renner, R. R.: Am. J. Roentgenol., vol. 78, 1957.)

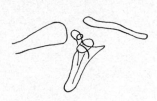

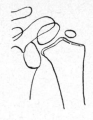

SHOULDER AT BIRTH

SHOULDER, MALE WHITE,
2 YEARS

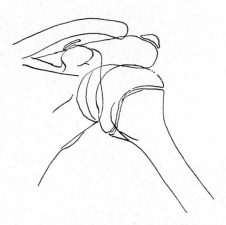

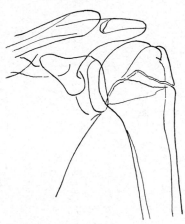

SHOULDER, FEMALE, II YEARS

SHOULDER, FEMALE, 16 YEARS

FIG. 4–4. Tracings of radiographs to illustrate the osseous changes which occur in the shoulder in different age groups.

centers of ossification for the margins of the glenoid cavity, the inferior angle, the vertebral border, and two centers for the acromion all appear about puberty, and fuse with the main body of the scapula between 20 and 25 years of age. Very occasionally, the epiphysis formed from the two acromial centers fails to fuse with the rest of the scapula, and remains a separate bone throughout life. When this occurs, the condition is usually bilateral, and must not be confused with a fracture.

ROUTINE RADIOGRAPHIC STUDIES OF THE SHOULDER REGION

1. **The Shoulder with the Arm in Rotation.** These views are particularly valuable for demonstration of the upper shaft of the humerus and the soft tissue structures in the vicinity of the shoulder joints. Thus, in addition to visualizing the greater and lesser tuberosities and intertubercular sulcus from different anatomic aspects, we are also permitted to demonstrate bursal abnormalities and occasionally joint capsules.

The views usually obtained in this regard are:

(*a*) NEUTRAL ANTERO-POSTERIOR VIEW OF THE SHOULDER (Fig. 4–5). In this position the patient is rotated approximately 15 degrees so that the shoulder

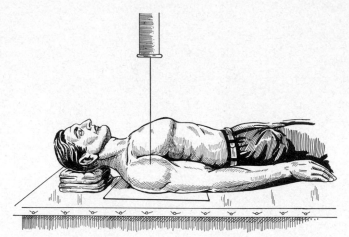

FIG. 4–5.   NEUTRAL ANTERO-POSTERIOR VIEW OF THE SHOULDER: **a,** Method of positioning patient

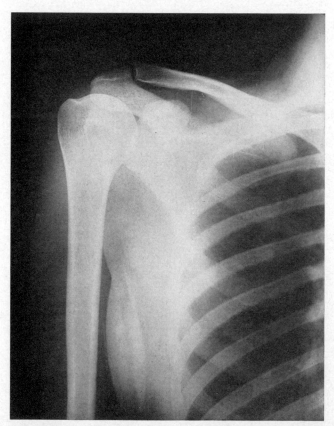

FIG. 4–5.   NEUTRAL ANTERO-POSTERIOR VIEW OF THE SHOULDER: **b,** Radiograph.

Points of Practical Interest with Reference to Figure 4–5:

1. The patient may be examined either in the erect position or supine as shown, and center midway between the summit of the shoulder and lower margin of the anterior axillary fold.
2. To produce better contact of the affected shoulder with the film, rotate the opposite shoulder away from the table top approximately 15 to 20 degrees, supporting the elevated shoulder and hip on sandbags.
3. When looking for faint flecks of calcium in the soft tissues, no-screen film and technique should be employed unless the shoulder is very muscular, in which case the Potter-Bucky apparatus may be employed in addition. When using the Potter-Bucky diaphragm (or grid cassette) it is best to position the cassette so that the central ray will pass through the center of the cassette and the coracoid process.

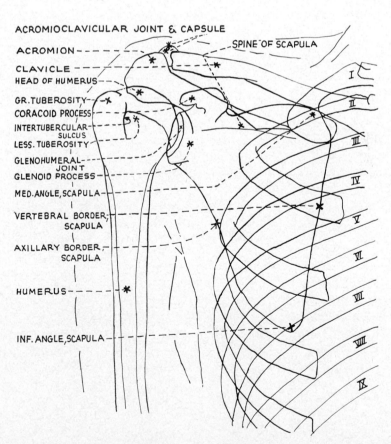

FIG. 4–5. NEUTRAL ANTERO-POSTERIOR VIEW OF THE SHOULDER: c, Labeled tracing of b.

being examined is flat against the table top (or film) and the opposite shoulder is slightly above the table top (or film). The arm is placed along the patient's side in a neutral position with the elbow somewhat obliquely placed. The technical factors will be varied depending upon what anatomic parts one wishes to emphasize.

If the soft tissues happen to be our major interest, and the shoulder is not too muscular, one would use a nonscreen technique with the film in a cardboard holder. This has the additional advantage of finer detail and less tendency to particulate artefacts. However, if the bony structures are to be investigated primarily, intensifying screen technique is more desirable.

In this view the greater tuberosity (tubercle) tends to be projected at the upper outer margin of the humerus, and the intertubercular sulcus is seen almost directly "en face." The lesser tuberosity is not seen to best advantage. The junction between the neck and the head of the humerus appears as an angular notch.

The anterior and posterior margins of the epiphyseal line are both seen, and are somewhat irregular. One must not confuse these with a fracture.

The glenoid fossa is not seen in complete profile, but its margins can be delineated with considerable clarity. It is particularly important to delineate the inferior margin of the glenoid cavity clearly, since this is the part that becomes roughened or hollowed out in repeated dislocations.

Occasionally, a thin semilunar radiolucent shadow is obtained between the head of the humerus and the glenoid cavity, particularly in children. It is probable that this represents a temporary vacuum in the glenohumeral joint.

The other structures of the scapula are seen in frontal view, but the posterior parts as well as the anterior may be identified. Thus, the coracoid process, spine, subscapular and infrascapular ridges may be seen. The scapula is projected behind the upper part of the thoracic cage, and thus there is some loss of detail.

The acromion process and its articulation with the clavicle are quite clear. Occasionally, the joint capsule is likewise delineated. The presence of the disk explains the wide separation of the acromioclavicular joint.

The clavicle in most of its length is also seen, and its various anatomic parts clearly delineated.

The bursal structures ordinarily blend with the other soft tissue structures and cannot be delineated. Under abnormal conditions of calcification or calcium deposition in the supraspinatus muscle tendon, these anatomic structures do attain radiographic significance.

(*b*) ANTERIOR-POSTERIOR VIEW OF THE SHOULDER WITH INTERNAL ROTATION OF THE HUMERUS (Fig. 4–6). The position of the patient is the same except that the entire arm (not just the forearm) is rotated inward. The greater tuberosity is projected along the medial margin of the upper shaft, and the lesser tuberosity is seen, but poorly. The intertubercular sulcus is likewise seen in profile and hence is difficult to identify clearly.

The other structures of the shoulder are essentially the same as previously described.

The bursal structures move with the head of the humerus, and if there be abnormal calcium within them, the rotation is apt to project this calcium away from the bony structures.

(*c*) ANTERO-POSTERIOR VIEW OF THE SHOULDER WITH EXTERNAL ROTATION OF THE HUMERUS (Fig. 4–7). Again the position of the patient is the same except that the entire arm is rotated externally. Here the lesser tuberosity is projected into silhouette along the upper outer margin of the shaft of the humerus. The other structures of the upper shaft of the humerus are not so clearly shown as in the neutral position.

This additional rotation affords another opportunity to demonstrate abnormal calcium in a bursa without interfence by the adjoining bones.

2. **View of the Shoulder for Greater Detail in Reference to the Glenoid Process** (Fig. 4–8). In order to see the glenoid process of the scapula in profile, the opposite shoulder must be rotated upward at least 45 degrees. This view is particularly important in cases of chronic dislocation of the shoulder, since in such abnormalities there is frequently erosion of the inferior margin of the glenoid process, seen only in profile in this projection.

3. **View of the Shoulder for Testing the Integrity and Degree of Separation of the Acromioclavicular Joint.** In order to demonstrate possible tear of the joint capsule of the acromioclavicular joint a special view must be obtained with the arm in traction (Fig. 4–9). This is done by taking an erect antero-posterior view of the shoulder with a heavy weight in the hand pulling down on the arm. Any latent separation of this joint thus becomes manifest when compared with the width of the joint space of the opposite side.

The comparison with the opposite side is most readily accomplished if both shoulders are filmed simultaneously as shown in Fig. 4–9.

4. **Lateral View of the Shoulder through the Axilla** (Fig. 4–10). In this view, the film is placed perpendicular to the table top and the central ray is directed horizontally into the axilla. The coracoid process is ordinarily projected anteriorly, and the acromion process posteriorly. The other structures are readily identified.

5 **Lateral View of the Shoulder Projected through the Body** (Fig. 4–11). It is frequently impossible to raise the arm when a shoulder has suffered injury. In order to obtain a lateral projection of the bones of this region, the arm on the affected side is placed against the film. The Bucky apparatus must be utilized to improve detail. The central ray is directed through the body at an upward angle of about 5 degrees. This view does not give the most accurate detail, but demonstrates the relative positions of the gross structures and the alignment of fragments.

6. **Lateral View of the Scapula** (Fig. 4–12). In this view, the scapula is placed perpendicular to the film, and the central ray strikes it in tangential fashion. The vertebral and axillary margins are projected over one another. Any disturbance in the main body of the scapula or its processes is readily detected in this manner.

7. **Special View of the Clavicle** (Figs. 4–13, 4–14). This is ordinarily an antero-posterior view of the clavicle with the central ray tilted about 5 degrees toward the head to project the clavicle away from the chest, and throw it into profile. Occasionally there is an anomalous articulation between the coracoid process and conoid tubercle of the clavicle; the sternoclavicular joint is not well shown in this view and will be further discussed under the thoracic cage.

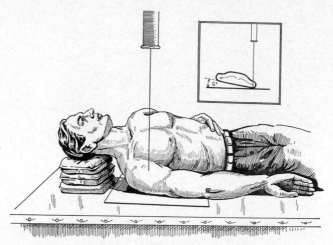

FIG. 4–6. ANTERO-POSTERIOR VIEW OF THE SHOULDER WITH INTERNAL ROTATION OF THE HUMERUS: **a,** Method of positioning patient.

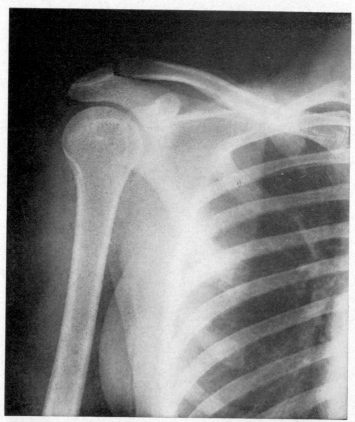

FIG. 4–6. ANTERO-POSTERIOR VIEW OF THE SHOULDER WITH INTERNAL ROTATION OF THE HUMERUS: **b,** Radiograph.

POINTS OF PRACTICAL INTEREST WITH REFERENCE TO FIGURE 4-6

1. One must make certain in this position that the entire humerus is rotated inward in addition to merely the forearm and hand.
2. The central ray may pass through the region of the coracoid process.
3. The angle of rotation of the body may be increased to 15 to 20 degrees instead of the 5 degrees as shown. This will produce a slightly better profile view of the glenoid process.
4. It is most important that sandbags be used on the hand and forearm to immobilize the patient. (These have been omitted for clarity in Fig. 4-6a.)

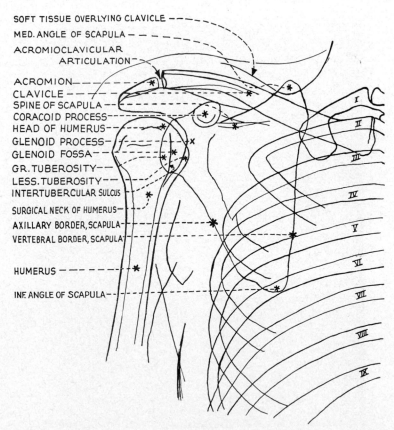

FIG. 4-6. ANTERO-POSTERIOR VIEW OF THE SHOULDER WITH INTERNAL ROTATION OF THE HUMERUS: c, Labeled tracing of b.

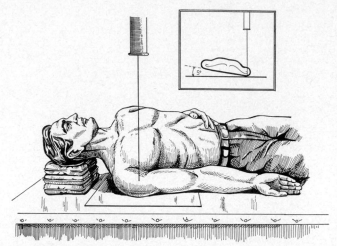

FIG. 4–7.   ANTERO-POSTERIOR VIEW OF THE SHOULDER WITH EXTERNAL ROTATION OF THE HUMERUS:
a, Method of positioning patient.

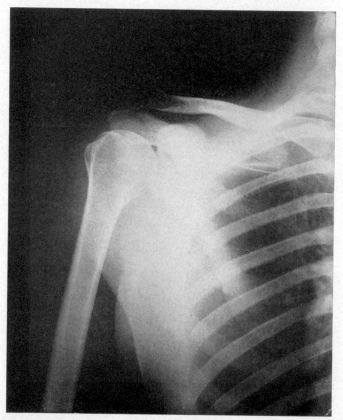

FIG. 4–7.   ANTERO-POSTERIOR VIEW OF THE SHOULDER WITH EXTERNAL ROTATION OF THE HUMERUS: **b,**
Radiograph.

POINTS OF PRACTICAL INTEREST WITH REFERENCE TO FIGURE 4–7.

1. One must make certain to rotate the entire arm externally in addition to the forearm and hand. (Sandbags as indicated for Fig. 4–6.)
2. In order to obtain a slightly better profile view of the glenoid process of the scapula, the angle of rotation may be increased from 5 degrees as shown to 15 or 20 degrees.
3. When looking particularly for small flakes of calcium deposit in the soft tissues of the shoulder, one must use a no-screen technique with or without the Potter-Bucky diaphragm. The central ray may be directed through the coracoid process rather than the centering as shown.

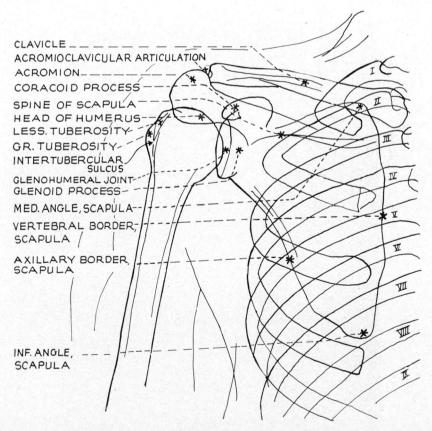

FIG. 4–7.   ANTERO-POSTERIOR VIEW OF THE SHOULDER WITH EXTERNAL ROTATION OF THE HUMERUS:
c, Labeled tracing of b.

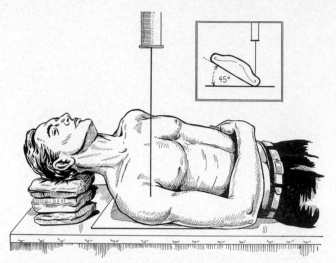

FIG. 4–8. VIEW OF SHOULDER FOR GREATER DETAIL WITH REFERENCE TO THE GLENOID PROCESS: a, Method of positioning patient.

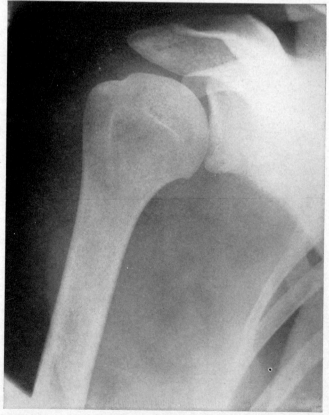

FIG. 4–8. VIEW OF SHOULDER FOR GREATER DETAIL WITH REFERENCE TO THE GLENOID PROCESS: b, Radiograph.

POINTS OF PRACTICAL INTEREST WITH REFERENCE TO FIGURE 4–8:

1. Adjust the degree of rotation to place the scapula parallel with the plane of the film, and the head of the humerus in contact with it. This will usually come to an angle of 45 degrees as shown.
2. The arm is very slightly abducted and internally rotated, and the forearm is rested against the side of the body.
3. For a more uniform density, respiration is suspended in the expiratory phase.
4. The central ray is directed to a point 2 inches medial and 2 inches distal to the upper-outer border of the shoulder.
5. This view is particularly valuable in cases suspected of chronic dislocation of the shoulder, since in the latter instance the inferior margin of the glenoid process is frequently eroded or contains spurs in contrast to the smooth contour shown.

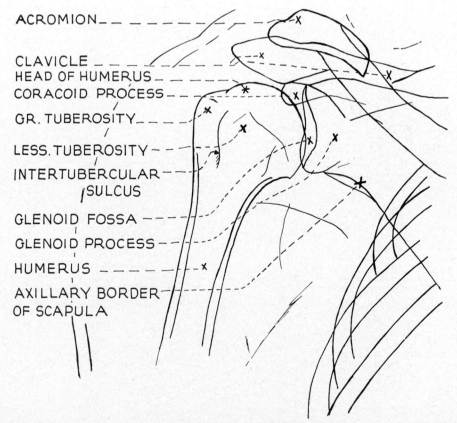

ACROMION

CLAVICLE
HEAD OF HUMERUS
CORACOID PROCESS

GR. TUBEROSITY

LESS. TUBEROSITY
INTERTUBERCULAR
SULCUS

GLENOID FOSSA

GLENOID PROCESS

HUMERUS

AXILLARY BORDER
OF SCAPULA

FIG. 4–8. VIEW OF SHOULDER FOR GREATER DETAIL WITH REFERENCE TO THE GLENOID PROCESS: c, Labeled tracing of b.

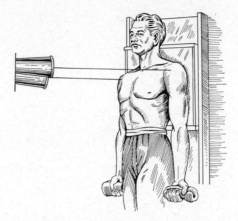

FIG. 4–9.   DETECTION OF INTEGRITY OF THE ACROMIOCLAVICULAR JOINT: **a,** Method of positioning patient. (In small individuals may be obtained as a single exposure as indicated in the illustrations
below; or in larger individuals two separate exposures may be required with the cone centering
over each joint separately without moving the patient.)

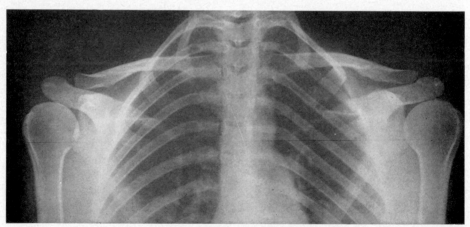

FIG. 4–9.   DETECTION OF INTEGRITY OF THE ACROMIOCLAVICULAR JOINT: **b,** Radiograph.

Points of Practical Interest with Reference to Figure 4–9:

1. When there is a tear in the acromioclavicular joint capsule, there is a tendency for the distal end of the clavicle to rise above the level of the adjoining acromion process. The two films must be so equivalent in the projection as to make it possible to measure not only the joint space between the clavicle and the acromion process, but also the difference in relation to a horizontal line which would connect the superior margins of the acromion processes.
2. The technique employed should be such as to demonstrate the acromioclavicular joint capsule on each side by soft tissue contrast. Hemorrhage and swelling of the joint capsule may thereby be detected as well.

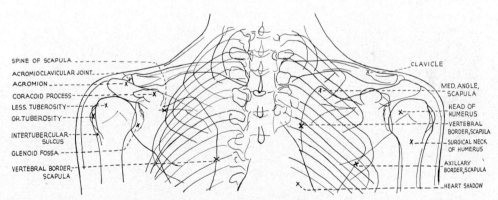

SPINE OF SCAPULA
ACROMIOCLAVICULAR JOINT
ACROMION
CORACOID PROCESS
LESS. TUBEROSITY
GR. TUBEROSITY
INTERTUBERCULAR SULCUS
GLENOID FOSSA
VERTEBRAL BORDER, SCAPULA

CLAVICLE
MED. ANGLE, SCAPULA
HEAD OF HUMERUS
VERTEBRAL BORDER, SCAPULA
SURGICAL NECK OF HUMERUS
AXILLARY BORDER, SCAPULA
HEART SHADOW

Fig. 4–9   View of the shoulder for detection of integrity of the acromioclavicular joint: c, Labeled tracing of b.

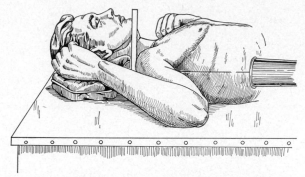

FIG. 4–10.   LATERAL VIEW OF SHOULDER WITH THE CENTRAL HORIZONTAL RAY PROJECTED THROUGH
THE AXILLA: **a,** Method of positioning patient.

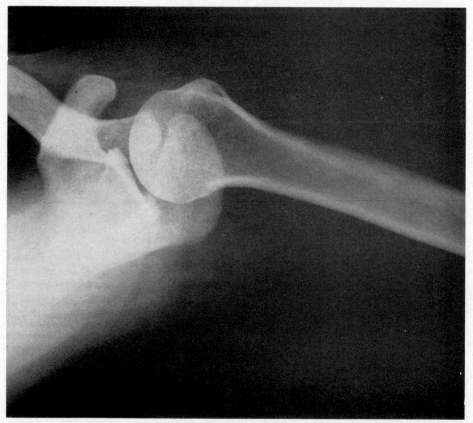

FIG. 4–10.   LATERAL VIEW OF SHOULDER WITH THE CENTRAL HORIZONTAL RAY PROJECTED THROUGH
THE AXILLA: **b,** Radiograph.

POINTS OF PRACTICAL INTEREST WITH REFERENCE TO FIGURE 4–10:

1. The arm is kept in external rotation, while the forearm and hand are adjusted and supported in a comfortable position.
2. The central ray is directed through the axilla to the region of the acromioclavicular joint.
3. The arm should be abducted as near as possible to a right angle with respect to the long axis of the body.
4. It is important to push the cassette against the patient's neck as far as possible to obtain maximal visualization of the scapula.

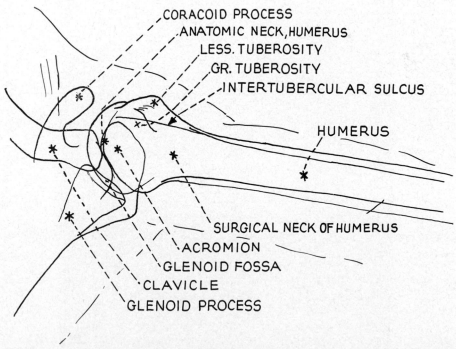

FIG. 4–10. LATERAL VIEW OF SHOULDER WITH THE CENTRAL HORIZONTAL RAY PROJECTED THROUGH THE THE AXILLA: **c,** Labeled tracing of **b.**

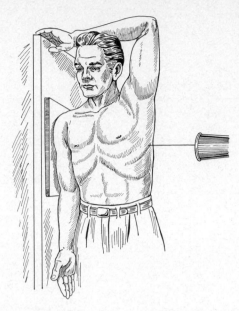

FIG. 4–11.   LATERAL VIEW OF SHOULDER WITH THE CENTRAL HORIZONTAL RAY PROJECTED THROUGH
THE ENTIRE BODY: **a,** Method of positioning patient.

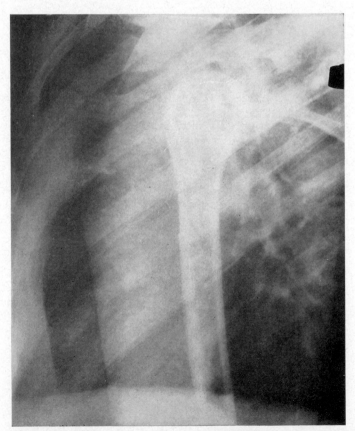

FIG. 4–11.   LATERAL VIEW OF SHOULDER WITH THE CENTRAL HORIZONTAL RAY PROJECTED THROUGH
THE ENTIRE BODY: **b,** Radiograph.

POINTS OF PRACTICAL INTEREST WITH REFERENCE TO FIGURE 4–11:

1. For best results one must employ a screen film, with a vertical Potter-Bucky diaphragm, or grid-front cassette.
2. The cassette is centered to the region of the surgical neck of the affected humerus, as is the central ray. The central ray may be angled cephalad 5 to 15 degrees.
3. The patient stands perfectly perpendicular to the film as shown, with the opposite shoulder raised out of the way by resting the patient's forearm upon his head and elevating the opposite scapula.
4. It is best to suspend respiration in full inspiration in this instance so that the lungs, being full of air, will improve the contrast of the bone and decrease the exposure necessary to penetrate the body.
5. This view may be the only method of obtaining a lateral view of the upper humerus in the event of a fracture in this location, where the patient is unable to abduct the arm.
6. While the erect position is shown, the recumbent position may also be employed, although it is less desirable.

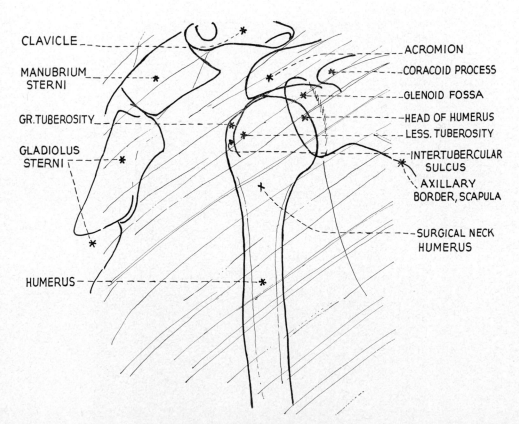

FIG. 4–11.   LATERAL VIEW OF SHOULDER WITH THE CENTRAL HORIZONTAL RAY PROJECTED THROUGH THE ENTIRE BODY: c, Labeled tracing of b.

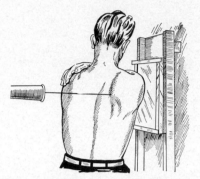

FIG. 4-12.   LATERAL VIEW OF SCAPULA: a, Method of positioning patient.

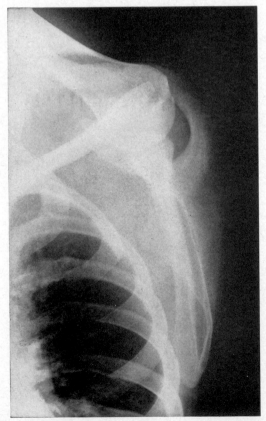

FIG. 4-12.   LATERAL VIEW OF SCAPULA: b, Radiograph.

Points of Practical Interest with Reference to Figure 4–12:

1. The Potter-Bucky diaphragm is necessary to obtain best results with this view.
2. The scapula is placed perpendicular to the film, rotating the opposite shoulder out of view, and one centers over the position of the spine of the scapula after palpating it.
3. To rotate the wing of the scapula outward to its maximum it is best to rest the forearm of the affected side on the opposite shoulder, bringing the arm of the affected side as close to the anterior chest wall as possible. Although the erect position is preferable, the recumbent position may also be employed in this instance.

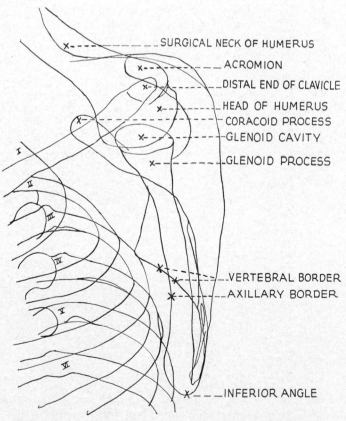

SURGICAL NECK OF HUMERUS
ACROMION
DISTAL END OF CLAVICLE
HEAD OF HUMERUS
CORACOID PROCESS
GLENOID CAVITY
GLENOID PROCESS
VERTEBRAL BORDER
AXILLARY BORDER
INFERIOR ANGLE

FIG. 4–12.   LATERAL VIEW OF SCAPULA: c, Labeled tracing of b.

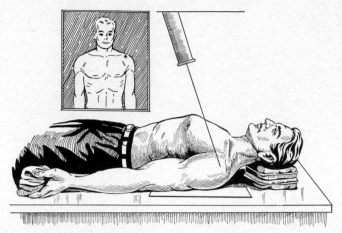

FIG. 4–13. SPECIAL ANTERO-POSTERIOR VIEW OF CLAVICLE ABD CORACOID PROCESS OF SCAPULA: a, Method of positioning patient.

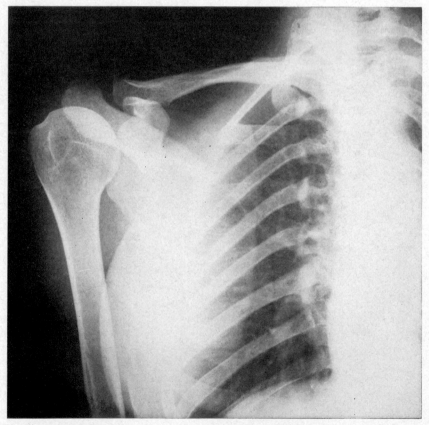

FIG. 4–13. SPECIAL ANTERO-POSTERIOR VIEW OF CLAVICLE AND CORACOID PROCESS OF SCAPULA: b, Radiograph.

Points of Practical Interest with Reference to Figure 4–13:

1. A 5 degree angulation of the tube is usually adequate to project the clavicle away from the rest of the thoracic cage in this view.
2. When interpreting this film, the physician must take into account a considerable element of projection and distortion, since the clavicle is a fair distance from the film.
3. The central ray should pass through the middle of the clavicle in this projection, or through the acromioclavicular articulation as shown.

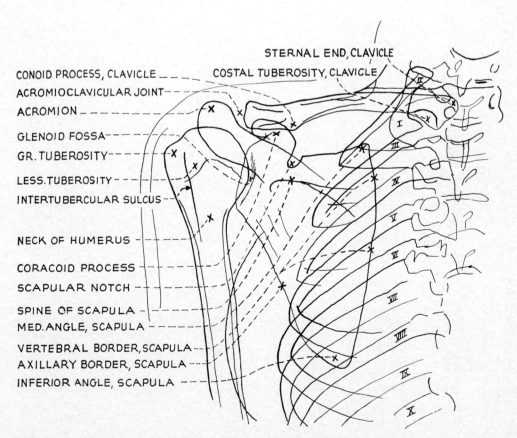

Fig. 4–13. SPECIAL ANTERO-POSTERIOR VIEW OF CLAVICLE AND CORACOID PROCESS OF SCAPULA: c, Labeled tracing of b.

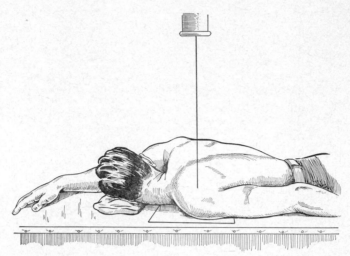

FIG. 4–14.   SPECIAL POSTERO-ANTERIOR VIEW OF CLAVICLE: **a,** Method of positioning patient.

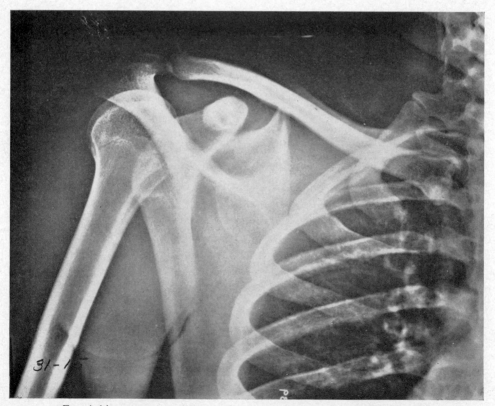

FIG. 4–14.   SPECIAL POSTERO-ANTERIOR VIEW OF CLAVICLE: **b,** Radiograph.

Points of Practical Interest with Reference to Figure 4–14:

1. This view may be employed with either the erect or the prone position as shown. The erect position is probably more readily obtained in the event of injury to the clavicle.
2. The central ray passes through the center of the clavicle in this instance; an angulation of 10 degrees toward the feet may be employed.
3. Approximately one half of the clavicle is projected over the bony thorax as shown, but there is less distortion and magnification in this view than in Figure 4–13, and hence it is more desirable in some instances.

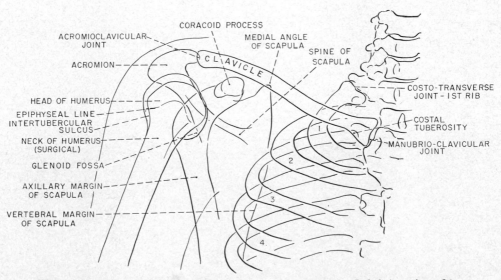

FIG. 4–14. SPECIAL POSTERIOR-ANTERIOR VIEW OF CLAVICLE: **c,** Labeled tracing of **b.**

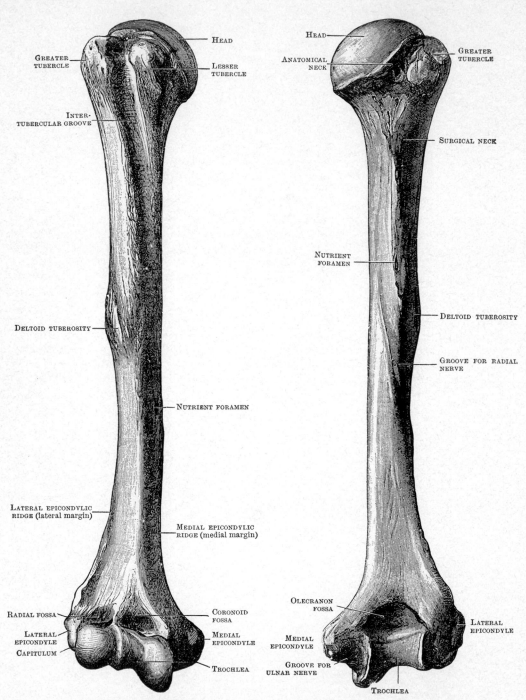

FIG. 4–15. Anterior and posterior views of the humerus. (From Cunningham's *Text-Book of Anatomy*, Edited by Arthur Robinson, Published by Oxford University Press.)

THE ARM

Related Gross Anatomy of the Humerus (Fig. 4–15). The humerus forms the bony support for the arm, and articulates with the glenoid process of the scapula. The head of the humerus is a hemispherical structure mounted obliquely on the upper metaphysis of the humerus. The anatomic neck, greater and lesser tuberosities and intertubercular groove are readily seen. The epiphyseal line at the base of the head of the humerus is very irregular in its contour and this must be differentiated from a fracture since it is visualized radiographically in its entire circumference.

Immediately below the two tuberosities, the bone becomes contracted and forms the surgical neck.

The shaft or body of the humerus is spiral in contour, being rather cylindrical superiorly and flattened inferiorly. The groove for the radial nerve accentuates this spiral appearance. The deltoid tubercle forms a prominence near the middle of the shaft laterally and anteriorly.

The flattened distal portion of the humerus tends to be thinner in the central region above the epiphysis. Anteriorly this forms the coronoid fossa, posteriorly the olecranon fossa. The medial and lateral margins or borders form the medial and lateral supracondylar ridges respectively.

The distal end of the humerus resembles a spool in outline, forming the capitulum, the trochlea, and the medial and lateral epicondyles.

The chief nutrient artery of the shaft of the humerus runs a course of over 2 inches. It is situated on the anteromedial surface or border below the insertion of the coracobrachialis muscle and is directed distally toward the elbow. This must not be confused with a fracture.

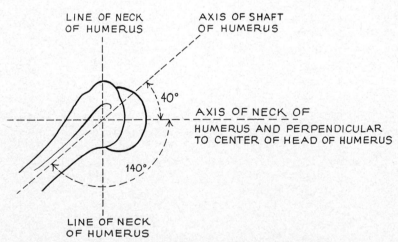

FIG. 4–16.   Axial relationships at the upper part of the humerus. (Modified from C. Toldt, *An Atlas of Human Anatomy.*)

Axial Relationships at the Upper Part of the Humerus.   The axial relationships of the head of the humerus to the anatomic neck and shaft are illustrated in Figure 4–15. When a line is drawn through the upper margin of the anatomic neck, it is perpendicular to the central axis of the head of the humerus. The latter axis is situated at an angle of approximately 140 degrees with respect to the axis of the shaft of the humerus.

Subdeltoid Bursa (Subacromial) (Fig. 4–17).   Beneath the deltoid muscle and overlying the head of the humerus there is a hemispherical pouchlike structure lined by synovial membrane called the "subdeltoid" or "subacromial" bursa. This is in close apposition with the supraspinatus tendon, and usually communicates with the glenohumeral joint. This bursa is particularly prone to calcification and inflammation.

There is a second bursa which frequently communicates with the shoulder joint under the tendon of the infraspinatus muscle.

Changes with Growth and Development (Fig. 4–4).   At birth, the main shaft of the humerus is ossified, but the ends are still cartilaginous. There are secondary centers of ossification for the head, greater tuberosity, lesser tuberosity, capitulum (and lateral part of trochlea), medial part of the trochlea, medial epicondyle and lateral epicondyle.

Only the secondary center for the head appears at birth or soon thereafter; the greater and lesser tuberosities appear between 3 and 5 years of age. The centers for the head and the tuberosities coalesce in about the sixth year to form one epiphysis but the center for the greater tuberosity may remain separate in about half of the cases until union with the shaft occurs. In all individuals with epiphyses, it is well to obtain comparison films of the opposite side, since it may be very difficult at times to assess normality.

ROUTINE RADIOGRAPHIC STUDIES OF THE ARM

1. **Antero-posterior View of the Arm** (Fig. 4–18).   The patient's arm is placed flat upon the film so that the anterior aspect of the humerus points directly upward. The central ray is allowed to pass through the center of the arm, and either the shoulder or the elbow joint, or both, are included in the film. Most of the anatomic parts of the humerus are readily identified: the head, anatomic neck, surgical neck, greater and lesser tubercles, the intertubercular groove or sulcus, the deltoid tubercle, the medial and lateral epicondyles, the olecranon fossa, the capitulum and the trochlea articulating with the radius and ulna respectively. Although no great effort is made to identify the soft tissue structures, the position of the radial nerve must always be borne in mind when viewing fractures of the arm.

2. **Lateral View of the Arm** (Fig. 4–19).   In this view, the medial border of the humerus is placed against the film, and the central ray is directed through the mid-shaft of the humerus on its lateral margin. The medial and lateral epicondyles are projected over one another, and the cubital fossa is seen in profile. The capitulum and the trochlea of the humerus are projected over one another also. There is a gentle concavity of the distal shaft of the humerus on its anterior aspect.

When we desire to demonstrate the anatomic or surgical neck of the humerus in the lateral projection, the view previously described as the lateral view of the shoulder taken through the body is taken (Fig. 4–11).

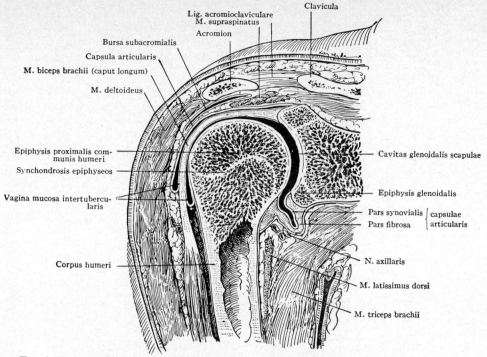

FIG. 4–17. **a,** Subdeltoid bursa and its anatomic relationships. (From Anson and Maddock, Callander's *Surgical Anatomy*.)

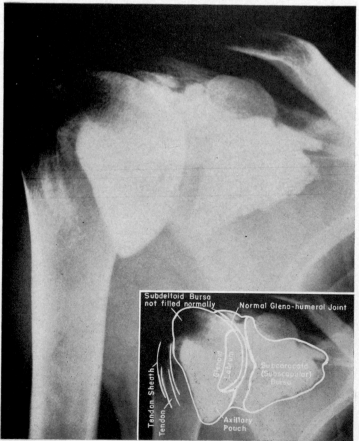

FIG. 4–17. **b,** Normal Hypaque arthrogram of an adult's shoulder demonstrating the normal joint, subscapularis bursa and dependent axillary pouch. (From Kernwein, G. A., Roseberg, B., and Sneed, W. R., Jr.: J. Bone & Joint Surg., vol. *39A*, 1957.)

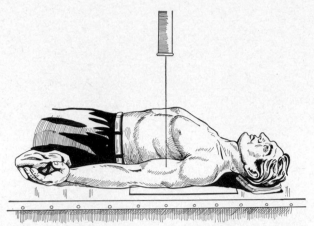

FIG. 4–18.   ANTERO-POSTERIOR VIEW OF THE ARM: **a,** Method of positioning patient.

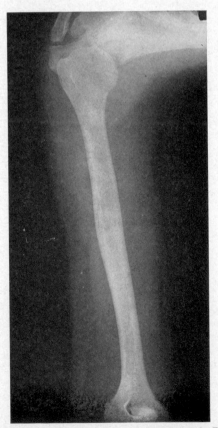

FIG. 4–18.   ANTERO-POSTERIOR VIEW OF THE ARM: **b,** Radiograph.

Points of Practical Interest with Reference to Figure 4–18:

1. The entire humerus from head to epicondyle should be included if at all possible.
2. One must make certain to supinate the hand sufficiently so that the epicondyles both lie flat on the film.
3. The central ray is directed through the mid-shaft of the humerus.
4. The opposite shoulder may be rotated up and supported by means of sandbags in order to facilitate placing the humerus in better contact with the film.

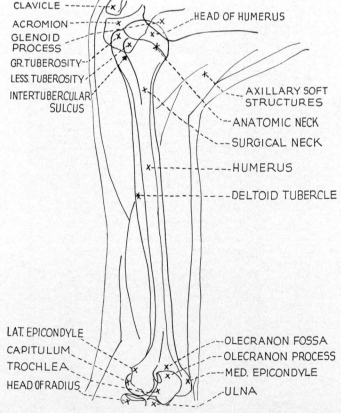

Fig. 4–18.   Antero-posterior view of the arm: c, Labeled tracing of b.

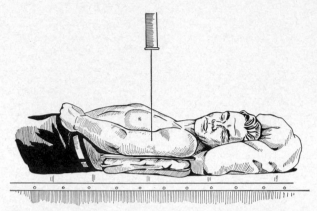

FIG. 4–19.   LATERAL VIEW OF THE ARM: **a,** Method of positioning patient.

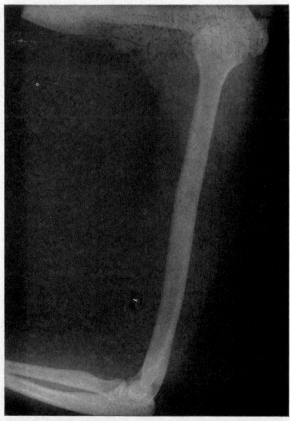

FIG. 4–19.   LATERAL VIEW OF THE ARM: **b,** Radiograph.

POINTS OF PRACTICAL INTEREST WITH REFERENCE TO FIGURE 4–19:

1. One must make certain that the film size chosen is adequate to include the entire shaft of the humerus from head to elbow joint.
2. The two epicondyles must be perfectly superimposed over one another and perpendicular to the film surface. To accomplish this, the physician may have to elevate the film on a sandbag as shown, and flex the forearm, resting the forearm upon the abdomen.
3. An alternative technique allows the patient to sit in a chair and extend the arm across the table, with the arm in perfect contact with the film, particularly in its lower two-thirds.

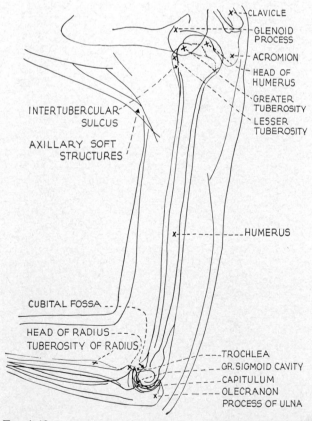

FIG. 4–19.   LATERAL VIEW OF THE ARM: c, Labeled tracing of b.

THE ELBOW

Related Anatomy of the Elbow Joint. The elbow joint is a hinge joint, with the trochlea of the humerus articulating with the greater sigmoid cavity of the ulna, the capitulum of the humerus with the head of the radius, and the head of the radius with the radial notch of the coronoid process of the ulna. The joint capsule is thickened medially and laterally by the ulnar and radial collateral ligaments.

Between the dense outer capsule and the inner synovial membrane are three masses of fat: (1) over the olecranon fossa; (2) over the coronoid fossa; and (3) over the radial fossa.

There are projections of the synovial membrane which tend to subdivide the joint into three communicating parts: (1) humeroradial; (2) humeroulnar; and (3) proximal radioulnar joints.

The annular ligament binds the head of the radius to the radial notch of the ulna; the integrity of this ligament prevents the constant subluxation of the head of the radius by flexion of the biceps brachii muscle.

Because of the obliquity of the trochlea with respect to the shaft of the radius, the forearm in flexion tends to move into a position lateral to the axis of the shaft of the humerus; in extension the "carrying angle" (Fig. 4–20) is maintained.

An accessory bone has been described over the anterior aspect of the joint.[2]

The Interosseous Membrane. The interosseous membrane is a broad thin fibrous sheet of tissue which extends between the interosseous crests of the radius and ulna (Fig. 4–28). It commences about 2.5 cm. beneath the tuberosity of the radius. Its purpose is to increase the extent of surface for attachment of the deep muscles of the forearm, and it aids in holding the radius and ulna together.

Its integrity is important from the standpoint of the supination and pronation movements of the forearm.

The Distal Radioulnar Articulation. The distal radioulnar articulation is separated from the radiocarpal or wrist joint by an articular disk or triangular fibrocartilage. The upper surface of this disk articulates with the head of the ulna, and its lower surface with the lunate and triangular carpal bones. The disk is attached at its apex to the junction of the styloid process and the head of the ulna, and at its base to the lower ridge of the ulnar notch of the radius.

In addition there are volar and dorsal radioulnar ligaments which maintain the capsular integrity of this joint.

The Bursae of the Elbow. Two bursae of the elbow (and sometimes three) are of clinical importance in that they are subject to inflammation: (1) the olecranon bursa; (2) the radiohumeral bursa; and (3) the bursa over the medial epicondyle of the humerus.

The olecranon bursa is subcutaneous and lies over the olecranon process. It ordinarily facilitates the movement of the triceps tendon over the bone at this point (The inflammation of this bursa gives rise to a condition known as "miners' elbow" or "students' elbow.")

The radiohumeral bursa is situated between the conjoined tendon of the extensor muscles and the radiohumeral joint. Inflammation of this bursa gives rise to a condition known as "tennis elbow."

An inconstant bursa may be found over the medial epicondyle of the humerus.

Axial Relationships at the Elbow (Fig. 4–20).   The axial relationships of the shaft of the humerus with respect to the forearm are such that an angle is formed measuring approximately 165 degrees, with the apex of the angle directed medially. This is called the "carrying angle." The axis of the trochlea forms an angle of about 80 degrees with the axis of the shaft of the humerus. The axis of the trochlea is parallel with that of the elbow joint, and both are perpendicular to the axis of the forearm.

A line through the epicondyles forms an angle of approximately 10 to 15 degrees with the axis of the elbow joint.

Structural Variations of the Elbow with Age (Fig. 4–21).   There are usually seven secondary centers of ossification in the elbow: (1) the capitulum and lateral part of the trochlea which appear at 1 to 1½ years of age; (2) the medial part of the trochlea which appears at 10 years of age; (3) the lateral epicondyle

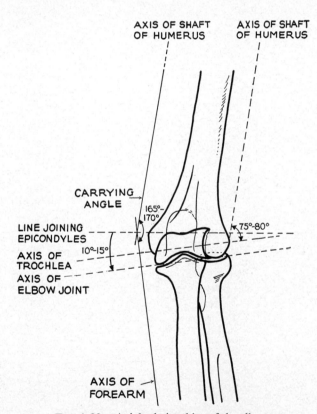

FIG. 4–20.   Axial relationships of the elbow.

The angles as given must not be regarded as absolute, but rather indicative of the type of carrying angle which usually occurs. The carrying angle may be measured directly from an antero-posterior view of the elbow provided that the two epicondyles are perfectly flat with respect to the film and that the elbow is completely extended. Both the distal humerus and proximal forearm must be in good contact with the film.

It will be noted that the axis of flexion of the forearm is perpendicular to the transverse axis of the trochlea rather than in line with the axis of the shaft of the humerus.

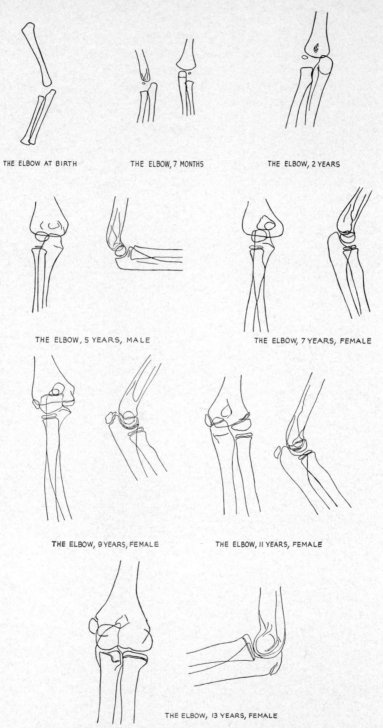

THE ELBOW AT BIRTH   THE ELBOW, 7 MONTHS   THE ELBOW, 2 YEARS

THE ELBOW, 5 YEARS, MALE   THE ELBOW, 7 YEARS, FEMALE

THE ELBOW, 9 YEARS, FEMALE   THE ELBOW, 11 YEARS, FEMALE

THE ELBOW, 13 YEARS, FEMALE

FIG. 4–21.   Tracings of radiographs to illustrate the osseous changes which occur in the elbow region in different age groups.

which appears at 14 years; (4) the medial epicondyle which appears in females between 5 and 6, and in males between 8 and 9 years; (5) the proximal end of the olecranon which appears at 11 years; (6) the head of the radius which appears between 5 and 6 years in females, and between 5 and 7 in males; and (7) occasionally the radial tuberosity which appears at puberty.

These for the most part fuse around 14 to 15 years of age in the female and between 18 to 21 years in the male, with the exception of the radial tuberosity which fuses very rapidly after it once appears (when it appears separately).

The centers for the capitulum and the trochlea coalesce to form one epiphysis at about 15 years in boys and 13 years in girls, and the lateral epicondyle usually joins the shaft independently. In about one third of the cases the latter does not appear as a separate center but appears to be ossified by extension from the capitulum.

It can thus be seen that the elbow furnishes good opportunity to help establish the so-called bone age of the growing individual, particularly between the ages of 5 and 14. The head of the radius appears after the capitulum and lateral part of the trochlea, which appear very early. The medial epicondyle, the trochlea, the olecranon and the lateral epicondyle appear sequentially in that order at the ages indicated. *In general, when determining bone age, it is advisable to take views of several areas rather than to rely completely on one.*

ROUTINE RADIOGRAPHIC STUDIES OF THE ELBOW REGION

1. **Routine Antero-posterior View of the Elbow** (Fig. 4–22). The patient is immobilized with the volar aspect of the forearm pointing directly upward and the central ray of the x-ray tube projected into the cubital fossa. The anatomic parts are indicated in Figure 4–22.

2. **Antero-posterior Views of Distal Humerus and Proximal Forearm.** *When the patient is unable to extend the forearm fully*, an antero-posterior view is first obtained of the distal humerus, and then another view is taken for the proximal forearm, each in proper turn being flat on the film cassette or cardboard film holder (Figs. 4–23, 4–24). Another means of overcoming this difficulty is to take the antero-posterior view, gauging an equal angle between the forearm and table top and arm and table top respectively.

Under such circumstances it may also be advisable to obtain a special view of the olecranon process by placing the olecranon process tangentially in the central x-ray beam (Fig. 4–25).

3. **Routine Lateral View of the Elbow** (Fig. 4–26). The elbow is partially flexed, and the forearm is so placed that the thumb points directly upward. The distal portion of the humerus as well as the proximal forearm are seen in lateral profile. The capitulum and trochlea overlap one another completely, and the head of the radius overlaps the coronoid process partially. The radial tubercle points anteriorly. The portion of the forearm adjoining the interosseous crest is also seen.

The student's attention is particularly directed to the practical points of interest in relation to Figures 4–22 to 4–26. Unless the technical details of positioning are accurately followed, considerable distortion and possible inaccuracy in interpretation of the anatomy may result.

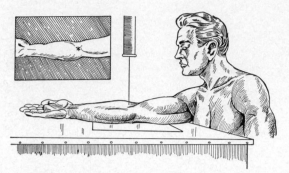

FIG. 4–22.   ANTERO-POSTERIOR VIEW OF ELBOW: **a,** Method of positioning patient.

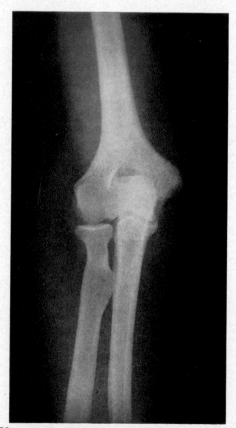

FIG. 4–22.   ANTERO-POSTERIOR VIEW OF ELBOW: **b,** Radiograph.

POINTS OF PRACTICAL INTEREST WITH REFERENCE TO FIGURE 4–22:

1. Note that the patient is seated low enough to place the shoulder joint and the elbow in approximately the same plane. This assures a good contact between the distal humerus and the film.
2. The anterior surface of the elbow and the plane passing through the epicondyles must be perfectly parallel with the film. To accomplish this the hand must be completely supinated and usually supported in this position by means of a sandbag. Occasionally also the patient must lean somewhat laterally.
3. The olecranon and coronoid fossae of the humerus, being superimposed and merely being a very thin plate of bone, will frequently appear as a foramen rather than as a bony plate, which may be misleading. A foramen in lieu of this bony plate does occur very rarely in anomalous conditions.

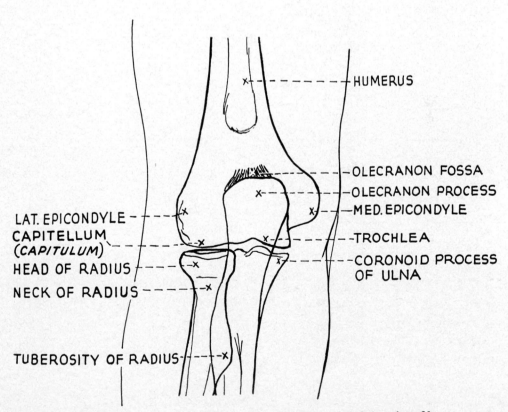

FIG. 4–22. ANTERIOR-POSTERIOR VIEW OF ELBOW: c, Labeled tracing of b.

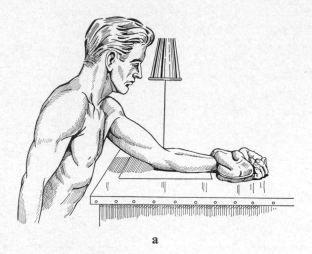

a

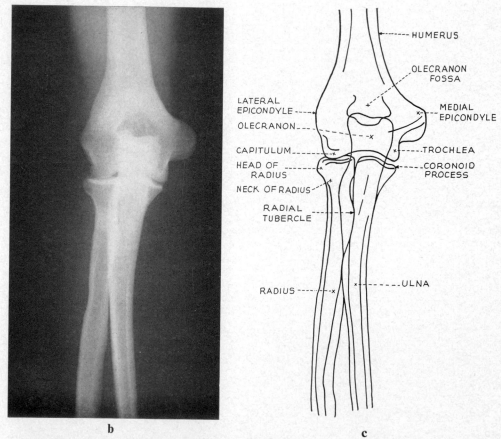

b   c

FIG. 4–23.   VIEWS OF THE ELBOW REGION WHEN THE ELBOW CANNOT BE FULLY EXTENDED. VIEW OF THE PROXIMAL FOREARM, WITH A DISTORTED VIEW OF THE DISTAL HUMERUS: a, Method of positioning patient. b, Radiograph. c, Labeled tracing of b.

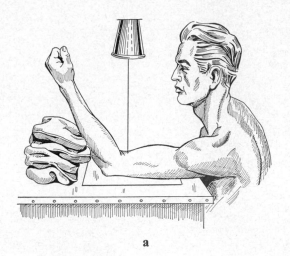

a

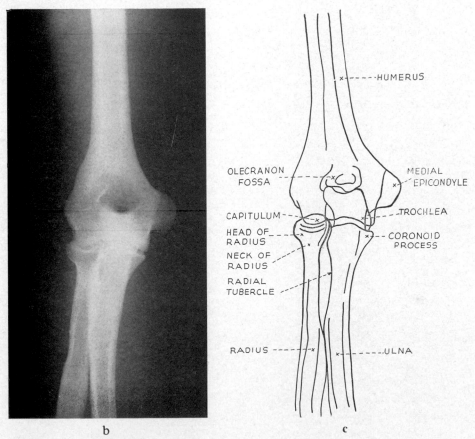

b   c

FIG. 4–24.   VIEWS OF THE ELBOW REGION WHEN THE ELBOW CANNOT BE FULLY EXTENDED. VIEW OF
DISTAL HUMERUS, WITH A DISTORTED VIEW OF THE PROXIMAL FOREARM: a, Method of positioning
patient. b, Radiograph. c, Labeled tracing of b.

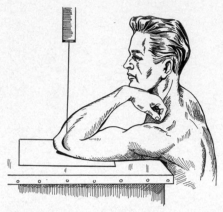

FIG. 4–25.   VIEWS OF THE ELBOW REGION WHEN ELBOW CANNOT BE FULLY EXTENDED. SPECIAL VIEW OF
THE OLECRANON PROCESS: **a,** Method of positioning patient.

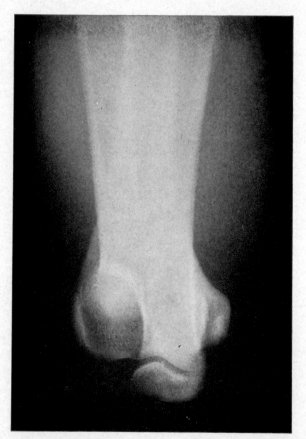

FIG. 4–25.   VIEWS OF THE ELBOW REGION WHEN ELBOW CANNOT BE FULLY EXTENDED. SPECIAL VIEW OF
THE OLECRANON PROCESS: **b,** Radiograph.

POINTS OF PRACTICAL INTEREST WITH REFERENCE TO FIGURE 4-25:

1. The patient must be seated in such a way as to allow the entire humerus to be placed in good contact with the table top and film.
2. The elbow is flexed as acutely as possible and the hand pronated.
3. It is important in this instance also to obtain a visualization of the soft tissues immediately outside the olecranon process in view of their frequent involvement by inflammatory process and calcium deposit.

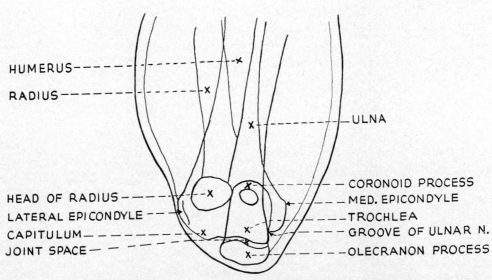

FIG. 4-25.   VIEWS OF THE ELBOW REGION WHEN ELBOW CANNOT BE FULLY EXTENDED. SPECIAL VIEW OF THE OLECRANON PROCESS: c, Labeled tracing of b.

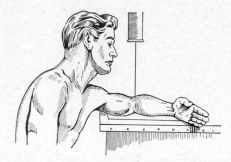

FIG. 4–26.   LATERAL VIEW OF ELBOW: **a,** Method of positioning patient.

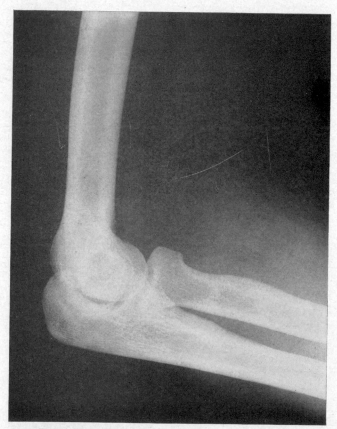

FIG. 4–26.   LATERAL VIEW OF ELBOW: **b,** Radiograph.

POINTS OF PRACTICAL INTEREST WITH REFERENCE TO FIGURE 4–26:

1. The patient is so placed with respect to the table that the arm is at the same level as the shoulder. Unless this is done the elbow joint proper will not be visualized clearly, and a rather oblique view of the head and neck of the radius will be obtained.
2. The elbow is ordinarily flexed approximately 90 degrees. The center of the film is placed immediately beneath the elbow joint and the central ray passes through the joint and center of the film, the epicondyles of the humerus being superimposed and perpendicular to the latter. The forearm is placed so that the thumb points directly upward and the palm of the hand is perpendicular to the table top surface. The fist may be clenched to facilitate maintenance of position. It is best to immobilize the forearm in this position by means of sandbags.
3. Since fractures of the head and neck of the radius are among the most frequently missed fractures in radiography, one must examine the contour and structure of these regions with extreme care to avoid such an error.

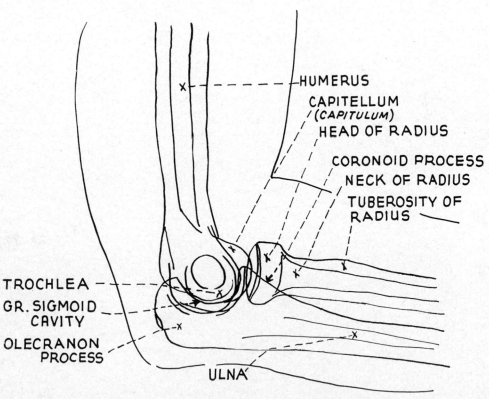

FIG. 4–26. LATERAL VIEW OF ELBOW: c, Labeled tracing of b,

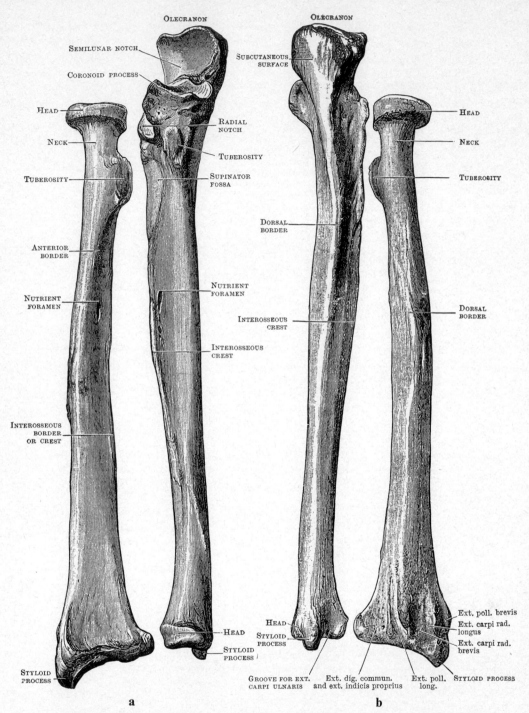

FIG. 4–27.   **a,** Volar aspect of the radius and ulna; **b,** Dorsal aspect of the radius and ulna. (From Cunningham's *Text-Book of Anatomy*, Edited by Arthur Robinson, published by Oxford University Press.)

THE FOREARM

Related Gross Anatomy of the Radius (Fig. 4–27). The head of the radius is a circular disk whose flat upper surface articulates with the capitulum of the humerus, and whose medial edge articulates with the radial notch of the ulna. The head is completely surrounded by a capsular or annular ligament. The neck is the constricted portion below the head. The radial tuberosity is situated anteromedially below the neck. The body gradually increases in size distally and is concave toward the ulna. The sharp medial edge below the radial tuberosity is known as the interosseous crest.

The distal portion of the dorsal surface of the shaft contains numerous grooves for the tendons of muscles, and for the attachment of ligaments. These grooves and irregularities must be recognized as normal.

The styloid process is the pointed distal extremity of the shaft of the radius. The distal articular surface articulates with both the navicular and lunate carpal bones and medially with the head of the ulna.

Related Gross Anatomy of the Ulna. The proximal portion of the ulna contains an articular surface which is concave in the long axis of the bone and convex from side to side. The proximal part is the olecranon and the anterior projection is the coronoid process. The concave portion is the greater sigmoid cavity or semilunar notch. This articulates with the trochlea of the humerus. The radial notch is the articular surface for the head of the radius and is situated on the lateral aspect of the coronoid process. There are several bony ridges for muscular attachment below the coronoid process. The interosseous crest is the sharp lateral edge which gives attachment to the interosseous membrane.

The lower portion of the ulna is small and consists of the head and styloid process, separated by a groove.

The head articulates with the ulnar notch of the radius, *but not with the carpus*, since it is separated from it by a triangular cartilaginous disk.

There is a very slight bowing of the distal half of the ulna medially. In the act of supination, the interosseous borders of the radius and ulna are posterior in position. In cross section, the anterior surfaces of the radius and ulna form almost a perfect semicircle with the interosseous membrane (Fig. 4–28), while

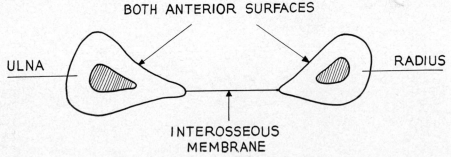

FIG. 4–28. Relationship of the interosseous membrane to the radius and ulna in cross section. (Modified from C. Toldt, *An Atlas of Human Anatomy*.)

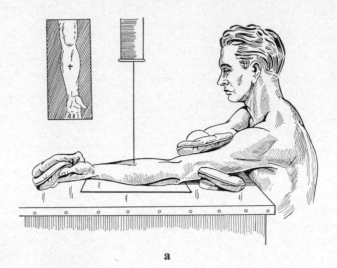

a

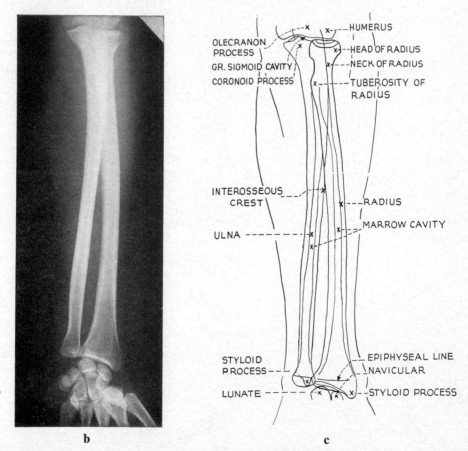

b

c

FIG. 4–29.   ANTERO-POSTERIOR VIEW OF FOREARM.   **a,** Method of positioning patient. **b,** Radiograph.
c, Labeled tracing of **b.**

POINTS OF PRACTICAL INTEREST WITH REFERENCE TO FIGURES 4–29 AND 4–30:

1. When the proximal two-thirds of the forearm are of greatest anatomic interest, the elbow joint is always included. The wrist joint is always included when the major anatomic interest is in the distal one-third of the forearm. Thus, the important technical adjuncts which apply to the elbow joint and wrist also apply here, with the exception that the forearm is always in a supinated position with the volar aspect uppermost in these views.

   In any case, it is well to seat the patient low enough to place the shoulder and the elbow in approximately the same plane, to assure good contact between the distal humerus and the film. A platform on the table top, with the patient's arm and the film on the platform, can achieve the same purpose.

2. In both of these views, it is important to obtain an accurate concept of the integrity of the interosseous membrane. The ability of the patient to pronate and supinate his forearm depends in greatest measure upon an adequacy of this membrane and the space between the two bones of the forearm throughout their lengths. With injury to the bones of the forearm, there is a tendency for the fragments of the radius and ulna to contact one another, and form a bony bridge between them across the interosseous membrane. This tendency must be recognized early and prevented.

---

the posterior surfaces form a flat surface. This configuration assists materially in the supination and pronation functions of the forearm, and every effort is made to preserve this configuration in the event of fracture.

The functions of supination and pronation are carried out exclusively by the radius with the ulna remaining in relatively constant position unless the humerus is also moved.

ROUTINE RADIOGRAPHIC STUDIES OF THE FOREARM

1. **Routine Antero-posterior View of the Forearm** (Fig. 14–29). The forearm is supinated so that the volar aspect is turned upward, and the central ray passes through the central portion of the forearm. It is important that the palm be turned perfectly upward to obtain the proper perspective.

   The various anatomic parts are illustrated in Figure 4–29.

2. **Routine Lateral View of the Forearm** (Fig. 4–30). It is helpful in this view to raise the elbow on a small platform into a horizontal position with respect to the shoulder. The elbow is flexed sufficiently to permit a perfect superposition of the proximal portions of the radius and ulna. This is best obtained by making certain that the thumb points straight upward, and the hand and wrist are perfectly perpendicular to the film and table top. The central ray passes through the center of the forearm. The anatomic parts are well illustrated in Figure 4–30.

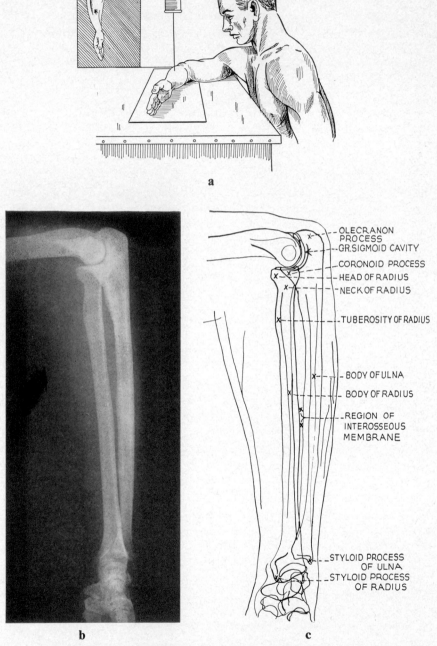

a

b

c

FIG. 4–30. LATERAL VIEW OF FOREARM: a, Method of positioning patient. b, Radiograph. c, Labeled tracing of b.

THE WRIST

Related Gross Anatomy of the Carpus or Wrist (Fig. 4–31). The carpus consists of eight bones, arranged in two rows. The proximal row is formed by the navicular, lunate, triquetral and pisiform; the distal row by the greater multangular, lesser multangular, capitate and hamate. A line joining the superior surfaces and margins of the bones is convex, whereas the volar aspect is concave. The margins of this concavity are formed by the tuberosity of the navicular and the ridge of the greater multangular laterally, and the pisiform and the hook of the hamate medially. The pisiform bone is attached to the volar surface of the triquetral, and stands out clearly in a lateral profile view of the wrist.

The proximal articulation with the radius is formed by the navicular and lunate bones only. The distal articular surfaces of the wrist bones which articulate with the metacarpals are very irregular.

The articular surface between the two rows of carpal bones is concavo-convex from side to side.

Each carpal bone except the pisiform (which is virtually a sesamoid bone) has six surfaces—with two to four articular surfaces depending upon whether the bone is an outer or inner one, and the remaining surfaces rough for the attachment of ligaments. These multiple surfaces are important from a radiographic standpoint since their numerous margins are all visualized and it is necessary to view all x-rays with a three-dimensional concept to aid in the interpretation of these lines.

The carpal bones articulate with one another by diarthrodial synovial joints, there being a similar joint between the pisiform and the triquetral bones. Each of the two rows of carpal bones moves as a unit so there are but three functional joints in the wrist: the radiocarpal, the intercarpal and the carpometacarpal.

Axial Relationships at the Wrist (Fig. 4–32). The axis of flexion of the hand is perpendicular to the axis of the forearm, and forms an angle of 10 to 15 degrees with the line connecting the styloid processes of the radius and ulna.

In the straight lateral view of the wrist, the midplane of the carpus is perpendicular to the plane of the radiocarpal joint. The midplane of the carpus forms an angle of 165 degrees with the axis of the forearm. The plane of the radiocarpal joint forms an angle of 75 degrees with the axis of the forearm.

ROUTINE RADIOGRAPHIC STUDIES OF THE WRIST

There are several special views in the case of the wrist which are employed for demonstration of certain anatomic features. In view of the curvature of the navicular carpal bone, a fracture through its midsection may escape detection unless this portion of the bone is brought into relief, and because of the great frequency of distressing symptoms in fracture of the navicular these special views assume considerable importance. It is also helpful to learn to recognize the navicular carpal bone on the straight lateral projection.

1. **Routine Postero-anterior View of the Wrist** (Fig. 4–33). In this view, the forearm is pronated, and the hand placed palm downward on the film. The palm may be spread out, or the fist clenched. In the latter case, there is somewhat less overlapping of articular margins in the carpometacarpal joints. The central ray is directed over the middle of the carpus.

The anatomic parts are illustrated in Figure 4–33.

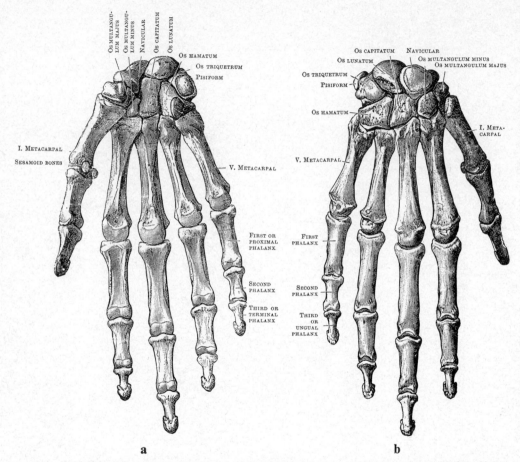

FIG. 4–31.   **a,** Volar aspect of the bones of the right hand and wrist; **b,** Dorsal aspect of the right hand and wrist. (From Cunningham's *Text-Book of Anatomy,* Edited by Arthur Robinson, published by Oxford University Press.)

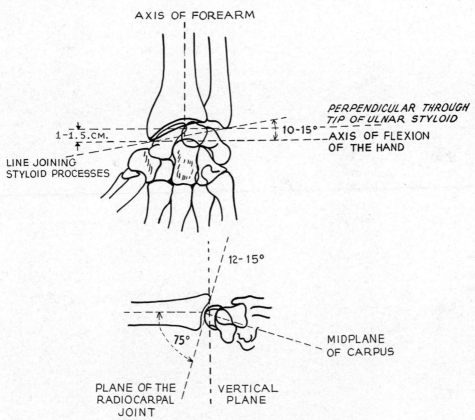

FIG. 4–32. Axial relationships of the wrist.

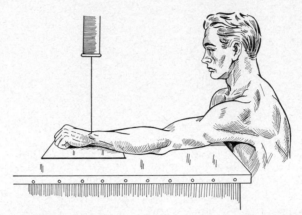

FIG. 4–33. POSTERO-ANTERIOR VIEW OF WRIST: **a,** Method of positioning patient.

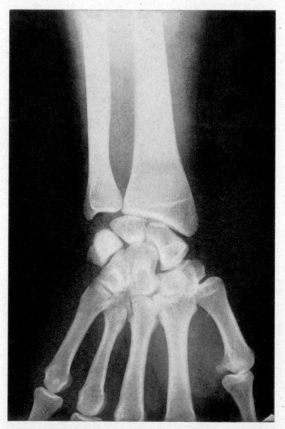

FIG. 4–33. POSTERIOR-ANTERIOR VIEW OF WRIST: **b,** Radiograph.

POINTS OF PRACTICAL INTEREST WITH REFERENCE TO FIGURE 4–33:

1. The postero-anterior projection of the wrist is usually preferable to permit better contact between the carpus and the film than is obtained in the reverse projection. In contrast to this, however, the antero-posterior view of the forearm is the more desirable since pronation of the hand would cause the two bones of the forearm to cross one another.
2. The central ray is projected immediately over the navicular carpal bone, midway between the styloid processes.
3. The clenched fist as shown places the wrist at a very slight angulation but the navicular carpal bone is at right angles to the central ray, so that it is usually projected without any superimposition, both by itself or adjoining structures.

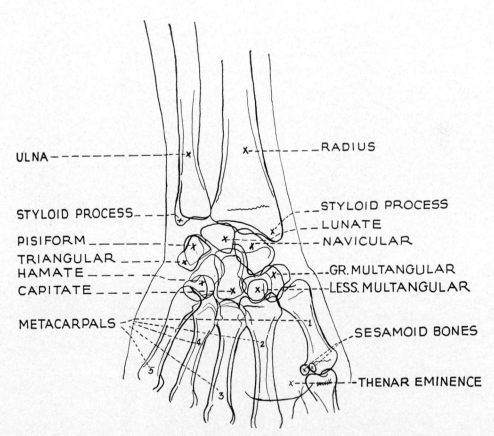

FIG. 4–33. POSTERO-ANTERIOR VIEW OF WRIST: c, Labeled tracing of b.

2. **Routine Lateral View of the Wrist** (Fig. 4–34).   The wrist is placed in the same position as was the case in the lateral view of the forearm, with the thumb upward and the hand and wrist perfectly perpendicular to the film. The central ray is directed over the carpus. The relationship of the carpus to the distal articular margin of the radius is of particular importance here.

3. **Special View for Demonstration of the Midsection of the Navicular Carpal Bone** (Fig. 4–35).   The palm is outstretched and placed on the film, spreading the thumb and the index finger. The axis of the central ray bisects the angle between the thumb and the index finger, at an angle of 45 degrees with the horizontal. The central ray is directed over the region of the navicular. A markedly distorted but good view of the midsection of the navicular is thus obtained.

4. **Oblique View of the Carpus** (Fig. 4–36).   In this projection, the wrist is placed to form an angle of 45 degrees with the horizontal, the palm downward, and the radial border of the wrist farthest from the film. The central ray is directed over the middle of the carpus. This view is of value also in obtaining a better perspective of the midsection of the navicular, and less distortion of the other carpal bones than in the markedly distorted view previously described.

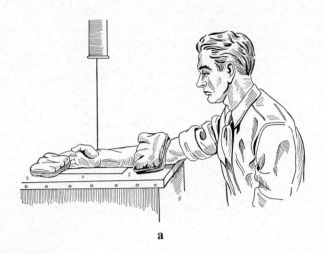

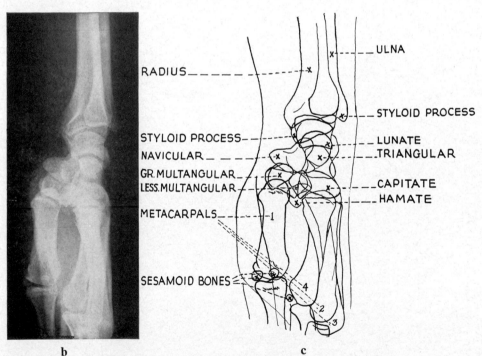

FIG. 4–34. LATERAL VIEW OF THE WRIST: **a**, Method of positioning patient. **b**, Radiograph. **c**, Labeled tracing of **b**.

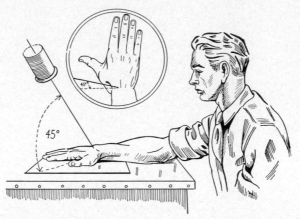

FIG. 4–35.   SPECIAL VIEW FOR DEMONSTRATING NAVICULAR CARPAL BONE: **a,** Method of positioning patient.

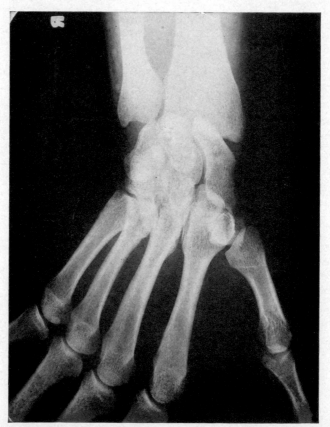

FIG. 4–35.   SPECIAL VIEW FOR DEMONSTRATING NAVICULAR CARPAL BONE: **b,** Radiograph.

POINTS OF PRACTICAL INTEREST WITH REFERENCE TO FIGURE 4–35:

1. This view is an application of the principle of distortion in order to provide increased clarity of a pathologic process within a bony structure. Actually a rather distorted and elongated view of the navicular carpal bone is obtained, but it will be noted that it is completely clear for the most part of adjoining structures, particularly in the area that is most prone to be fractured, namely its midsection. Also its own structure is not superimposed upon itself.
2. This view is also of some value with reference to the base of the first metacarpal, but is of very little value with reference to the rest of the carpus.

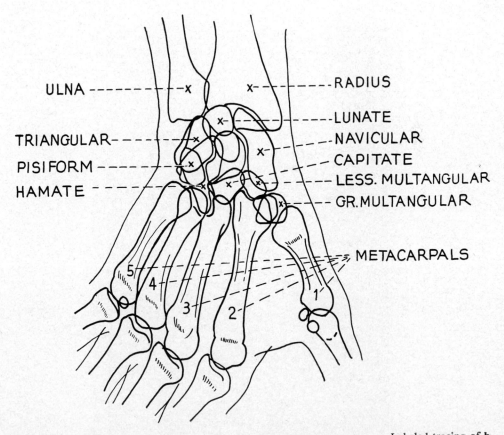

FIG. 4–35. SPECIAL VIEW FOR DEMONSTRATING NAVICULAR CARPAL BONE: c, Labeled tracing of b.

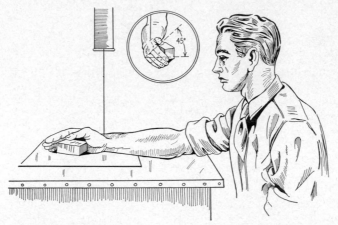

FIG. 4–36.   OBLIQUE VIEW OF WRIST: **a,** Method of positioning patient.

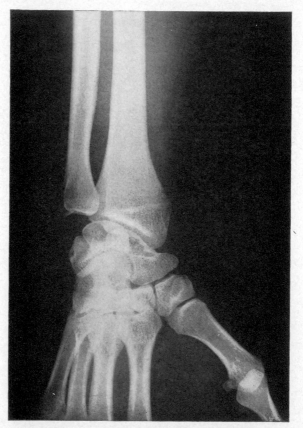

FIG. 4–36.   OBLIQUE VIEW OF WRIST: **b,** Radiograph.

POINTS OF PRACTICAL INTEREST WITH REFERENCE TO FIGURE 4–36:

1. The film is placed under the wrist so that the center of the film is approximately 3 to 4 cm. anterior to the carpal bones. This will place the film immediately under the navicular carpal bone when the wrist is slightly pronated to about 45 degrees from the lateral position. The hand is supported on a balsa wood block or sandbag as shown, and the forearm may be immobilized by an additional sandbag.
2. The central ray is directed immediately over the navicular carpal bone.
3. This view is also particularly valuable in obtaining a clear perspective of the joint between the greater multangular and the first metacarpal.

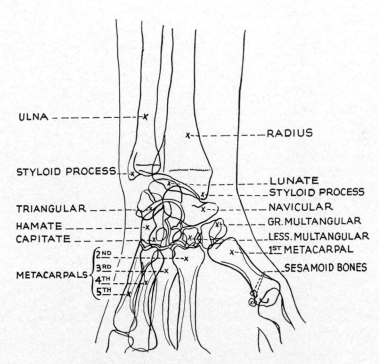

NOTE: IT IS NECESSARY FOR THE STUDENT TO DEVELOP A THREE-DIMENSIONAL CONCEPT, IN THAT ONE VISUALIZES BOTH THE ANTERIOR AND THE POSTERIOR MARGIN OF A SURFACE RIGHT THROUGH ANY INTERVENING STRUCTURE.

FIG. 4–36. OBLIQUE VIEW OF WRIST: c, Labeled tracing of b.

THE HAND

Related Gross Anatomy of the Metacarpals (Fig. 4–31). These consist of five "long bones in miniature" articulating with the carpus proximally and the phalanges distally. When considered as a group, they form a concavity deep in the palm of the hand. With the exception of the first metacarpal, they are usually triangular in cross section, the apex of the triangle being a palmar ridge. The nutrient canal (Fig. 3–6) is usually in the middle of the shaft and is directed away from the wrist with the exception of the thumb which runs proximally. The head is a rounded articular surface distally, and on each side of the head is a prominent tubercle. The second metacarpal is usually the longest, whereas the first is the shortest and widest. The first metacarpal also differs in other respects. Its epiphysis is at its base instead of its head; its concavity and ridge are medial rather than palmar.

The other metacarpals differ from one another largely at their bases, which have angular and irregular articular margins and facets. A three-dimensional "mind's eye concept" is of the utmost importance here also.

Related Gross Anatomy of the Phalanges (Fig. 4–31). The thumb has two phalanges, and each of the other four fingers has three, distinguished as proximal, middle and distal, respectively.

The proximal phalanges are semicylindrical in cross section, the flat aspect being on the palmar side. The base is a concave articular surface, whereas the distal articular surface is "half dumbbell-shaped," with a central groove and two condyle-like structures on either side.

The middle phalanx is lacking in the thumb and in the case of the other fingers is distinguished from the first phalanx by having a ridge in its proximal articular surface to correspond with the groove in the adjoining distal articular surface of the first phalanx. The distal end of the second phalanx resembles that of the proximal phalanx. The palmar surface contains a tendinous impression.

The distal phalanges differ by having a club-shaped end known as the ungual *tuberosity* or *tuft*.

The nutrient canals tend to be in the midshaft on the radial side and they are directed distally.

With advancing age there is a tendency for the margins of the shafts to become more and more irregular, particularly in the areas of muscular attachment. These irregularities must not be misinterpreted as periostitis.

Sesamoid Bones (Fig. 4–37). The sesamoid bones are small, rounded bones which are embedded in certain tendons. In the hand the following sesamoid bones are of almost constant occurrence: (1) two over the metacarpophalangeal joints of the thumb (flexor pollicis brevis muscle); (2) one over the interphalangeal joint of the thumb; and (3) one over the metacarpophalangeal joint of the fifth finger.

Other supernumerary bones which may occur are shown in Figure 4–38.

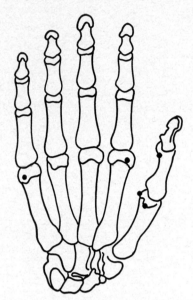

FIG. 4–37. The most frequent sites of sesamoid bones of the hand.

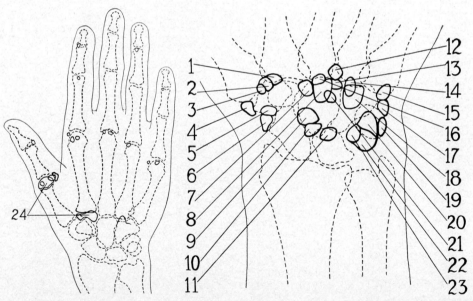

FIG. 4–38. SUPERNUMERARY BONES OF THE HAND. (From C. McNeill: *Roentgen Technique*, Charles C Thomas, Publisher.) 1, Os trapezoides secundarium; 2, trapezium secundarium; 3, praetrapezium; 4, paratrapezium; 5, epitrapezium; 6, radiale externum; 7, styloid; 8, subcapitatum; 9, os centrale; 10, hypolunatum; 11, epilunatum; 12, ossiculum gruberi; 13, os capitatum secondarium; 14, os hamuli proprium; 15, os vesalianum; 16, parastyloid; 17, ulnare externum; 18, hamulare basale; 19, pisiforme proprium; 20, triquetrum ulnare; 21, metastyloid; 22, triquetrum radiale; 23, epipyramis.

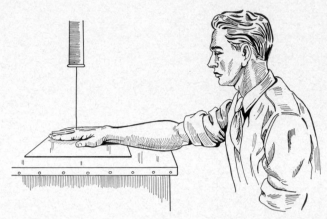

FIG. 4–39.   POSTERO-ANTERIOR VIEW OF HAND: **a,** Method of positioning patient.

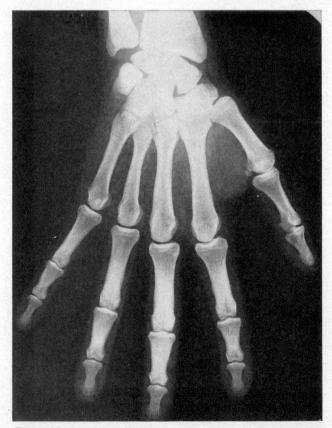

FIG. 4–39.   POSTERO-ANTERIOR VIEW OF HAND: **b,** Radiograph.

POINTS OF PRACTICAL INTEREST WITH REFERENCE TO FIGURE 4–39:

1. The fingers should be spread slightly, and completely extended and in good contact with the film.
2. The central ray should pass through the third metacarpophalangeal joint.
3. It is well to immobilize the forearm just above the wrist by means of a sandbag.
4. The greatest care must be exercised to obtain a clear view, particularly of the tufted ends of the distal phalanges as well as the shafts of the phalanges, since many of the pathologic processes of a systemic type will produce minute and very important changes in these structures. The student should obtain a very clear mental concept of the normal appearance of the phalanges and metacarpals.
5. If a single finger is in question a lighter exposure technique is employed and usually four views of that finger from all perspectives are taken.
6. All the structures are shown in straight postero-anterior projection except the thumb, in which case an oblique view is obtained.

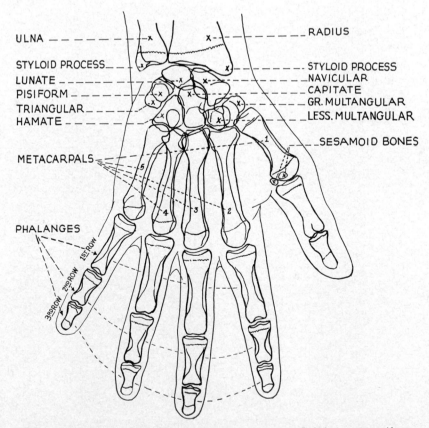

FIG. 4–39. POSTERO-ANTERIOR VIEW OF HAND: c, Labeled tracing of b.

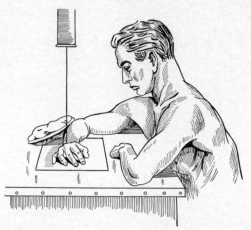

FIG. 4–40.   OBLIQUE VIEW OF HAND: **a,** Method of positioning patient.

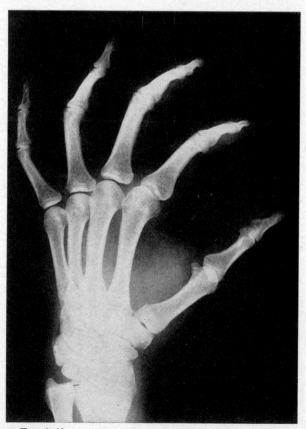

FIG. 4–40.   OBLIQUE VIEW OF HAND: **b,** Radiograph.

PRACTICAL POINTS OF INTEREST WITH REFERENCE TO FIGURE 4-40:

1. One should adjust the obliquity of the hands so that the metacarpophalangeal joints form an angle of approximately 45 degrees with the film.
2. The central ray is directed vertically through the third metacarpophalangeal joint.
3. Cotton pledgets may be employed to spread the fingers. A 2-inch square of balsa wood placed under the thumb makes an excellent immobilization device.

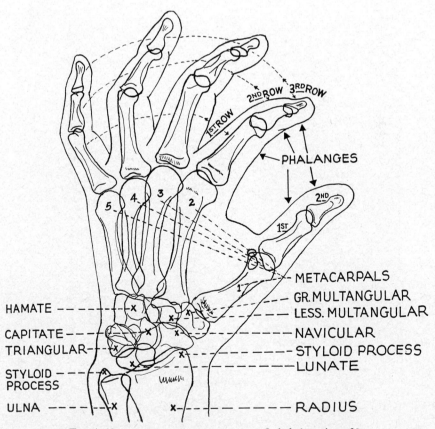

FIG. 4-40.   OBLIQUE VIEW OF HAND: c, Labeled tracing of b.

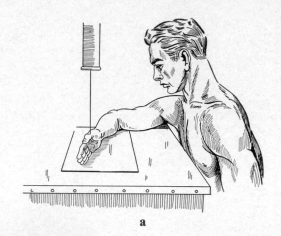

a

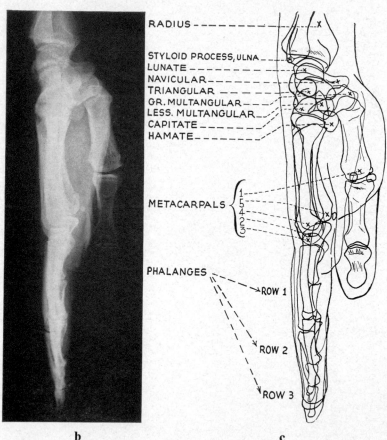

RADIUS

STYLOID PROCESS, ULNA
LUNATE
NAVICULAR
TRIANGULAR
GR. MULTANGULAR
LESS. MULTANGULAR
CAPITATE
HAMATE

METACARPALS
1
5
4
2
3

PHALANGES
ROW 1

ROW 2

ROW 3

b   c

FIG. 4–41.   STRAIGHT LATERAL VIEW OF THE HAND: a, Method of positioning patient. b, Radiograph.
c, Labeled tracing of b.

ROUTINE RADIOGRAPHIC STUDIES OF THE HAND

1. **Routine Postero-anterior View of the Hand** (Fig. 4–39). The hand is placed palm downward on the film, and the central ray passes through the head of the third metacarpal. In view of the fact that there may be considerable variation in density between the metacarpal and phalangeal areas of the hand, special views are frequently employed to obtain better detail of the fingers. If a single finger is in question, multiple views of the one finger are usually in order.

2. **Routine Oblique View of the Hand** (Fig. 4–40). The hand is placed palm downward on the film, with the thumb and thenar portion of the hand raised about 45 degrees from the film, and the hypothenar portion of the hand in contact with it. The central ray is once again made to pass through the head of the third metacarpal. This view has the advantage over the direct lateral in that the various anatomic parts do not overlap so much, but exact degree of displacement is impossible to describe except in the straight lateral.

3. **Straight Lateral View of the Hand** (Fig. 4–41). The hand is placed perpendicular to the film with the thumb pointing upward. The central ray is made to pass through the line of the heads of the metacarpals. It is important to note the normal curvature of the metacarpals in this projection with their concavity on the palmar aspect of the hand. Various sesamoid bones, particularly at the metacarpophalangeal junctions, will be demonstrated clearly.

Points of Practical Importance. The overlapping articulations of the distal row of carpal bones with the bases of the metacarpals are of particular importance. These overlapping surfaces frequently give rise to the impression of fracture unless they are carefully delineated.

The tufted ends (ungual tufts) of the distal phalanges alter their appearance both from injury and metabolic disease. They must be studied carefully from this aspect.

In view of the fact that in the straight lateral view of the hand many of the bones are projected over one another, the oblique view of the hand is more frequently employed. The lateral view is taken particularly if a knowledge of the exact degree of antero-posterior displacement is of importance.

REFERENCES

1. Moore, R. D., and Renner, R. R.: The Coraco-Clavicular Joint. Am. J. Roentgenol., *78:* 86–88, 1957.
2. Simril, Wayne, and Trotter, Mildred: An Accessory Bone and Other Skeletal Anomalies of the Elbow. Radiology, *53:* 97–100, 1949.

CHAPTER 5

The Pelvis and
Lower Extremity

THE ANATOMIC GROUPS that are considered radiographically in the examination
of pelvis and lower extremity are: pelvis, hip, thigh, knee, leg, ankle and foot.
Considered also are special examinations for some of the component parts of
these regions such as the patella and the calcaneus.

THE PELVIS

Gross Anatomy with Radiographic Significance. THE OS COXAE, INNOMI-
NATE OR HIP BONE (Figs. 5–1, 5–2). This bone, together with its fellow of the
opposite side, forms the anterior and lateral walls of the bony pelvis. It articulates posteriorly with the sacrum, and the two hip bones articulate anteriorly to
form the pubic symphysis.

The hip bone is formed by three separate bones which are firmly united at
the acetabulum in the adult: the ilium, ischium and pubis, each contributing
two-fifths, two-fifths and one-fifth respectively to the deep hemispherical socket
which articulates with the head of the femur.

The trabecular pattern of the ilium suggests a moderately cancellous type
of bone, with the major direction toward the acetabulum, except at the iliac
crest, where the trabeculae tend to run parallel with the crest. There is a rough-
ness visualized on the surfaces of the ilium related to the areas of attachment
of the heavy gluteal muscles and the iliacus muscle. The following anatomic
parts of the ilium can be identified radiographically: the anterior superior iliac
spine; the anterior inferior iliac spine; the posterior superior iliac spine; the
posterior inferior iliac spine; the iliac crest; the iliopectineal eminence, which
indicates the point of union of the ilium and pubis; the iliac fossa; the auricular
surface, for articulation with the sacrum; and the auricular tuberosity or tuberosity of the ilium. There are two notches in the contour of the ilium just above
the acetabulum: the posterior notch below the articular auricular surface is
the greater sciatic notch; and the anterior is situated between the anterior inferior iliac spine and the acetabulum and is known as the inferior iliac notch.

The important anatomic landmarks with regard to the ischium are the following: the body of the ischium; the ischial spine, below the greater sciatic
notch; the lesser sciatic notch, below the ischial spine; the ischial tuberosity;
the superior ramus, which ultimately fuses with the superior ramus of the pubis;

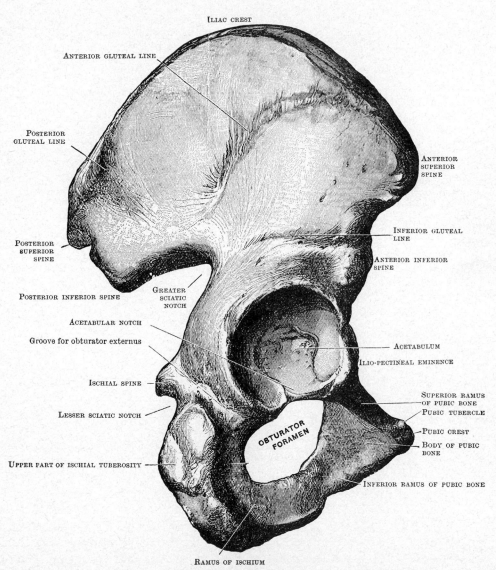

Fig. 5–1.   Os coxae or hip bone from the lateral aspect. (From Cunningham's *Text-Book of Anatomy* Edited by Arthur Robinson, published by Oxford University Press.)

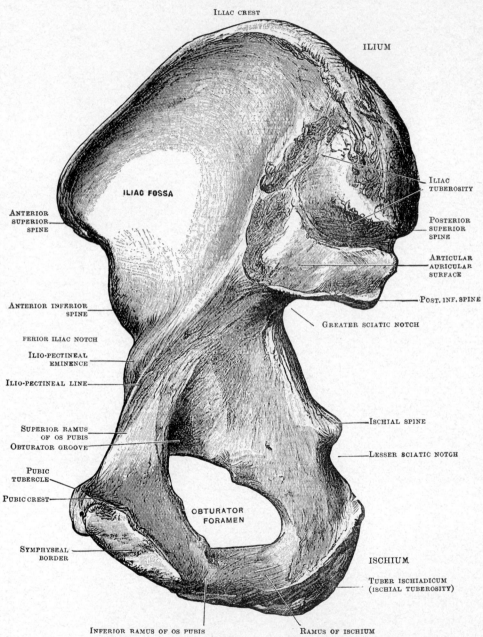

ILIAC CREST

ILIUM

ILIAC FOSSA

ILIAC
TUBEROSITY

ANTERIOR
SUPERIOR
SPINE

POSTERIOR
SUPERIOR
SPINE

ARTICULAR
AURICULAR
SURFACE

ANTERIOR INFERIOR
SPINE

POST. INF. SPINE

FERIOR ILIAC NOTCH

GREATER SCIATIC NOTCH

ILIO-PECTINEAL
EMINENCE

ILIO-PECTINEAL LINE

ISCHIAL SPINE

SUPERIOR RAMUS
OF OS PUBIS

LESSER SCIATIC NOTCH

OBTURATOR GROOVE

PUBIC
TUBERCLE

PUBIC CREST

OBTURATOR
FORAMEN

SYMPHYSEAL
BORDER

ISCHIUM

TUBER ISCHIADICUM
(ISCHIAL TUBEROSITY)

INFERIOR RAMUS OF OS PUBIS   RAMUS OF ISCHIUM

FIG. 5-2.   Os coxae from the medial aspect. (From Cunningham's *Text-Book of Anatomy*, Edited by
Arthur Robinson, published by Oxford University Press.)

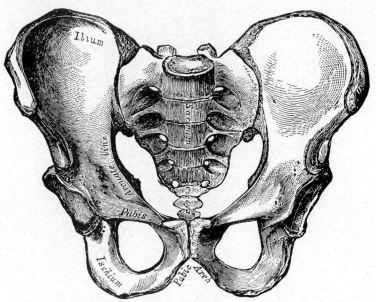

Fig. 5–3.   The bony pelvis (male). (From Gray, *Anatomy of the Human Body*, Edited by C. M. Goss, courtesy of Lea & Febiger.)

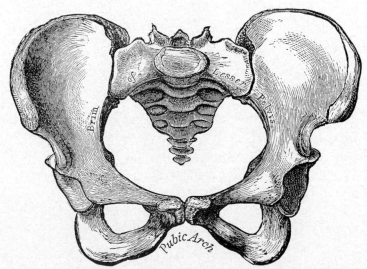

Fig. 5–4.   The bony pelvis (female). (See Chap. 17 for significance in relation to obstetrical radiology.) (From Gray, *Anatomy of the Human Body*, Edited by C. M. Goss, courtesy of Lea & Febiger.)

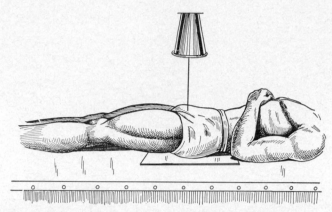

FIG. 5–5. ANTERO-POSTERIOR VIEW OF PELVIS: **a,** Method of positioning patient. (The cassette would ordinarily be within the Bucky tray underneath the table top, and not visible.)

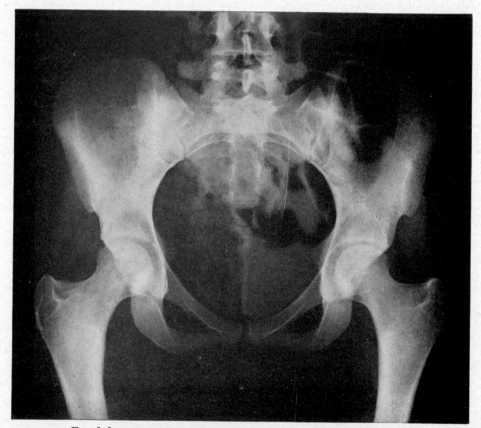

FIG. 5–5. ANTERO-POSTERIOR VIEW OF PELVIS: **b,** Radiograph (female).

POINTS OF PRACTICAL INTEREST WITH REFERENCE TO FIGURE 5–5:

1. Center the patient to the median line of the table with the center of a 14 x 17 inch cassette placed crosswise 1½ inches above the superior margin of the pubic symphysis. This will place the upper border of the film above the iliac crest and the lower border of the film well below the lesser trochanters of the femurs.
2. In order to project the necks of the femurs in their full lengths it is well to invert the feet about 15 degrees and immobilize them with sandbags in this position.
3. The entire pelvis must be symmetrical. This may necessitate placing a folded sheet or balsa wood block under one side.
4. There are various special views for the ilium, the acetabulum, the anterior pelvic bones and the pubes which have not been included in this text. These special views need be employed only on rare occasions.

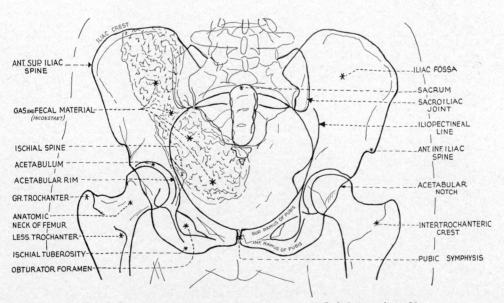

FIG. 5–5.   ANTERO-POSTERIOR VIEW OF PELVIS: c, Labeled tracing of b.

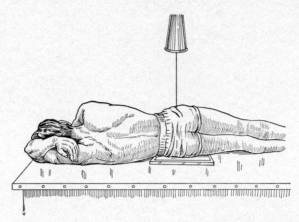

FIG. 5–6.   Lateral view of pelvis for sacrum: **a,** Method of positioning patient.

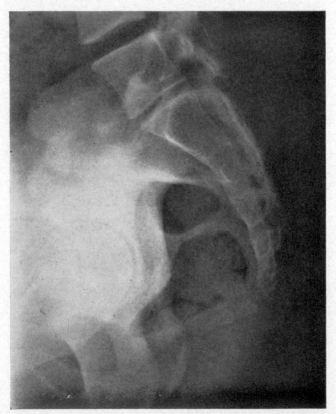

FIG. 5–6.   LATERAL VIEW OF PELVIS FOR SACRUM: **b,** Radiograph.

POINTS OF PRACTICAL INTEREST WITH REFERENCE TO FIGURE 5–6:

1. The patient is placed in the lateral position, either erect or recumbent, and the film is placed in the Potter-Bucky diaphragm. The knees and hips are slightly flexed to facilitate maintenance of position.
2. The gluteal cleft is placed parallel with the film.
   Immobilization with a compression band is frequently very helpful. This is applied across
3. the trochanteric region of the pelvis.
   Center in the midaxillary plane over the depression between the iliac crest and the greater
4. trochanter of the femur.
   There should be almost perfect superposition of the ischial spines as well as the acetabula in
5. this projection.

FIG. 5–6.   Lateral view of pelvis for sacrum: c, Labeled tracing of b.

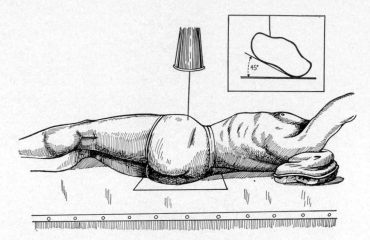

FIG. 5–7. OBLIQUE VIEW OF THE SACROILIAC JOINTS AND LOWER LUMBAR SPINE: **a,** Method of positioning patient.

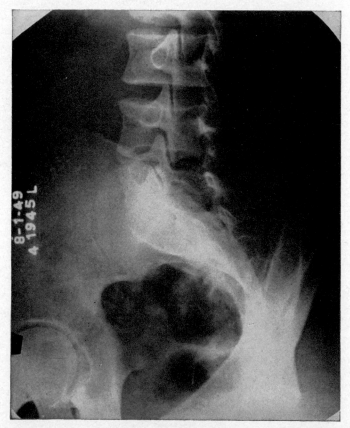

FIG. 5–7. OBLIQUE VIEW OF THE SACROILIAC JOINTS AND LOWER LUMBAR SPINE: **b,** Radiograph.

POINTS OF PRACTICAL INTEREST WITH REFERENCE TO FIGURE 5–7:

1. Elevate the side being examined approximately 45 degrees and support the shoulder and the upper thigh on sandbags, making certain that the sandbags do not appear on the radiograph.
2. The sacroiliac joint which is farthest from the film will appear most clearly and it is this sacroiliac joint which is being examined. The two articular surfaces of the sacroiliac joint closest to the film are superimposed over one another, and hence this point is not shown to best advantage.
3. A somewhat similar oblique view of the sacroiliac joints may be obtained in the posteroanterior projection by placing the patient obliquely prone instead of supine as noted above.
4. Oblique views of both sacroiliac joints are always obtained in that one joint offers some comparison for analysis of the other.
5. The central ray may be angled 5 degrees cephalad. In some patients this improves visualization of the sacroiliac and lumbar apophyseal joints.

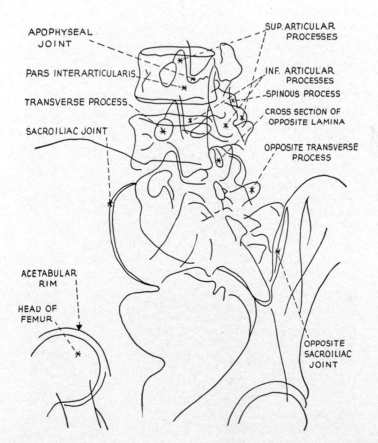

FIG. 5–7. OBLIQUE VIEW OF THE SACROILIAC JOINTS AND LOWER LUMBAR SPINE: **c**, Labeled tracing of **b**.

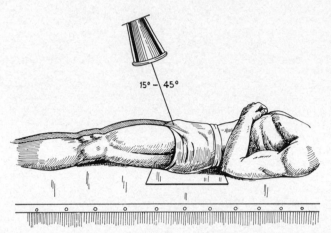

FIG. 5–8.   DISTORTED VIEW OF SACRUM: **a,** Method of positioning patient.

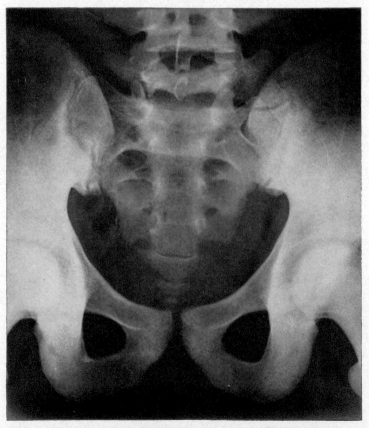

FIG. 5–8.   DISTORTED VIEW OF SACRUM: **b,** Radiograph.

Points of Practical Interest with Reference to Figure 5–8:

1. For more marked distortion angulation up to 45 degrees of the tube cephalad may be employed.
2. The central ray is adjusted so that it enters the body just above the pubic symphysis and so that it will leave the body at approximately the upper margin of the sacrum or at the level of the fifth lumbar segment. Care is exercised to center the x-ray film to the central ray of the x-ray tube, otherwise one will not obtain the anatomic structures depicted.
3. This view is particularly valuable for demonstrating sacralization of the last lumbar transverse processes as is indicated in the accompanying diagram. Also defects in the neural arch of the fifth lumbar vertebra are well demonstrated in this view.

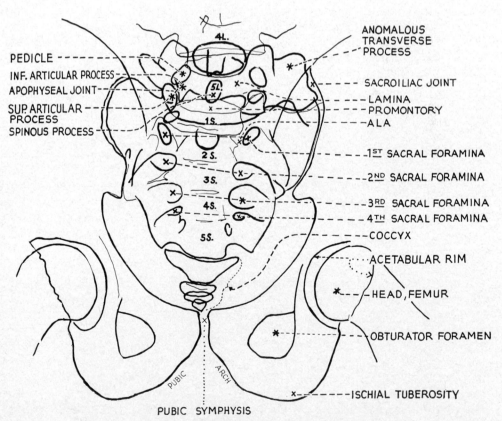

FIG. 5–8. DISTORTED VIEW OF SACRUM: c, Labeled tracing of same.

and the inferior ramus which fuses with the inferior ramus of the pubis. The ischial and pubic rami and the bodies of the ischium and pubis enclose an opening called the obturator foramen. Antero-superiorly it is deeply grooved for passage of the obturator vessels and nerves.

The pubis consists of a body and two rami, and is united with its fellow of the opposite side at the pubic symphysis. The lines of union of the pubis and ischium (ischio-pubic synchondrosis) are frequently readily evident on the radiograph, and care must be exercised to differentiate these from fracture.

The acetabulum contains both an articular and a nonarticular portion, the acetabular fossa and lunate surface respectively. The nonarticular portion is formed mainly by the ischium, and is continuous with the margin of the obturator foramen. The margins of this socket, although thick, are subject to fracture. In order to visualize the posterior margin of the acetabulum, this structure must be viewed through the head of the femur. The shelving portion of the acetabulum is also of considerable importance, and when defective in development, congenital dislocation of the hip may result. The articular portion resembles a semilunar-shaped cartilage with its concavity directed toward the obturator foramen and it extends in irregular fashion around the ligamentum teres, excluding the latter structure from the synovial cavity. The outer edge of the articular portion is rough and uneven and gives attachment to the glenoidal labrum which deepens the socket. There is a ligament, the transverse ligament, which connects the opposite extremities of this lunate cartilage, forming the acetabular foramen. A nerve and vessels enter the joint through this foramen.

THE BONY PELVIS (Figs. 5–3, 5–4).   The bony pelvis is formed by the two hip bones together with the sacrum and coccyx. The iliopectineal line divides the pelvis into two areas, the one above being known as the greater or false pelvis and the one below as the true pelvis. These bony structures are very firmly bound together, and it ordinarily requires considerable trauma to injure this bony cage. The most vulnerable portion is the region of the pubis and its rami. An injury in this location will frequently be accompanied by a "contrecoup" fracture of the opposite wing of the sacrum. Urinary bladder or urethral injury is not infrequently found when the bony pelvis is injured.

The female bony pelvis is of particular importance from its obstetric implications. The true pelvis is described as having an inlet, a cavity and an outlet. The contour and dimensions of these are carefully studied in relation to the fetal head (see Chap. 17), and although other factors such as uterine tone are of great importance in this regard, one must also consider the simpler anatomic details of pelvic structure. Apart from actual measurements, the concavity of the sacrum, the pubic angle, the size of the ischial spines, and the mobility and position of the coccyx all play an essential part in conversion of the pelvis to a birth canal.

The sacroiliac articulations are synovial (diarthrodial) joints and are normally obliquely situated at an angle of approximately 45 degrees to the sagittal plane. It is significant that the sacroiliac joints are perpendicular to the plane of the intervertebral or apophyseal joints, and thus constitute structural supports for one another. When viewing the sacroiliac joints, the obliquity produces an irregular antero-posterior appearance, and for their interpretation one must visualize these joints in three dimensions. For that reason the oblique projection of the sacroiliac joints has considerable value.

ROUTINE VIEWS OF THE PELVIS AND LOWER EXTREMITY

1. **Antero-posterior View of the Pelvis** (Fig. 5–5). A 14 x 17 inch cassette is placed crosswise to the table, and the central ray is directed perpendicular to a point about 1 inch superior to the pubic symphysis.

2. **Lateral View of the Pelvis** (Fig. 5–6). The patient is turned on one side, and the central ray is directed over the highest part of the convexity at about the level of the second sacral segment. The thighs and knees are usually slightly flexed. The lumbar spine is supported with towels or any radiolucent material so that it is horizontal and parallel with respect to the table top. One tries to visualize the pubic symphysis, ischial spines and tuberosities, as well as the entire sacrum and coccyx in this projection.

3. **Oblique View of the Sacroiliac Joints** (Fig. 5–7). The patient lies on his back with the side in question turned obliquely away from the table top at an angle of about 45 degrees, and the central ray is made to pass through the sacroiliac joint farthest from the film. The apophyseal joints which are closest to the film are shown in best relief, but the sacroiliac joint farthest from the film is the one shown in profile when the pelvis is placed obliquely with respect to the film.

4. **Distorted View of the Sacrum** (Fig. 5–8). In the straight antero-posterior projection of the pelvis, the lower segments of the sacrum and the coccyx are seen to underlie the pubic symphysis and thus are partially obscured. By tilting the tube about 15 degrees toward the head and flexing the thighs so that the sacrum is flat against the table, a somewhat distorted view of the sacrum is obtained, but the sacrum is completely visualized. The sacroiliac joints are also distorted, but shown to good advantage in this projection. This view will also reveal a possible articulation of the transverse process of the last lumbar vertebra with the superior surface of the wing of the sacrum or medial portion of the iliac crest to better advantage. The special view of the pelvic inlet and views for pelvic mensuration are described in Chapter 17.

THE THIGH

Correlated Gross Anatomy. As in the case of the upper extremity, our main radiographic interest concerns the bony structure, although the supportive soft tissues are always studied with equal thoroughness. The femur (Figs. 5–9, 5–10), or thigh bone, is the largest and longest bone in the skeleton, and supports the entire weight of the skeleton between the legs (the locomotor organs) and the pelvis. It curves somewhat medially and posteriorly.

The head of the femur is a smooth, hemispherical structure which articulates with the acetabulum, and contains a small depression a little behind and below its center called the fovea centralis, for the ligamentum teres. The neck is mounted at an angle with respect to the shaft of the femur in two planes (Fig. 5–11):

(*a*) The medio-lateral angle which the neck forms with the shaft of the femur measures about 160 degrees at birth; in the adult, it varies between 110 and 140 degrees (approximately 125 degrees on the average).

(*b*) The neck is anteverted with respect to the shaft, which likewise varies with the age of the individual as indicated in Table 5–1. This angle may meas-

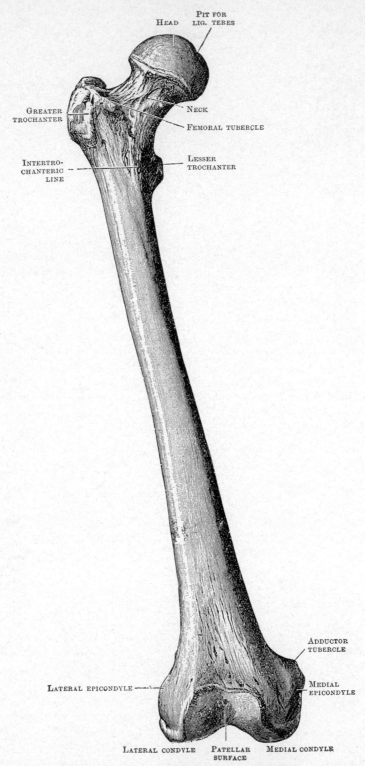

FIG. 5-9.   Femur, anterior aspect. (From Cunningham's *Text-Book of Anatomy*, Edited by Arthur Robinson, published by Oxford University Press.)

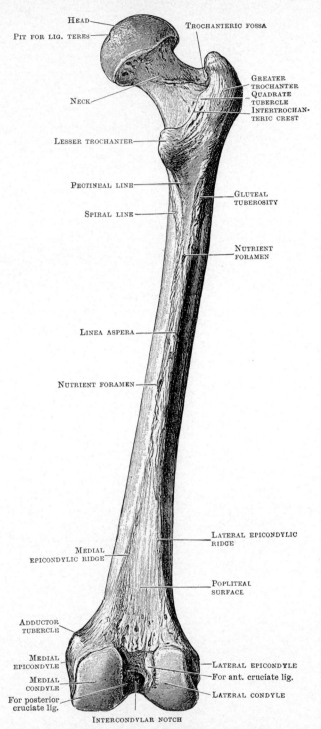

FIG. 5–10.   Femur, posterior aspect. (From Cunningham's *Text-Book of Anatomy*, Edited by Arthur Robinson, published by Oxford University Press.)

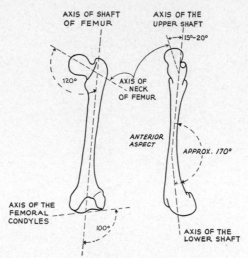

FIG. 5-11. **a,** Axial relationships of the shaft of the femur. (Angles are approximations and not invariable. See text.)

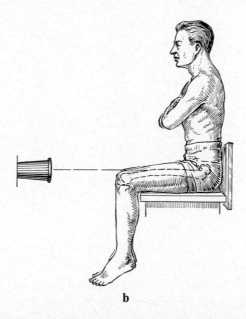

b

FIG. 5-11. **b,** Special view designed to measure the degree of anteversion of the neck of the femur with respect to the shaft. Position of patient. Note that the central ray strikes the middle of the shaft of the femur, and not the knee joint proper. As noted in Figure 5–11, **a,** the shaft of the femur arches posteriorly. It is the *proximal* one-half of the femoral shaft which is horizontal and actually the distal one-half of the femur dips downward toward the floor slightly. It is this expedient which will permit a diagnostic film to be obtained using lumbosacral spine technical factors. Otherwise, detail procured will be inadequate for measurement.

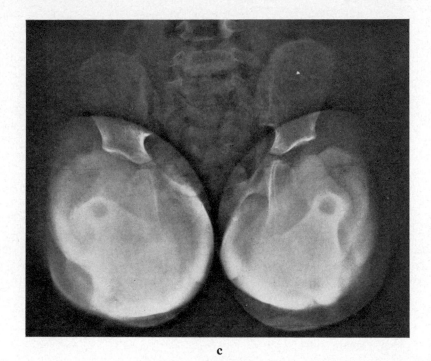

c

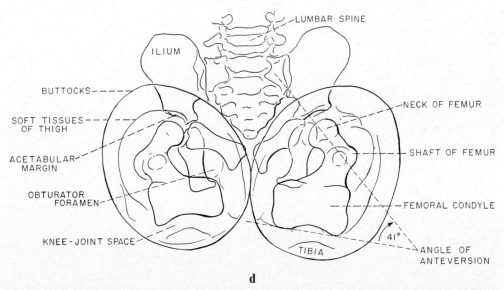

d

FIG. 5–11. Special view designed to measure the degree of anteversion of the neck of the femur with respect to the shaft. **c,** The film so obtained (intensified). The detail is poor, but adequate to draw the angle of anteversion as indicated in **d. d,** Tracing of c. One line is drawn along the inferior margins of the femoral condyles; the other is drawn through the axis of the neck of the femur. The angle between may then be measured.

Table 5–1.   Normal Degrees of Anteversion of the Femoral Neck
(Averages Adapted from Several Investigators[2, 4])

AGE	ANTEVERSION (IN DEGREES)
Birth to 1 year	30–50
2 years	30
3–5	25
6–12	20
12–15	17
16–20	11
Greater than 20	8

ure as much as 50 degrees at birth, and diminishes to about 8 degrees in the adult. A method of measuring this angle for clinical application is important, and is shown in Figure 5–11 **b, c, d.** The diagnosis of anteversion of the hip in the growing child must be made with considerable caution and parallels the diagnosis of congenital dislocation of the hip on the basis of the angle for measuring the shelving portion of the acetabulum (alpha angle for acetabular dysplasia, Fig. 5–17).

The neck of the femur is demarcated from the shaft by a ridge called the intertrochanteric line. This line furnishes the attachment anteriorly for the capsule of the hip joint (Fig. 5–14). The posterior surface of the neck of the femur tends to be concave, and only its medial two-thirds is enclosed within the joint cavity. The superior border of the neck is perforated by large nutrient foramina, although much of the bony nutrition also comes from the capsular attachment. The greater and lesser trochanters form the projections at the extremities of the intertrochanteric line.

The anteversion and the usual elements in radiography causing distortion and magnification (see Chapter 1) make it difficult for the orthopedic surgeon to anticipate the true length of the neck of the femur for purposes of choosing an appropriate nailing and fixation device for repair of a fracture of the neck of the femur. A method of measurement of the neck of the femur to overcome this difficulty has been devised,[9] but is considered outside the scope of this text.

The shaft of the femur is rather cylindrical but a rough longitudinal ridge in its middle third posteriorly spreads out distally to enclose the popliteal surface of the bone. The lateral ridge terminates in the lateral epicondyle, whereas the medial ridge ends in the adductor tubercle just above the medial epicondyle. The nutrient foramen is situated on the posteromedial aspect of the shaft of the femur at the junction of its middle and distal one thirds, and is directed toward the hip.

The intercondyloid fossa separates the two articular condyles posteriorly, but they are continuous in front, forming a smooth trochlear surface for articulation with the patella. In the lateral projection, each condyle appears to consist of a fusion of the segments of two spheres giving the condyles a "figure 3" appearance (or reverse "3" for the left femur). The medial condyle is more prominent, thinner and longer than its lateral fellow which compensates for the obliquity of the femur.

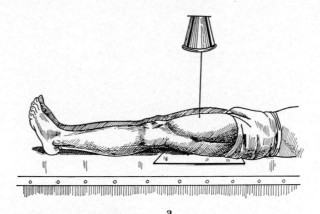

a

b   c

FIG. 5–12.   ROUTINE ANTERO-POSTERIOR VIEW OF FEMUR: **a,** Method of positioning patient; **b,** radio-graph; **c,** labeled tracing of **b.**

The following labels appear in part **c:**

CORTEX

MEDULLA

SHAFT OF FEMUR

FUSED EPIPHYSEAL LINES

LAT. EPICONDYLE

LAT. CONDYLES

INTERCONDYLOID FOSSA

PATELLA

MED. EPICONDYLE

MED. CONDYLES

INTERCONDYLOID EMINENCE

TIBIAL TUBEROSITY

FIBULA

TIBIA

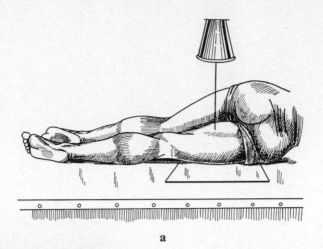

a

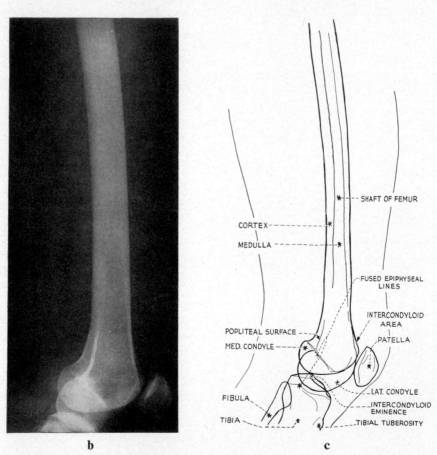

b　　　　　　　　　　　　　　　　　　　　　**c**

FIG. 5–13.　ROUTINE LATERAL VIEW OF THIGH:　**a,** Method of positioning patient; **b,** radiograph; **c,** labeled tracing of **b.**

The distal epiphysis of the femur during its development may take on a very markedly irregular appearance (Figs. 5–54 and 3–11). This must not be taken for abnormal. Also, this epiphysis may appear radiolucent in part; this likewise is a normal variant.

The Fabella. The fabella is a frequent sesamoid bone situated in the lateral head of the gastrocnemius muscle, and is projected on the posterior aspect of the lateral femoral condyle (Fig. 5–27, **d**). Its usual measurement is about 8 mm. in diameter, and it tends to be spherical in shape.

Axial Relationships of the Shaft of the Femur (Fig. 5–11). 1. The axis of the shaft of the femur forms an angle of 110 to 140 degrees with the axis of the neck of the femur.

2. A line drawn through the lowermost margins of the femoral condyles forms an angle of 10 degrees with the perpendicular (or 100 degrees with the axis of the shaft). There is thus a slight genu varum deformity which is normal.

3. There is a slight anterior bowing of the shaft of the femur, so that the axis of the upper two thirds of the shaft of the femur forms an angle of 170 degrees with the axis of the lower one third of the shaft of the femur, and this latter axis is continuous with that of the leg in the extended position.

4. The axis of the neck of the femur in the true lateral perspective forms an angle of 8 to 50 degrees with the axis of the upper shaft of the femur. Table 5–1 lists the degrees of anteversion, showing regression with age.

RADIOGRAPHIC EXAMINATION OF THE THIGH

1. **Routine Antero-posterior View of the Femur** (Fig. 5–12). The patient lies flat on his back, with the film beneath his thigh. The central ray passes through a point just below the midsection of the thigh, and the knee joint (or hip joint) is always included.

2. **Routine Lateral View of the Thigh** (Fig. 5–13). The patient lies on the affected side and the knee is slightly flexed. The opposite thigh is placed so that it will not interfere with the projection. The thigh is placed perpendicular to the film and the central ray passes through a point just distal to the midsection of the thigh. The knee joint is included in this view.

THE HIP JOINT

Correlated Gross Anatomy of Importance. The line of attachment of the hip joint capsule is illustrated in Figure 5–14, being attached anteriorly at the intertrochanteric line and posteriorly at the junction of the middle and distal thirds of the neck of the femur. The joint capsule of the hip is usually readily identified in the radiograph (Fig. 5–20, **c**) and is of considerable importance. Not infrequently the earliest manifestation of hip joint disease will be found in a swelling of this structure.

The bursal structures surrounding the hip joint are also of considerable importance. As in the case of the shoulder, these are subject to calcium deposit and inflammation. Thus, there may be four or more bursae adjoining the greater trochanter and one adjoining the ischial tuberosity, some larger than others.

There is also frequently a small extra ossicle adjoining the superior lip of the acetabulum (Fig. 5–15), called the os acetabuli. This may not be symmetrical on the two sides and must be carefully differentiated from fracture.

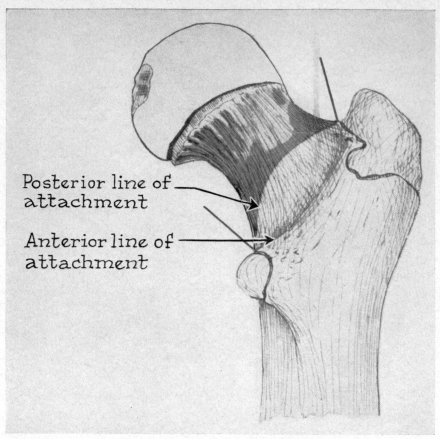

Posterior line of
attachment

Anterior line of
attachment

FIG. 5–14. The line of attachment of the capsule of the hip joint. (Modified from Perry, in Morris
Human Anatomy, The Blakiston Co., Publishers.)

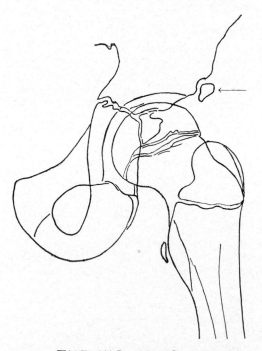

THE HIP AT 12 YEARS

FIG. 5–15. Tracing of radiograph to show os acetabuli (indicated by ←).

Axial Relationships of the Hip (Fig. 5–16). Some of the more useful axial and angular relationships of the hip joint region which assist in the evaluation of the hip joint from a functional point of view are as follows:

1. The angle formed by the axis of the neck of the femur with the axis of the shaft of the femur usually exceeds 120 degrees.

2. A horizontal line drawn perpendicular to the axis of the shaft of the femur through the uppermost margin of the greater trochanter should pass through or below the fovea centralis of the head of the femur (Skinner's line).

3. The inferior margin of the neck of the femur forms a continuous arc with the superior and medial margin of the obturator foramen (Shenton's line).

4. A line indicating the slope of the iliac portion of the acetabulum forms an angle of 33 degrees or less (Fig. 5–17) with the horizontal in the preambulatory period of a child. An angle greater than this indicates congenital absence of the shelving portion of the acetabulum and a probable predisposition to congenital dislocation of the hip.

5. Since the various measurements given in Figure 5–17 are fraught with some latitude and uncertainty, Andren and von Rosen[1] have worked out a simple method for demonstrating congenital dislocation of the hip in newborns, by keeping the hips dislocated during the x-ray exposure. This is accomplished by forcible abduction, *to at least 45 degrees, with appreciable inward rotation of the femora* (Fig. 5–18). If the hip is normal, the line of femoral shaft will be directed toward the upper edge of the bony acetabular wall, but in the presence of congenital dislocation of the hip, it will point to the anterior superior iliac spine. It should be stressed that the abduction must be at least 45 degrees, or the results will be misleading. Also, owing to the marked anteversion of the femoral necks of the newborn (Table 5–1) a fair degree of inward rotation of the femora is necessary.

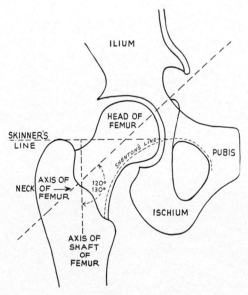

FIG. 5–16.   Axial relationships of the hip joint.

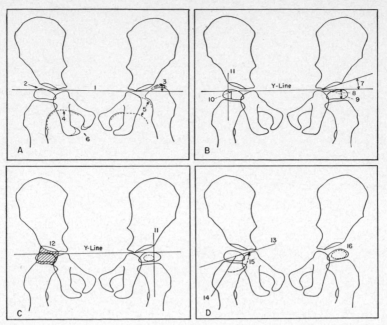

FIG. 5–17. CRITERIA FOR CONGENITAL DISLOCATION OF HIP. *1*, Y-Symphyseal line. *2* and *3*, Normally are equal. *4*, Shenton's line unbroken—normal. *5*, Shenton's line broken—dislocation or fracture. *6*, Fusion delayed, with dislocation. *7*, Not greater than 34° in newborn, normally; not greater than 25° after 1 year. *8*, Not less than 6 mm. normally. *9*, Less than 16 mm. normally. *10*, Less than one-half of epiphyseal width, normally. *11*, Should cross epiphysis lateral to center normally. *12*, Right angled cylinder, normally. *13*, Line: center of acetabulum to center of head. *14*, Axis of neck of femur. *15*, Angle 120° normally. (Modified from Kohler, A., and Zimmer, E. A.: *Border-lands of the Normal and Early Pathologic in Skeletal Roentgenology*, Grune and Stratton, 1956.)

6. Klein et al.[6] have described the roentgenographic features of a slipped capital femoral epiphysis in some detail and have proposed the lining technique illustrated in Figure 5–19. The technique consists of the following: The antero-posterior and lateral views of both hips are obtained simultaneously on one film for each view using the straight AP view and frog-leg AP views as illustrated in Figure 5–5 and Figure 5–22. The centering point is about 1½ inches above the pubic symphysis. A line is drawn along the superior margin of the neck of the femur on each hip region. Normally this line transects the head of the femur on both views. When this is not present slipping may be diagnosed and measured, particularly if there is one normal hip on the opposite side.

7. The axial relationships of the neck of the femur to the shaft in regard to anteversion have already been described, and do not deserve further attention here (Fig. 5–11, **b, c, d**).

RADIOGRAPHIC METHODS OF EXAMINATION OF THE HIP JOINT

1. **Routine Antero-posterior View of the Hip** (Fig. 5–20). The patient is placed flat on his back with the *toe of his foot pointing somewhat to the median plane*. This latter measure is of importance so that the neck of the femur is not foreshortened. The central ray passes through a point 1 inch below the center of the inguinal ligament.

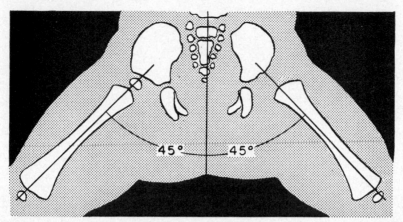

FIG. 5–18. Tracing of roentgenograms (post mortem) of newborn with femur abducted and rotated inwards. Right side: Normal hip, femoral shaft directed towards edge of acetabular wall. Left side: Dislocation, femoral shaft directed towards anterior superior iliac spine. (Ortolani's "click" could be elicited on this side but not on the right.) (Modified from Andren and Von Rosen, Acta Radiologica, vol. 49, 1958.)

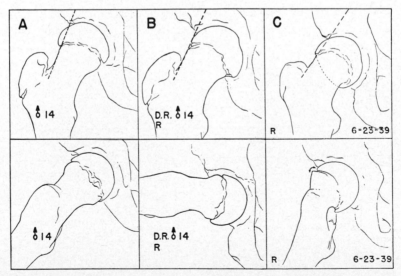

FIG. 5–19. MEDIAL AND POSTERIOR SLIPPING. A, Normal hip for comparison. B, Medial slipping· In this case slipping is detectable only in the antero-posterior view where the head is not transected by the prolongation of the superior neck line. C, Posterior slipping. In the antero-posterior view the posteriorly displaced head is projected through the proximal portion of the neck. In the lateral view the amount of posterior slipping is denoted by the curved arrow. (From Klein, A. et al., Am. J. Roentgenol., vol. 66, 1951.)

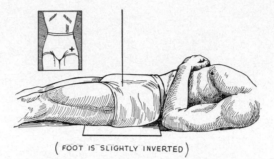

(FOOT IS SLIGHTLY INVERTED)

Fig. 5–20.   ROUTINE ANTERO-POSTERIOR VIEW OF HIP: **a,** Method of positioning patient.

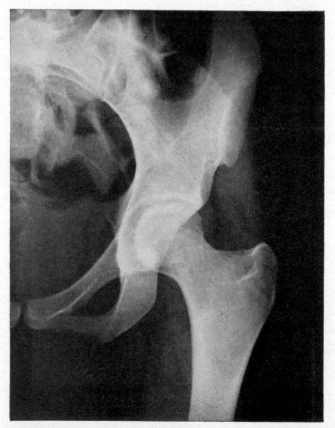

Fig. 5–20.   ROUTINE ANTERO-POSTERIOR VIEW OF HIP: **b,** Radiograph.

Points of Practical Interest with Reference to Figure 5–20:

1. The patient is placed in the perfectly supine position. The entire pelvis must be symmetrical even though only one side is considered.
2. For maximum elongation and detail with regard to the femoral neck the foot is inverted approximately 15 degrees and immobilized by means of a small sandbag in that position.
3. A line is drawn between the anterior-superior iliac spine and the superior margin of the pubic symphysis. The centering point is taken as the point 1 inch distal to the midpoint of this line. This point will ordinarily fall immediately over the hip joint proper.
4. If the foot is everted instead of inverted the lesser trochanter will be shown in maximum detail and the neck of the femur will be completely foreshortened.
5. For maximum detail with regard to both the greater and the lesser trochanter the foot should point directly upward and remain perpendicular to the table top at time the film is obtained.

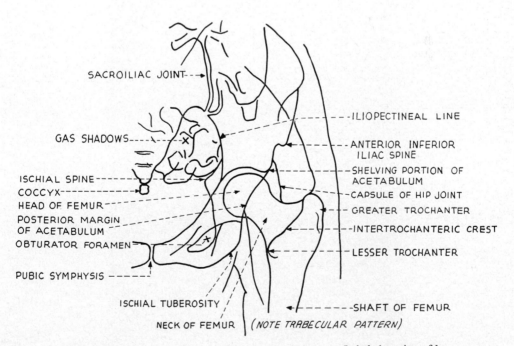

Fig. 5–20. Routine antero-posterior view of hip: c, Labeled tracing of b.

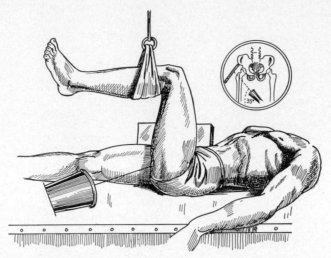

Fig. 5–21. ROUTINE LATERAL VIEW OF HIP, EMPLOYING A HORIZONTAL X-RAY BEAM: a, Method of positioning patient.

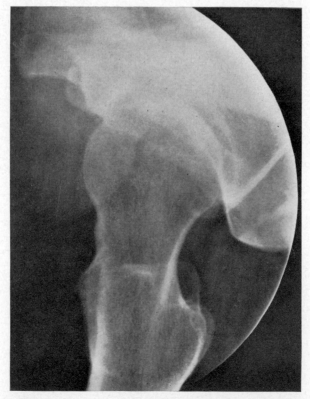

Fig. 5–21. ROUTINE LATERAL VIEW OF HIP, EMPLOYING A HORIZONTAL X-RAY BEAM: b, Radiograph.

POINTS OF PRACTICAL INTEREST WITH REFERENCE TO FIGURE 5–21:

1. The patient is placed in a supine position and the pelvis is elevated on a firm pillow or folded sheets, sufficiently to raise the ischial tuberosity approximately 3 cm. from the table top. This support of the gluteus must not extend beyond the lateral margin of the body so that it will not interfere with the placement of the cassette directly on the table top.
2. To localize the long axis of the femoral neck: (a) Draw a line between the anterior-superior iliac spine and the upper border of the pubic symphysis and mark its center point. (b) Next draw a line approximately 4 inches long perpendicular to this midpoint, extending down to the anterior surface of the thigh. This latter line represents the long axis of the femoral neck.
3. Adjust the central ray so that it is perpendicular to the midpoint of this long axis and adjust the film perpendicular to the table top so that the projection of this long axis will fall entirely upon the film
4. If the foot is maintained in a vertical position the anteversion of the neck with respect to the shaft of the femur will be demonstrated. If the foot of the affected side is inverted approximately 15 degrees the plane of the neck will be parallel with the film and form a straight line with the axis of the shaft of the femur.
5. The unaffected side may be supported over the x-ray tube or by a sling from above as shown.
6 The thickness of the part traversed by the central ray is comparable with that of a lateral lumbar spine, and the same technical factors as for a lateral lumbar spine film should ordinarily be employed.
7. A grid cassette is a very desirable adjunct for this projection.

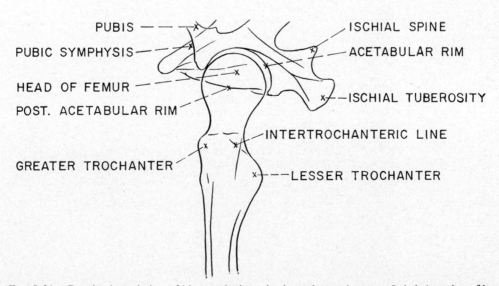

FIG. 5–21. Routine lateral view of hip, employing a horizontal x-ray beam: c, Labeled tracing of b

2. Routine Lateral View of the Hip Employing a Horizontal X-ray Beam (Fig. 5–21). This view may be obtained in either of two ways: The central ray may be directed from the medial aspect of the thigh, or from the lateral aspect of the hip. It is usually advisable to mark the probable position of the neck of the femur on the patient before proceeding. The central ray is made to pass as nearly perpendicular to this line and central to it as possible. If the medial position of the tube is employed, the film is placed perpendicular to the table top, and parallel with the neck of the femur, if possible. A close film-target distance must usually be employed in view of the fact that this part of the body is so thick. Actually a longer film-target distance in this instance would be more desirable from the standpoint of eliminating distortion and magnification as much as possible. If the central ray is directed from the lateral aspect of the thigh, usually a curved cassette is required in the groin. In this projection, it is important to visualize the entire acetabulum along with the ischial tuberosity and neck of the femur. The pubic symphysis is frequently seen also.

3. Lateral View of the Hip Employing the "Frog-leg" Position (Fig. 5–22). The patient lies flat on his back and places the heel of the affected side on the opposite knee, and everts the thigh so that it lies as nearly flat on the table top as possible. Alternately, he may place both thighs in this position and allow the soles of both feet to touch one another. The central ray passes through a point about 1 inch below the center of the inguinal ligament. When views of both hips are obtained simultaneously in this projection, the central ray passes through the pubic symphysis.

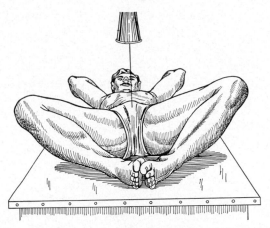

Fig. 5–22. LATERAL VIEW OF BOTH HIPS, EMPLOYING THE "FROG-LEG" POSITION: a, Method of positioning patient.

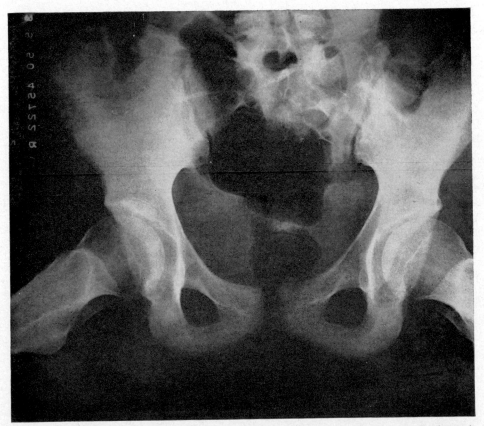

Fig. 5–22. LATERAL VIEW OF BOTH HIPS, EMPLOYING THE "FROG-LEG" POSITION: b, Radiograph.

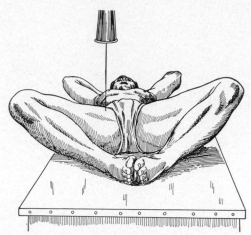

Fig. 5–22. LATERAL VIEW OF ONE HIP, EMPLOYING THE "FROG-LEG" POSITION: **c**, Method of positioning patient.

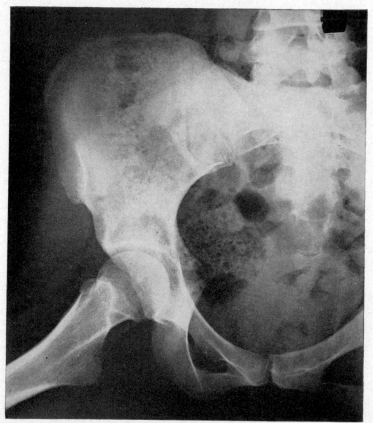

Fig. 5–22. LATERAL VIEW OF ONE HIP, EMPLOYING THE "FROG-LEG" POSITION: **d**, Radiograph.

Points of Practical Interest with Reference to Figure 5–22:

1. The "frog-leg" lateral view of the hip is actually a useful but imperfect lateral perspective of the head, neck, and upper shaft of the femur. The acetabulum remains in an antero-posterior relationship, and the normal anteversion of the neck of the femur with respect to the shaft is not shown. Moreover, this technique cannot be employed following most injuries where the hip joint motion is very limited and painful. Nevertheless, it is particularly useful in analysis of suspected hip abnormalities in children, and in other circumstances where acetabular lateral perspectives are unnecessary. Technically, this view is easier to obtain than is the true lateral shown in Figure 5–21.

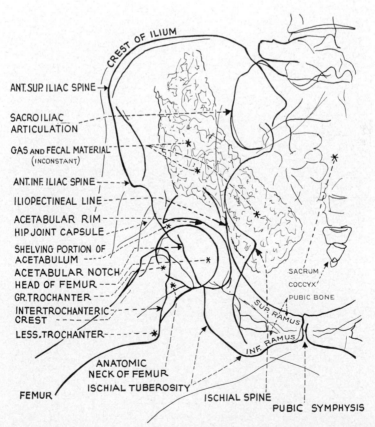

FIG. 5–22.   LATERAL VIEW OF ONE HIP, EMPLOYING THE "FROG-LEG" POSITION: e, Labeled tracing of d.

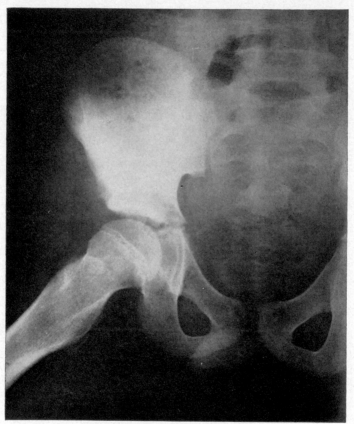

FIG. 5–22.   LATERAL VIEW OF ONE HIP, EMPLOYING THE "FROG-LEG" POSITION: f, Radiograph showing epiphyseal relationship of head of femur.

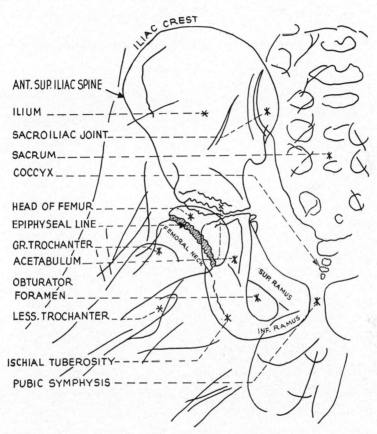

FIG. 5–22.   LATERAL VIEW OF ONE HIP, EMPLOYING THE "FROG-LEG" POSITION: g, Labeled tracing of **f**.

THE KNEE JOINT

Correlated Gross Anatomy (Fig. 5–23).   The knee joint is composed of the articular margins of the condyles and trochlear surface of the femur, the condyles of the tibia, the patella, and several bursal structures encased by numerous external and internal ligaments, joined by an articular capsule. The internal ligaments extend obliquely between the middle of the articular surface of the tibia to that of the femur, and are known as the anterior and posterior crucial (or cruciate) ligaments.

There are two semilunar cartilages which rest upon the upper surface of the tibial plateau, which are known as the medial and lateral menisci respectively; these deepen the upper surface of the tibia for articulation with the femur. The peripheral border of each is thick and convex, and is attached to the edge of the tibial condyles by the coronary ligaments, which are actually thickened areas in the joint capsule.

The medial meniscus is intimately connected with the tibial collateral ligament but the lateral is separated from the fibular collateral ligament by synovial tissue. Their inner borders are concave, thin and free, their cross sections triangular, and they are composed of fibrocartilage. The lateral meniscus has a smaller diameter and is thicker than the medial. Their extremities are known as the cornua. The anterior cornu of the medial meniscus is reflected down toward the tibial tuberosity.

The synovial membrane of the knee bulges upward from the patella to form the suprapetallar bursa, situated beneath the tendon of the extensor muscles on the front of the distal femur. This bursa frequently contains folds of synovia producing communicating compartments. There are two additional pouches at the back of the knee joint posterior to the femoral condyles, and beneath the origin of the gastrocnemius muscle. The reader is referred to Figure 5–24 which demonstrates soft tissue structures around the knee joint.[7]

An inconstant posterior pouch extends into the popliteal space in about 13 per cent of knees. When the stalk-like communication of this pouch with the knee is obstructed, or when this bursa becomes inflamed, this popliteal bursa is called a "Baker's cyst."

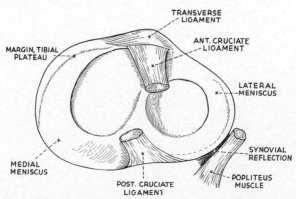

FIG. 5–23.   The condyles of the tibia seen from above showing a top view of the medial and lateral menisci and the synovial reflexion around the popliteus muscle. The latter casts a definite shadow on the pneumoarthrogram.

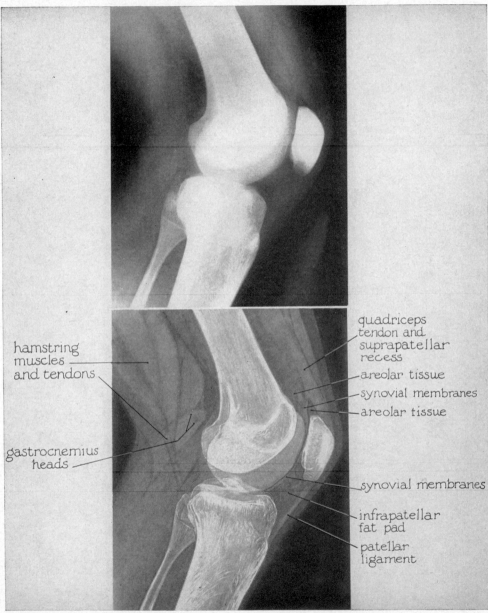

FIG. 5–24.   A normal lateral view of the knee with the associated soft tissue anatomy which can sometimes be identified by either routine views or viewing the film with a bright light. (From Lewis, R. W., Am. J. Roentgenol., vol. 65, 1951.)

There is a large process of synovial membrane containing a layer of fat within it that projects into the knee on the anterior inferior aspect of the patella known as the patellar synovial fold (ligamentum mucosum), and infrapatellar fat pad respectively. This extends upward and posteriorly to the intercondyloid notch of the femur where it is attached in front of the anterior crucial ligament and lateral to the posterior crucial ligament.

Since the cartilaginous structures of the knee are of the same order of radiolucency as the surrounding soft tissue structures, special contrast media must be introduced into the knee joint to demonstrate them. The most successful medium in this regard is a negative contrast type such as air or oxygen, and a special technique of spreading the knee has been devised to accomplish this end most successfully. The technique of this procedure will be described later (Fig. 5–29). It is most valuable in demonstrating the bursae, menisci, crucial ligaments, reflection of synovia over the popliteus muscle, the infrapatellar fat pad and the cartilage covering the articular margins of the femur, tibia and patella.

Without special contrast, the infrapatellar fat pad can usually be demonstrated since its fatty tissue produces a triangular radiolucent area. The bursae are not ordinarily identified without contrast media, unless they are distended abnormally by fluid.

Axial Relationships of the Knee (Fig. 5–25).   1. In the antero-posterior projection, the axis of the femoral shaft forms an angle of 100 degrees on the medial side (or 80 degrees on the lateral side) with the plane of the knee joint.

2. In the lateral projection when the knee is fully extended, the axis of the lower one third of the shaft of the femur forms a continuous line with the axis of the shaft of the tibia.

3. The line through the lowermost margins of the femoral condyles is parallel to the line drawn through the upper articular margins of the tibia.

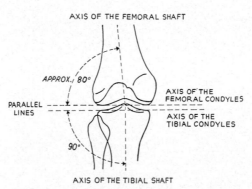

FIG. 5–25.   Axial relationships of the knee joint.

RADIOGRAPHIC METHODS OF EXAMINATION

1. **Routine Antero-posterior View of the Knee** (Fig. 5–26). The patient lies flat on his back and the film is placed under his knee. The central ray passes through a point about ½ inch below the tip of the patella, so that it will pass directly through the knee joint space.

2. **Routine Lateral View of the Knee** (Fig. 5–27). The knee is partially flexed, and its lateral aspect placed next to the film. The central ray passes through the knee joint space approximately in the midcondylar plane. In order to superimpose the two tibial condyles, 5 degree tube angulation of the shaft of the femur may be employed.

3. **Special View of the Intercondyloid Fossa of the Femur** (Fig. 5–28). This projection is employed to obtain a clear visualization of the knee joint space. The knee is bent over a curved cardboard film holder or curved cassette and the central ray is directed into the intercondyloid fossa of the femur as shown. This view may reveal a loose opaque body in the knee when other views fail to show it clearly because of overlying bone.

4. **Routine Views in Pneumoarthrography of the Knee** (Fig. 5–29). The postero-anterior views of the knee are most valuable in this regard, but occasionally antero-posterior views give additional information. The spreading of one side and then of the other is most important, since this permits the negative contrast medium to enter the space so created, and allows the internal structures of the knee on that side to be delineated. Occasionally oblique views are found to be helpful, but this can be determined at the time the knee is fluoroscoped.

Special devices are available for "spreading the knee" (Fig. 5–30).

A routine lateral view of the knee is also obtained.

For further detailed illustrations of many of the variations of normal and abnormal with regard to pneumoarthrography of the knee, the reader is referred to a comprehensive review of the subject by Meschan and McGaw: Radiology *49:* 675–710, 1947.

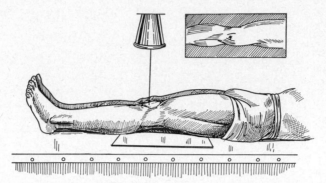

FIG. 5–26.   ROUTINE ANTERO-POSTERIOR VIEW OF KNEE: **a,** Method of positioning patient.

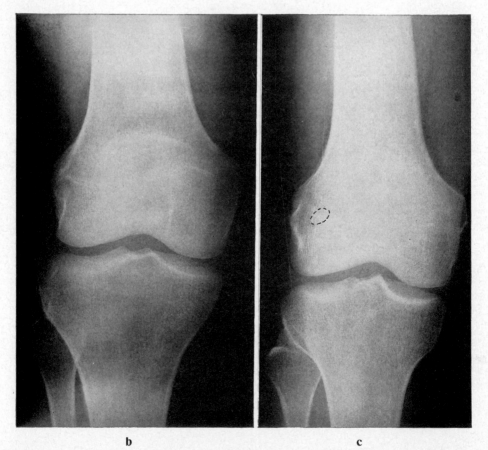

b   c

FIG. 5–26.   ROUTINE ANTERO-POSTERIOR VIEW OF KNEE: **b,** Radiograph. **c,** Radiograph demonstrating fabella.

POINTS OF PRACTICAL INTEREST WITH REFERENCE TO FIGURE 5–26:

1. The knee should be completely extended with the patient in the supine position. If unable to extend the knee completely, the postero-anterior projection is preferable.
2. Alternately, if the knee cannot be fully extended the cassette should be elevated on sandbags to bring it into closer contact with the popliteal space. If the degree of flexion of the knee is great, a curved cassette or curved film holder should be employed.
3. The leg is adjusted in the true antero-posterior position and the distal apex of the patella is noted.
4. Center the cassette and the central ray of the x-ray tube approximately 1 cm. below the patellar apex.
5. When radiographing the joint space it may be helpful to tilt the tube approximately 5 degrees cephalad. This expedient will help give a clear view of the knee joint space in that it superimposes the anterior and posterior margins of the tibial plateau somewhat more satisfactorily.

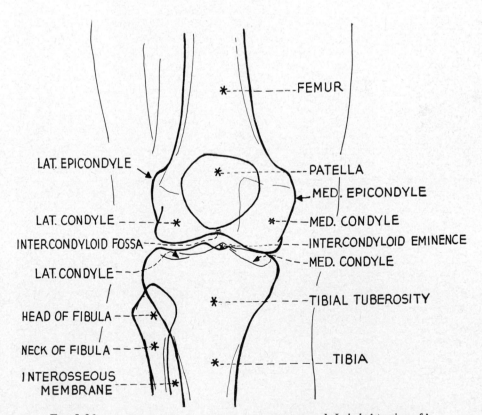

FIG. 5–26. ROUTINE ANTERO-POSTERIOR VIEW OF KNEE: **d,** Labeled tracing of **b.**

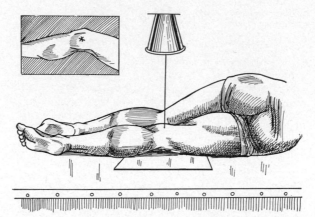

Fig. 5–27. ROUTINE LATERAL VIEW OF KNEE: **a.** Method of positioning patient.

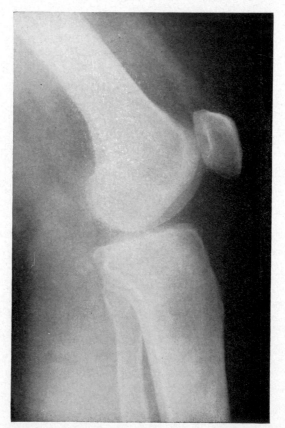

Fig. 5–27. ROUTINE LATERAL VIEW OF KNEE: **b,** Radiograph.

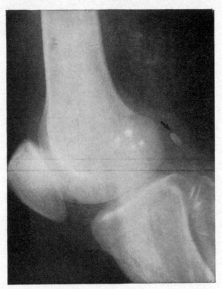

FIG. 5–27. ROUTINE LATERAL VIEW OF KNEE: c, Radiograph demonstrating fabella.

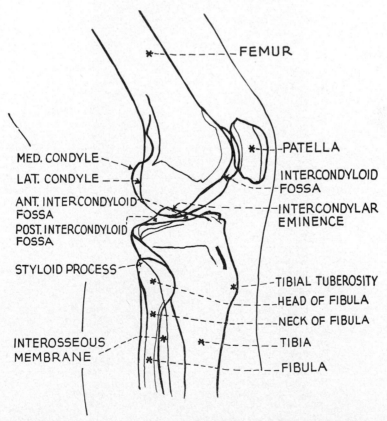

FIG. 5–27. ROUTINE LATERAL VIEW OF KNEE: d, Labeled tracing of b.

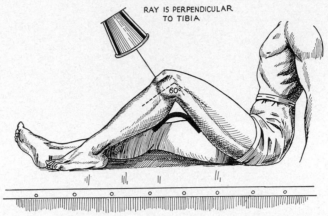

RAY IS PERPENDICULAR
TO TIBIA

60°

FIG. 5–28.   SPECIAL VIEW OF INTERCONDYLOID FOSSA OF FEMUR: **a,** Method of positioning patient.

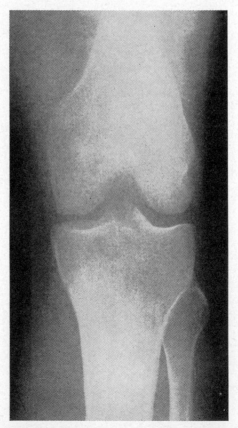

FIG. 5–28.   SPECIAL VIEW OF INTERCONDYLOID FOSSA OF FEMUR: **b,** Radiograph.

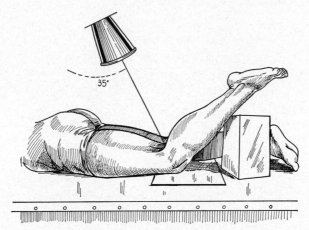

FIG. 5–28. SPECIAL VIEW OF INTERCONDYLOID FOSSA OF FEMUR: **c,** Alternate method of positioning patient. A very similar radiograph is obtained.

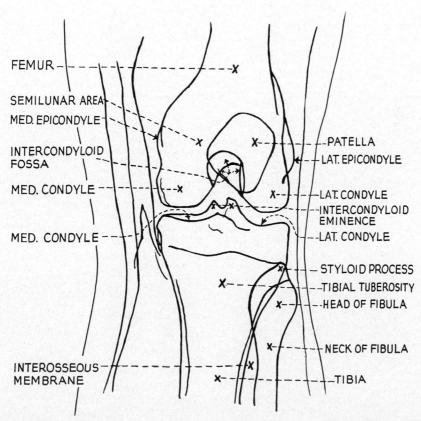

FIG. 5–28. SPECIAL VIEW OF INTERCONDYLOID FOSSA OF FEMUR: **d,** Labeled tracing of **b.**

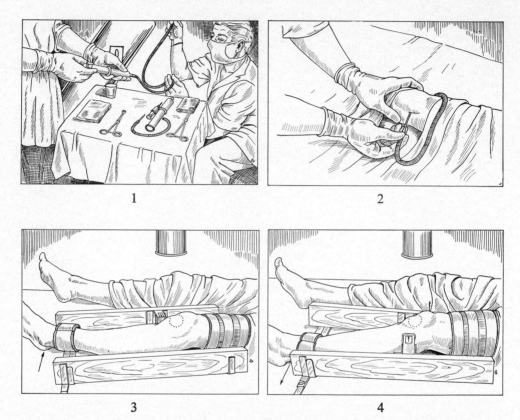

FIG. 5–29.   PNEUMOARTHROGRAPHY OF THE KNEE: **a,** Routine technique. **1,** Method of loading
the 50 cc. syringes from the oxygen tank under sterile technique. **2,** Method of inserting needle under
the superior margin of the patella into the suprapatellar bursa where 80 to 120 cc. of oxygen is thereafter injected. **3,** Method of positioning the patient for the antero-posterior view of the lateral meniscus. Note the lateral side of the knee joint is being spread by the special spreader device. **4,** Method of
positioning patient for the antero-posterior view of the medial meniscus, spreading the medial side
of the knee joint.

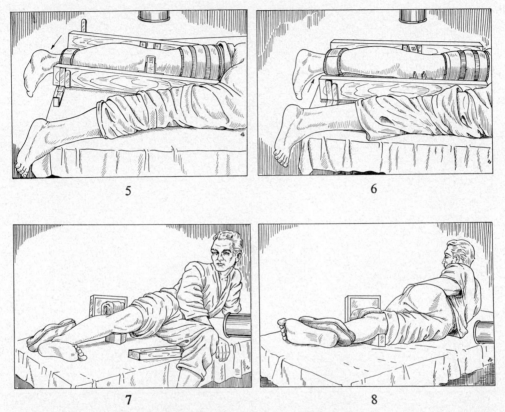

FIG. 5–29. PNEUMOARTHROGRAPHY OF THE KNEE: a, Routine technique (continued). 5, Method of positioning patient for postero-anterior view of the lateral meniscus. 6, Method of positioning patient for postero-anterior view of the medial meniscus. 7, Method of positioning patient for a horizontal or decubitus view of the lateral meniscus in the antero-posterior projection. 8, Method of positioning patient employing a horizontal x-ray beam spreading the medial joint space. In both of these latter projections the oxygen rises to the top, giving one a maximum delineation of the topmost portion of the knee, still obtaining a spread visualization of the knee

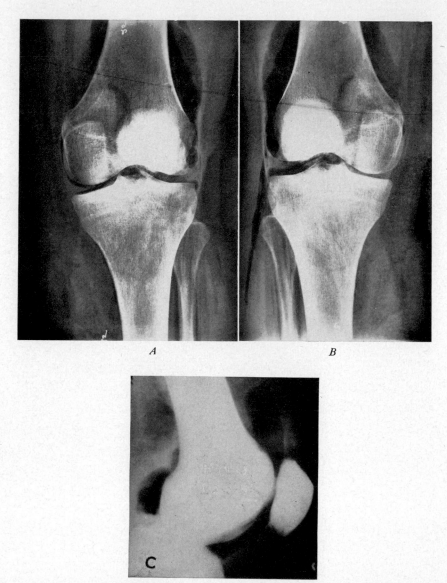

FIG. 5–29.   PNEUMOARTHROGRAPHY OF THE KNEE: **b,** Radiographs. *A* and *B*, Radiographs obtained in the postero-anterior projection, first with the medial knee joint spread, and next with the lateral knee joint spread. *C*, Radiograph of the knee in a straight lateral projection.

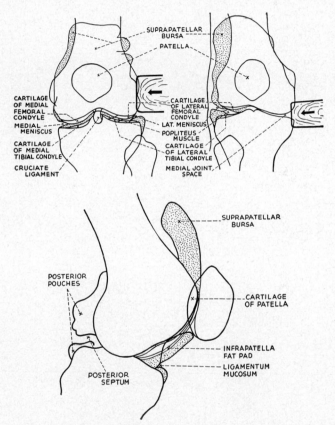

FIG. 5–29. PNEUMOARTHROGRAPHY OF THE KNEE: **c,** Labeled tracings of **b.**

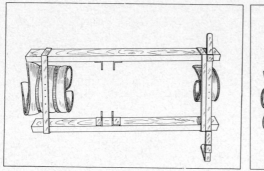
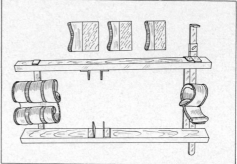

a   b

FIG. 5–30.   SPECIAL DEVICE FOR SPREADING THE KNEE FOR PNEUMOARTHROGRAPHY.   a, Top view; b, bottom-side up. The blocks of wood are adjusted in the slots and act as a fulcrum against the knee while the ankle in its brace is moved in one or the other direction, depending upon which side of the knee joint is being spread.

THE PATELLA

The patella is a triangular sesamoid bone developed in the tendon of the quadriceps femoris muscle (Fig. 5–31). Its anterior surface is perforated by many small openings which transmit nutrient vessels, and this roughened appearance must be recognized as a normal condition. Its anterior surface is covered by one or more bursae, and its posterior surface is articular, articulating with the anterior aspects of both femoral condyles.

Ossification of the patella begins about the third year of life, and is usually completed about the age of puberty.

Occasionally a segmentation of the patella persists throughout life, separating the upper outer quadrant on the articular aspect of the bone from the rest of the patella. This is called a bipartite patella (Fig. 5–32). More rarely, there may be a third segment which remains separate on the outer lower aspect of the bone; this constitutes a tripartite patella. These entities are important from the standpoint of differentiation from fracture.

In view of the distance of the patella from the film in the antero-posterior projection, a certain amount of distortion is obtained of the patella in this view. Also, projection may produce some confusion as to the exact position of the patella with relation to the distal femur. This is overcome by obtaining the postero-anterior view of the patella which furnishes considerably greater detail regarding patellar structure and position.

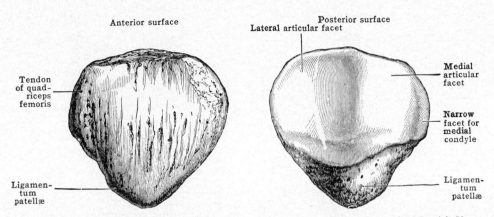

Anterior surface

Tendon
of quad-
riceps
femoris

Ligamen-
tum
patellæ

Posterior surface
Lateral articular facet

**Medial
articular
facet**

Narrow
facet for
medial
condyle

Ligamen-
tum
patellæ

FIG. 5–31.   The patella, anterior, posterior and superior views. (From Terry, in Morris' *Human Anatomy*, The Blakiston Co., Publishers.)

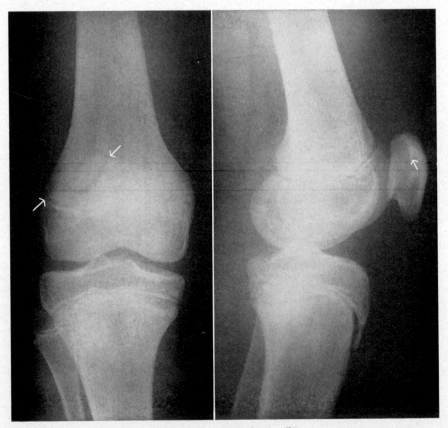

FIG. 5–32.   Bipartite patella.

RADIOGRAPHIC METHODS OF EXAMINATION OF PATELLA

1. Postero-anterior View of the Patella (Fig. 5–33).　The patient lies prone with the film beneath the patella. *A relatively short film-target distance is employed* so that most of the knee will be distorted, and the patella will be more clearly defined since it is close to the film. The central ray in this instance can pass either through the knee joint proper as illustrated, or it may pass through the patella.

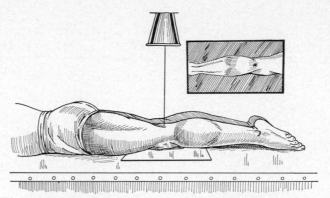

FIG. 5–33.　POSTERO-ANTERIOR VIEW OF PATELLA:　**a**, Method of positioning patient.

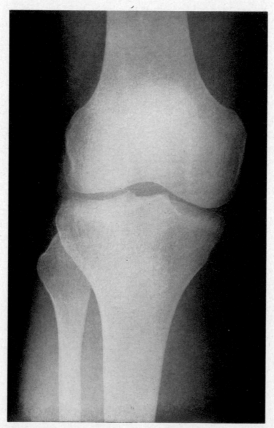

FIG. 5–33.　POSTERO-ANTERIOR VIEW OF PATELLA:　**b**, Radiograph.

POINTS OF PRACTICAL INTEREST WITH REFERENCE TO FIGURE 5–33:

1. The patient is placed in the prone position with the ankles and the feet ordinarily supported by sandbags.
2. The film is centered to the patella and the central ray so adjusted as to pass through the center of the patella. The heel may have to be rotated outward slightly to accomplish this.
3. Ordinarily, it is desirable to use a telescopic cone and bring the cone fairly close to the knee in order to produce a distortion of the superimposed femoral condyles and a clearer concept of the patella which lies next to the film.
4. This view definitely gives better detail of the patella than can be obtained in the anteroposterior projection.

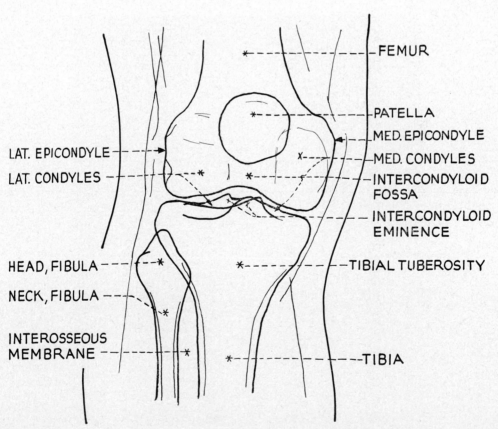

FIG. 5–33. POSTERO-ANTERIOR VIEW OF PATELLA: c, Labeled tracing of b.

2. **Special Tangential View of the Patella** (Fig. 5–34). The two views usually employed in this connection are illustrated in the accompanying diagrams. One frequently finds the anterior margin of the patella to be quite irregular owing to the fact that it is penetrated by several nutrient vessels from its anterior aspect. This imparts a very serrated appearance to the patella.

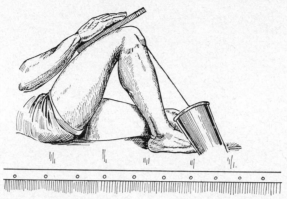

Fig. 5–34.   SPECIAL TANGENTIAL VIEW OF PATELLA: **a,** Method of positioning patient.

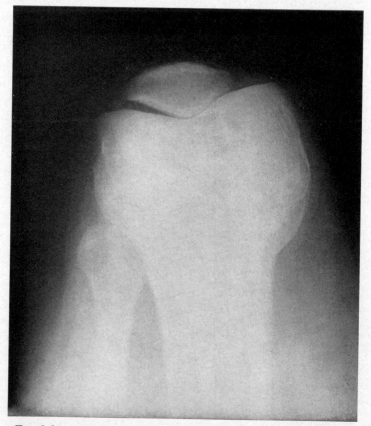

FIG. 5–34.   SPECIAL TANGENTIAL VIEW OF PATELLA: **b,** Radiograph.

POINTS OF PRACTICAL INTEREST WITH REFERENCE TO FIGURE 5–34:

1. This view may be obtained with the patient either prone or supine. If prone, the thigh is placed flat against the table and the leg flexed by means of a band wrapped around the ankle and the ends held by the patient's hand. If the patient is supine, the film is placed along the distal aspect of the thigh as shown.
2. The central ray is directed at right angles to the joint space between the patella and the femoral condyles, and the degree of central ray angulation will depend upon the degree of flexion of the knee. Ordinarily the central ray should be parallel with the articular margin of the patella.
3. The outer margin of the patella as projected in this view frequently presents a rather serrated and irregular appearance which must not be interpreted as abnormal. This serrated appearance is due to points of tendinous attachments to the bony substance of the patella, as well as penetration by nutrient vessels.

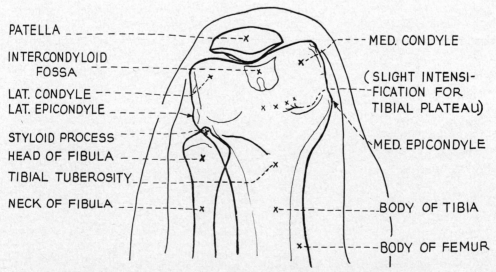

FIG. 5–34. SPECIAL TANGENTIAL VIEW OF PATELLA: c, Labeled tracing of b.

THE LEG

Correlated Anatomy of the Tibia.   The upper end of the tibia (Figs. 5–35, 5–36) contains the medial and lateral condyles which articulate with the corresponding condyles of the femur. Anteriorly, the condyles meet to form the tuberosity of the tibia, which receives an attachment of the ligamentum patellae. Between the ligament and the anterior upper aspect of the tuberosity, there is a prominent, more superficial bursa. (This bursa is subject to inflammation in individuals who must rest their weight upon this structure for one reason or another, such as frequent kneeling or scrubbing floors.)

The shaft of the tibia has a prominent crest (the anterior crest) anteriorly in its upper two thirds, which gradually extends medially towards the medial malleolus. The lateral border of the tibia forms the interosseous crest, which gives attachment to the interosseous membrane.

The lower end of the tibia presents the medial malleolus on the medial aspect, a smooth anterior aspect, and a roughened posterior aspect. The posterior surface contains two grooves—the medial receiving the tendons of the tibialis posterior and flexor digitorum longus muscle, and the lateral the flexor hallucis longus muscle. The lateral aspect is indented for its articulation with the fibula. The distal articular surface extends along the lateral aspect of the medial malleolus, and the entire surface articulates with the talus tarsal bone.

There are several items of particular radiographic interest in this bone. The tibial tuberosity is a rather variable structure in its appearance, and is subject to degenerative changes during the growth period. Not infrequently, the tuberosity will appear different on the two sides.

The upper margin of the interosseal crest is frequently of a lesser density than the remainder of this ridge, and simulates a periosteal elevation or thickening. This appearance is normal, however, and should not be interpreted as a periostitis.

There is a slight normal curvature of the tibia, both laterally and anteriorly. On the other hand, the fibula tends to curve somewhat posteriorly, producing an ovoid aperture in the interosseal region in the lateral view. These slight curvatures must be considered in studying the lines of weight bearing in the leg.

Correlated Anatomy of the Fibula.   The fibula (Figs. 5–35, 5–36) in man bears none of the weight of the trunk, and is important only from the standpoint of its muscular attachments and its participation in the formation of the ankle joint. The head of the fibula is rather a bulbous structure which rises to a pointed apex known as the styloid process which is considerably roughened for attachment of muscles and ligaments. Medially, it articulates with the lateral condyle of the tibia. The shaft of the fibula contains numerous longitudinal and oblique grooves which furnish muscular attachment; the interosseous crest on the medial aspect gives attachment to the interosseous membrane. The lateral malleolus is particularly important because of its frequent participation in injuries to the ankle area. The upper medial surface articulates with the talus tarsal bone, and is smooth, but the rest of the malleolus is very roughened and grooved. It gives attachment to numerous ligaments around the ankle and is grooved posteriorly for the peronei tendons. The tip of the lateral malleolus affords attachment to the calcaneofibular ligament of the ankle which is particularly subject to tear and strain in inversion injuries.

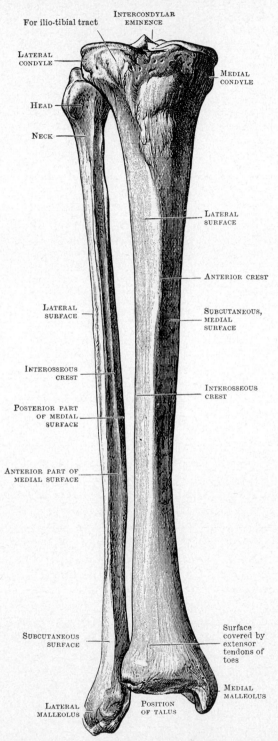

For ilio-tibial tract

INTERCONDYLAR
EMINENCE

LATERAL
CONDYLE

MEDIAL
CONDYLE

HEAD

NECK

LATERAL
SURFACE

ANTERIOR CREST

LATERAL
SURFACE

SUBCUTANEOUS,
MEDIAL
SURFACE

INTEROSSEOUS
CREST

INTEROSSEOUS
CREST

POSTERIOR PART
OF MEDIAL
SURFACE

ANTERIOR PART OF
MEDIAL SURFACE

Surface
covered by
extensor
tendons of
toes

SUBCUTANEOUS
SURFACE

MEDIAL
MALLEOLUS

LATERAL
MALLEOLUS

POSITION
OF TALUS

FIG· 5–35. Tibula and fibula, anterior aspect. (From Cunningham's *Text-Book of Anatomy*, Edited
by Arthur Robinson, published by Oxford University Press.)

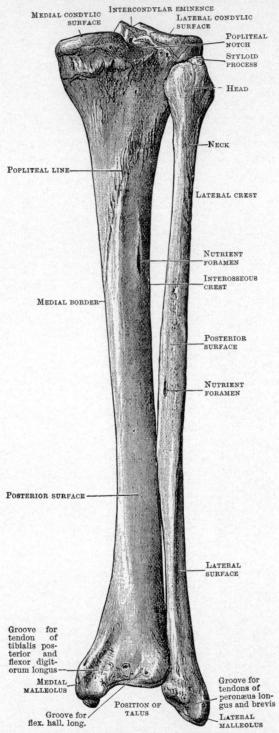

FIG. 5-36.   Tibia and fibula, posterior aspect. (From Cunningham's *Text-Book of Anatomy*, Edited by Arthur Robinson, published by Oxford University Press.)

In view of the great importance of the malleoli, special views of these structures from several perspectives are obtained, and minute abnormalities require the closest inspection. The irregularities which may occur normally must be understood; only then can abnormal irregularities be recognized.

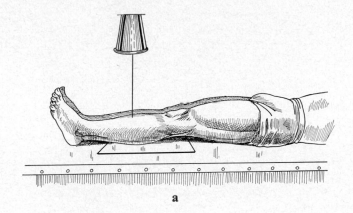

a

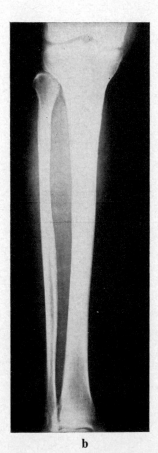

b

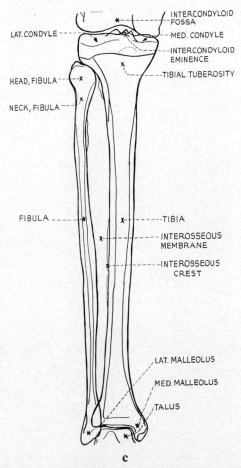

c

FIG. 5-37. ROUTINE ANTERO-POSTERIOR VIEW OF LEG: **a,** Method of positioning patient; **b,** radiograph; and **c,** labeled tracing of **b.**

RADIOGRAPHIC METHODS OF EXAMINATION OF THE LEG

1. **Routine Antero-posterior View.**
2. **Lateral View** (Figs. 5–37, 5–38).   The diagrams are self-explanatory. It is only important to emphasize that in the antero-posterior projection the toes point slightly medially. If possible, both the knee joint and joint between the tibia and talus should be included so that the line of weight bearing can be accurately drawn. In any event, one of these joints should always be shown.

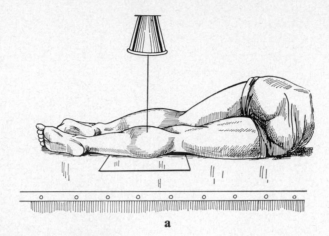

a

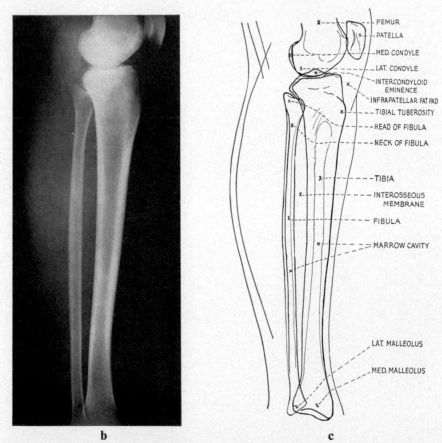

b   c

Fig. 5–38.   ROUTINE LATERAL VIEW OF LEG: a, Method of positioning patient; b, radiograph; and c, labeled tracing of b.

THE TARSUS

Correlated Gross Anatomy (Figs. 5–39, 5–40). There are seven tarsal bones—the calcaneus, talus, navicular, cuboid, and three cuneiform bones. Each has approximately six surfaces, some surfaces being articular and others roughened by ligamentous attachments.

The talus supports the tibia, articulating with the malleoli on either side, the calcaneus below, and the navicular in front. Anteriorly, the head of the talus articulates with the navicular. Inferiorly, there are two separate articular surfaces for the calcaneus—one which articulates with the sustentaculum tali, and the other which is larger which articulates with the calcaneus proper. Occasionally, there is a separate ossicle along the posterior margin of the larger calcaneal articular surface known as the *os trigonum*. Its primary radiographic importance is the necessity for differentiating it from a fracture.

The calcaneus is the largest tarsal bone, and forms the heel of the foot. Superiorly and anteromedially it articulates with the talus. Anteromedially where it supports the talus there is a well-marked process known as the sustentaculum tali. Anteriorly, it articulates with the cuboid. Unlike the other tarsal and carpal bones, there is a secondary epiphysis situated on the heel aspect of the calcaneus which begins to ossify in the sixth to the tenth year, and unites with the body of the bone between the thirteenth to the twentieth year. This ossification varies considerably in different individuals, and even on the two feet of a single individual. *The bone of this epiphysis tends to be somewhat more compact than that of most epiphyses, and any interpretations of abnormality in this epiphysis, either with regard to its irregularity or its density, must be entertained with considerable caution.*

Boehler's[3] *angle for the normal calcaneus* (Fig. 5–41) is a line drawn from the posterior superior margin of the talocalcaneal joint through the posterior superior margin of the calcaneus, making an angle of approximately 35 to 40 degrees with a second line drawn from the posterior superior margin of the talocalcaneal joint to the superior articular margin of the calcaneocuboid joint. Less than 28 degrees is quite definitely abnormal and poor position from the functional standpoint.

The navicular bone is situated between the talus behind and the three cuneiforms in front. Its tuberosity is a prominent eminence on its medial aspect. Its superior surface is somewhat variable in appearance, and rather irregular. There is not infrequently a small extra ossicle adjoining the tuberosity known as the *accessory navicular* which, like the os trigonum, owes its importance to the fact that it must not be confused with a fracture in this region.

The three cuneiform bones are wedge-shaped bones situated between the navicular behind and the first three metatarsals in front. Although they are in the same line posteriorly, the first and third project farther anteriorly than does the second. This forms a recess into which the base of the second metatarsal is received.

The cuboid, as its name indicates, is an irregular cube in shape and is situated between the calcaneus behind, and the fourth and fifth metatarsals in front. In addition, it also articulates with the third cuneiform, and occasionally also with the navicular and talus.

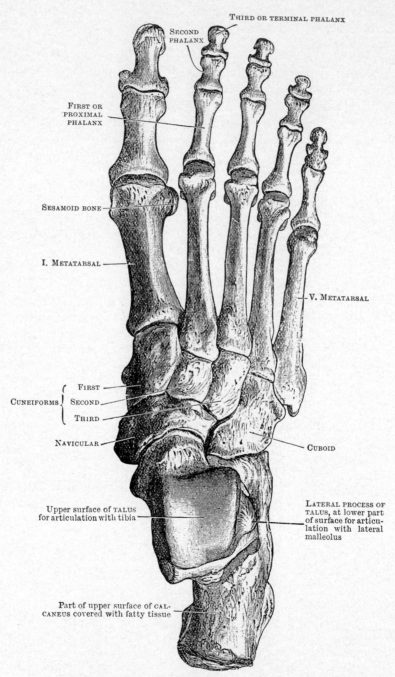

THIRD OR TERMINAL PHALANX

SECOND PHALANX

FIRST OR PROXIMAL PHALANX

SESAMOID BONE

I. METATARSAL

V. METATARSAL

FIRST

CUNEIFORMS { SECOND

THIRD

NAVICULAR

CUBOID

Upper surface of TALUS for articulation with tibia

LATERAL PROCESS OF TALUS, at lower part of surface for articulation with lateral malleolus

Part of upper surface of CAL-CANEUS covered with fatty tissue

FIG. 5–39. Dorsal view of foot. (From Cunningham's *Text-Book of Anatomy*, Edited by Arthur Robinson, published by Oxford University Press.)

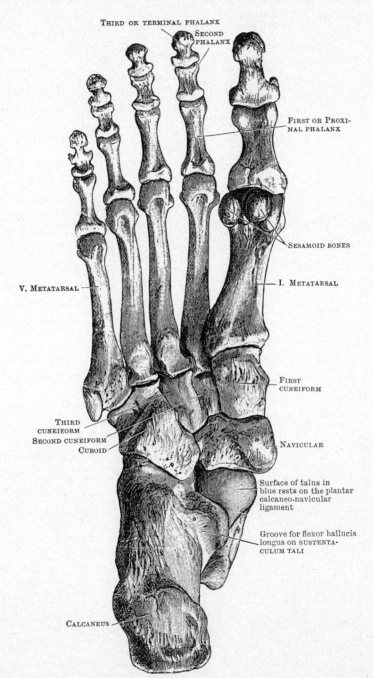

THIRD OR TERMINAL PHALANX

SECOND PHALANX

FIRST OR PROXI- MAL PHALANX

SESAMOID BONES

I. METATARSAL

V. METATARSAL

FIRST CUNEIFORM

THIRD CUNEIEORM

SECOND CUNEIFORM

CUBOID

NAVICULAR

Surface of talus in blue rests on the plantar calcaneo-navicular ligament

Groove for flexor hallucis longus on SUSTENTA- CULUM TALI

CALCANEUS

FIG. 5–40. Plantar view of foot. (From Cunningham's *Text-Book of Anatomy*, Edited by Arthur Robinson, published by Oxford University Press.)

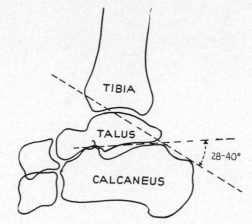

FIG. 5–41.   The criteria for a normal calcaneus (Boehler).

One of the most frequent sesamoid bones of this region is the *peroneal sesamoid* which is situated between the cuboid and the base of the fifth metatarsal, in the tendon of the peroneus longus muscle. An accessory first cuneiform is another frequent extra ossicle arising from the separate ossification of the plantar and dorsal aspects of the first cuneiform, and is situated in the tendon of the tibialis anterior muscle.

The most frequent sesamoid bone of the ankle area is the os trigonum situated over the medial surface of the head of the talus in the tendon of the tibialis posterior muscle (see Fig. 5–48).

The Ankle Joint (Fig. 5–42).   The ankle joint is formed by the lower ends of the tibia and fibula and the upper surface of the talus, apart from ligamentous structures. The synovial membrane of this joint is very extensive, being very loose, and extending beyond the actual articulation. Since the medial and lateral malleoli are subject to frequent injury, this joint is of considerable importance in traumatic medicine. Since a portion of the lateral malleolus is obscured by the talus, oblique views are necessary to show the lateral malleolus clearly in its entirety. The so-called trimalleolar fracture is actually a clinical misnomer since there are not three malleoli in this region; the term, however, refers to a combined fracture of the posterior articular margin of the tibia and medial malleolus which may or may not be continuous, as well as a coexisting fracture of the lateral malleolus. The ankle joint space is a very regular structure, with a parallelism of the articular margins which is demonstrated in Figure 5–43.

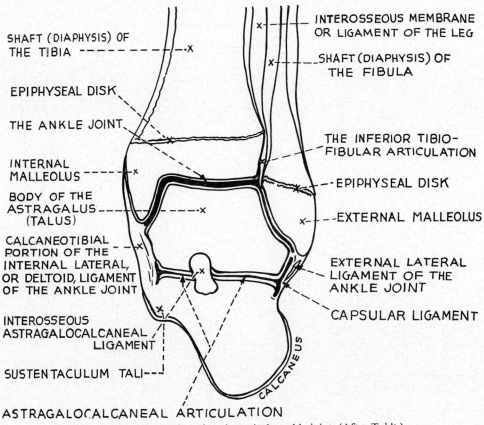

SHAFT (DIAPHYSIS) OF
THE TIBIA -------- -x

INTEROSSEOUS MEMBRANE
OR LIGAMENT OF THE LEG

SHAFT (DIAPHYSIS) OF
THE FIBULA

EPIPHYSEAL DISK

THE ANKLE JOINT

THE INFERIOR TIBIO-
FIBULAR ARTICULATION

INTERNAL
MALLEOLUS

EPIPHYSEAL DISK

BODY OF THE
ASTRAGALUS
(TALUS)

EXTERNAL MALLEOLUS

CALCANEOTIBIAL
PORTION OF THE
INTERNAL LATERAL,
OR DELTOID, LIGAMENT
OF THE ANKLE JOINT

EXTERNAL LATERAL
LIGAMENT OF THE
ANKLE JOINT

CAPSULAR LIGAMENT

INTEROSSEOUS
ASTRAGALOCALCANEAL
LIGAMENT

SUSTENTACULUM TALI---

CALCANEUS

ASTRAGALOCALCANEAL ARTICULATION

FIG. 5–42.   Coronal section through the ankle joint. (After Toldt.)

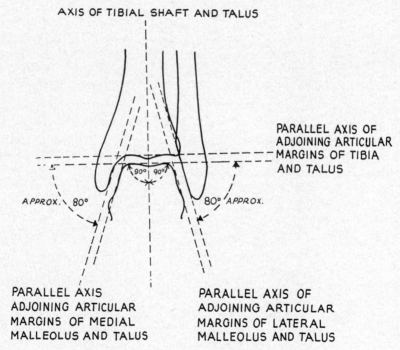

FIG. 5–43.   Axial relationships of the ankle joint.

Axial Relationships of the Ankle (Fig. 5–43). 1. The axis of the shaft of the tibia is perpendicular to the horizontal plane of the ankle joint.

2. The axes of the articular margins of the distal extremity of the tibia and the proximal talus are parallel.

3. The axes of the malleolotalar joints form angles of 80 degrees on either side with the axis of the tibiotalar joint.

4. The articular margins of both malleoli and the distal tibia are equidistant from the proximal articular margin of the talus.

5. The axis of the shaft of the tibia is continuous with the vertical axis of the talus.

6. Less than 50 per cent overlap of the fibula by the lateral tibial tubercle in the straight antero-posterior projection indicates tibiofibular diastasis from torn tibiofibular ligament. This in turn strongly suggests that a search be made for fracture of the fibular shaft about 6 cm. above the lateral malleolus.

The Tarsal Joints. The tarsal joints, together with the tarsometatarsal, metatarsophalangeal and interphalangeal joints, constitute the joints of the foot.

RADIOGRAPHIC METHODS OF EXAMINATION OF THE ANKLE

1. **Routine Antero-posterior View of the Ankle** (Fig. 5–44). The patient lies flat, with the toe pointing slightly medially. The central ray passes through the center of the talotibial joint. The lateral malleolus is partially obscured on this view, and the tarsal bones distal to the talus are not shown to good advantage.

2. **Routine Lateral View of the Ankle** (Fig. 5–45). The ankle is placed against the film so that the lateral malleolus is in the central ray. The foot is perpendicular to the film, and the two malleoli should be projected directly over one another. This view shows the lateral relation of the talotibial joint, the anterior and posterior lips of the medial malleolus, and the lateral malleolus through the medial.

3. **Oblique View of the Ankle** (Fig. 5–46). This view is illustrated in the accompanying diagram. Its main purpose is to show the lateral malleolus and tibiofibular joint to better advantage.

4. **Special Tangential View of the Calcaneus** (Fig. 5–47). This view demonstrates the posterior two thirds of the calcaneus in excellent, though distorted, profile. Fracture of the body of the calcaneus and of its posterior aspect will be shown in this projection.

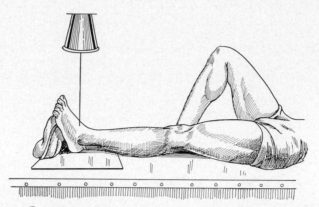

FIG. 5–44. ROUTINE ANTERO-POSTERIOR VIEW OF ANKLE: **a,** Method of positioning patient.

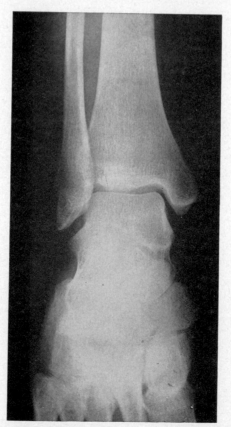

FIG. 5–44. ROUTINE ANTERO-POSTERIOR VIEW OF ANKLE: **b,** Radiograph.

Points of Practical Interest with Reference to Figure 5–44:

1. If less overlapping of the distal tibia and fibula is desired, the foot should be inverted slightly. This expedient will increase the clarity of the lateral malleolus particularly, but will interfere with the measurement of the distance between the talal articular margin and the malleoli.
2. In young individuals, in whom the distal epiphyses of the tibia and fibula are not yet united to their respective shafts, it is particularly important to obtain comparison films of the opposite normal side. It may otherwise be very difficult to be certain regarding the absence of a slight fracture through the epiphyseal disk.
3. Although the ligaments around the ankle are not visualized radiographically, it is important to know their relationships accurately. Often the more important aspect of trauma and injury to the ankle concerns the ligamentous rather than the bony abnormality.

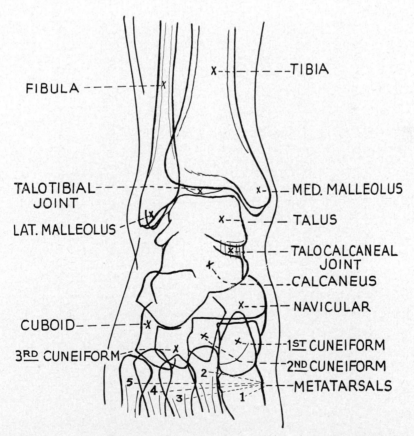

FIG. 5–44. ROUTINE ANTERO-POSTERIOR VIEW OF ANKLE: c, Labeled tracing of b.

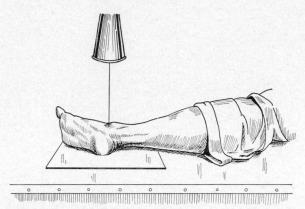

Fig. 5–45.   ROUTINE LATERAL VIEW OF ANKLE: **a,** Method of positioning patient.

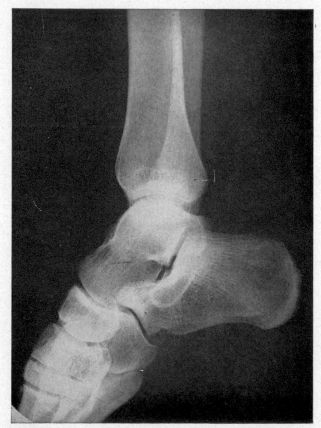

Fig. 5–45.   ROUTINE LATERAL VIEW OF ANKLE: **b,** Radiograph.

POINTS OF PRACTICAL INTEREST WITH REFERENCE TO FIGURE 5–45:

1. The affected leg and ankle are so placed that the sagittal plane of the leg is perfectly parallel with the table top and film. The film holder and central ray are centered to a point approximately 2 cm. proximal to the tip of the lateral malleolus. A sandbag or balsa wood block placed under the distal one third of the foot facilitates true alignment.
2. The unaffected side is sharply flexed and placed in a comfortable position forward so that no movement will be obtained during the x-ray exposure.

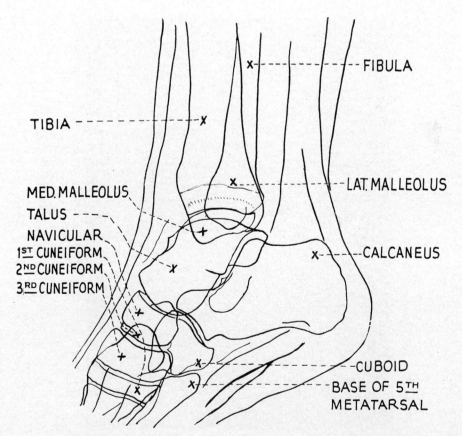

FIG. 5–45. ROUTINE LATERAL VIEW OF ANKLE: c, Labeled tracing of b.

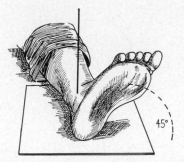

FIG. 5–46.   OBLIQUE VIEW OF ANKLE: **a,** Method of positioning patient.

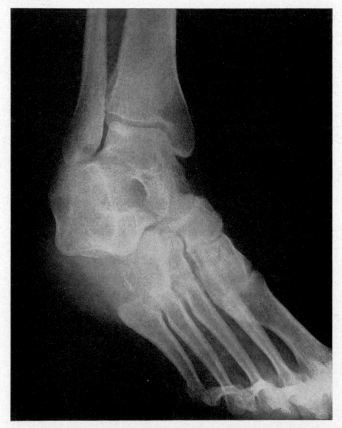

FIG. 5–46.   OBLIQUE VIEW OF ANKLE: **b,** Radiograph.

POINTS OF PRACTICAL INTEREST WITH REFERENCE TO FIGURE 5–46:

1. As much as possible the leg is kept in the antero-posterior position while inverting the foot approximately 45 degrees. Immobilize with sandbags placed across the leg and against the plantar surface of the foot.
2. The central ray is directed to the middle of the talotibial joint.
3. This view permits an unobstructed projection of the lateral malleolus and of the space between the talus and malleolus where so frequently injury may be manifest.

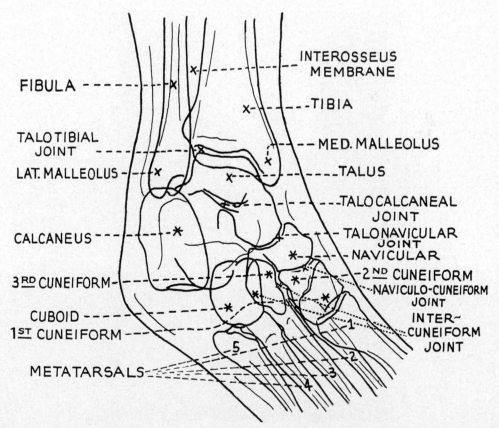

FIBULA

INTEROSSEUS MEMBRANE

TIBIA

TALOTIBIAL JOINT

MED. MALLEOLUS

LAT. MALLEOLUS

TALUS

TALOCALCANEAL JOINT

CALCANEUS

TALONAVICULAR JOINT

NAVICULAR

3RD CUNEIFORM

2ND CUNEIFORM

NAVICULO-CUNEIFORM JOINT

CUBOID

INTER-CUNEIFORM JOINT

1ST CUNEIFORM

METATARSALS

FIG. 5–46. OBLIQUE VIEW OF ANKLE: c, Labeled tracing of b.

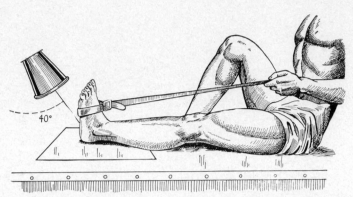

FIG. 5–47.   SPECIAL TANGENTIAL VIEW OF CALCANEUS: **a,** Method of positioning patient.

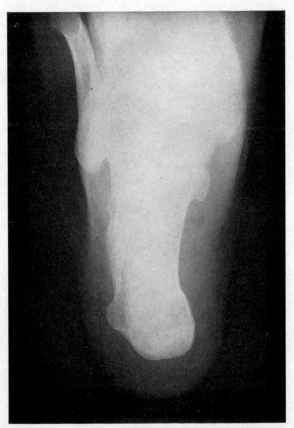

FIG. 5–47.   SPECIAL TANGENTIAL VIEW OF CALCANEUS: **b,** Radiograph.

POINTS OF PRACTICAL INTEREST WITH REFERENCE TO FIGURE 5–47:

1. The ankle is placed over the film so that the talotibial joint falls over the central portion of the film.
2. The plantar surface of the foot should be as near to right angles with the table top and film as possible in acute flexion.
3. The central ray should be centered to the midpoint of the film. It will usually enter the plantar surface at the level of the bases of the fifth metatarsals and emerge in the region of the upper tarsus.
4. Ordinarily all portions of the calcaneus are included between the tuberosity and the susten-taculum tali.
5. An alternate view may be used by placing the patient prone, film perpendicular to the table top in contact with the sole of the foot, directing the central ray through the heel with 45 degree caudad angulation.

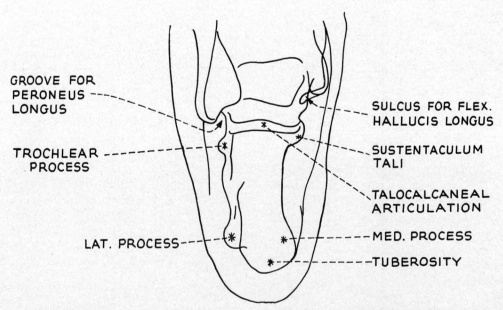

FIG. 5–47. SPECIAL TANGENTIAL VIEW OF CALCANEUS: c, Labeled tracing of b.

THE METATARSALS

Correlated Gross Anatomy. There are five metatarsal bones articulating with the tarsus behind, and the phalanges in front. They are slightly convex on their dorsal, and concave on their ventral aspects. The bases are wedge-shaped, and the heads semicircular. On each side of the head, there is a depression surmounted by a tubercle. The inferior surfaces of the heads are grooved to allow passage of the flexor tendons.

The first metatarsal is the shortest and thickest of the series, while the second metatarsal is the longest.

The fifth metatarsal articulates with the cuboid by means of a long triangular facet, which may on occasion be separate from the rest of the base as an ununited extra ossicle. Also in younger individuals where this basilar epiphysis has not united with the shaft of the fifth metatarsal, differentiation from fracture may be difficult. A fracture line in this location is usually transverse, but the epiphyseal line is oblique.

There is a normal slight medial angulation of the first metatarsophalangeal joint, which may on occasion become excessive, in which case the abnormality of hallux valgus results. There is a bursa which adjoins the head of the first metatarsal which is prone to become inflamed in this condition.

The Phalanges of the Foot. Except for the great toe, there are three phalanges for each digit, which tend to be considerably smaller than the phalanges of the hand. The great toe, like the thumb, has two phalanges which tend to be moderately stout bones.

Since the toes tend to have a plantar curvature and concavity, the phalanges may be foreshortened and partially projected over one another in the radiographs. If one wishes to obtain accurate detail regarding the phalanges of the third, fourth and fifth toes particularly, it is necessary to straighten the toes manually to obtain an undistorted, full-length view.

Although the phalanges of the foot are very small replicas of the phalanges of the hand, the structure of the two bears close resemblance.

Sesamoid Bones of the Foot (Fig. 5–48). A pair of sesamoid bones which begin to ossify about the fifth year is constant under the metatarsophalangeal joint of the great toe in the tendons of the flexor hallucis brevis. Occasionally there are three sesamoid bones in this location, or one of them may be bivalved and appear fractured (bipartite sesamoids). Additional sesamoids occur over the interphalangeal joint of the great toe, the metatarsophalangeal joints of the second and fifth toes, and less frequently, of the third and fourth.

The sesamoid and supernumerary bones of the foot are actually very numerous and the most common of these are illustrated in Figure 5–48.

The Interrelationship of the Bones of the Foot. The foot contains two arches, the longitudinal, and the transverse, which serve to increase the elasticity of the foot, and provide a hollow for the protection of the plantar soft tissues. The longitudinal arch extends between the calcaneus and the heads of the metatarsals, while the transverse arch is situated under the metatarsals, and is supported medially and laterally by the first and the fifth metatarsals respectively. Weight-bearing films, as described later, are necessary to demonstrate these arches.

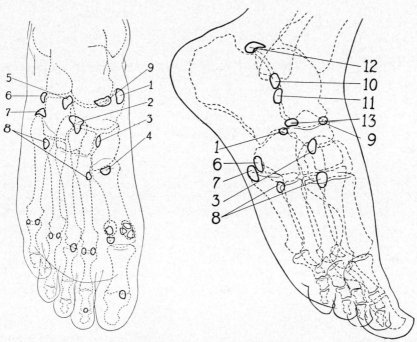

FIG. 5–48. Schematic diagram to show sesamoid bones and supernumerary bones of the foot. 1, Os tibiale externum; 2, processus uncinatus; 3, intercuneiforme; 4, pars peronea metatarsalia I; 5, cuboides secundarium; 6, os peroneum; 7, os vesalianum; 8, intermetatarseum; 9, accessory navicular; 10, talus accessorius; 11, os sustentaculum; 12, os trigonum; 13, calcaneus secundarius. (From McNeill, *Roentgen Technique*, Charles C Thomas, Publisher.)

The most common of these are: 1, 6, 7, 9 and 12.

RADIOGRAPHIC METHODS OF EXAMINATION OF THE TARSUS AND FOOT

1. **Antero-posterior View of the Foot** (Fig. 5–49).
2. **Lateral View of the Foot** (Fig. 5–50).
3. **Oblique View of the Foot** (Fig. 5–51). These projections are designed to show the tarsus as well as the metatarsals and phalanges of the foot. The exposure factors will vary slightly, depending upon whether it is desired to show the phalanges or the tarsus to best advantage. The accompanying diagrams show the positions in which these views are obtained. The lateral view is frequently obtained in the standing position, particularly if one is interested in demonstrating the integrity of the longitudinal arch. Occasionally one may obtain coned-down films of the great toe, since it is so frequently the area of major interest. The oblique view of the foot is of more value than the lateral, since the configuration of the metatarsal bones and phalanges is obscured in the latter, owing to the fact that they are projected over one another.

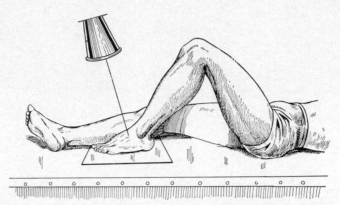

Fig. 5–49. ANTERO-POSTERIOR VIEW OF FOOT: **a,** Method of positioning patient.

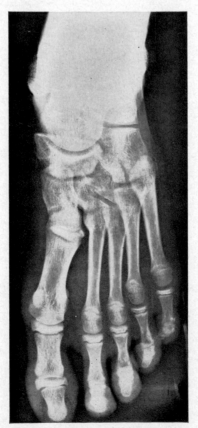

Fig. 5–49. ANTERO-POSTERIOR VIEW OF FOOT: **b,** Radiograph.

Points of Practical Interest with Reference to Figure 5–49:

1. It will be noted that for visualization of the entire tarsus, both this view and the antero-posterior view of the ankle (Fig. 5–44) are necessary. The talus is not shown to good advantage in this projection, whereas the more distal tarsal bones are not presented clearly on the antero-posterior view of the ankle.
2. This view may also be required for special problems with the patient standing and bearing his weight.

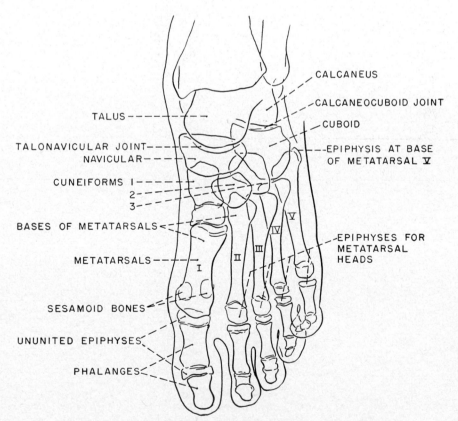

Fig. 5–49. ANTERO-POSTERIOR VIEW OF FOOT: c, Labeled tracing of b.

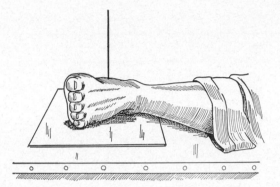

FIG. 5–50. LATERAL VIEW OF FOOT: **a,** Method of positioning patient.

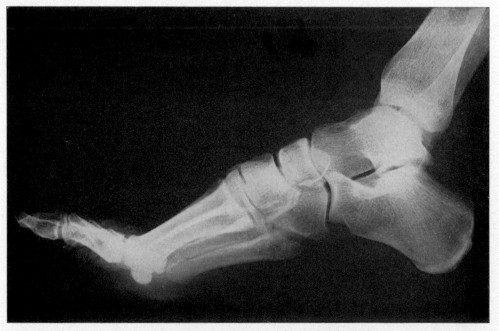

FIG. 5–50. LATERAL VIEW OF FOOT: **b,** Radiograph.

POINTS OF PRACTICAL INTEREST WITH REFERENCE TO FIGURE 5–50:

1. The knee may be elevated slightly on a sandbag so that the sagittal plane of the foot is perfectly parallel with the table top and film. The center of the tarsus is placed over the center of the film.
2. The ankle is immobilized by means of a sandbag.
3. The recumbent position is utilized to demonstrate the bony structure particularly. If one is desirous of showing the longitudinal arch under weight-bearing conditions an erect film is obtained with the patient standing, but in rather similar fashion.
4. If it is desired to obtain a coned-down lateral view of the body of the calcaneus, the foot is positioned similarly, but the central ray passes through the central portion of the calcaneus rather than through the center of the tarsus. The latter view of the calcaneus is particularly valuable for demonstration of Boehler's critical angle (see text).

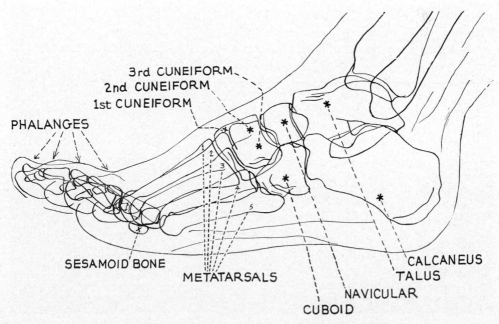

FIG. 5–50. LATERAL VIEW OF FOOT: **c**, Labeled tracing of **b**.

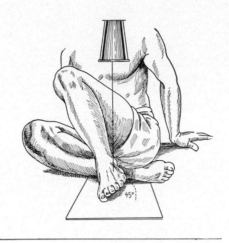

FIG. 5–51. OBLIQUE VIEW OF FOOT: **a,** Method of positioning patient.

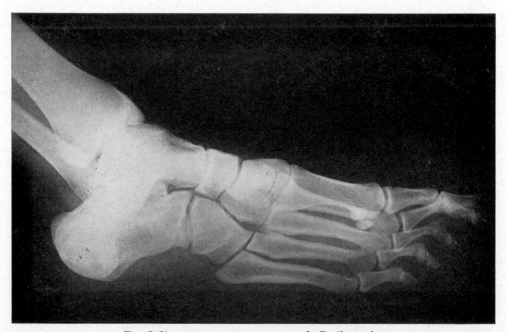

FIG. 5–51. OBLIQUE VIEW OF FOOT: **b,** Radiograph.

POINTS OF PRACTICAL INTEREST WITH REFERENCE TO FIGURE 5–51:

1. This view is particularly valuable (*a*) to demonstrate the intertarsal joints; (*b*) to outline the various tarsal bones more clearly; (*c*) to demonstrate the joint between the tarsus and the fourth and fifth metatarsals as well as the structural detail of the base of the fifth metatarsal.
2. This oblique projection is employed where structural detail of the bones of the foot is of paramount interest. It is ordinarily employed along with the antero-posterior projection of the foot. When, however, we desire to localize a foreign body accurately, it is the true lateral projection of the foot which is employed instead of this oblique projection.

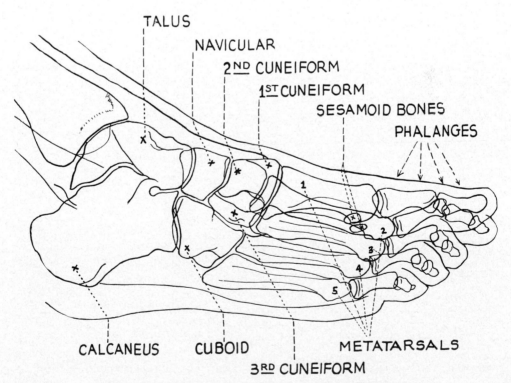

FIG. 5–51. OBLIQUE VIEW OF FOOT: **c,** Labeled tracing of **b.**

CHANGES WITH GROWTH AND DEVELOPMENT (Figs. 5–52 to 5–56)

At birth the larger part of the bony pelvis is ossified, including a part of the acetabulum, but the upper part of the ilium, the greater part of the acetabulum, the lower end of the ischium, the medial part of the pubis and the conjoined rami are still cartilaginous.

By the tenth year, most of the cartilage is ossified in the innominate bone, and the acetabular junction of the three bones appears as a triradiate strip. The conjoined rami are completely fused together and ossified. Secondary centers of ossification appear in the triradiate strip at about 12 years of age, and in the other parts of the innominate bone *at puberty.* The acetabular epiphyses usually unite about 17 years of age, but the others do not fuse until the early twenties.

At birth, in both sexes, the pelvis is relatively small, but as the lower limbs grow the pelvis keeps pace with its growth. The pelvic organs gradually descend into the pelvis minor by the sixth year. The growth is similar in both boys and girls until puberty, when the growth is modified according to the sex of the individual.

There is also a change in the lumbosacral angle, and the sacrum tends to sink in between the two innominate bones. The acetabula become deeper and thus tend to stabilize the hip joints.

The pelvis of a woman differs from that of a man, preparatory to the child-bearing function in the woman, unless there is an abnormal aberration in the female pelvis. The female pelvis minor is larger in all diameters, and the cavity tends to be less funnel-shaped, and is shorter. The female pubic arch is wide and the angle blunt. The midpelvic measurements approach a sphere, and the pelvic inlet in the so-called gynecoid pelvis is circular. Any abnormalities in this contour become of considerable importance during parturition.

The main body of the femur is ossified at birth (Figs. 5–53, 5–54), and usually the epiphysis for the distal end is also just beginning to ossify. This is the most reliable evidence of the fetus being full-term. Ossification extends into the neck after birth. The epiphysis of the head of the femur begins to ossify between 6 months and 1 year of age. The epiphysis for the greater trochanter appears between 4 and 5 years of age, and that of the lesser trochanter between 9 and 11 years. All of these secondary epiphyses fuse between 16 and 17 years in the female, and around 18 years in the male.

The patella is cartilaginous at birth, and ossification usually begins about the third year, and is completed about puberty. During this period, it is usually quite irregular in outline.

At birth only the ends of the tibia are still cartilaginous (Figs. 5–54, 5–55), and occasionally the proximal epiphysis has begun to calcify. The epiphyseal line extends downward in front to include the tibial tubercle. The ossification in this tongue of cartilage begins about 10 years of age, and this is the last part of the epiphysis to unite with the shaft. The medial malleolus is largely cartilaginous until the eighth year, when it begins to ossify rapidly, but the distal epiphysis usually begins to ossify by 1 year of age. These secondary epiphyses usually fuse in the female by 16 or 17 years of age and in the male by 18 or 19.

The proximal and distal epiphyses of the fibula (Fig. 5–55) are still cartilaginous at birth. The distal epiphysis begins to ossify first at about 1 or 2 years of age, and the proximal epiphysis by 3 or 4 years, somewhat earlier in the female than the male. They fuse by 16 in the female and 18 in the male.

The fibula is thicker in the child than in the adult when compared with the comparable tibia, and once it begins to ossify it grows distally more rapidly than does the medial malleolus, which ultimately accounts for the fact that it is slightly more distal then the medial malleolus.

Ossification begins at birth in the following tarsal bones (Fig. 5–56): the calcaneus, the talus, and occasionally the cuboid. Thereafter, the third cuneiform begins to ossify by the first year, the navicular by the third year, and rapidly thereafter the second cuneiform and first cuneiform (third and fourth years).

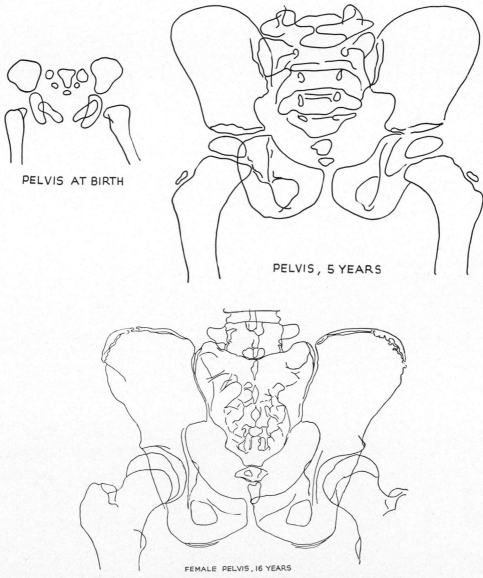

PELVIS AT BIRTH

PELVIS, 5 YEARS

FEMALE PELVIS, 16 YEARS

FIG. 5–52. Change in growth and development as seen in pelvis.

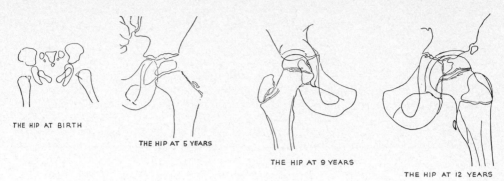

THE HIP AT BIRTH

THE HIP AT 5 YEARS

THE HIP AT 9 YEARS

THE HIP AT 12 YEARS

Fig. 5–53.   Change in growth and development as seen in hip.

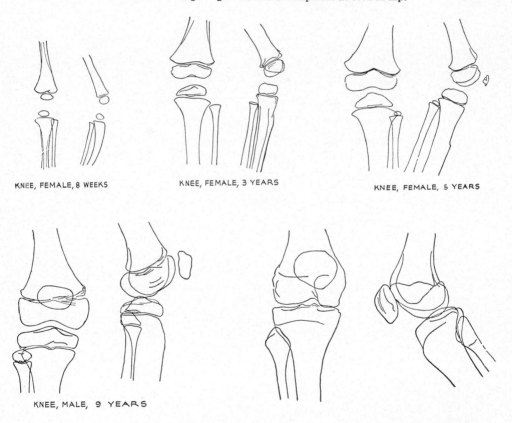

KNEE, FEMALE, 8 WEEKS

KNEE, FEMALE, 3 YEARS

KNEE, FEMALE, 5 YEARS

KNEE, MALE, 9 YEARS

KNEE, FEMALE, 17 YEARS

Fig. 5–54.   Change in growth and development as seen in knee.

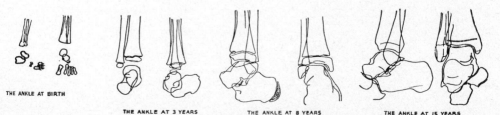

THE ANKLE AT BIRTH

THE ANKLE AT 3 YEARS

THE ANKLE AT 8 YEARS

THE ANKLE AT 15 YEARS

Fig. 5–55.   Change in growth and development as seen in ankle.

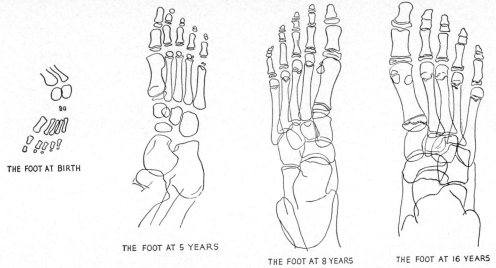

THE FOOT AT BIRTH

THE FOOT AT 5 YEARS

THE FOOT AT 8 YEARS

THE FOOT AT 16 YEARS

FIG. 5–56. Change in growth and development as seen in foot.

The centers for the navicular may be multiple but rapidly fuse into one. The calcaneus is the only tarsal bone with a secondary center of ossification. That part of this bone which ultimately forms the medial and lateral tubercles is ossified at 8 years in girls and 10 years in boys and unites at 15 years and 18 years respectively. Otherwise, ossification of all the tarsal bones is complete by puberty or shortly thereafter. The posterior tubercle of the talus may develop as a separate bone called the os trigonum.

The main shafts of the metatarsals are ossified at birth, and the epiphysis for the base of the first and heads of the others appear at 2 years in females and 3 years in males, and they fuse at 15 and 18 respectively.

The base of each of the phalanges ossifies from separate centers of ossification which appear at 2 years in females and 3 years in males, and fuse at 15 and 18 years respectively (see Figs. 3–7, 3–8, 3–9, 3–10, 3–11, and Tables 3–1 and 3–2).

REFERENCES

1. Andren, L., and von Rosen, S.: The Diagnosis of Dislocation of the Hip in Newborns and the Primary Results of Immediate Treatment. Acta radiol., 49: 89–95, 1957.
2. Billing, L.: Roentgen Examination of Proximal Femur End in Children and Adolescents. Acta radiol., Supplement 110, pp. 1–80, 1954.
3. Boehler, L: Diagnosis, Pathology and Treatment of Fractures of the Os Calcis. J. Bone & Joint Surg., 13: 75–89, 1931.
4. Budin, E., and Chandler, E.: Measurement of Femoral Neck Anteversion by a Direct Method. Radiology, 69: 209–213, 1951.
5. Caffey, J., Ames, R., Silverman, W., Ryder, C. T., and Hough, G.: Congenital Dislocation of the Hip. Pediatrics, 17: 632–641, 1956.
6. Klein, A., Joplin, R. J., Reidy, J. A., and Haneline, J.: Roentgenologic Features of Slipped Capital Femoral Epiphysis. Am. J. Roentgenol., 66: 361–374, 1951.
7. Köhler, A., and Zimmer, E. A.: Borderlands of the Normal and Early Pathologic in Skeletal Roentgenology. English translation by J. T. Case. New York, Grune and Stratton, 1956, pp. 491–494.
8. Lewis, R. L.: A Roentgen Study of Soft Tissue Pathology in and about the Knee Joints. Am. J. Roentgenol., 65: 200–219, 1951.
9. van Brunt, E.: A Method of Measuring the Femoral Neck in Surgical Treatment of Fractures. Am. J. Roentgenol., 76: 1163–1165, 1956.

CHAPTER 6

The Skull

THE RADIOGRAPHIC ANATOMY of the skull can be conveniently divided into three parts:

Part   I: General survey of the skull (Chap. 6)
Part II: Detailed consideration of certain areas of the skull of importance radiographically (Chap. 7)
Part III: The radiographic study of the brain by pneumoencephalography, ventriculography, and angiography (Chap. 8)

GENERAL SURVEY OF THE SKULL

There are twenty-two bones in the skull, including the mandible, which are firmly bound together at immovable joints called sutures or primary cartilaginous joints (with the exception of the temporomandibular joints).

These are subdivided into the bones of the calvarium (or brain case), and the bones of the face and mandible (Fig. 6–1, **a** and **b**).

The calvarium or cranium is composed of eight bones: the paired parietal and temporal bones, and the frontal, occipital, sphenoid and ethmoid bones, which are single. The temporal bones contain the ossicles of the ear.

The cranial cavity lodges the brain, and is formed by the frontal, parietal, occipital, temporal, sphenoid and ethmoid bones. The roof of the cranial cavity is composed of the frontal, parietal, occipital, squamous portions of the temporal bones, and the greater wings of the sphenoid bone. These bones are largely flat bones composed of a dense outer layer of bone known as the outer table, a less dense middle zone known as the diploe, and another dense inner zone known as the inner table. In the white race, each of these layers averages approximately 2 mm. in thickness; in some individuals, and in the Negro race particularly, these layers are thicker and denser than is usual in the white races, and the diploe is more difficult to distinguish. The total thickness of the calvarium in Negroes is sometimes as much as 15 mm., and this is apparentlywithout any pathologic significance.

THE BONES OF THE CALVARIUM

The *frontal bone* anteriorly forms the forehead and the anterosuperior portion of the cranial vault, the roof of the orbits, and the greater part of the floor of the anterior cranial fossa. The frontal sinuses are air spaces contained within the frontal bones, and these will be described in detail later.

220

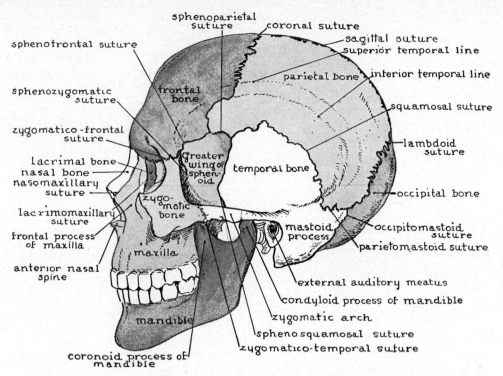

FIG. 6–1. a, Lateral view of the skull showing the bones of the calvarium, face and mandible. (From *The Head and Neck in Roentgen Diagnosis*, by Pendergrass, Schaeffer, and Hodes, Charles C Thomas, Publisher.)

The *parietal bones* form the greater portion of both sides of the skull. These meet superiorly in the midline to form the sagittal suture, articulate with the frontal bone anteriorly to form the *coronal suture*, posteriorly with the occipital to form the *lambdoid suture*, and inferiorly they adjoin the temporal bone at its squamous portion to form the *squamous suture*.

The *occipital bone* (Fig. 6–2) is situated at the posterior and lower portion of the skull. It forms the posterior portion of the roof of the brain, as well as the greater part of the floor of the posterior cranial fossa. It contains a large oval aperture, the foramen magnum, which permits communication between the cranial cavity and the vertebral column. The foramen magnum divides the bone into three sections: (*a*) the squamous portion which articulates with the parietal and temporal bones at the lambdoid suture; (*b*) the pars lateralis, lateral to the foramen magnum, which contains the condyles for articulation with the first cervical vertebra; and (*c*) the basilar portion anterior to the foramen for articulation with the basilar portion of the sphenoid bone at the basisphenoid suture. Unlike other sutures at the base of the skull, this basisphenoid suture is open at birth, and remains so for several years.

The *temporal bone* (Fig. 7–17) forms the side of the skull below the parietal bones, and the base of the skull in front of the occipital bone. This bone contains the internal ear, the middle ear, the bony part of the external ear, a small cavity adjoining the middle ear called the tympanic antrum, and numerous air cells throughout. The following major parts of the temporal bone are identified:

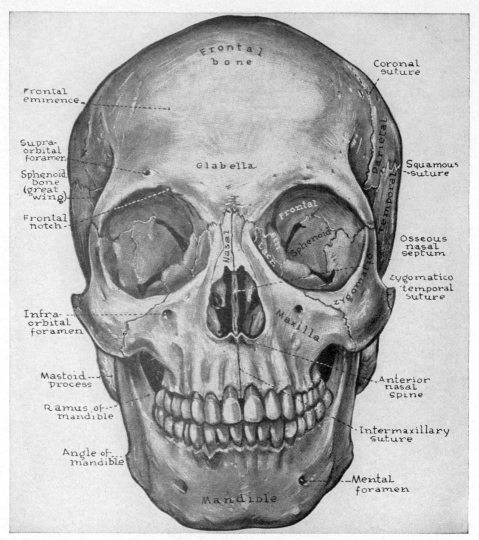

FIG. 6–1. **b,** Skull viewed from its frontal aspect. (From *The Head and Neck in Roentgen Diagnosis* by Pendergrass, Schaeffer and Hodes, Charles C Thomas, Publisher.)

squamous, mastoid, tympanic, petrous, the styloid process and temporomandibular fossa (Fig. 7–17). This bone has considerable clinical significance in view of its association with the auditory and vestibular mechanisms and must be studied exhaustively radiographically. A more detailed consideration will be given in Chapter 7.

The *sphenoid bone* lies in the floor of the cranial cavity posterior to the orbits. It encloses air spaces beneath the sella turcica called the sphenoid sinuses. It is a bone shaped somewhat like a bird, having a body, greater and lesser wings (both of which form portions of the superior and lateral walls respectively of the orbit), and paired downward projections called the pterygoid process or plates.

The *ethmoid bone* is situated between the orbits and below the frontal bone. This contains numerous small air cells called the ethmoid sinuses; the superior and middle nasal conchae project from its medial aspect and participate in the formation of the nasal turbinates.

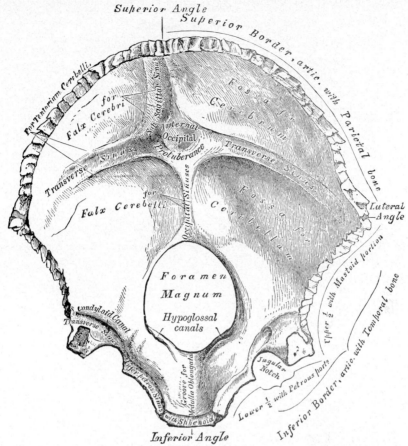

Fɪɢ. 6–2. The occipital bone, inner surface. (From Gray, *Anatomy of the Human Body,* Edited by C. M. Goss, Lea & Febiger, Publishers.)

THE FACIAL BONES

The skeleton of the face is composed of fourteen bones (including the mandible); the nasal bones, maxillae, lacrimals, zygomata, palatine and inferior nasal conchae are paired, and the vomer and the mandible are single.

The face also contains numerous cavities, namely, the orbits, the nasal cavities, the paranasal sinuses (contained within the maxillary, frontal, ethmoid and sphenoid bones), as well as the mouth.

The nose and nasal cavity and the paranasal sinuses are anatomic subdivisions that require special radiographic techniques for demonstration, and will be considered subsequently (Chap. 7).

The bones which contribute most significantly to the contour of the face are the maxillae, the zygomatic bones and the mandible.

The Maxillae. The two maxillae form the upper jaw. Each maxilla has a body and four processes. The body encloses a large pyramidal air space called the maxillary sinus. The processes extend upward to the frontal bone and medial wall of the orbit, laterally to the zygoma, downward to form the alveolus and upper dental arch, and medially to form the anterior larger part of the hard palate on its own side.

The maxilla articulates with the frontal bone at the maxillofrontal suture between the frontal process of the maxillary bone and the frontal bone; with the nasal bones at the nasomaxillary suture; with the lacrimal bone at the lacrimomaxillary suture; with the maxilla of the opposite side of the palate at the intermaxillary suture; with the zygoma at the maxillozygomatic suture; and with the ethmoidal bone between the orbital processes of the ethmoid and the maxillary bone at the maxillo-ethmoidal suture.

The Zygomatic Bone. The zygomatic bone forms the anterior part of the zygomatic arch and unites with the frontal and sphenoid bones above, and the zygomatic process of the temporal bone behind to form the zygomatic arch. It forms the so-called malar prominence of the face, and is particularly subject to injury around the orbit. It articulates with the maxilla below at the maxillo-zygomatic suture.

Radiographically, the maxillae and zygomatic bones must be demonstrated both from the frontal projection and the supero-inferior projection to determine accurately any displacement of a bony fragment that may be present. Because of the marked swelling over these areas which accompanies injuries, such displacement is not demonstrable by clinical means.

The zygomatic arches are thin segments of bone formed by the fusion of the zygomatic processes of the zygomatic and the temporal bones. Special views are usually required to demonstrate the arch in its entirety in the so-called axial projection. The remainder of the skull must be "under-penetrated" by the x-ray exposure to show the zygomatic arches clearly (Fig. 6–29).

The Lacrimal Bone. The lacrimal bone lies below the inner canthus of the eye in the medial wall of the orbit and helps form the groove in which the lacrimal sac lies. It is the smallest bone of the face and the most fragile. It is surrounded by the following sutures: the lacrimo-ethmoidal, the lacrimofrontal and the lacrimomaxillary.

The Inferior Nasal Concha. This bone helps form the inferior nasal turbinate and is best described with the nasal cavity.

The Vomer. The vomer forms the posterior and postero-inferior part of the nasal septum, and is best seen in the view of the base of the skull (Fig. 6–13).

The Palatine Bones. These bones are likewise best outlined in the view of the base of the skull. They form the posterior quarter or one-third of the corresponding part of the hard palate (Fig. 6–13) and contribute to the formation of the nasal cavity also.

The Mandible (Fig. 6–3). The mandible is the lower jaw bone and is composed of two bodies united in the midline at the symphysis, and two rami at either end of the body. Two processes project upward from each ramus—the coronoid anteriorly, the condyloid posteriorly—and the sigmoid notch lies between. The condyloid process is composed of an articular head and a neck. The mandibular foramen on the medial aspect of the ramus leads to the mandibular canal, the foramen transmitting the inferior alveolar vessels and nerve, and the canal their mylohyoid branches. The mental foramen is anterior on the lateral aspect of the body of the mandible and transmits the mental vessels and nerve.

The mylohyoid groove (which parallels the mandibular canal) and mylohyoid line on the mandible frequently impart a sclerotic appearance to the mandible which is normal. These markings, in contrast with the areas of diminished density produced by the mandibular and mental foramina, may lead to an erroneous impression of bone destruction for the student.

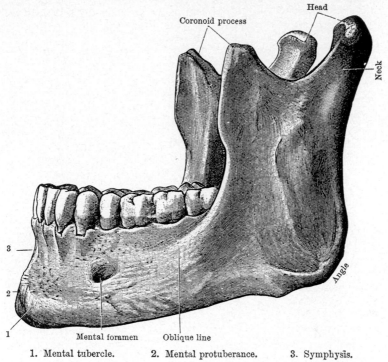

Head

Coronoid process

Neck

3

2

1

Mental foramen   Oblique line

Angle

1. Mental tubercle.   2. Mental protuberance.   3. Symphysis.

a

Coronoid
process

Head

Mandi-
bular
foramen

Mylo-
hyoid
groove

Lingula

Alveolar margin

2

Angle

1

Submaxillary fossa

Digastric fossa   Mylo-hyoid line

1. Mental spine divided   2. Above sublingual fossa.
   into genial tubercles.

b

FIG. 6–3. **a,** Mandible, seen from the left side. **b,** Medial surface of the right half of the mandible;
(From Cunningham's *Text-Book of Anatomy*, Edited by Arthur Robinson, published by Oxford
University Press.)

The Teeth[5] (Figs. 6–4, 6–5).   We have considered the teeth out of the scope of this text. Ordinarily, for accurate visualization of the teeth, special intraoral films are taken of each region. The integrity of the periodontal membrane is most important in this regard. Moreover, in the young individual one must learn to differentiate the normal dental anlage from an abnormality such as a periapical abscess and granuloma.

There are several types of intraoral dental films (Fig. 6–5), each with its own purpose. Small intraoral films are most accurate for visualization of the apex and periapical structures; occlusal films (approximately 2½ x 3½ inches) are larger and are placed between the teeth and are employed to obtain an infero-superior perspective of one alveolus or an associated abnormality of the jaw. Bite-wing films are used particularly for demonstration of dental crown abnormalities, and show the relationship of the upper and lower rows of teeth to one another.

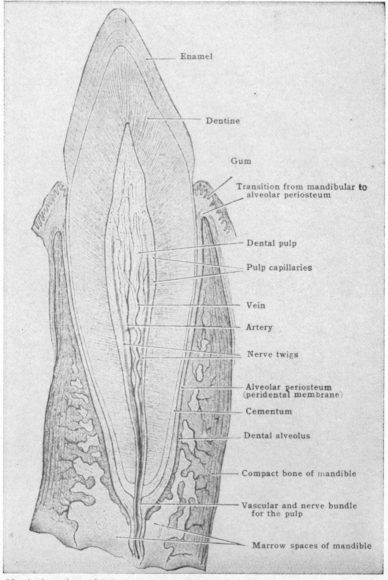

Enamel

Dentine

Gum

Transition from mandibular **to**
alveolar periosteum

Dental pulp

Pulp capillaries

Vein

Artery

Nerve twigs

Alveolar periosteum
(peridental membrane)

Cementum

Dental alveolus

Compact bone of mandible

Vascular and nerve bundle
for the pulp

Marrow spaces of mandible

FIG. 6–4.   Vertical section of inferior canine tooth in situ. (From Jackson, C. M. Morris' *Human Anatomy*, The Blakiston Co., Publishers.)

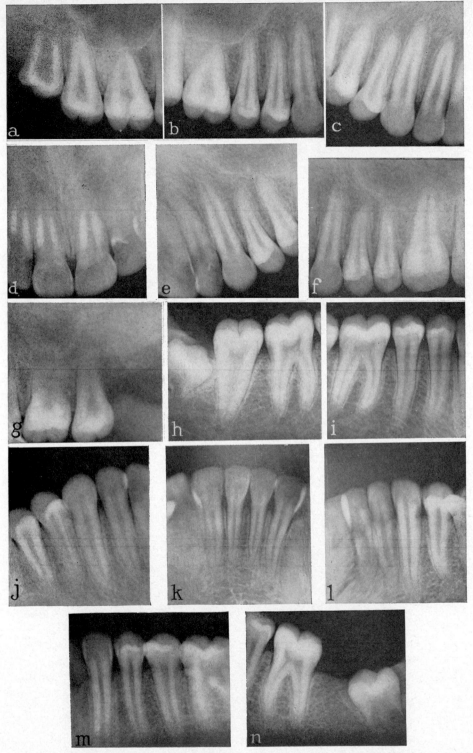

FIG. 6–5. Representative intraoral dental films: **a,** Right upper molar area; **b,** right upper bicuspid area; **c,** right upper cuspid area; **d,** upper incisor area; **e,** left upper cuspid area; **f,** left upper bicuspid area; **g,** left upper molar area; **h,** right lower molar area; **i,** right lower bicuspid area; **i,** right lower cuspid area; **k,** lower incisor area; **l,** left lower cuspid area; **m,** left lower bicuspid area; **n,** left lower molar area.

The Mandibular Joint (Fig. 6–6). The mandible articulates with the temporal bone at the temporomandibular fossa and is the only freely movable bone of the face. The range of motion is free in all directions. The condyles move forward to the articular tubercles when the mouth is opened. Subluxation must therefore be interpreted with caution.

There is a plate of fibrocartilage interposed between each articular margin of the mandible and temporal bone. This cartilage or disk is connected with the articular capsule throughout its circumference. Thus, there are two synovial sacs or spaces in the one joint, and they do not communicate unless the disk is perforated.

No examination of the temporomandibular joints is complete unless an effort is made to demonstrate the extent and character of movement of the condyloid process with relation to its articulating fossa when the mouth is opened. Occasionally we have found the view of the skull in Towne's position (Fig. 6–25) of particular value for demonstration of the articular tubercles and the necks of the condyloid processes.

Body section radiographs of the temporomandibular joint are also of considerable value (Fig. 6–33, **d**).

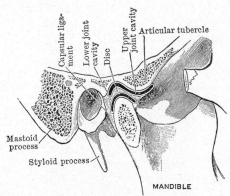

FIG. 6–6. Antero-posterior section through the temporomandibular joint. (From Cunningham's *Text-Book of Anatomy*, Edited by Arthur Robinson, published by Oxford University Press.)

LINES, IMPRESSIONS, CHANNELS AND SUTURES OF THE CRANIAL VAULT OF RADIOGRAPHIC SIGNIFICANCE

There are various lines and impressions on the cranial vault which are of great radiographic significance.

1. **Granular Pits or Arachnoidal (Pacchionian) Granulation Impressions** (Fig· 6–7). These are small irregular parasagittal impressions which lodge the arachnoidal granulations. They are usually found in the parasagittal region of the vault adjoining the superior sagittal sinus. Occasionally, however, they are found in a more lateral situation, and not infrequently give even the experienced observer considerable difficulty in distinguishing them from abnormal areas of bone absorption. They are occasionally also found in the occipital bone. Ordinarily, the impression involves only the inner bony table, and minute channels can be identified leading into them in stellate fashion.

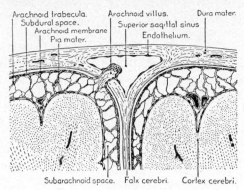

FIG. 6–7. Schematic diagram of a coronal section of the meninges and cerebral cortex. (Weed Am. J. Anat.; courtesy of Wistar Institute.)

2. **Arterial Grooves.** The arterial grooves (Fig. 6–8) are narrow branching grooves for the meningeal vessels—the middle meningeal being the largest. The main groove begins at the foramen spinosum, traverses the squamous temporal bone, and divides into an anterior and posterior branch which are clearly visible on the parietal bones. These meningeal vessels are so closely applied to the bone that they are likely to be torn when the skull over them is injured (especially the veins, which lie between the arteries and the skull and have thinner walls). The inner table here is very thin and brittle, and may crack even if the outer table remains intact.

The margins of these grooves usually have a slightly denser appearance than the surrounding bone, and the course of the arteries is relatively smooth and undulating, and never sharply angled as in a fracture. This characteristic appearance together with their usual location is their distinguishing feature.

3. **Venous Plexuses Within the Diploe.** The venous plexuses within the diploe (Fig. 6–9) are impressions within the diploe found in each of the frontal, parietal and occipital bones, giving the skull a mosaic appearance on the radiograph. In the parietal bones particularly, they have been referred to as the "parietal star" or "spider." At times these appear unusually accentuated. It is usually hazardous, however, to interpret any abnormality on the appearance of the venous diploe alone.

4. **Venous Sinuses.** The venous sinuses (Fig. 8–30) produce their impression on the inner table of the skull so that they appear as radiolucent channels bounded by curved bony ridges. The lateral sinus (or transverse sinus) is the largest of these, and has its origin near the internal occipital protuberance, passing forward around the occipital bone with a slight upward convexity to the pneumatic portion of the mastoid bone. Here it curves downward to become the sigmoid sinus.

The sphenoparietal sinus is another commonly prominent venous sinus. It begins in connection with the anterior parietal diploic vein, just posterior to the coronal suture, and then courses along the inferior surface of the lesser wing of the sphenoid to become a tributary of the cavernous sinus.

The point of junction of the lateral sinuses and the superior sagittal sinus is virtually the point of confluence of all the major dural sinuses, and hence is called the sinus confluens. It has a variable appearance, resembling a crossroad with or without a bony island contained within it (Fig. 6–10).

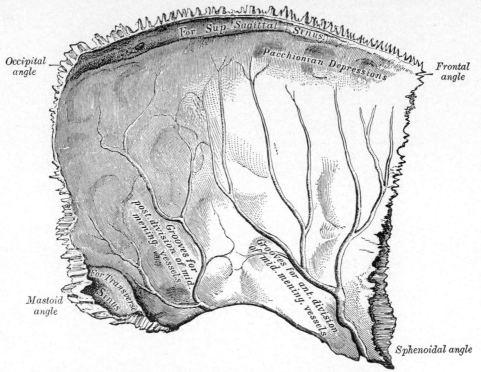

FIG. 6–8.   The left parietal bone, inner aspect showing vascular grooves. (From Gray, *Anatomy of the Human Body*, Edited by C. M. Goss, Lea & Febiger, Publishers.)

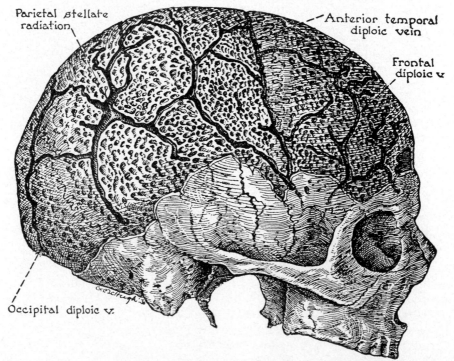

FIG. 6–9.   Diploic venous plexuses of the calvarium. (From Bailey, *Intracranial Tumors*, Charles C Thomas, Publisher.)

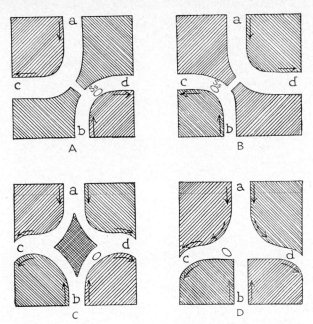

FIG. 6-10. Schematic illustration of the sinus confluens, showing variations in its appearance. (From *The Head and Neck in Roentgen Diagnosis*, by Pendergrass, Schaeffer and Hodes, Charles C Thomas, Publisher.)

5. **Emissary Veins.** Some of the emissary veins achieve considerable size and serve to connect the venous blood channels outside the calvarium with those inside. One of the most significant of these is the mastoid emissary vein which is situated near the sigmoid sinus and can be identified posterior to the pneumatized portion of the mastoid.

Also, and quite distinct from the thinning-out of the parietal bones to be described, the parietal bone may contain enlarged *parietal foramina* (Fig. 6-15). These are ordinarily extremely small (not greater than 1 mm.), and transmit an emissary vein. Abnormally large foramina occasionally occur, and this tendency to enlarged parietal foramina is apparently inherited. These are ordinarily situated close to the sagittal suture, about 1 to 1½ inches above the lambdoid suture just medial to the parietal tuberosity.

6. **The Sutures.** A number of important sutures marks the superior portion of the skull: The *sagittal suture* marks the junction of the two parietal bones superiorly, and extends from the bregma, which is its junction with the coronal suture, to the lambda, which is its junction with the lambdoid suture. The *coronal suture* is situated between the parietal bones posteriorly and the frontal bone anteriorly. It ends by joining the sphenoid bone laterally, and this point of union is known as the *pterion* on either side. The *lambdoidal suture* is situated between the parietal bone anteriorly and the interparietal portion of the occipital bone posteriorly. Its point of junction with the squamosal suture is known as the *asterion*. When the interparietal portion of the occipital bone exists as an independent element (the *inca* bone), a *transverse occipital suture* is formed between it and the occipital bone proper.

The two halves of the frontal bone normally fuse by the fifth or sixth year of childhood, and this line of fusion disappears; however, in about 10 per cent of cases this suture persists, and is called the *metopic suture* (Fig. 6–11), and extends from the frontonasal suture to the coronal suture. Occasionally this suture may persist incompletely, and lead to an erroneous interpretation of skull fracture.

On the lateral aspect of the skull, the *sphenofrontal, sphenoparietal* and *squamosal sutures* form a continuous irregular line outlining the upper outer margin of the greater wing of the sphenoid and the squamous temporal bone. These extend from the posterior margin of the frontal bone to the occipital bone. There are several important variations in the interrelationship of the frontal, temporal, sphenoid and parietal bones. Occasionally, the sphenoparietal suture is lacking, and the coronal suture is directly continuous with the suture between the greater wing of the sphenoid and with the squamous temporal bone. On other occasions, there is an extra bone at this crossing, known as the *epipteric* bone (example of sutural or wormian bone). Other variations are shown in Figure 6–12. The *sphenozygomatic suture* is situated between the zygomatic bone and the greater wing of the sphenoid. The *zygomaticofrontal suture* is situated between the frontal process of the zygoma and the inferolateral portion of the frontal bone.

Extending horizontally from the squamosal suture to the lambdoid suture is a small irregular suture which remains rather prominent throughout life, known as the *parietomastoid suture*. It is situated between the mastoid process of the

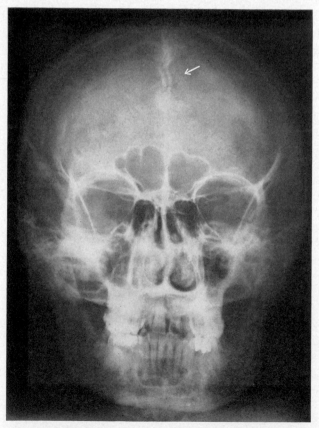

FIG. 6–11.   Film to demonstrate metopic suture.

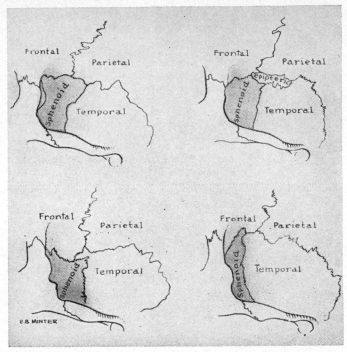

FIG. 6–12. Variations in the interrelationship of the frontal, temporal, sphenoid and parietal bones. (From *The Head and Neck in Roentgen Diagnosis*, by Pendergrass, Schaeffer and Hodes, Charles C Thomas, Publisher.)

temporal bones and the parietal bone. On the posterior aspect of the mastoid process and between the latter and the occipital bone is the *occipitomastoid* suture. The *zygomaticotemporal suture* is the suture which joins the zygomatic processes of the zygomatic and temporal bones. This is usually situated at the junction of the anterior and middle thirds of the zygomatic arch.

The superior and inferior temporal lines are muscular and fascial attachment ridges situated 2 to 3 cm. above the squamosal sutures in the parietal bones, and should not be confused with sutures.

On the basilar aspect (Fig. 6–13), the occipital bone articulates with the mastoid process at the occipitomastoid suture, and with the petrous temporal bone at the *occipitopetrosal suture*. The basilar portion of the occipital bone articulates with the body of the sphenoid at the *basisphenoid suture*. The spheno-squamosal suture can be identified once again between the sphenoid and the squamous temporal bone medial to the mandibular fossa for articulation with the mandible; the *sphenopetrosal suture* is situated anteriorly between the sphenoid and the petrous temporal bone. The *median palatine suture* is situated between the two palatine processes of the maxillae, and the *transverse palatine suture* between the palatine processes of the maxilla and the palatine bone. The vomer articulates with six bones: two of the cranium—the sphenoid and the ethmoid; and four of the face—the two maxillae and the two palatine bones. It also joins with the septal cartilage of the nose.

Sutural (or wormian) bones are occasionally found to lie within a suture, particularly at its junction with another suture. This is particularly true of the lambdoid suture, and in the region of the pterion.

The sutures ordinarily present a very irregular appearance and follow the rather definite anatomic pattern described above and illustrated. Under the age of 6, the sutures are considerably wider than they are in the adult, beginning with the relatively widespread appearance in the newborn (Fig. 6–22). The posterior fontanel is frequently closed at birth, or at least by the age of 6 months to 1 year. The anterior fontanel rarely ever closes before 1 year of age, and sometimes not before 2 or 3. The appearance of the normal degree of separation at the various age levels must be well recognized so that diastasis of a suture can be diagnosed in the child and the adult following trauma.

7. **The Digitate or Convolutional Markings** (Fig. 6–14). These are irregular areas of increased and decreased density throughout the skull due to thinning of the inner table as the result of pressure produced by the convolutions or gyri of the brain. In individuals under approximately 16 years of age, these may be moderately marked, and readily detectable normally. Beyond this age, or when unduly accentuated in the younger age groups, these may indicate increased intracranial pressure, and are of pathologic significance.

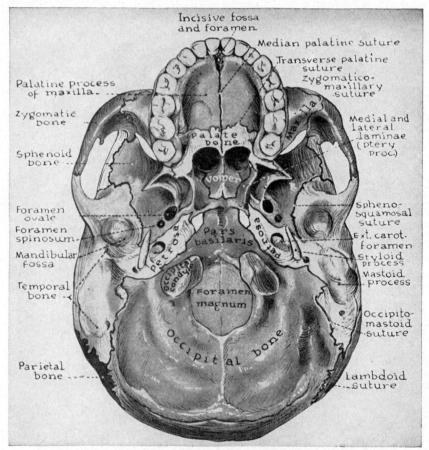

FIG. 6–13. The skull viewed from below. (From *The Head and Neck in Roentgen Diagnosis*, by Pendergrass, Schaeffer and Hodes, Charles C Thomas, Publisher.)

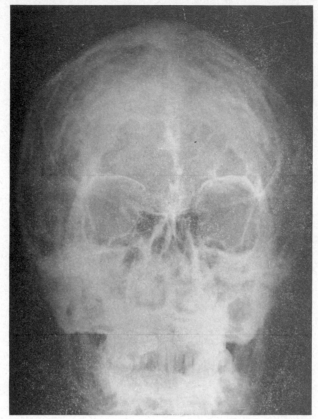

FIG. 6–14.   Radiograph to show accentuated convolutional markings in a normal skull (child)

8. **Thinning of the Bones of the Calvarium.**   The parietal bone superiorly and laterally may on occasion be unusually thin owing to a lack of development of the diploe. There may be a bony dehiscence, the inner table being less affected than the outer. This thinning is usually bilateral, but occasionally is unilateral. This is usually a normal variant but on occasion does have pathoogic significance.[7]

9. **Thickened Areas of the Calvarium.**   The internal and external occipital protuberances ordinarily project inward and outward respectively from the occipital bone, forming thickened areas of bone in these locations. Occasionally, the external protuberance is a considerable process of bone.

There is not infrequently thickened bone immediately above the frontal sinuses, and in the vicinity of the junction of sutures.

There is occasionally also a small exostosis in the external acoustic meatus which may be a minute nodule, or large enough to fill the entire meatus. These are usually bilateral, and when unilateral tend to be more frequent on the left side.

10. **Depressions in the Contour of the Calvarium.**   There may be normal depressions in the contour of the calvarium in the region of the bregma or lambda. When greatly accentuated these may be an indication of developmental deficiency or abnormality, but otherwise may be considered a normal variant.

A CORRELATED ANATOMIC AND RADIOGRAPHIC SURVEY OF THE EXTERNAL ASPECT OF THE BASE OF THE SKULL

Viewed from the external aspect, the base of the skull (Fig. 6–13) is divisible into three portions.

1. The anterior portion consists principally of the palatine processes of the maxillary bone, palatine bone, and the upper alveolus bearing the teeth.

2. The middle portion lies between the posterior edge of the hard palate and the anterior margin of the foramen magnum. This contains the basilar portion of the occipital bone, the petrous portions of the temporal bone, the body and greater wings and laminae of the sphenoids, and the vomer. The foramen lacerum is an irregular aperture which is situated at the junction of the petrous apex with the basilar occipital bone and the sphenoid. Within the petrous ridge posterolateral to the foramen lacerum is the entrance opening for the carotid canal, and still more laterally is the stylomastoid foramen from which the facial nerve emerges from the skull. The jugular foramen is formed between the apex of the petrous temporal bones and the occipital and is slightly larger on the right than the left. Within the sphenoid bone, just anterior to the petrous portion of the temporal bone, are three major orifices (from before backward): the foramen rotundum (concealed), the foramen ovale and the foramen spinosum. The foramen rotundum is somewhat hidden under the pterygoid processes of the sphenoid. The pterygoid processes together with the vomer and the palatine bone form the choanae, or posterior nares, which open into the nasal cavity. Lateral to the choanae are the pterygoid fossae and the internal auditory or eustachian tubes which connect with the middle ear. The foramen rotundum transmits the maxillary nerve; the foramen ovale, the mandibular nerve; and the foramen spinosum, the middle meningeal vessels.

3. The third portion is the posterior portion which contains the foramen magnum. On either side of this area are the occipital condyles, and immediately anterolateral to these condyles are the jugular and hypoglossal foramina. The jugular foramen transmits the internal jugular vein, the ninth, tenth and eleventh cranial nerves, and the lateral and inferior petrosal dural venous sinuses. The hypoglossal foramen transmits the hypoglossal nerve (twelfth cranial nerve),

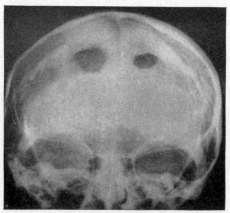

FIG. 6–15. Roentgenograph of a patient with enlarged parietal foramina. (*The Head and Neck in X-Ray Diagnosis*, by Pendergrass, Schaeffer and Hodes. Charles C Thomas, Publisher.)

and a small artery. The lateral margin of this portion is formed by the mastoid process of the temporal bone on either side. A line drawn from one external acoustic meatus to the other would pass through the following parts: the stylomastoid foramen, the root of the styloid process, the jugular foramen, the hypoglossal canal, the anterior margin of the occipital condyle, and the anterior margin of the foramen magnum, in that order lateromedially.

In the lateral roentgenogram (Fig. 6–26), the base of the skull appears as a steplike, irregular structure which descends from the frontal sinuses to the upper margin of the cervical spine. Each succeeding step represents a separate subdivision of the inside of the cranium which will be described in greater detail when considering the internal aspect of the cranial cavity.

A CORRELATED ANATOMIC AND RADIOGRAPHIC CONSIDERATION OF THE INTERNAL ASPECT OF THE CRANIAL CAVITY

The floor of the cranial cavity is divided into three fossae (Fig. 6–16) called the anterior, middle and posterior respectively.

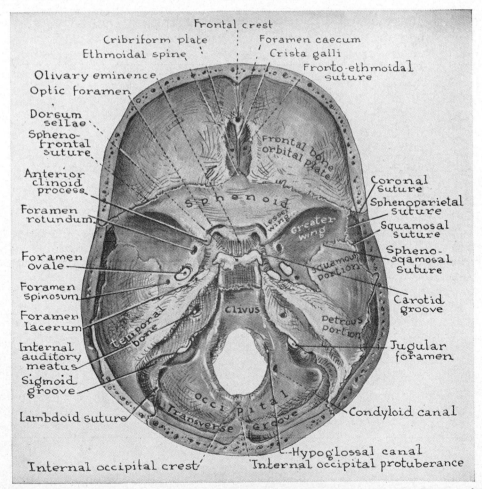

FIG. 6–16.   Internal aspect of the base of the skull. (*The Head and Neck in Roentgen Diagnosis,* by Pendergrass, Schaeffer and Hodes, Charles C Thomas, Publisher.)

The *anterior cranial fossa* extends between the frontal bone and the sharp posterior margins of the lesser wings of the sphenoid. It is located over the nasal cavity and the orbits, and houses the frontal lobes of the brain. It is formed by the orbital plate of the frontal bone, the cribriform plate of the ethmoid, the lesser wings of the sphenoid, and the ventral part of the body of the sphenoid. The tuberculum sellae and the anterior clinoid processes of the sella turcica form part of the posterior boundary of the fossa centrally. The crista galli rises from the cribriform plate, which ordinarily is depressed. The frontal and ethmoidal air sinuses encroach to a variable extent on the anterior cranial fossa in front and below.

The posterior margin of the lesser wings of the sphenoid marks the locations of the anterior part of the lateral cerebral fissure (sylvian fissure), and hence helps to demarcate the position of the frontal from the temporal lobes of the brain (see Fig. 8–4, *b*).

In the lateral view of the skull, the floor of this fossa has a very irregular appearance related to the impressions formed by the convolutions of the brain. A mind's eye impression of this irregularity must be retained by the student if he is to interpret fractures or abnormalities in bony structure such as occur with some brain tumors in this area.

The *middle cranial fossa* is at a slightly lower level than the anterior, and resembles a bird with outstretched wings. The midportion, formed by the body of the sphenoid, is elevated above the lateral parts and contains the sella turcica, the optic foramina united by the chiasmatic groove, and the carotid grooves. The front elevation of the sella turcica is composed of the tuberculum sellae and the anterior clinoid processes, whereas the back of the sella is composed of the dorsum sellae and the posterior clinoid processes. The curved hollow between the two is called the hypophyseal fossa since it houses the pituitary body of the brain. The carotid groove begins at the medial side of the irregular foramen lacerum and ends medial to the anterior clinoid processes. The cavernous venous sinus lies at the side of the carotid groove and the internal carotid artery is virtually embedded in this sinus.

The lateral portions of the middle cranial fossa are formed by the temporal bone in great part, but also by the great wing of the sphenoid and a small portion of the parietal bones. This houses the temporal lobes of the brain. The posterior margin of the fossa is grooved and contains the superior petrosal venous sinus.

The more important foramina of the middle cranial fossa are: (1) the optic foramen for the optic nerve and ophthalmic artery; (2) the superior orbital fissure, for passage of the ophthalmic nerve, the third, fourth and sixth cranial nerves, several small arteries and sympathetic nerves; (3) the foramen rotundum, which transmits the maxillary nerve; (4) the foramen ovale, which transmits the mandibular nerve, the lesser superficial petrosal nerve, and the accessory meningeal artery; (5) the foramen spinosum, which transmits the middle meningeal artery, and the recurrent branch of the mandibular nerve; and (6) the foramen lacerum, which is crossed by the internal carotid artery and its sympathetic plexus as it emerges from the carotid canal.

In the lateral radiograph of the skull, the superposition of the mastoid and petrous portions of the temporal bone between the middle and posterior cranial fossae may cause some confusion. Various special views are employed to demonstrate these structures clearly and these special anatomic studies will be described later (Chap. 7).

The *posterior cranial fossa* is at a still lower level than the middle fossa and lodges the cerebellum, pons and medulla oblongata. It is bounded posteriorly by the transverse sulcus of the occipital bone, and roofed over by the tentorium cerebelli. This tentorium is an arched lamina which covers the superior surface of the cerebellum and supports the occipital lobes of the cerebrum. In the median part of the posterior cranial fossa is the foramen magnum which divides the occipital bone into three parts as already mentioned. The hypoglossal canal is seen on the medial aspect of its thickened anterior margin above the occipital condyle for articulation with the first cervical vertebra. The internal occipital crest is the ridge between the foramen magnum and the internal occipital protuberance. The clivus or basiocciput is the broad extension of the occipital bone forward to its junction with the basisphenoid. The transverse sinus sweeps around the occipital bone to the margin of the sigmoid groove at the lateral margin of the petrous temporal bone and curves forward to the jugular foramen. This latter leads downward to the lower surface of the skull and there is situated opposite the lower margin of the external acoustic meatus, separated from it by the styloid process. The jugular foramen transmits the large venous sinuses (inferior petrosal and lateral) and the ninth, tenth and eleventh cranial nerves as well as meningeal branches from the occipital and accessory pharyngeal arteries. The internal acoustic meatus, which is situated in the anterior wall of the posterior cranial fossa, is a short canal in the petrous portion of the temporal bone and is separated laterally by thin bone from the internal ear. It transmits the auditory and facial nerves.

Towne's position (Fig. 6–25) affords an excellent opportunity to study many structures in the middle and posterior fossae. The posterior two thirds of the foramen magnum are shown quite clearly, and very frequently the neural arch of the first cervical vertebra is seen through it. The spinous process of the second cervical vertebra may also be seen. The dorsum sellae is frequently seen faintly identified along with the posterior clinoid processes. The petrous portion of the temporal bone extends laterally from the foramen magnum. In this structure, the internal acoustic meatus, the arcuate eminence (under which lie the semicircular canals), the tegmen tympani and the mastoid process can be identified. The occipital bone extends above these ridges on either side. Extending from the region of the tegmen tympani is a rather broad suture, the occipitomastoid suture, which intersects the parietomastoid suture. Extending inward from this intersection is the lambdoid suture. The junction of these three sutures is the asterion. In the midline the lambdoid suture meets the sagittal suture at the lambda. The grooves for the venous sinuses in the occipital bone, and the increased density in the region of the internal occipital protuberance have already been described.

NORMAL CALCIFICATION WITHIN THE CALVARIUM WHICH MAY BE SEEN RADIOGRAPHICALLY

The Pineal Gland. The pineal gland (Fig. 6–17) is calcified in about 50 per cent of normal adults beyond the age of 20, and occasionally it may be calcified in younger individuals also. It is a perfectly midline structure, and is very centrally placed in the skull. It is frequently closely associated with calcification in the posterior commissure, which gives it a multicentric appearance. Vastine and Kinney have plotted the position of the pineal gland on the lateral projection of the skull in many normal individuals (Fig. 6–17, **e**) and have established normal limits for its position (Fig. 6–17, **b, c** and **d**), deviations from which prove very valuable for detection of a space-occupying lesion within the skull.

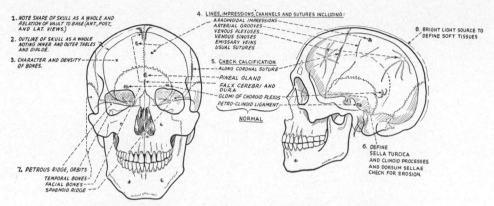

Routine method of study of radiographs of skull—frontal and lateral perspectives.

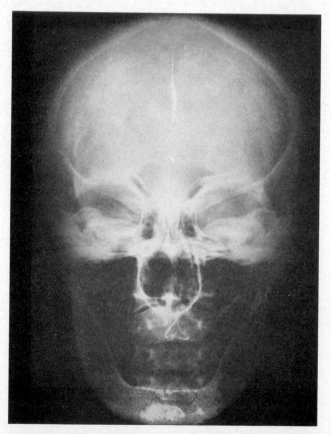

Fig. 6–17.   pineal gland: **a,** Radiograph to show calcification in pineal gland and falx cerebri.

Note on Routine of Study of Skull:

1. The student should become thoroughly familiar with a routine method for studying films of each region of the body. The routines shown in the text need not be arbitrarily followed, but a somewhat similar procedure is necessary to avoid missing important observations.

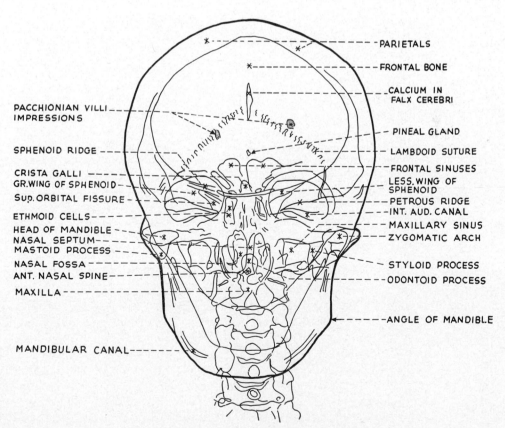

FIG. 6–17.PINEAL GLAND: **b,** Labeled tracing of **a.**

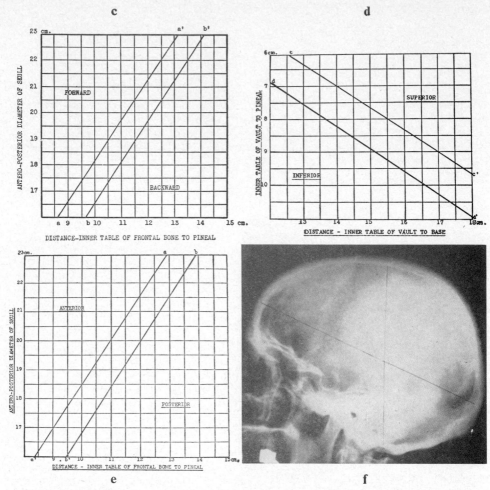

FIG. 6–17. PINEAL GLAND: **c**, Vastine-Kinney graph for localization of the pineal body in antero-posterior plane. Pineals that fall between the lines a-a′ and b-b′ are in the normal zone, while those that fall anterior to this zone are displaced forward, and those posterior to it are displaced backward. **d**, Vastine-Kinney graph for localization of the pineal body in the vertical plane. Normal zone lies between lines c-c′ and d-d′. When the pineal falls above, it is displaced superiorly, and below, it is displaced inferiorly. **e**, Dyke's modification of the Vastine-Kinney graph in the antero-posterior plane. The normal zone is 4 mm. anterior to the comparable Vastine-Kinney graph. **f**, Lateral view of the skull, indicating points from which measurements are made to determine position of pineal body, by Vastine-Kinney method: (1) Inner table of frontal bone and (2) inner table of occipital bone at their most distant points; (3) inner table of the vault, and (4) inner table of the cerebellar fossa at the foramen magnum. (From Golden's *Diagnostic Roentgenology*, Thomas Nelson and Sons, Publishers.)

Other Areas of Calcification.   *Habenular calcification*[6] can be recognized in lateral roentgenograms of the skull as a "C" shaped calcification in the pineal region. It represents calcification in the taenia habenulae and is separated from the pineal body by the habenular commissure. This calcification was identified in 89 out of 187 normal skull roentgenograms showing pineal calcification. Its position averages 5.8 mm. anterior to the center of the pineal calcification.[5] The *falx cerebri* (Fig. 6–17, **a**) is also frequently calcified in the adult and may be seen on the antero-posterior or postero-anterior projection as a thin stripe-like shadow. Unless the calcium is very extensive, this cannot be detected with accuracy on the lateral projections of the skull, but may appear as a faint plaque-like structure. It is such a rigid structure that it is not readily displaced by a space-occupying lesion, and thus has less value than the pineal gland in assisting the radiologist.

The *glomera of the choroid plexuses* (Fig. 6–18) at the junction of the posterior and temporal horns of the lateral ventricles frequently undergo calcification, and are to be found symmetrically on either side of the midline in the antero-posterior projections and behind and superior to the pineal gland in the lateral projections. Occasionally they will be displaced by a space-occupying lesion, and in that case permit an accurate diagnosis of that condition. Slight asymmetries, however, must be interpreted with caution.

The *petro-clinoid ligament* (Fig. 6–19) situated posterior to the sella turcica may also be calcified, and appears as a thin shadow extending from the dorsum sellae to the petrous ridge.

Very occasionally there is a *calcific bridge between the anterior and posterior clinoid processes of the sella turcica,* but usually this overbridged appearance of the sella turcica is due to the overlapping shadows of the anterior and posterior clinoids (since the interclinoid distance of the anterior clinoids is considerably greater than that of the posterior) on the lateral roentgenogram of the skull, and not actually to a true bridging of the bone.

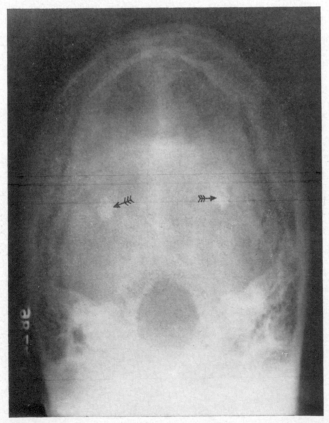

FIG. 6–18. ROENTGENOGRAM TO SHOW CALCIFICATION IN THE GLOMERA OF THE CHOROID PLEXUSES: a, Towne's position.

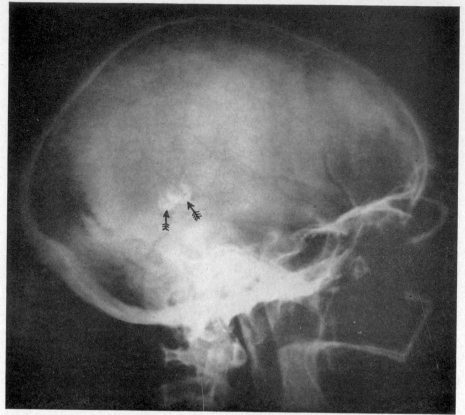

FIG. 6–18. ROENTGENOGRAM TO SHOW CALCIFICATION IN THE GLOMERA OF THE CHOROID PLEXUSES:
b, Lateral view.

There may be *calcium deposit* in the wall of the *superior sagittal venous sinus within the dura*. This may occur adjoining the parietal bone, or near its junction with the sinus confluens particularly. This is without pathologic significance.

Occasionally small *granular calcified areas may appear in the basal ganglia*.[3] They are situated on either side of the midline largely within the middle cranial fossa. It is not completely certain that patients may not suffer from this calcium deposit, since the patients in whom this calcification was found had variable abnormalities which might or might not be related to it.

Calcification may occur *in the cerebral arteries*, particularly the internal carotid artery adjoining the sella turcica. This entity is outside the scope of normal calcium deposit.

THE BLOOD SUPPLY OF THE CALVARIUM AND ITS VENOUS DRAINAGE

The bones of the calvarium do not have single nutrient arteries as do the bones of the extremities, but most of their arterial supply is derived on the deeper surfaces from the meningeal arteries in the depths of the meningeal grooves. A few other small arterioles penetrate the outer surface of the occipital bone and temporal bones, especially near the attachment of the temporal muscles.

Actually most of the circulation of the calvarium is of a venous nature in the diploe, and in general there is one major diploic channel for each cranial bone (Fig. 6–9). This tends to branch in stellate fashion, with a very irregular course. Usually the diploic veins lie closer to the inner table than the outer.

Thus the following diploic channels can be identified: The frontal diploic veins (which may open exteriorly into the veins in the vicinity of the supraoribital notch); the parietal diploic vein, which seems to be in the shape of a star, and hence is referred to as the "parietal star"; the temporal diploic vein, which anastomoses freely with the middle meningeal veins; the occipital diploic veins; and numerous anastomoses with the venous channels in the dura mater.

THE SKULL AT BIRTH AND ITS GROWTH AND DEVELOPMENT

The Skull at Birth. The cranial vault at birth (Fig. 6–20) is quite large in relation to the bones of the face, since the teeth and air sinuses are so rudimentary. The bones of the cranial vault are also quite widely separated and filled with fibrous tissue. The edges of these are not yet serrated as they are in the adult. Strictly speaking there are *seven* fontanels: In addition to the *anterior frontal* and *posterior occipital* fontanels, there are the paired *sphenoidal* fontanels, at the junction of the squamous portions of the temporal bones with the coronal suture, the paired *mastoid* fontanels between squamous portions of the temporal bones and the lambdoid suture on either side, and the *sagittal*

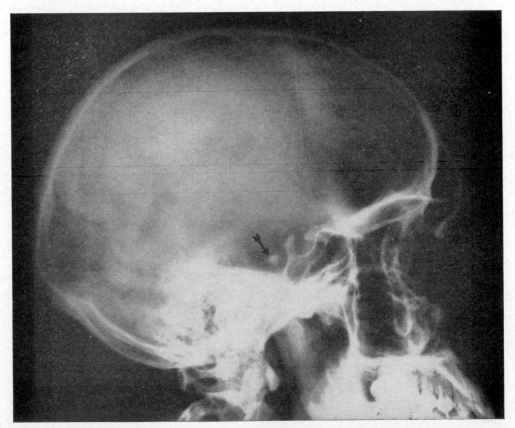

FIG. 6–19. Radiograph to show calcification in the petro-clinoid ligament.

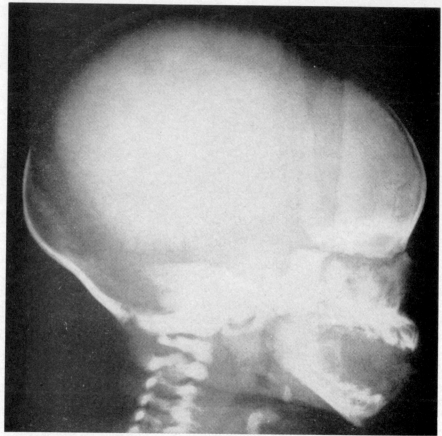

FIG. 6–20   NORMAL NEONATAL SKULL: a, Roentgenogram, lateral view. (From Caffey, *Pediatric X-Ray Diagnosis*, Year Book Publishers.)

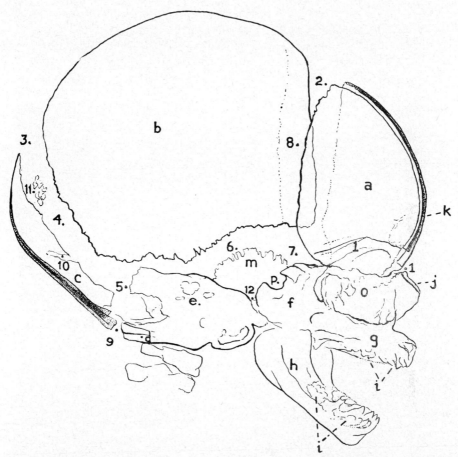

FIG. 6–20.   NORMAL NEONATAL SKULL :   **b,** Labeled tracing of **a.** *a,* Frontal bone; *b,* parietal bone; *c,* squamous portion of occipital bone; *d,* exoccipital portion of occipital bone; *e,* superimposed petrous pyramids of temporal bone; *f,* body of sphenoid; *g,* upper maxilla; *h,* mandible; *i,* partially mineralized deciduous teeth, and dental crypts; *j,* nasal bone; *k,* squamosa of the frontal bone; *l,* horizontal plates of the frontal bone; *m,* squamosa of the temporal bone; *o,* orbit; *p,* pituitary fossa; *1,* frontonasal suture; *2,* anterior fontanel; *3,* posterior fontanel; *4,* lambdoidal suture; *5,* postero-lateral fontanel; *6,* squamosal suture; *7,* anterolateral fontanel; *8,* coronal suture; *9,* synchondrosis between exoccipitals and supraoccipital portions of occipital bone; *10,* mendosal suture; *11,* multiple ossification centers (wormian bones) in lambdoidal suture; *12,* occipitosphenoid synchondrosis. (From Caffey, *Pediatric X-Ray Diagnosis,* Year Book Publishers.)

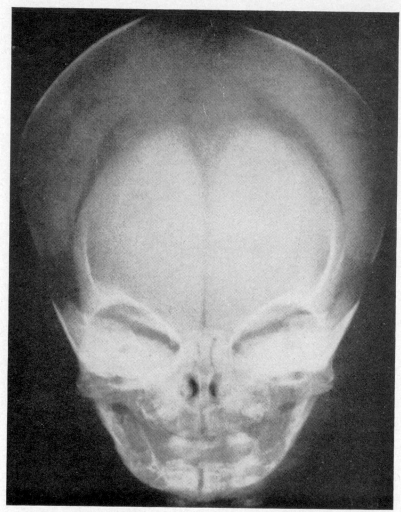

FIG. 6–20. NORMAL NEONATAL SKULL: **c,** Roentgenogram, postero-anterior view. (From Caffey, *Pediatric X-Ray Diagnosis*, Year Book Publishers.)

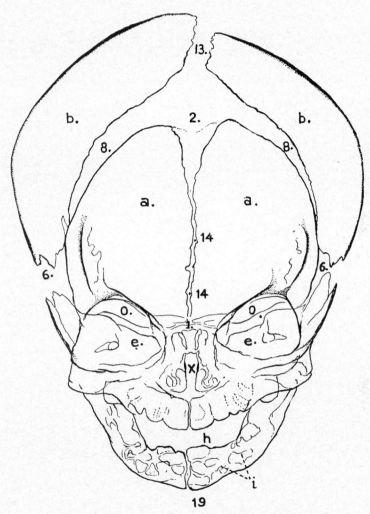

FIG. 6–20. NORMAL NEONATAL SKULL: **d,** Labeled tracing of **c.** *a,* Frontal bone; *b,* parietal bone; *e,* superimposed petrous pyramids of temporal bone; *h,* mandible; *i,* partially mineralized deciduous teeth, and dental crypts; *o,* orbit; *x,* nasal septum; *2,* anterior fontanel; *6,* squamosal suture; *8,* coronal suture; *13,* sagittal suture; *14,* metopic suture dividing the frontal bone; *19,* symphysis of mandible. (From Caffey, *Pediatric X-Ray Diagnosis,* Year Book Publishers.)

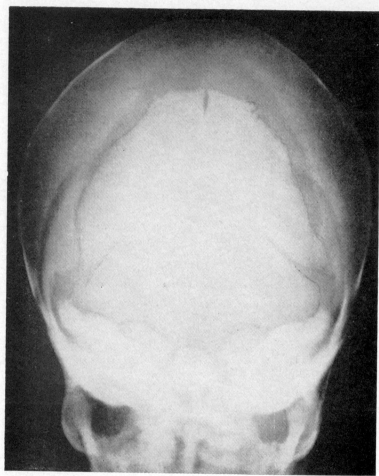

Fig. 6–20.   NORMAL NEONATAL SKULL: e, Roentgenogram, antero-posterior view. Modified Towne's
projection. (From Caffey, *Pediatric X-Ray Diagnosis*, Year Book Publishers.)

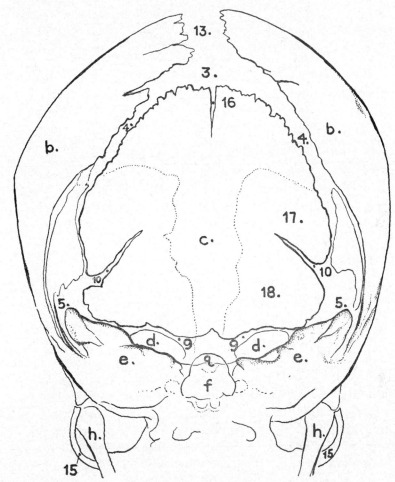

FIG. 6–20. NORMAL NEONATAL SKULL: f, Labeled tracing of e. b, Parietal bone; c, squamous portion of occipital bone; d, exoccipital portion of occipital bone; e, superimposed petrous pyramids of temporal bone; f, body of sphenoid; h, mandible; q, basioccipital portion of occipital bone; 3, posterior fontanel; 4, lambdoidal suture; 5, posterolateral fontanel; 9, synchondrosis between exoccipitals and supraoccipital portions of occipital bone; 10, mendosal suture; 13, sagittal suture; 15, zygomatic arch; 16, superior median fissure of occipital bone; 17, interparietal portion of occipital bone; 18, supraoccipital portion of occipital bone. (From Caffey, *Pediatric X-Ray Diagnosis*, Year Book Publishers.)

fontanel situated at the obelion just above the lambda. These are usually all closed by the age of 2, the posterior and sphenoidal fontanels closing shortly after birth or at least by 6 months of age, and the mastoid fontanels closing by the first year. When closure of the fontanels occurs, irregularities in the bony structure may form the sutural bones already mentioned.

At birth the occipital bone is divided into four parts: There is an incomplete cleft between the interparietal and supraoccipital portions of the bone, which may be misinterpreted as a fracture if one is not familiar with this developmental phenomenon; there are also the two lateral parts on either side of the foramen magnum, and the basilar part in the center anteriorly. The two lateral parts fuse with the supraoccipital portion during the third year, and with the basilar portion during the fourth or fifth year. The basisphenoid suture (suture between the sphenoid and the basilar part of the occipital bone) does not fuse until about the age of 25. A knowledge of these sutural developments is of paramount importance when interpreting skull radiographs.

The sphenoid bone is formed in five separate parts: a median and two lateral portions, in addition to the two sphenoidal conchae. The median part consists of the body and the small wings; each lateral part consists of the pterygoid process and a great wing. The dorsum sellae is still cartilaginous in large part at birth, and ossifies slowly. It therefore appears considerably elongated and shallow. The sphenoid sinuses are not aerated, but their rudiments are present in the conchae. Extension of the rudimentary sinus by absorption of the spongy bone does not begin until the sixth or seventh year, and fusion of the concha with the sphenoid does not occur until the eighth or ninth year.

The temporal bone is divided into four parts—the petromastoid, the squamous, the tympanic and the styloid process. The mastoid process has not yet begun to develop at birth, and the osseous portion of the external auditory meatus is lacking. (The tympanic membrane therefore lies near the surface of the head and its obliquity is different from that of the adult.) The mandibular fossa is shallow and large, and looks laterally as well as downward.

The ethmoid bones at birth already contain the sinuses in each labyrinth, but the perpendicular plate and the cribriform plate are not yet completely formed or ossified. The ossification of the perpendicular plate is not complete before the fifth or sixth year, and the cribriform plate is ossified usually during the second year. Fusion of the ethmoid and sphenoid does not occur until about 25 years of age.

The inferior nasal concha is already ossified at birth, and arises as a separate bone.

The frontal bone at birth is divided into halves by the frontal suture, which, when it persists into adult life is called the "metopic" suture. The frontal and parietal eminences or tuberosities are more convex and relatively prominent in the child than in the adult. Obliteration of the frontal suture usually occurs by the fifth or sixth year of life. The superciliary arch becomes prominent with growth. The supraorbital notch is more centrally placed in the newborn child than in the adult.

The maxillae are vertical and of small height, accounting for the short distance between the palate and the orbits. The maxillary sinus at this time is a mere groove in the lateral wall of the middle meatus. The alveolar process is also very small and hollowed out for the dental sacs. The maxillary sinus is ordinarily not significantly aerated before 2 or 3 years of age, and its growth (Fig. 6–21) contributes considerably to the growth of the face in general. Sometimes there are septae in the maxillary sinus which persist throughout life.

The vertical plates of the palatine bones are short at birth; the nasal bones are low and flat, and the nasal cavity is situated almost entirely between the orbits. At this time the orbital opening is large and nearly circular, and has sharp margins; the orbital fissures are wide, and the lacrimal fossa is deep and looks forward instead of in a lateral direction.

Growth and Age Changes of the Skull (Fig. 6–21).   The growth of the facial bones exceeds the growth of the cranial vault. The capacity of the cranium at birth is fully two thirds that of the adult, and in the adult the volume occupied by the face roughly equals that occupied by the cranium. The volume of the face in the newborn infant is only one eighth that of the entire skull. The growth of the face and skull in general is most rapid in the first six or seven years— the facial growth occurring largely in the air sinuses, nose and the alveolar processes of the maxilla and mandible.

The accompanying radiographs (Fig. 6–22) demonstrate the type of growth which occurs in the face. The mastoid process begins to be well pneumatized by the age of 6, and the frontal sinuses likewise tend to develop air cells. The frontal sinuses are really outgrowths from the ethmoidal labyrinth, and have a similar origin to the ethmoid air cells.

The growth of the alveolar processes parallels the dental growth, and after old age, owing to the loss of the teeth, there is a diminution in the size of the jaws owing to the absorption of the walls of the alveoli; the chin protrudes and the angle of the mandible becomes more obtuse.

At approximately the age of 7 the orbits, the laminae cribrosae of the ethmoids, the body of the sphenoid, the petrous part of the temporal bones and the foramen magnum have reached their adult size.

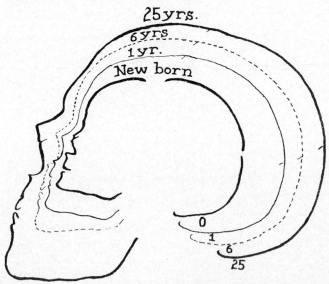

FIG. 6–21.   Proportionate growth of the facial bones and calvarium during infancy, childhood and early manhood, shown in medial longitudinal section of the skull. (From Caffey, *Pediatric X-ray Diagnosis*, Year Book Publishers.)

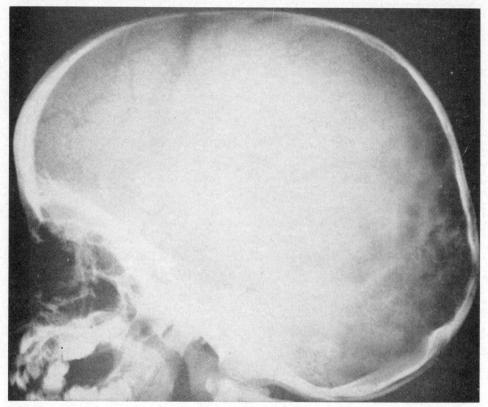

Fig. 6–22. NORMAL SKULL AT 2 YEARS: a, Radiograph, lateral view. (From Caffey, *Pediatric X-Ray Diagnosis*, Year Book Publishers.)

POINTS OF PRACTICAL INTEREST WITH REFERENCE TO RADIOGRAPHY OF THE SKULL:

'. The position of the patient's body is most important in radiography of the skull. At all times the patient's body should be so situated that:

(*a*) The sagittal plane of the skull is perfectly parallel with the table top and film when lateral views are obtained.

(*b*) In the direct antero-posterior or postero-anterior view a line drawn between the outer canthus of the eye and the tragus of the ear or external acoustic meatus (cantho-meatal line) must be perfectly perpendicular to the table top.

2. When it is necessary for the skull to be raised away from the table top, as in the case with an obese patient, the sagittal plane must still be parallel with the film, but this increase in part-to-film relationship must be compensated for by a corresponding increase in focal-film distance.

3. When it is impossible to manipulate the patient freely, lateral views may be obtained by utilizing a horizontal x-ray beam and placing a grid-cassette perpendicular to the table top against the lateral aspect of the head.

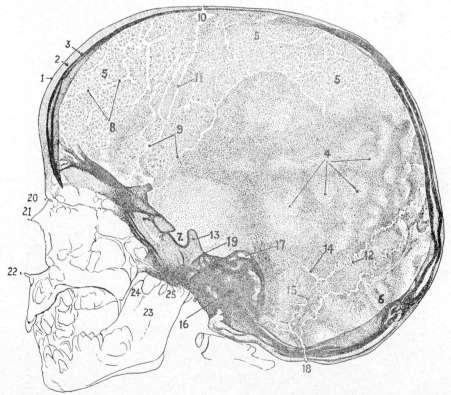

FIG. 6–22.   NORMAL SKULL AT 2 YEARS: **b,** Labeled tracing of **a.** *1,* Outer table; *2,* diploic space; *3,* inner table; *4,* convolutional markings; *5,* fine honeycomb of diploic structure; *6,* internal occipital protuberance; *7,* pituitary fossa; *8,* diploic veins; *9,* vascular grooves; *10,* anterior fontanel; *11,* coronal suture; *12,* lambdoidal suture; *13,* dorsum sellae; *14,* parietomastoid suture; *15,* occipito-mastoid suture; *16,* petrous pyramids; *17,* small temporal pneumatic cell; *18,* synchondrosis between exoccipital and supraoccipital; *19,* spheno-occipital synchondrosis; *20,* nasofrontal suture; *21,* nasal bone; *22,* anterior nasal spine; *23,* mandible; *24,* coronoid process of mandible; *25,* articular process of mandible. (From Caffey, *Pediatric X-Ray Diagnosis,* Year Book Publishers.)

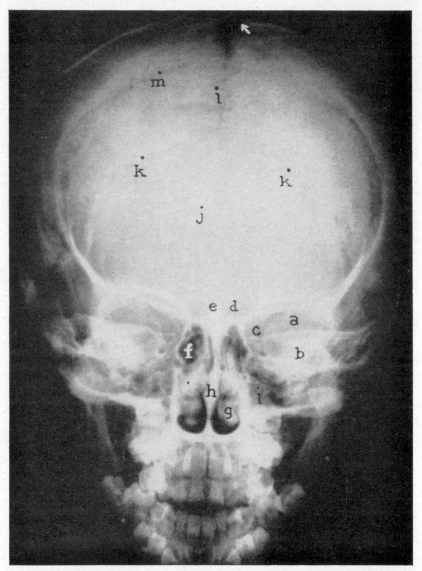

Fig. 6–22. Normal skull at 6 years: c, Radiograph, postero-anterior view. *a*, Orbit; *b*, petrous pyramid; *c*, superior orbital fissure; *d*, frontal sinus; *e*, crista galli; *f*, ethmoid cells; *g*, inferior turbinate; *h*, nasal septum; *i*, maxillary sinus; *j*, frontal bone; *k*, lambdoidal suture; *l*, sagittal suture; *m*, coronal suture. (From Caffey, *Pediatric X-Ray Diagnosis*, Year Book Publishers.)

At puberty there is another rapid increase in the rate of growth in all directions, especially in the frontal and facial regions, owing to a further increase in the size of the air sinuses, and the skull and face begin to take on a more definitive appearance.

Closure of the sutures of the cranial vault begins variably between 30 and 40 years of age. Usually the coronal, sagittal and lambdoidal sutures close in that order, and usually the process begins on the inner surface of the suture about ten years sooner than on the outer surface.

The nasal septum is also different in the child from that of the adult. It is thick and pale in color compared with that seen in adults. On each side, the posterior ends of the middle conchae are conspicuous. Just above the soft palate, the posterior ends of the inferior nasal conchae are visible. The superior nasal conchae may be seen high in the nasal cavity adjoining the nasal septum.

ROUTINE RADIOGRAPHIC POSITIONS FOR STUDY OF THE SKULL

So many positions have been described for radiographic study of the that usually one has to compromise on certain ones, depending on the anatomic part or parts which one wishes to demonstrate to best advantage. We have been very arbitrary in choosing these projections, depending on their anatomic indications.

Routine Survey of the Bones of the Calvarium. To accomplish this end, we ordinarily obtain:

1. POSTERO-ANTERIOR VIEW WITH A 15 DEGREE TILT OF THE TUBE CAUDALLY (CALDWELL'S PROJECTION) (Fig. 6–23). This has the advantage over the straight postero-anterior projection (Fig. 6–24) in that it permits visualization of the orbital structures unobstructed by the petrous ridges. It permits the visualization of the superior orbital fissure with the surrounding lesser and greater wings of the sphenoid to better advantage (Fig. 7–14). On the other hand, the petrous ridge is obscured to a greater extent behind the maxillary antra and ethmoids. The other bones of the cranial vault are well visualized in either case.

2. STRAIGHT POSTERO-ANTERIOR VIEW OF THE SKULL (Fig. 6–24). In this view the bones of the calvarium are visualized in undistorted frontal projection. The petrous ridges are projected into the orbits.

3. ANTERO-POSTERIOR VIEW WITH A 30 DEGREE TILT OF THE TUBE CAUDALLY (TOWNE'S POSITION) (Fig. 6–25). This view demonstrates the entire occipital bone, foramen magnum and dorsum sellae, along with a clear view of the petrous ridges. Often these structures are partially or completely obscured.

4. BOTH LATERAL PROJECTIONS OF THE SKULL (Fig. 6–26), FIRST WITH ONE SIDE CLOSE TO THE FILM, AND THEN WITH THE OTHER SIDE. These views demonstrate the bones of the calvarium and base of the skull in the lateral perspective. The best visualization of the sella turcica is also obtained at this time.

5. THE AXIAL VIEW OF THE SKULL (VERTICO-SUBMENTAL) (Fig. 6–27). This projection allows a direct visualization of the base of the skull, and the various foramina contained therein. It also shows another view of the petrous ridges, the ethmoid and sphenoid, along with the facial bones and orbit.

Any or all of these projections may be obtained stereoscopically.

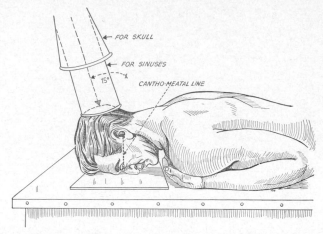

FIG. 6–23. CALDWELL'S PROJECTION OF THE SKULL: **a,** Positioning of patient. Note cantho-meatal line is perpendicular to the film. (The original Caldwell projection for sinuses was 23 degrees with respect to the glabello-meatal line, which is the same as 15 degrees with respect to the cantho-meatal line, but somewhat more variable and hence a less accurate designation.)

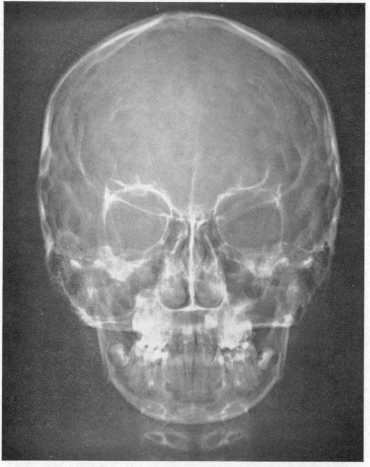

FIG. 6–23. CALDWELL'S PROJECTION OF THE SKULL: **b,** Radiograph.

Points of Practical Interest with Reference to Figure 6–23:

1. The patient's head is adjusted so that the sagittal plane is perfectly perpendicular to the table top and so that the cantho-meatal line (outer canthus of the eye to the tragus of the ear or external acoustic meatus) is perpendicular to the plane of the film also. It may be necessary to support the patient's chin on either his fist or on a folded towel.
2. The central ray is centered to the glabella and angled toward the feet approximately 15 degrees with respect to the cantho-meatal line.
3. It will be noted that in this view the petrous ridges are projected near the inferior margins of the orbits and hence a clearer concept of the orbits is obtained than would be possible without the 15 degree angulation. Also the lesser and greater wings of the sphenoid bone are projected in the orbits. In the straight postero-anterior view of the skull these are obscured by the petrous ridges which are for the most part projected into the orbits.
4. If the frontal bone in itself is the point of major interest, a straight postero-anterior view of the frontal bone is obtained without angulation of the tube.

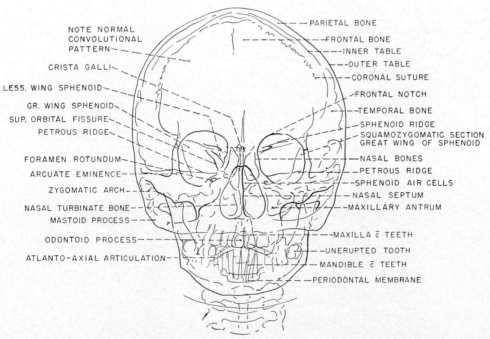

Fig. 6–23. Caldwell's projection of the skull: c, Labeled tracing of b.

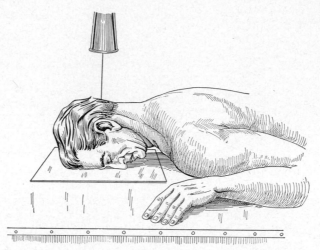

FIG. 6–24.   STRAIGHT POSTERO-ANTERIOR VIEW OF SKULL: **a,** Positioning of patient.

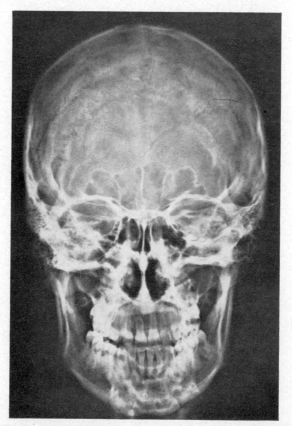

FIG. 6–24.   STRAIGHT POSTERO-ANTERIOR VIEW OF SKULL: **b,** Radiograph.

POINTS OF PRACTICAL INTEREST WITH REFERENCE TO FIGURE 6–24:

1. It will be noted that this view differs from the Caldwell position in that the central ray of the x-ray tube is perpendicular to the film and coincides with the cantho-meatal line. It will be noted that the petrous ridges are projected into the orbits, completely obscuring the orbital contents. The sphenoid ridges are projected over the petrous ridges and likewise are considerably obscured.
2. The posterior instead of the anterior cells of the ethmoidal sinuses are shown, and the dorsum sellae is seen as a curved line extending between the orbits just above the ethmoids.

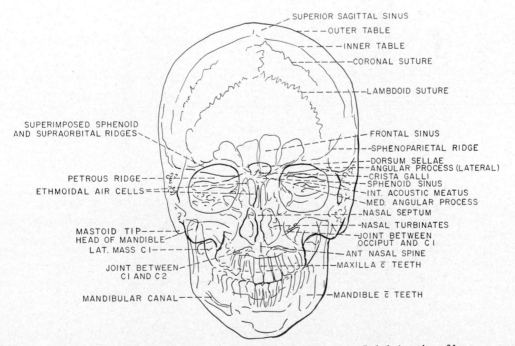

FIG. 6–24. STRAIGHT POSTERO-ANTERIOR VIEW OF SKULL: c, Labeled tracing of b.

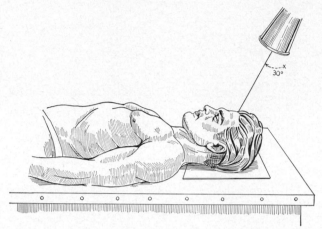

FIG. 6–25.   TOWNE'S PROJECTION OF THE SKULL: **a,** Positioning of patient.

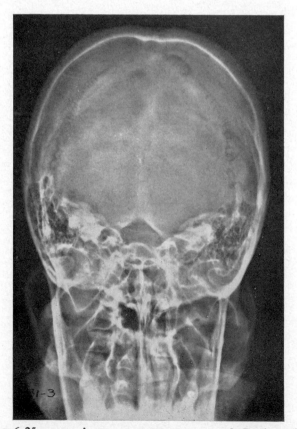

FIG. 6–25.   TOWNE'S PROJECTION OF THE SKULL: **b,** Radiograph.

POINTS OF PRACTICAL INTEREST WITH REFERENCE TO FIGURE 6–25:

1. The sagittal plane of the patient is placed perpendicular to the table top and along the midline of the table.
2. The head is adjusted so that the cantho-meatal line is approximately perpendicular to the table top. This will require that the chin be somewhat depressed upon the neck.
3. The central ray is adjusted at an angle of 30 degrees toward the feet so that it enters the forehead ordinarily at the hairline, and leaves the posterior portion of the cranium in the region of the external occipital protuberance.
4. For better projection of the dorsum sellae into the foramen magnum a somewhat greater angle than 30 degrees may be employed (up to 45 degrees).
5. A view which is of similar value may be obtained with the patient prone and with the tube angled 30 degrees toward the head rather than toward the feet. In the latter instance the central ray would enter the head in the region of the external occipital protuberance and leave the cranium in the region of the forehead approximately 4 cm. above the superciliary arches. This is called the *"reverse Towne's projection."*

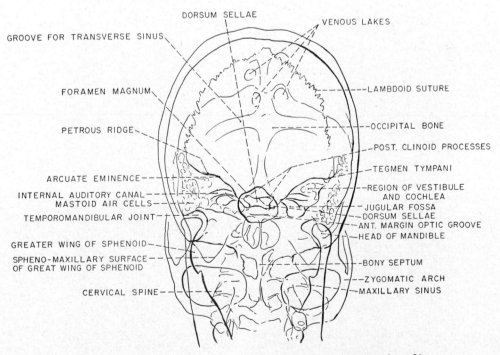

FIG. 6–25.   TOWNE'S PROJECTION OF THE SKULL: c, Labeled tracing of b.

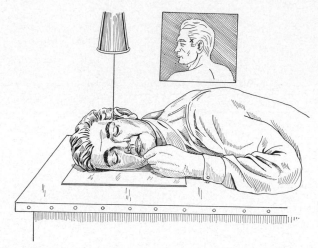

FIG. 6–26.   LATERAL VIEW OF SKULL: **a,** Positioning of patient.

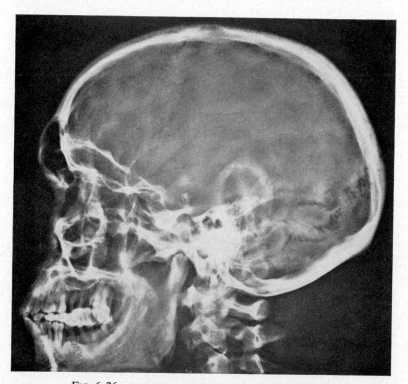

FIG. 6–26.   LATERAL VIEW OF SKULL: **b,** Radiograph.

POINTS OF PRACTICAL INTEREST WITH REFERENCE TO FIGURE 6–26:

1. The position of the head is adjusted so that its sagittal plane is parallel with the table top and with the film. Its coronal plane is centered to the longitudinal axis of the table. The film is placed transversely in the Potter-Bucky diaphragm beneath the skull.
2. A support is placed under the chin; usually the clenched fist of the patient is adequate in this regard.
3. The central ray passes through a point one inch above the midpoint of the line joining the outer canthus of the eye with the tragus of the ear (cantho-meatal line). This will ordinarily fall immediately over the sella turcica.
4. To evaluate a good lateral projection the two halves of the mandible should be almost perfectly superimposed over one another. If the two rami of the mandible are obliquely projected at fair distances from each other, the projection of the skull is too oblique and should be repeated.
5. It is to be noted that a rather oblique and distorted view of the upper cervical spine is obtained in this lateral view of the skull. This view must not be used routinely for examination of this segment of cervical spine.

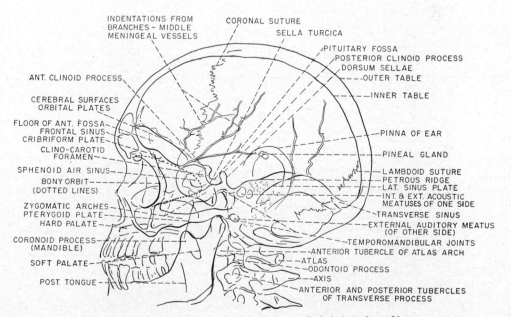

FIG. 6–26.   LATERAL VIEW OF SKULL: c, Labeled tracing of b.

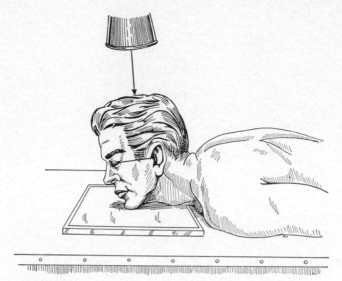

FIG. 6–27.   AXIAL VIEW OF SKULL: **a,** Positioning of patient.

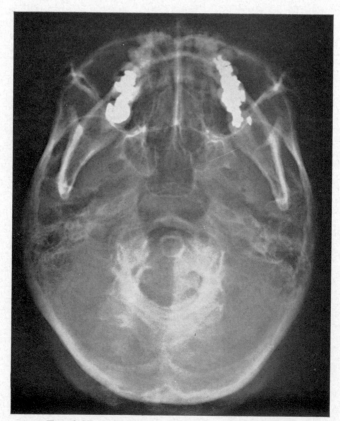

FIG. 6–27.   AXIAL VIEW OF SKULL: **b,** Radiograph.

Points of Practical Interest with Reference to Figure 6–27:

1. The head should be rested on the fully extended chin. The more closely perpendicular the line of the face is to the film the more satisfactory will be this projection.
2. If possible, the cantho-meatal line should be parallel with the table top and film.
3. The central ray should pass through the sagittal plane of the skull perpendicular to the cantho-meatal line at its midpoint. It may be necessary to angle the central ray caudally to maintain this relationship if the patient is unable to extend the chin sufficiently.
4. This view is particularly valuable for visualization of the facial bones in tangential projection. It is used along with the frontal view of the facial bones in every instance.
5. This view is also of value for visualization of the posterior ethmoid and sphenoid cells.

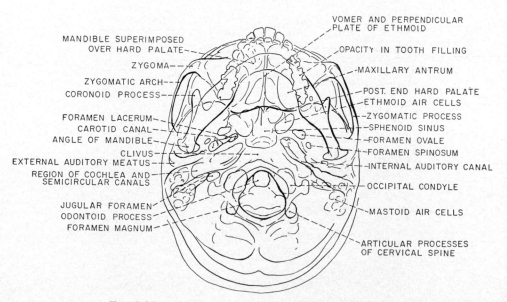

FIG. 6–27. AXIAL VIEW OF SKULL: c, Labeled tracing of b.

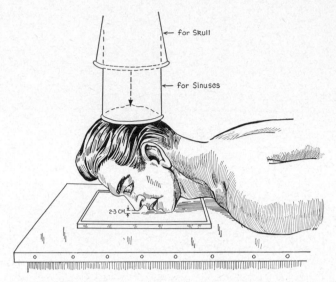

FIG. 6–28.   POSTERO-ANTERIOR VIEW OF FACE (Water's projection):   **a,** Positioning of patient.

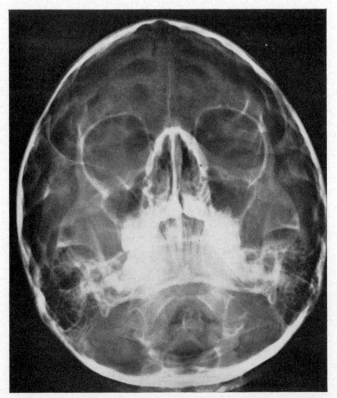

FIG. 6–28.   POSTERO-ANTERIOR VIEW OF FACE (WATER'S PROJECTION): **b,** Radiograph.

Special Study of the Facial Bones Apart from the Nose. To accomplish this end, the following projections may be obtained:

1. POSTERO-ANTERIOR VIEW OF THE FACE (Fig. 6–28), WITH THE NOSE RAISED OFF THE FILM ABOUT 2 TO 3 CM., AND THE CHIN ON THE FILM (WATER'S PROJECTION). This view affords an excellent opportunity to study the maxillae, zygomata, orbits and nasal cavity.

2. SUBMENTO-VERTICAL VIEW OF THE SKULL (AXIAL VIEW) (Fig. 6–29). This view resembles the vertico-submental view closely, in that it permits visualization of the foramina at the base of the skull, the petrous ridges, and the ethmoid and sphenoid bones. It allows a somewhat more satisfactory tangential perspective of the maxillary bones, zygomata, zygomatic arches, orbits and nasal cavity than does the other.

3. LATERAL VIEW OF THE FACE (Fig. 6–30). This is a straight lateral projection of the face, obtained in similar fashion to the lateral view of the sphenoid, except we make certain to include the entire face. For the anatomic description of this view, the student should also note the lateral sphenoid sinus view (Fig. 7–12).

Routine Study of the Zygomatic Arches (Fig. 6–28). This very frequently is part of a facial bone survey, and actually can be seen on the routine films if a bright light source is employed in viewing the submento-vertical film. However, if a special further study is desirable, it is well to obtain a vertico-submental projection (Fig. 6–27), employing soft tissue technique so that the zygomatic arches are not "burned out." Other oblique projections may also be employed.

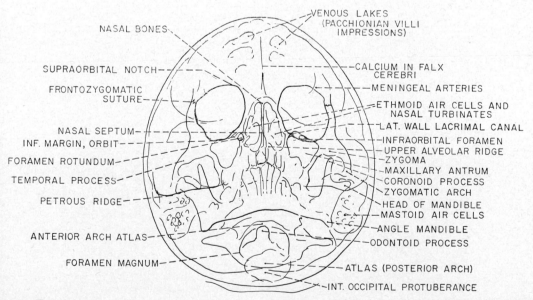

FIG. 6–28. POSTERO-ANTERIOR VIEW OF FACE (WATER'S PROJECTION): **c,** Labeled tracing of **b.**

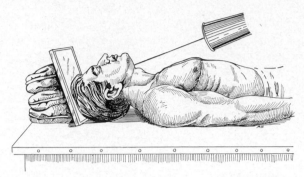

FIG. 6–29.   AXIAL VIEW OF FACE (SUBMENTO-VERTICAL VIEW):   **a,** Positioning of patient. This view using slightly "lighter" exposure technique is utilized for visualization of the zygomatic arches in the infero-superior projection.

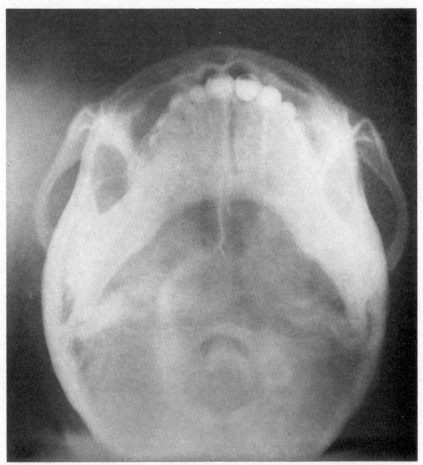

FIG. 6–29.   AXIAL VIEW OF FACE (SUBMENTO-VERTICAL VIEW):   **b**, Radiograph.

POINTS OF PRACTICAL INTEREST WITH REFERENCE TO FIGURE 6–29:

1. The film and the patient's head are placed so that the cantho-meatal line is parallel with the surface of the film.
2. The central ray is directed perpendicular to the midpoint of he cantho-meaal line in he sagittal plane of the patient's skull.
3. A similar view may be obtained in the sitting posture with the patient's head leaned backward against a firm support; or in the supine position by placing a pillow under the upper back. Wherever possible a grid cassette or Potter-Bucky diaphragm should be employed.
4. In this view a clearer concept of the anterior ethmoidal cells is obtained and ordinarily the facial bones and mandible are projected over one another.
5. This view is also of value for visualization of the zygomatic arches, since they are thrown into bold relief by means of this projection. However, a lighter exposure technique must be employed for this purpose.

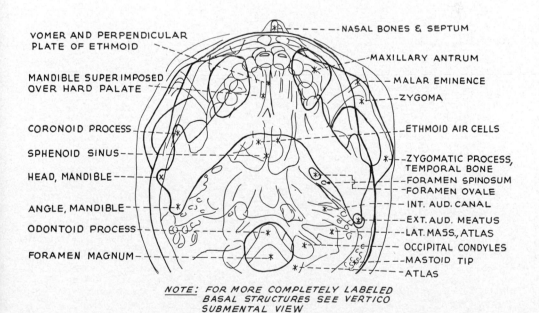

FIG. 6–29. AXIAL VIEW OF FACE (SUBMENTO-VERTICAL VIEW): c, Labeled tracing of b.

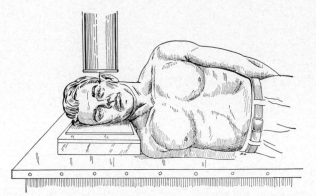

FIG. 6–30.   LATERAL VIEW OF FACE: **a,** Positioning of patient.

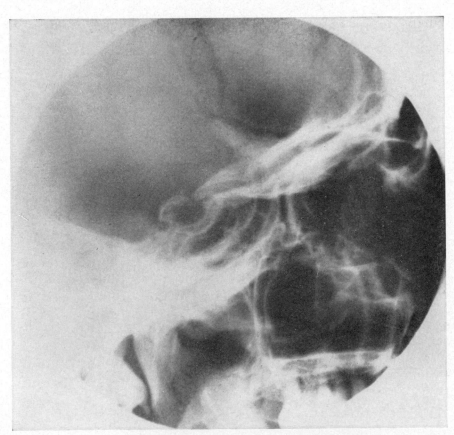

FIG. 6–30.   LATERAL VIEW OF FACE: **b,** Radiograph.

POINTS OF PRACTICAL INTEREST WITH REFERENCE TO FIGURE 6-30:

1. The sagittal plane of the head is adjusted so that it is perfectly parallel with the film and the table top.
2. The cassette may be placed directly under the head without utilizing the Potter-Bucky diaphragm provided that the extended cone is likewise placed directly in contact with the opposite side of the head.
3. Center to the region of the sella turcica over a point 2.5 cm. anterior to and 2 cm. above the external acoustic meatus. Alternately one may center at a point about 2 cm. above the midpoint of the cantho-meatal line.

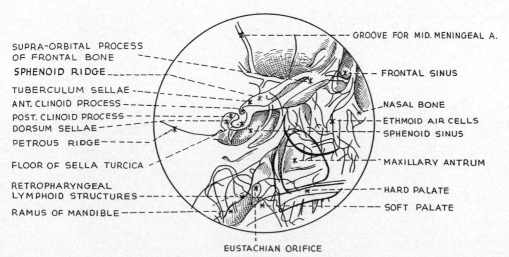

FIG. 6–30.   LATERAL VIEW OF FACE: **c,** Labeled tracing of **b.**

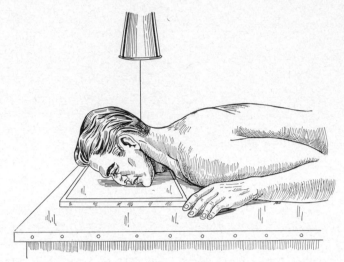

FIG. 6–31.   POSTERO-ANTERIOR VIEW OF MANDIBLE: **a,** Positioning of patient.

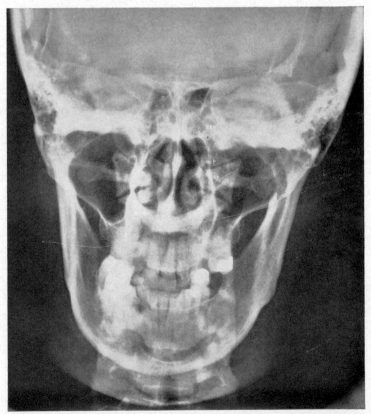

FIG. 6–31.   POSTERO-ANTERIOR VIEW OF MANDIBLE: **b,** Radiograph.

Routine Study of the Mandible.   One can obtain various obliquities depending upon whether one wishes to demonstrate the body or the ramus to better advantage.

1. STRAIGHT POSTERO-ANTERIOR VIEW OF THE MANDIBLE (Fig. 6–31). The chin is flexed on the neck, and the mandible is placed flat on the film. A short film-target distance is employed so as to avoid loss of detail caused by the cervical spine.

2. OBLIQUE PROJECTION OF EACH MANDIBLE (Fig. 6–32). This is obtained by placing both the mandible and the tube in the oblique position as shown and thus obtaining an unobstructed view.

3. SPECIAL VIEW OF THE TEMPOROMANDIBULAR ARTICULATION (Fig. 6–33). Law's position is employed as for demonstration of the mastoid process, except that in this instance *two views* are obtained of each temporomandibular joint, with the *mouth open on the one*, and the *mouth closed on the other*. This allows a proper perspective of the apparent normal subluxation which occurs when the mouth is opened, as well as the structural appearance of the joint.

4. INTRAORAL VIEW OF THE BODY OF THE MANDIBLE (Fig. 6–34). This is obtained by placing an occlusal film in the mouth as far back as possible, and directing the central ray through the submental region.

5. INTRAORAL VIEWS OF THE TEETH (Fig. 6–5).[5] Small contact films of the incisor, canine, premolar and molar areas are obtained of both sides (both upper and lower dental arches). Emphasis in these views is on the apical and periapical structure of the teeth, although a fairly good perspective of the crowns of the teeth is also obtained. For better demonstration of the crowns of the teeth, so-called bite-wing views are obtained.

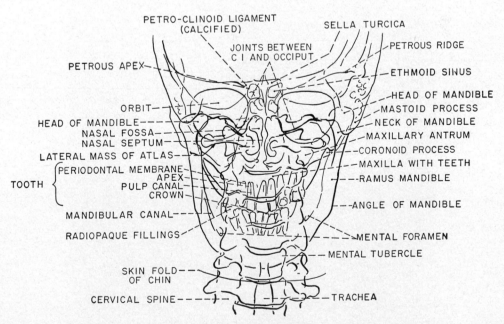

FIG. 6–31.   POSTERO-ANTERIOR VIEW OF MANDIBLE: c, Labeled tracing of b.

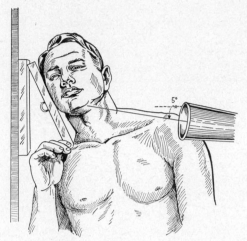

FIG. 6–32.   OBLIQUE VIEW OF MANDIBLE: **a,** Positioning of patient.

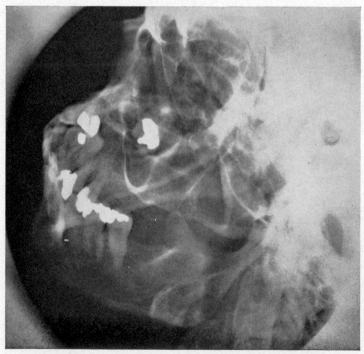

FIG. 6–32.   OBLIQUE VIEW OF MANDIBLE: **b,** Radiograph.

POINTS OF PRACTICAL INTEREST WITH REFERENCE TO FIGURE 6–32:

1. The film is placed against the patient's cheek at an angle of approximately 15 degrees with the vertical.
2. The broad surface of the mandibular body is placed parallel with the plane of the film.
3. To avoid distortion a long target-to-film distance may be employed.
4. For better detail with regard to the ramus of the mandible the central ray may be directed inward, centering over the ramus of the mandible, and the ramus of the mandible may be brought into a position more directly parallel with the plane of the film.
5. If more information is desired regarding the body of the mandible near the symphysis, the head is rotated so that this area is nearer the film.
6. It is ordinarily easier to obtain an erect position of the injured mandible than the recumbent, although the recumbent view may be obtained in somewhat similar fashion.

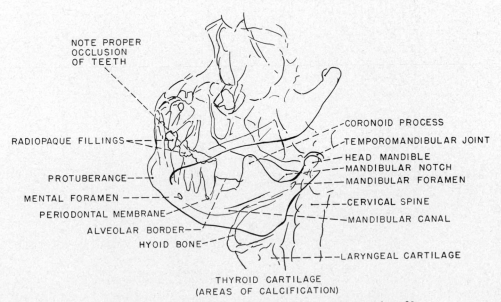

NOTE PROPER
OCCLUSION
OF TEETH

CORONOID PROCESS
RADIOPAQUE FILLINGS
TEMPOROMANDIBULAR JOINT
HEAD MANDIBLE
MANDIBULAR NOTCH
PROTUBERANCE
MANDIBULAR FORAMEN
MENTAL FORAMEN
CERVICAL SPINE
PERIODONTAL MEMBRANE
MANDIBULAR CANAL
ALVEOLAR BORDER
HYOID BONE
LARYNGEAL CARTILAGE

THYROID CARTILAGE
(AREAS OF CALCIFICATION)

FIG. 6–32. OBLIQUE VIEW OF MANDIBLE: c, Labeled tracing of b.

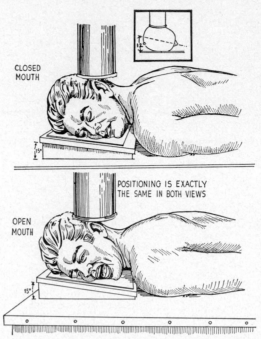

FIG. 6–33.   VIEWS OF TEMPOROMANDIBULAR JOINT WITH THE MOUTH OPEN AND CLOSED: **a,** Positioning of patient.

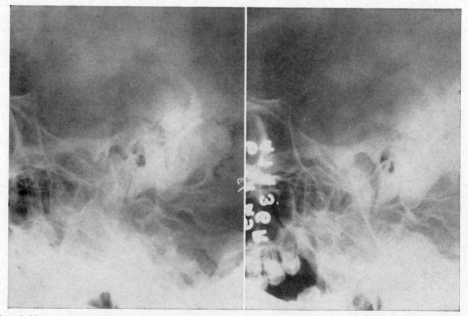

FIG. 6–33.   VIEWS OF TEMPOROMANDIBULAR JOINT WITH THE MOUTH OPEN AND CLOSED: **b,** Radiograph.

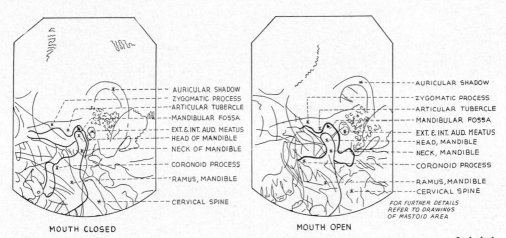

FIG. 6–33. VIEWS OF TEMPOROMANDIBULAR JOINT WITH THE MOUTH OPEN AND CLOSED: **c,** Labeled tracings of **b.**

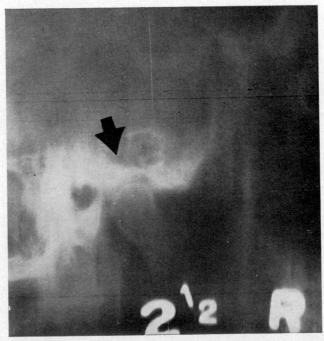

FIG. 6–33. VIEWS OF TEMPOROMANDIBULAR JOINT WITH THE MOUTH OPEN AND CLOSED: **d,** Body section radiograph—mouth closed.

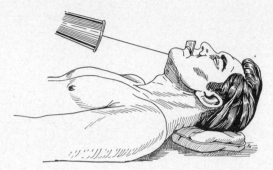

FIG. 6–34.　OCCLUSAL VIEW OF MANDIBLE (INTRAORAL):　**a,** Positioning of patient.

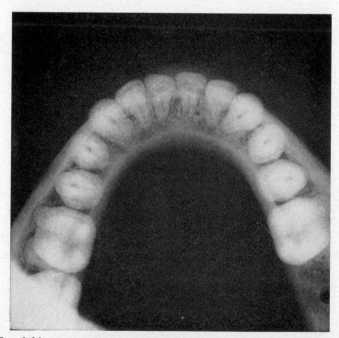

FIG. 6–34.　OCCLUSAL VIEW OF MANDIBLE (INTRAORAL):　**b,** Radiograph.

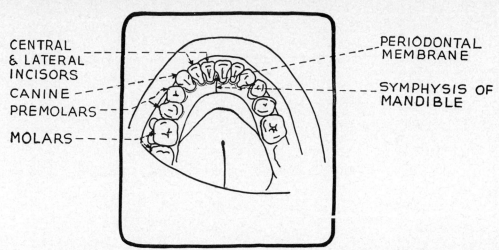

FIG. 6–34.   OCCLUSAL VIEW OF MANDIBLE (INTRAORAL):   **c,** Labeled tracing of **b.**

REFERENCES

1. Caffey, John: Accessory Ossicles of the Supraoccipital Bone. Am. J. Roentgenol., *70:* 401–412, 1953.
2. Etter, Lewis: Atlas of Roentgen Anatomy of the Skull. Charles C Thomas, Springfield, Illinois, 1955.
3. Love, J. G., Camp, J. D., and Eaton, L. M.: Symmetrical Cerebral Calcification, Particularly of Basal Ganglia, Demonstrable Roentgenologically, Associated with Cyst of Cavum Septi Pellucidi and Cavum Vergae. Proc. Staff. Meet., Mayo Clin., *13:* 225–232, 1938.
4. Pendergrass, E. P., Schaeffer, J. P., and Hodes, P. J.: The Head and Neck in Roentgen Diagnosis. 2nd Ed. Charles C Thomas, Springfield, Illinois, 1956.
5. Stafne, C. S.: Oral Roentgenographic Diagnosis. W. B. Saunders Co., Philadelphia, 1958.
6. Stauffer, H., Snow, L., and Adams, A.: Roentgenographic Recognition of Habenular Calcification as Distinct from Calcification in the Pineal Body: Its Applications in Cerebral Localization. Am. J. Roentgenol., *70:* 83–92, 1953.
7. Steinbach, H., and Obota, W.: The Sign of Thinning of the Parietal Bones. Am. J. Roentgenol., *78:* 39–45, 1957.

CHAPTER 7

Detailed Consideration
of Certain Areas
of the Skull

THERE ARE certain regions of the skull which require special radiographic techniques for demonstration of anatomic detail, in addition to the usual routine examination obtained for a survey of the calvarium or face.

These may be subdivided into the following: (1) the nose and nasal cavities; (2) the paranasal sinuses (which are intimately related to the nasal cavities); (3) the mouth and hard palate (see Chap. 13); (4) the orbits; (5) the temporal bone, its contents, subdivisions and development; and (6) the sella turcica.

THE NOSE

There are three anatomic divisions of the nose: (1) the external skeleton; (2) the nasal cavity; and (3) the paranasal sinuses.

The External Skeleton of the Nose (Fig. 7–1).   The lower part of the framework of the nose is formed by cartilages. These cartilages are not individually identifiable radiographically, although with soft tissue technique they can be readily demonstrated. Cartilage also participates in the formation of the anterior portion of the nasal septum, and here too the radiographic examination is not of much value.

The rest of the framework of the nose, however, is osseous, and as such can be demonstrated with considerable accuracy radiographically. The two nasal bones meet in the midline to form the dorsum and the bridge of the nose, and together form the upper portion of the pyriform aperture. Laterally, this aperture is bounded by the maxillae, which are continued inferiorly and anteriorly to form the nasal spine. The nasal bones articulate superiorly with the frontal bone, laterally with the frontal processes of the maxillae, and internally with the nasal septum (perpendicular plate of the ethmoid). Occasionally, because of extra centers of ossification, vertical and/or transverse sutures are found which must not be misinterpreted as fractures. The deep surface of each nasal bone is largely covered by mucoperiosteum and is grooved for the anterior ethmoidal nerve (external nasal branch of the nasociliary nerve). There is also a vascular foramen in the nasal bones which may lead to confusion.

282

Injuries to the nose are frequently accompanied by injuries to adjoining structures, particularly the nasal septum and lacrimal bones. In the routine examination of this region one should be cognizant of these close relationships.

Since the nasal bones are projected over one another, and since the usual skull exposure overpenetrates the nasal bones, special views to demonstrate the nose are employed as will be described below.

The Nasal Cavity (Fig. 7–2).   The nasal cavity extends from the nares in front to the choanae behind. It is divided into two halves or nasal fossae by the nasal septum and its base is formed by the roof of the mouth, consisting of the palatine processes of the maxilla anteriorly and the horizontal processes of the palate bone posteriorly. The nasal septum is formed by cartilage anteriorly and by the perpendicular plates of the ethmoid and vomer posteriorly. The lateral wall of each nasal fossa is subdivided into three or four regions called meatuses by the corresponding nasal conchae or turbinate bones. The superior and middle conchae are part of the ethmoid bone whereas the inferior concha is a separate bone. The superior, middle and inferior meatuses are those regions which lie under their respective conchae. A fourth and very small meatus may lie above the superior meatus (spheno-ethmoidal recess). The following openings are found in the nasal cavity (Fig. 7–3): (1) opening into the *inferior meatus* is the nasolacrimal duct; (2) the *middle meatus* contains openings from the middle ethmoidal air cells, the maxillary sinus, the anterior ethmoidal cells and the frontal sinus; (3) the *superior meatus* contains the orifice which communicates with the posterior ethmoidal cells; and (4) the sphenoid cells open into the *spheno-ethmoidal recess.*

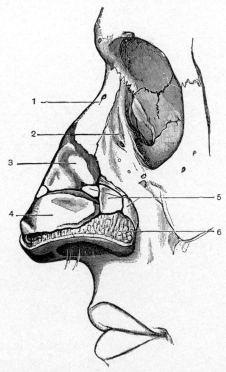

FIG. 7–1.   Diagram to illustrate bones and cartilages of external nose. *1*, Nasal bone; *2*, frontal process of maxilla; *3*, lateral cartilage; *4*, greater alar cartilage; *5*, lesser alar cartilage; *6*, fatty tissue of ala nasi. (From C. M. West in Cunningham's *Text-Book of Anatomy*, Oxford University Press.)

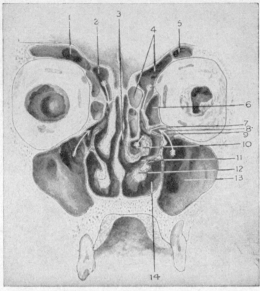

Fig. 7–2. Coronal section through nasal cavities and ethmoid sinuses. *1*, Left frontal sinus; *2*, left anterior ethmoidal cell; *3*, olfactory sulcus; *4*, right anterior ethmoidal cells; *5*, right frontal sinus; *6*, ethmoidal bulla; *7*, hiatus semilunaris; *8*, infundibulum; *9*, uncinate process; *10*, middle conchal cell; *11*, middle meatus; *12*, inferior concha; *13*, maxillary sinus; *14*, inferior meatus. (Guthrie, D., and Scott, C. E., in Turner's *Diseases of the Nose, Throat, and Ear*, published by John Wright & Sons, Ltd., Bristol, England.)

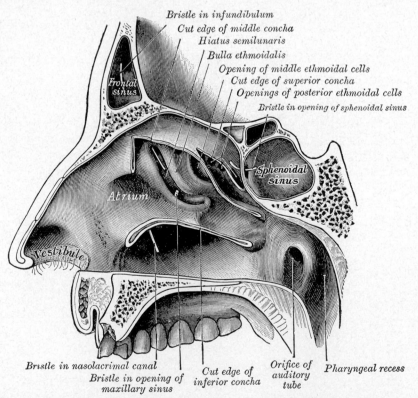

Fig. 7–3. **a**, Lateral wall of nasal cavity to demonstrate apertures leading into it. (Gray, *Anatomy of the Human Body*, Edited by C. M. Goss, Courtesy of Lea & Febiger, Publishers.)

The nasolacrimal passageways are occasionally investigated radiographically, but will not be considered in detail in this text. The reader is referred to the detailed summary of this subject by Pendergrass, Schaeffer and Hodes[3] (Fig. 7–3, **b**).

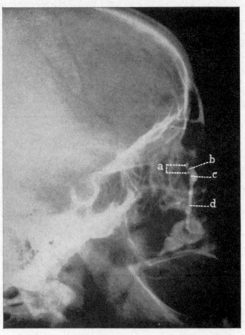

FIG. 7–3. **b,** Lateral view of nasolacrimal system: *a,* lacrimal puncta; *b,* canaliculi; *c,* lacrima sac; *d,* lacrimal duct. Contrast medium: 1 to 2 cc. warmed Beck's bismuth and oil paste. (From Pendergrass, Schaeffer and Hodes, *Head and Neck in Roentgen Diagnosis,* Charles C Thomas.)

ROUTINE RADIOGRAPHIC STUDY OF THE NOSE

Much of the nose is cartilaginous; although this can be moderately well visualized using soft tissue technique, most of the radiologist's study in this regard centers about the nasal bones, nasal cavity and bony nasal septum.

1. **Both Lateral Views of the Nasal Bones** (Fig. 7–4). A small film is placed as close to the side of the nose as possible, perpendicular to the central ray. Soft tissue technique is employed. The anterior nasal spine is also usually included. The various sutures, vascular foramen and groove for the anterior ethmoidal nerve are carefully differentiated from any anatomic abnormality.

2. **Tangential Supero-inferior View of the Nasal Bones** (Fig. 7–5). A film is placed in the mouth between the teeth, and the central ray is directed tangentially to the nasal bones, and perpendicular to the film from a superior vantage point. This permits a supero-inferior perspective of these bones, provided the glabella does not protrude too far forward.

3. **Postero-anterior View of the Nose with a 15 Degree Tilt of the Tube Caudally (Caldwell's Projection)** (Fig. 7–10). This is an identical technique to that employed in paranasal sinus survey, and in this instance is employed to show the bony nasal septum to best advantage. It also demonstrates the nasal cavity moderately well.

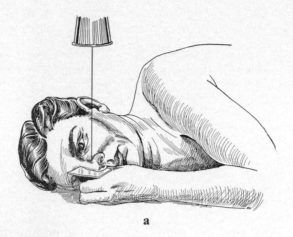

a

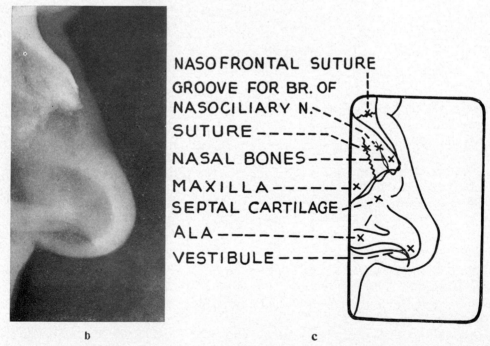

b   c

FIG. 7–4. LATERAL VIEW OF NASAL BONES: **a,** Positioning of patient; **b,** radiograph; **c,** labeled
tracing of **b.**

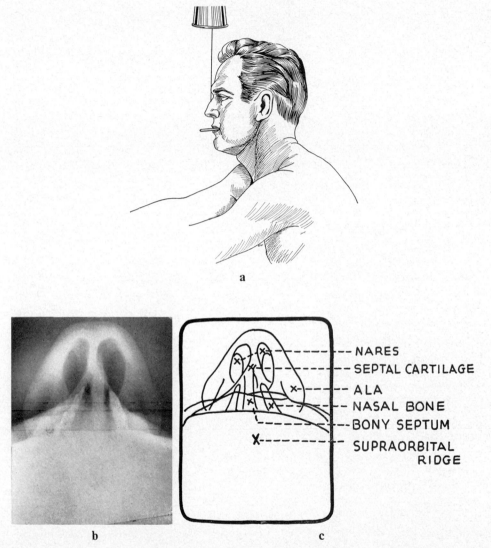

FIG. 7–5. TANGENTIAL SUPERO-INFERIOR VIEW OF NASAL BONES: **a,** Positioning of patient; **b,** radiograph; **c,** labeled tracing of **b.**

THE PARANASAL SINUSES

The radiographic anatomy of the paranasal sinuses is particularly complex because of two factors: (1) The sinuses are projected over one another to a great extent and anatomic detail is thus obscured; and (2) there is a great range of normal variants of the sinuses among different individuals in various age groups, as well as in the same age groups.

The paranasal sinuses have already been identified as paired cavities in the frontal, maxillary, ethmoid and sphenoid bones. They communicate with the nasal cavity and are lined by mucous membrane continuous with that of the nose. In the adult sinuses there are numerous complete and incomplete membranous and bony septa, some of which communicate independently with the nasal cavity.

The frontal sinus communicates with the middle meatus anteriorly through an orifice in the inferior portion of the sinus; the posterior ethmoid cells open into the superior meatus of the nose; the sphenoid sinuses communicate with the nose by means of an orifice in the spheno-ethmoidal recess; the maxillary sinuses and the nasal cavity are continuous through an opening which lies in the middle meatus; this orifice is situated high in the wall of the antrum so that emptying of the antrum cannot occur in the erect position except by overflow, or unless the head is inverted. These details are of considerable clinical importance. It has already been indicated that the orifice of the nasolacrimal duct is situated in the inferior meatus.

The Maxillary Sinuses (Fig. 7–6).   The maxillary sinuses are the first of the sinuses to be pneumatized, and each unaerated sinus containing myxomatous tissue measures approximately 8 x 4 x 6 mm. at birth.[3] The greatest diameter is directed antero-posteriorly. Prior to the fifth year the entire sinus is medial to the infraorbital foramen.

Since pneumatization of the alveolar process ordinarily *does not begin before 6 years of age*, and usually is not evident until the tenth or eleventh year, the relationship of the teeth to the floor of the maxillary sinuses is not so important in children as in adults. In the adult, usually the roots of the molars and second premolar are embedded just outside the floor of the maxillary antrum, and are important in that any inflammatory process of these teeth may transmit inflammation to the closely adjoining antrum and sinus.

In the frontal projection on the radiograph, the maxillary sinus is rather triangular in outline, with the apex situated medially between the orbit and the nasal aperture. The shape is very variable, and there are numerous irregular septa which are projected over the sinus. Most of these represent folds or incomplete partitions, but not infrequently there are complete divisions of the antra into separate chambers. Occasionally there are accessory ostia opening into the nose apart from those already described. The base of the maxillary sinus is formed by the alveolar process and this margin is constant compared with the variability of the antrum as a whole.

The mucoperiosteal lining of the cavity of the sinus is sufficiently dense in outline to be seen and is arbitrarily regarded as normal when it is not over 1 mm. in thickness. Normally no fluid is visible in the sinus in the erect position. The mucous membrane is particularly well demonstrated after the injection of iodized oil (Fig. 7–13) into the maxillary antrum, and any thickened areas are more accurately demonstrated in this manner than in conventional radiographs.

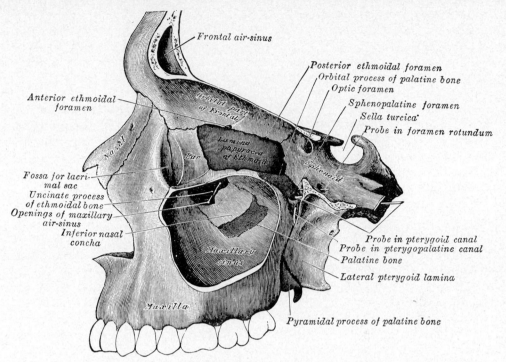

Frontal air-sinus

Posterior ethmoidal foramen
Orbital process of palatine bone
Optic foramen

Anterior ethmoidal foramen

Sphenopalatine foramen
Sella turcica·
Probe in foramen rotundum

Fossa for lacrimal sac
Uncinate process of ethmoidal bone
Openings of maxillary air-sinus
Inferior nasal concha

Probe in pterygoid canal
Probe in pterygopalatine canal
Palatine bone
Lateral pterygoid lamina

Pyramidal process of palatine bone

FIG. 7–6. Left maxillary sinus opened from lateral side. (Gray, *Anatomy of the Human Body*, Edited by C. M. Goss, Lea & Febiger.)

The projections which are most valuable for demonstration of the maxillary antra are: (1) Water's projection (Fig. 7–11), with the mouth open or closed; (2) a similar projection obtained in the erect position (Fig. 7–11, **c**) for demonstration of any fluid levels; and (3) the axial (Figs. 6–27, 6–29) or vertico-submental view, which gives one a supero-inferior perspective of the antra.

In the Water's projection, the shadows of the upper lips are projected over the antra, and may lead to confusion unless one is aware of their presence.

The Ethmoidal Sinuses. The ethmoidal sinuses or cells form the medial wall of each orbit on the one hand, and the lateral wall of the upper one half of the nose on the other. The cells may vary in number and size—there may be eighteen or more small ones or a few large cavities. The anterior ethmoidal cells open into the middle nasal meatus, whereas the posterior ethmoidal cells located in the dorsal portion of the nasal fossa open into the superior or supreme meatus.

There is a great tendency for the ethmoidal cells to grow into and encroach upon the surrounding bony structures such as the frontal bone, the maxillary bones, the sphenoid and the ethmoidal conchae. In the great majority o cases the frontal sinus is developed from a frontal anterior ethmoidal cell, which gradually grows into the frontal bone.

In infancy, it is extremely difficult to interpret lack of aeration of ethmoidal cells on the radiograph, since they are so poorly pneumatized. In the adult, the cells are of variable size and location and overlap one another and the sphenoid sinuses, so that again they are difficult to see very clearly.

In the postero-anterior view, the upper half of the cells of the ethmoid area represent the anterior cavities and those of the lower half represent the posterior cells.

The usual radiographs which demonstrate these cells to best advantage are: (1) Caldwell's position (Fig. 7–10); (2) straight lateral view of the face (Fig. 7–12); (3) the special view of the optic foramina, which is best taken stereoscopically (Fig. 7–16); and (4) the axial or vertico-submental view already described in the case of the base of the skull and the maxillary antra (Figs. 6–27, 6–29).

The Frontal Sinuses (Fig. 7–7).   The frontal sinuses are situated above the bridge of the nose between the inner and outer tables of the frontal bone. They vary greatly in size, but tend to be pyriform in shape. There is usually one sinus on each side, and they are usually asymmetrical. Not infrequently,

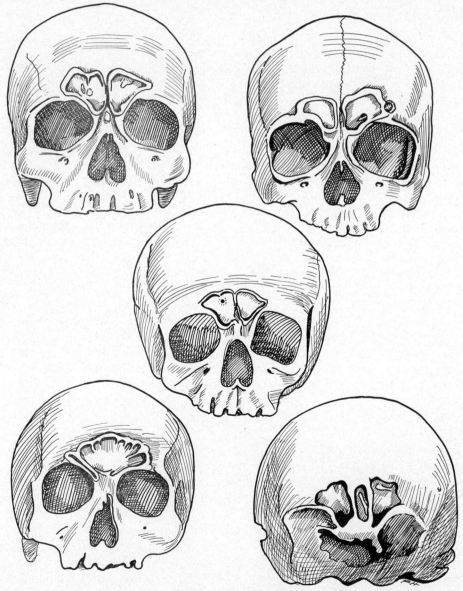

FIG. 7–7.   Variations in configuration of the frontal sinuses.

they extend into the orbital plate of the frontal bone, and fractures of this plate allow free air to escape into the orbital soft tissues, giving rise to an important radiographic sign of this injury.

Ordinarily, the frontonasal duct is a short tortuous channel which enters the middle meatus. This may be encroached upon by the frontal anterior ethmoidal cells to a variable extent.

Radiographically it is not possible to identify the frontal sinuses until about 2 years of age, and their development may be minimal before 6. They do not reach the level of the roofs of the orbits until about the eighth year of life. They may be entirely lacking in some people.

Although the frontal sinuses may be demonstrated by any of the sinus views, the most valuable views in this regard are: (1) Caldwell's projection (Fig. 7–10); and (2) straight lateral view of the face (Fig. 7–12).

The Sphenoidal Sinuses (Fig. 7–8). The sphenoid sinuses are two cavities situated in the body of the sphenoid bone, frequently extending into the contiguous structures. They are often so closely intermingled with the ethmoid sinuses that they cannot be clearly distinguished. The, two cavities are usually asymmetrical, and contain incomplete osseous septa, giving the impression of multiple sinuses.

The sphenoidal sinuses communicate with the spheno-ethmoidal recess, which is situated above the highest ethmoidal concha in the most posterior and superior portion of the nasal cavity.

The anatomic relationships of the sphenoid sinuses are of the utmost importance. The sella turcica, which houses the pituitary gland and hypophyseal stalk, is situated above them, and not infrequently pneumatization is present in the dorsum sellae or clinoid processes. The optic chiasma is situated immedi-

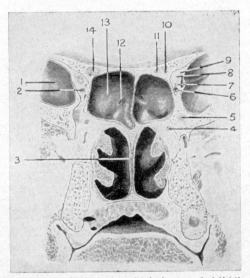

Fig. 7–8. Coronal section through the sphenoidal sinuses. *1*, Middle cranial fossa; *2*, oculomotor nerve, iii; *3*, nasal septum; *4*, nerve of the pterygoid canal (vidian nerve); *5*, maxillary (superior maxillary) nerve, v; *6*, internal carotid artery; *7*, abducens nerve, vi; *8*, ophthalmic nerve, v; *9*, trochlear nerve, iv; *10*, ophthalmic artery; *11*, right optic nerve, ii; *12*, sphenoidal ostium; *13*, left sphenoidal sinus; *14*, left optic nerve, ii. (From Guthrie, D., and Scott, C. E., in Turner's *Diseases of the Nose, Throat and Ear*, published by John Wright & Sons, Ltd., Bristol, England.)

ately anterior to the hypophyseal stalk. Lateral to the sphenoid air cells are the cavernous venous sinuses, through which course the internal carotid artery and the third, fourth, sixth, and ophthalmic and maxillary branches of the fifth cranial nerves. There may actually be an impression upon the sphenoid sinus by the optic nerve. The petrous apex may be in very close association with the sphenoid sinus, and occasionally directly contiguous with it. The vidian nerve, which supplies sympathetic and parasympathetic fibers to the spheno-palatine ganglion, lies close to the floor of the sphenoid sinus. These various relationships become of particular significance in the event of any pathologic process contained within these sinuses.

The sphenoid sinus does not begin to be pneumatized until the third or fourth year of life, and its gradual growth backward is illustrated in Figure 7–9*B*.

The radiographic positions which we find most useful for evaluation of the sphenoid sinuses are: (1) Water's position (Fig. 7–11) with the mouth open (both erect and recumbent); (2) lateral view of the face (Fig. 7–12), which projects both sinuses over one another; (3) the axial, or vertico-submental view (Figs. 6–27, 6–29).

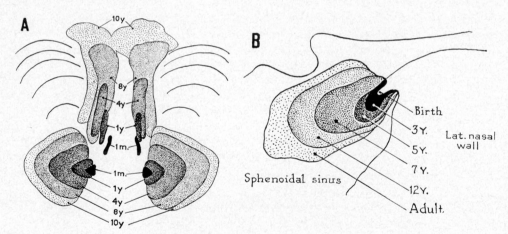

Fig. 7–9.   Diagrams to illustrate growth of frontal, maxillary and sphenoid sinuses. (From Caffey, *Pediatric X-Ray Diagnosis*, Year Book Publishers.)

ROUTINE PROJECTIONS FOR STUDY OF THE PARANASAL SINUSES

Every effort is made to see the paranasal sinuses as clearly as possible, and certain projections are more valuable for some of the sinuses than for others.

1. Postero-anterior Nose-Forehead Position with 15 Degree Tilt of the X-ray Tube Caudally (Caldwell's Projection) (Fig. 7–10). Since we are primarily interested in the paranasal sinuses here, the cone may be placed directly on the head, and it is then unnecessary to utilize the Potter-Bucky diaphragm. This view shows the frontal and ethmoid sinuses to best advantage, while the maxillary sinuses are obscured by the petrous ridges. The sphenoid sinuses are likewise obscured by the ethmoid bones.

2. **Postero-anterior View with the Chin on the Film, and the Nose Raised 2 or 3 cm. from the Film (Water's Projection)** (Fig. 7–11). This view allows the maxillary antra to be clearly seen and projects the petrous ridges beneath them. The frontal and ethmoid sinuses are only moderately visualized. A good view of the sphenoid sinuses is obtained through the open mouth. Also *it is well to obtain this view in both the recumbent as well as the erect positions* for demonstration of possible fluid levels within the maxillary antra.

3. **Lateral Projection of the Paranasal Sinuses** (Fig. 7–12). A straight lateral view of the sinuses is obtained which shows the sphenoid air cells to best advantage, and also allows another perspective of the frontal sinuses. The maxillary and ethmoid sinuses are not shown clearly in this view because of the considerable bony trabeculae lying in the central ray pathway. Nevertheless some further visualization of these structures is thus obtained.

4. **Use of Iodized Oil in the Maxillary Antra** (Fig. 7–13). Occasionally it is desirable to demonstrate the thickness of the mucous membrane of the antra as accurately as possible. To do so, iodized oil is introduced either through trocar puncture or through the natural ostium into each antrum, and erect and recumbent Water's views are taken, along with oblique views of each antrum. Occasionally a 24-hour study is obtained to test the ciliary function in the removal of this foreign material. The greater part of the iodized oil would be removed in this interval under normal conditions.

The Proetz technique for the displacement method of sinus diagnosis and treatment is as follows:[4]

1. The patient is placed in the supine position, and the head is extended backward so that a line drawn between the chin and the external auditory meatus is perpendicular to the examining table.
2. The iodized oil (such as Lipiodol or Brominol) is instilled into the nose through the nostril. Usually 4 to 8 cc. suffices.
3. Negative pressure is applied first to one nostril while the other is closed, and then the other. The pharynx is closed off at the same time by the patient's elevating the soft palate voluntarily.
4. The patient is then placed in the erect position.
5. Postero-anterior and both oblique views are thereafter made of the sinuses in both the erect and recumbent positions. In the recumbent positions, it is usually advisable to obtain these views in both the supine and prone positions.
6. An exposure of the sinuses is made in seventy-two hours, at which time they should be practically empty under normal conditions.

In this method there is only partial filling of the various sinuses, since the air is never permitted to escape completely, and hence if it is desired to demonstrate the structure of an entire sinus, a horizontal x-ray beam must be employed for several views while rotating the patient in various positions.

For best filling and visualization of the maxillary antra, it is probably best to inject the sinuses directly rather than by this indirect means.

Proetz places considerable emphasis on the emptying time of the sinuses in this method of examination also, in that a delay in emptying beyond seventy-two hours implies impaired ciliary function and probable inflammation.

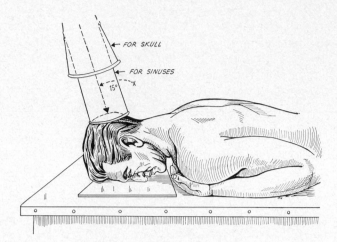

FIG. 7–10.   CALDWELL'S PROJECTION FOR THE PARANASAL SINUSES: **a,** Positioning of patient. (See comments, page 259, Figure 6–23.)

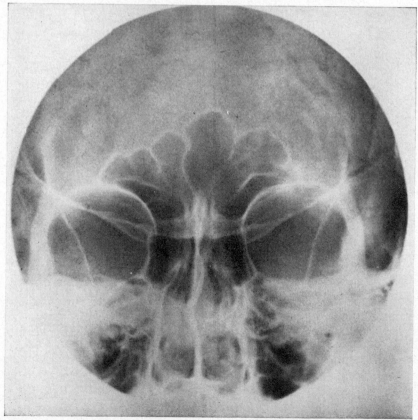

FIG. 7–10.   CALDWELL'S PROJECTION FOR THE PARANASAL SINUSES: **b,** Radiograph.

POINTS OF PRACTICAL INTEREST WITH REFERENCE TO FIGURE 7–10:

1. In this view, the petrous ridge is projected along the inferior margin of the orbit. The anatomic structures of major interest here are: the frontal sinuses; the ethmoid sinuses; the bony nasal septum; and the orbital contents, not including the optic foramina, however. The superior orbital fissure, with the bony structures immediately surrounding it, is seen to maximum advantage. These margins must be clearly identified.
2. Although the maxillary antra can be delineated here, they are not seen to good advantage because they are obscured by the projection of the petrous ridges.
3. The degree of aeration of the nasal air passages is also of importance, and can be evaluated in this projection. The middle and superior nasal turbinates can usually be identified. When these latter structures are swollen or hypertrophied, interference with aeration may result.

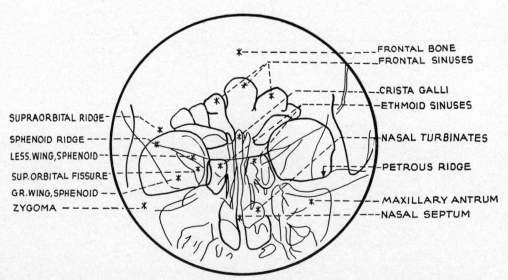

FIG. 7–10. CALDWELL'S PROJECTION FOR THE PARANASAL SINUSES: c, Labeled tracing of b.

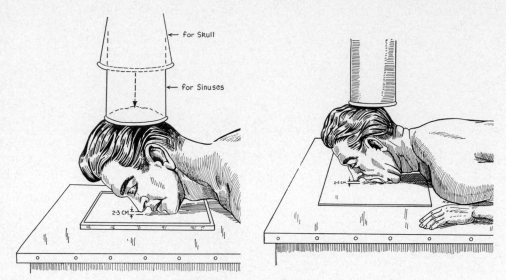

FIG. 7–11.   WATER'S PROJECTION FOR THE PARANASAL SINUSES: **a,** Positioning of patient: mouth
closed left; mouth open right.

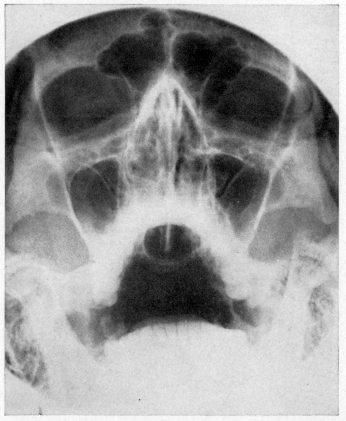

FIG. 7–11.   WATER'S PROJECTION FOR THE PARANASAL SINUSES: **b,** Radiograph, mouth open.

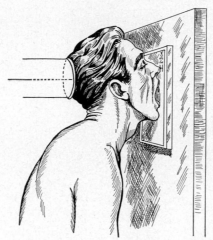

FIG. 7–11. WATER'S PROJECTION FOR THE PARANASAL SINUSES: **c,** Positioning of patient for erect film

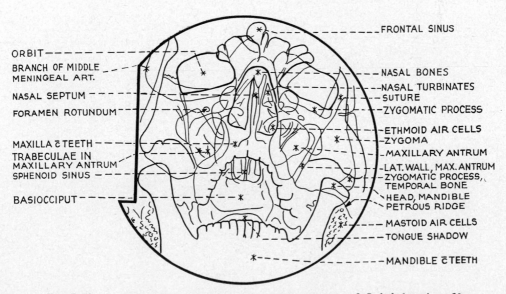

FIG. 7–11. WATER'S PROJECTION FOR THE PARANASAL SINUSES: **d,** Labeled tracing of **b.**

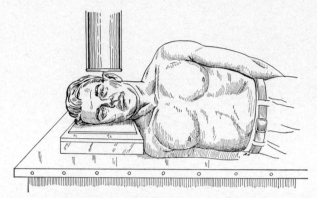

FIG. 7–12.   LATERAL PROJECTION OF PARANASAL SINUSES: **a,** Positioning of patient.

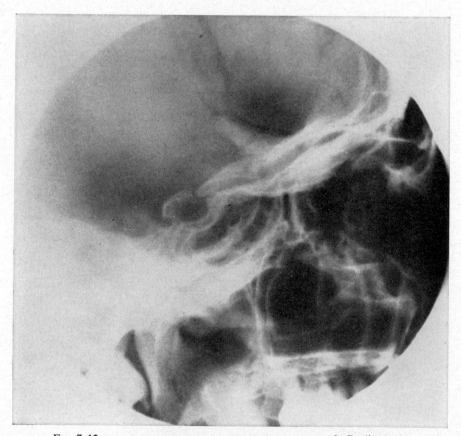

FIG. 7–12.   LATERAL PROJECTION OF PARANASAL SINUSES: **b,** Radiograph.

Points of Practical Interest with Reference to Figure 7–12:

1. The structures which must be clearly identified in this view are: the frontal sinuses; the sphenoid sinuses; the sella turcica; the retropharyngeal lymphoid structures and adjoining air space.
2. The maxillary antra and ethmoids may have confusing appearances, since so many anatomic structures are projected over one another in these planes. The nasal turbinates especially may simulate the appearance of a tumor within the maxillary antra.
   The walls of the orbits are considerably obscured, but some effort should be made to delineate these as well as is possible.

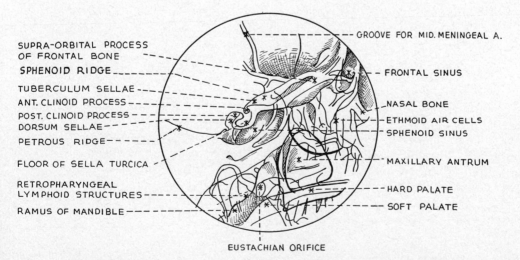

FIG. 7–12. LATERAL PROJECTION OF PARANASAL SINUSES: c, Labeled tracing of b.

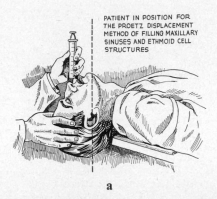

a

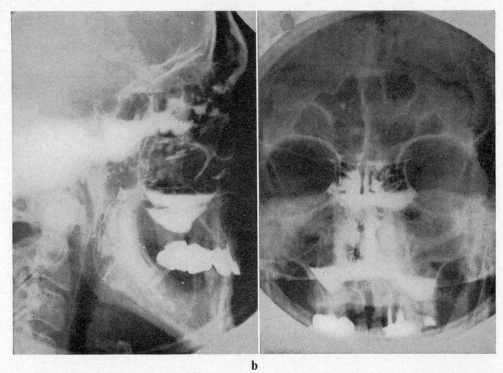

b

FIG. 7–13.   THE PROETZ DISPLACEMENT METHOD OF SINUS DIAGNOSIS: **a,** Positioning of patient.
b, Radiographs. (From *Applicability of Lipiodol in Roentgenography and the Technique of Its Use,*
E. Fougera & Company, Inc.)

THE ORBIT

The orbit is shaped like a four-sided pyramid with its base directed toward the face and its apex directed backward and medially. It contains the eyeball and its associated muscles, vessels and nerves and other structures (Fig. 7–14).

The apex of the orbit corresponds with the optic foramen which transmits the optic nerve and ophthalmic artery.

The bones which enter into the formation of the orbit are as follows:

The roof is formed by the orbital plate of the frontal bone and posteriorly by the lesser wing of the sphenoid. At the lateral angle the fossa for the lacr mal gland is situated.

The floor is formed by the orbitai processes of the maxilla, zygomatic and palatine bones. The nasolacrimal canal lies at its medial angle, containing the nasolacrimal duct. There is a groove on its surface which terminates anteriorly in the infraorbital canal through which the infraorbital artery and maxillary nerve emerge on to the face.

The lateral wall is formed by the great wing of the sphenoid and the zygomatic bone. Between the greater and lesser wings of the sphenoid at the posterior portion of this wall is the superior orbital or sphenoidal fissure connecting the orbit and the cranium. The inferior orbital fissure lies between the lateral wall and the floor (Fig. 7–15).

The medial wall is formed by the frontal process of the maxilla, the lacrimal bone, the lamina papyracea of the ethmoid and the body of the sphenoid. Anteriorly lies a hollow which contains the lacrimal sac; posteriorly, at the junction of the medial wall with the roof, lie the anterior and posterior ethmoidal canals.

The base of the pyramid which is seen as the facial boundary is quadrilateral in shape. It is bounded superiorly by the supraorbital margin of the frontal bone, and above this margin the superciliary arch extends medially to the glabella. The zygomatic and maxillary bones form the sharp infraorbital margin, the frontal process of the maxilla and the inferior angular process of the frontal bones form the medial. The zygomatic bone and the zygomatic process of the frontal bone form the lateral margin.

The axis of each orbit is directed forward and in a lateral direction, but the axes of the eyeballs are antero-posterior and parallel.

The sutures seen in the orbit are: the sutures around the lacrimal bone—the lacrimo-ethmoidal, lacrimofrontal, lacrimomaxillary; the sphenofrontal, between the lesser wing of the sphenoid and the frontal bone; the sphenozygomatic, between the greater wing of the sphenoid and the zygomatic; and the maxillo-ethmoidal, between the orbital process of the maxillary bone and the ethmoid.

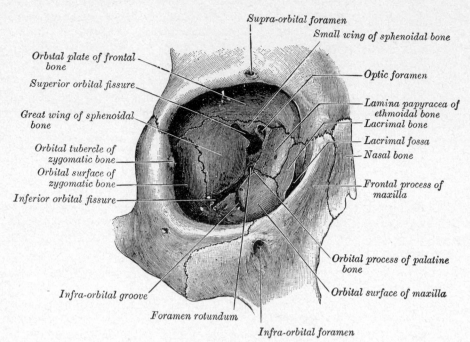

FIG. 7–14. The anatomy of the orbit. (From Gray, *Anatomy of the Human Body*, edited by C. M. Goss, courtesy of Lea & Febiger.)

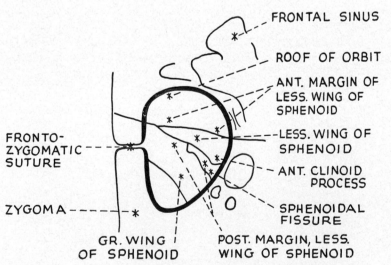

FIG. 7–15.   Tracing of orbital projection obtained by Caldwell's position.

ROUTINE RADIOGRAPHIC STUDY OF THE ORBITS

This study will vary somewhat, depending upon the anatomic relationship one wishes to demonstrate. The consideration for localization of foreign bodies in the eye is out of the scope of this text, and may be obtained from any manual of radiographic technique.

1. **Caldwell's Projection.** Ordinarily, Caldwell's projection (Figs. 7–10, 7–15) (postero-anterior view with a caudal 12 to 15 degree tilt of the tube) permits the least interrupted postero-anterior view of the orbit.

2. **Lateral View of Each Orbit Employing a Short Film-target Distance So As to Obscure the More Distant Orbit** (Fig. 7–12). This permits a lateral perspective, although it is not very satisfactory since there is too much interference between the two sides.

3. **Special View of the Optic Foramina** (Fig. 7–16). In view of the medial and inferior position of the optic foramen, it is not seen clearly except in the oblique projection demonstrated. An oblique view of the ethmoid air cells is also obtained in the same film study.

4. **Demonstration of Foreign Bodies Within the Orbit or Eye.** Special techniques are employed which are outside the scope of this normal anatomic consideration. Suffice it to say that tangential views of the anterior segment of the eyeball on dental films are very valuable adjuncts in this regard, particularly if obtained with the eye looking upward, downward, to each side, and straight ahead—each on a separate dental-type film. These dental film views are utilized in addition to Sweet localization films, or views of the orbit with a special disk on the anesthetized eye.

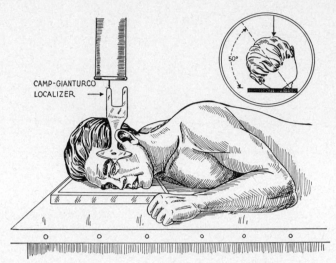

FIG. 7–16. SPECIAL VIEW OF OPTIC FORAMINA: **a,** Positioning of patient. (A 12 degree tilt of the tube toward the feet centered over the orbit may also be used.)

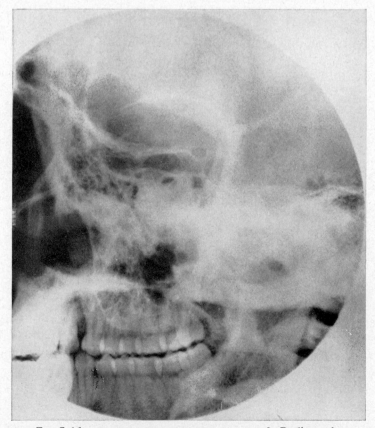

FIG. 7–16. SPECIAL VIEW OF OPTIC FORAMINA: **b,** Radiograph.

POINTS OF PRACTICAL INTEREST WITH REFERENCE TO FIGURE 7–16:

1. The position of the patient in this view is identical to that of Stenvers' view of the petrous ridges. The central ray of the x-ray beam, however, is directed 12 degrees *toward the feet*, if the angulated beam is employed, instead of 12 degrees *toward the head* (Stenvers' view).
2. When one studies optic foramina, the two sides are compared with one another; hence, equivalent views of the two sides must be obtained.
3. The ethmoid air cells are also clearly delineated here to best advantage.

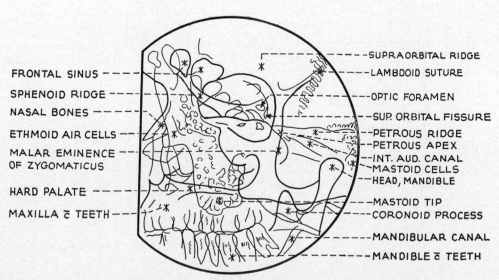

FRONTAL SINUS

SPHENOID RIDGE

NASAL BONES

ETHMOID AIR CELLS

MALAR EMINENCE
OF ZYGOMATICUS

HARD PALATE

MAXILLA c̄ TEETH

SUPRAORBITAL RIDGE

LAMBDOID SUTURE

OPTIC FORAMEN

SUP. ORBITAL FISSURE

PETROUS RIDGE
PETROUS APEX
INT. AUD. CANAL
MASTOID CELLS
HEAD, MANDIBLE

MASTOID TIP
CORONOID PROCESS

MANDIBULAR CANAL

MANDIBLE c̄ TEETH

FIG. 7–16. SPECIAL VIEW OF OPTIC FORAMINA: e, Labeled tracing of b.

THE TEMPORAL BONE

The temporal bone is usually divided into three portions: (*a*) the squamous portion; (*b*) the mastoid portion; and (*c*) the petrous portion (Fig. 7–17). These are practical subdivisions in the adult bone, but do not represent separate portions developmentally.

The *squamous portion* is largely a bony plate which helps form the calvarium laterally.

The *mastoid portion* is formed from both the squamous and petrous portions and this junction is indicated by the petrosquamous suture, which is somewhat variable in appearance and must not be misconstrued as a fracture.

The mastoid process itself is perforated by numerous foramina—the largest being the mastoid foramen which transmits the mastoid branch of the occipital artery, and a vein to the transverse sinus. The sigmoid groove for the transverse sinus is found on the inner aspect of the mastoid process.

The interior of the mastoid process contains numerous air cells which open into a common chamber—the mastoid or tympanic antrum. The latter communicates with the upper part of the tympanic cavity or epitympanic recess. There are three groups of cells in the mastoid portion: (1) the anterosuperior; (2) the middle; and (3) the apical. These have been further subdivided according to position into: (1) eustachian; (2) zygomatic; (3) cells along floor of middle fossa; (4) sublabyrinthine; (5) squamous; (6) lateral sinus cells; (7) marginal; (8) retrofacial; and (9) mastoid tip cells (Fig. 7–18).

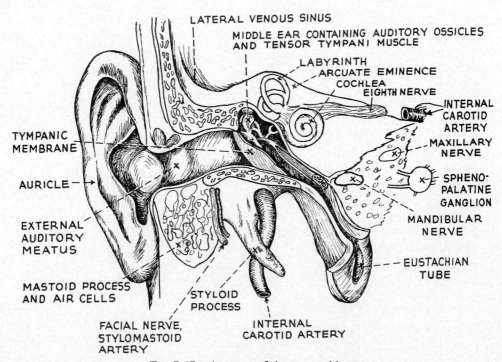

Fig. 7–17. Anatomy of the temporal bone.

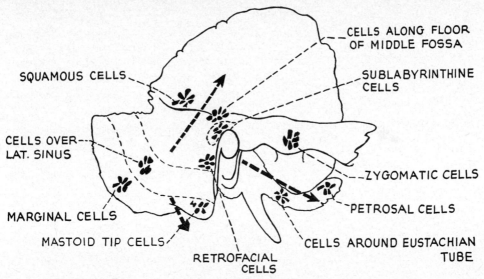

CELLS ALONG FLOOR OF MIDDLE FOSSA

SQUAMOUS CELLS

SUBLABYRINTHINE CELLS

CELLS OVER LAT. SINUS

ZYGOMATIC CELLS

MARGINAL CELLS

PETROSAL CELLS

MASTOID TIP CELLS

RETROFACIAL CELLS

CELLS AROUND EUSTACHIAN TUBE

Fig. 7–18. Cellular groups within the temporal bone. (Modification of Tremble, Arch. Oto-laryng. vol. 19, 1934.)

Their degree of pneumatization is very variable.

The *petrous portion* is a pyramid with two surfaces contained within the cranial cavity and one directed downward at the base of the skull.

On its *posteromedial surface* is situated the internal auditory meatus. At the bottom of this meatus (or canal) is a plate of bone pierced by numerous foramina known as the lamina cribrosa. This canal transmits the facial (seventh), auditory (eighth) and glossopalatine nerves and the internal auditory artery.

The anterosuperior surface of the pyramid contains: (1) an impression for the semilunar ganglion of the trigeminal nerve near the apex; (2) the hiatus of the facial canal; (3) the arcuate eminence, under which the superior semi-circular canal of the vestibular mechanism lies; and (4) the tegmen tympani laterally, which is a thin bony roof over the tympanic cavity.

The basilar surface of the pyramid is very irregular and presents important structures such as the carotid canal, jugular fossa, stylomastoid process and foramen. (The medial and posterior walls of the tympanic cavity of the temporal bone are sometimes described as a fourth surface.)

The tympanic cavity or middle ear is an air space about 2 to 4 mm. by 15 mm., lined with modified mucous membrane, situated between the external and internal ear (Fig. 7–17). It contains three small movable bones—the malleus, incus and stapes—and their attached ligaments and muscles which form a chain connecting the tympanic membrane and internal ear. It has an air space superiorly and posteriorly which is continuous with the mastoid antrum, and another anteriorly and inferiorly whereby it communicates with the eustachian tube and nasopharynx. It is in close proximity antero-inferiorly with the internal carotid artery and jugular vein. Medially, the tympanic cavity has a minute opening communicating with the vestibule (fenestra vestibuli). There is another minute opening covered by a membrane communicating with the cochlea (fenestra cochleae)—both parts of the internal ear. The internal ear is the essential organ of hearing and consists of a cavity known as the osseous labyrinth, and membrane-like structures which fit snugly into the bony shell. The osseous labyrinth which can be identified radiographically[2] is divided into the following portions: (1) the cochlear (containing the cochlea); (2) the semicircular canal-icular (containing the semicircular canals); and (3) the vestibular, containing two sacs, called the utricle and saccule respectively. There is a fluid substance filling all the remaining space (perilymph), and a similar but separate fluid substance within the membranous structures proper (endolymph).

The apex of the pyramid (of the petrous bone) presents the medial opening of the carotid canal through which the internal carotid artery passes into the skull.

The external auditory meatus is formed partly by the tympanic and partly by the squamous portions. It is an elliptical bony canal which is continuous with a cartilaginous tube to the nasopharynx.

The Development of the Temporal Bone. Developmentally, there are three parts which differ slightly from the adult subdivisions: The petromastoid portion contains the internal ear; the tympanic portion partially encloses the external auditory canal—with the middle ear lying between the petromastoid and tympanic portions; the squamozygomatic division forms part of the side wall of the skull and the roof of the external auditory canal. In the infant, the petro-squamosal suture has considerable clinical significance because it opens directly into the tympanic cavity and affords a pathway for the extension of infections from the middle ear to the meninges and brain. This suture closes slowly until 5 years of age when it is obliterated in about one half of the cases.

The mastoid process is not present at birth, and at this time the tympanic portion is a thin bony ring incomplete superiorly, and the squamosa is very thin and smooth. At birth, the cavities of the auditory tube, tympanic cavity and mastoid antrum are filled with mucoid material which is discharged through the auditory tube (eustachian tube) with respiration. Thereafter, pneumatization of the mastoid and petrous pyramids results by evaginations of epithelium from the primary cavities, and they all communicate directly or indirectly with the mastoid antrum, middle ear or eustachian tube. Thus, any infection of the one almost invariably involves the entire temporal bone if it is pneumatized.

The greater part of the process of formation of the air cells occurs in childhood, prior to adolescence, but this is very variable, and may be different on the two sides in the same individual. Thus, a middle ear infection may retard pneumatization on the one side considerably; also, it may allow the development of diploic cells only, rather than cells of a mixed type, such as occur normally when the development is uninterrupted.

ROUTINE STUDY OF THE PETROUS RIDGES AND MASTOID PROCESSES

This is usually a complete study of the temporal bone, and involves a study of the mastoid process from at least two vantage points, as well as the petrous ridge from at least two different perspectives.

1. **Lateral Projection of the Mastoid Process (Law's Position)** (Fig. 7–19). The various cellular groups are quite clearly delineated, along with a superposition of the internal and external acoustic meatuses, the lateral sinus plate, and the emissary vein posterior to the mastoid process.

2. **Tangential View of the Mastoid Tips** (Fig. 7–20).   This is virtually an antero-posterior view of the mastoid processes, but shows the mastoid air cells in the projecting portion of the mastoid in particular in unobstructed fashion. Other structures of the petrous ridge can also be identified if the exposure is sufficiently heavy, but ordinarily separate views are obtained for this purpose.

3. **Postero-anterior View of the Petrous Ridge with the Ridge Placed Parallel to the Film (Stenvers' Position)** (Fig. 7–21).   This is an unobstructed view of the petrous ridge obtained by placing the skull so that the petrous ridge is parallel with the film. An unobstructed view is obtained of the petrous apex, and the entire bone stands out as a pyramidal structure. Usually the bony labyrinth (semicircular canals, vestibule and cochlea) can be identified together with the internal auditory meatus and canal. The cellular structure is also clearly seen.

4. **Supero-inferior Projection of the Petrous Ridges** (Fig. 6–25).   This is obtained by means of Towne's position already described. This is the antero-posterior projection with 30 to 35 degree tilt of the tube caudally. As previously indicated, an excellent perspective of both petrous ridges is obtained, along with the view of the occipital bone, foramen magnum and dorsum sellae.

5. **Mayer's Position of the Mastoids** (Fig. 7–22).   This view is especially useful in separation of the anatomic structures of the middle ear as a prerequisite for fenestration operations. It is difficult to duplicate this view from patient to patient and hence the anatomic depiction is somewhat variable.

THE SELLA TURCICA

Deformity of the sella turcica is often the only clue that abnormality exists within the cranium, and hence a familiarity with its anatomy and radiologic appearance is essential.

The sella turcica is the superior saddle-shaped formation on the intracranial aspect of the body of the sphenoid bone. It is bounded anteriorly and posteriorly by the anterior and posterior clinoid processes respectively. The following parts of the sella are differentiated (Fig. 7–23): (1) the dorsum sellae; (2) the tuberculum sellae; (3) the hypophyseal fossa; (4) the anterior clinoid processes; and (5) the posterior clinoid processes.

The Dorsum Sellae.   This is a square-shaped plate of bone which is situated on the posterior aspect of the sella turcica and which terminates in the two posterior clinoid processes which project laterally and upward. This segment of bone is usually about 1 mm. in thickness when viewed on the lateral radiograph of the skull, with only a slight concavity on its anterior superior aspect, and another slight posterior concavity as it merges into the clivus. Abnormal erosion of the dorsum sellae is of great pathologic significance.

The Tuberculum Sellae.   The tuberculum sellae is a prominence on the anterosuperior wall of the sella turcica. It lies immediately beneath a prominent variable ridge known as the limbus sphenoidalis. There is usually a groove for the optic chiasma just anterior to the tuberculum sellae, and the optic foramina are situated on either side of it, immediately beneath and medial to the anterior clinoid processes.

The Hypophyseal Fossa.   This is the basal concavity of the sella turcica which houses the pituitary gland. In a straight lateral projection, it appears to

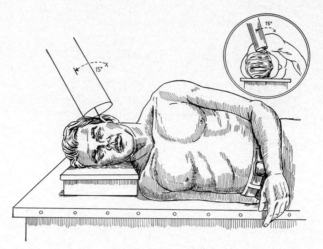

FIG. 7–19.   LATERAL PROJECTION OF MASTOID PROCESS: **a**, Positioning of patient.

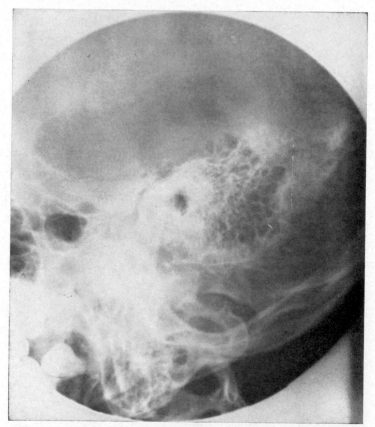

FIG. 7–19.   LATERAL PROJECTION OF MASTOID PROCESS: **b**, Radiograph.

POINTS OF PRACTICAL INTEREST WITH REFERENCE TO FIGURE 7-19:

1. There are actually two different ways of obtaining this projection—both acceptable. The alternative to the one shown is by placing a 15 degree angle board under the patient's head and utilizing a central ray that is perpendicular to the table top and centered to the mastoid process which is closest to the film. Thus, instead of angling the tube as shown here, the patient's head is angled an equivalent amount instead.

2. The routine recommended for study of this projection is as follows:

   (a) Note the degree of pneumatization, and whether the cells are diploic, small, mixed or large.

   (b) Note the relative radiolucency of the cells, and the integrity of their walls.

   (c) Trace the integrity of the lateral sinus plate.

   (d) Locate and state the size of the emissary vein.

   (e) Study the auditory meatuses for erosion or enlargement.

   (f) Note the integrity of the temporomandibular joint.

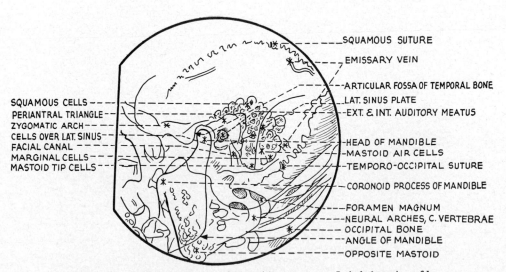

FIG. 7-19. Lateral projection of mastoid process: c, Labeled tracing of b.

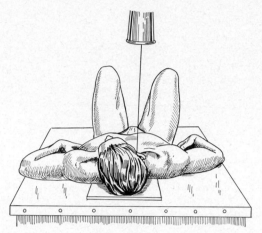

Fig. 7–20.   TANGENTIAL VIEW OF MASTOID TIPS.   **a,** Positioning of patient.

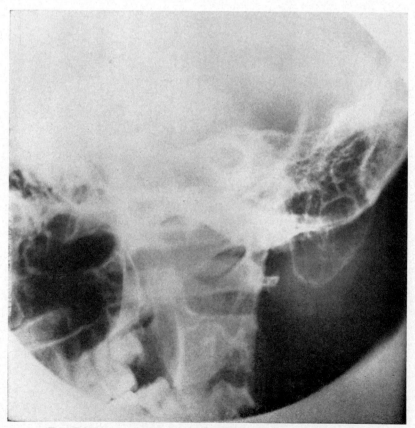

FIG. 7–20.   TANGENTIAL VIEW OF MASTOID TIPS: **b,** Radiograph.

Points of Practical Interest with Reference to Figure 7–20:

1. The auricles of the ears should be folded forward to avoid the projection of the pinna over the mastoid structures.
2. The smallest possible cone should be employed at a fairly close target-to-film distance (25 to 30 inches). The head is rotated 45 degrees away from the side being radiographed, and the tube is angled 15 degrees caudally, centering over the midpoint of the cantho-meatal line.
3. In this view the mastoid process is projected away from the rest of the calvarium, and the mastoid cells in the tip of the process are shown to best advantage. A somewhat lighter exposure technique must be employed to gain this view. This same projection, however, may also be used to visualize the petrous portion of the temporal bone if a somewhat heavier exposure technique is employed.
4. Comparison films between the two mastoids are always obtained.

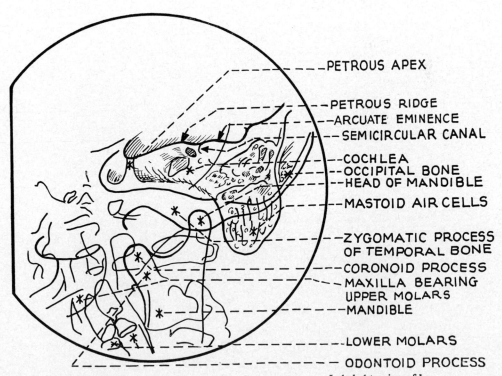

FIG. 7–20. TANGENTIAL VIEW OF MASTOID TIPS: c, Labeled tracing of b.

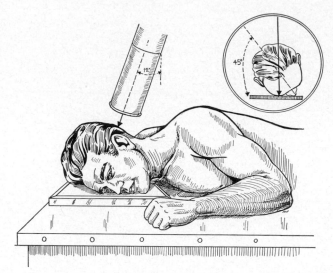

FIG. 7–21. STENVERS' VIEW OF PETROUS RIDGE: **a,** Positioning of patient.

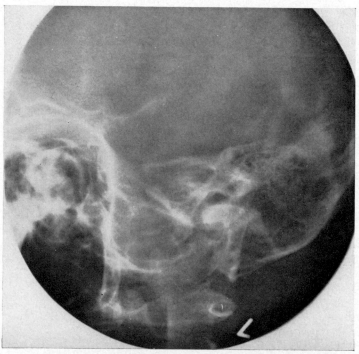

FIG. 7–21. STENVERS' VIEW OF PETROUS RIDGE: **b,** Radiograph.

POINTS OF PRACTICAL INTEREST WITH REFERENCE TO FIGURE 7–21:

1. Position the patient's head so that the tip of the nose, the point of the chin, and the outer canthus of the eye are all in contact with the plane of the film. This will place the head at an angle of approximately 45 degrees with respect to the film.
2. Adjust the central ray so that it passes to the midpoint of the film at an angle of 12 degrees.
3. In this position the petrous ridge is parallel with the plane of the film and its longest axis is shown to best advantage.
4. This view may also be utilized for visualization of the tips of the mastoid cells if a lighter exposure technique is employed. However, when satisfactory exposure factors are utilized to see the innermost aspect of the petrous ridge, the mastoid air cells and the tips of the mastoids will not be seen to good advantage except in an extremely bright light.

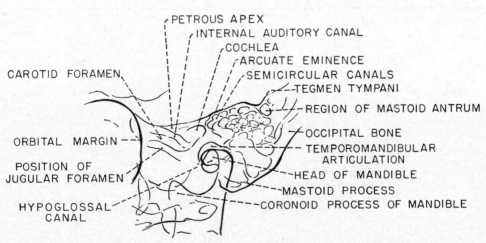

FIG. 7–21. STENVERS' VIEW OF PETROUS RIDGE: c, Labeled tracing of b.

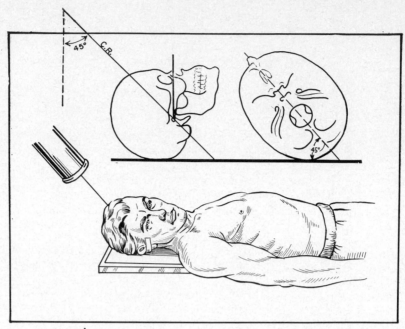

MAYER'S POSITION *(FOR PETROUS RIDGE AND MASTOIDS)*

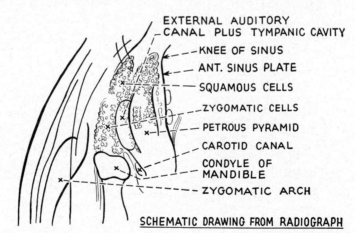

EXTERNAL AUDITORY
CANAL PLUS TYMPANIC CAVITY
KNEE OF SINUS
ANT. SINUS PLATE
SQUAMOUS CELLS
ZYGOMATIC CELLS
PETROUS PYRAMID
CAROTID CANAL
CONDYLE OF MANDIBLE
ZYGOMATIC ARCH

SCHEMATIC DRAWING FROM RADIOGRAPH

FIG. 7–22.   Mayer's position for examination of petrous ridge and mastoids.

form a dense single curved line which lies above the sphenoid sinus. In infants, it tends to be shallow, and somewhat prolonged in its antero-posterior dimension owing to the incomplete formation and ossification of the structures in the immediate vicinity of the tuberculum sellae. When the floor of the hypophyseal fossa takes on a double-contoured appearance, this manifestation may have considerable pathologic significance.

The Anterior Clinoid Processes.   The posterior border of the lesser wing of the sphenoid is prolonged medially as the anterior clinoid process on either side. Between the anterior clinoid process and the tuberculum sellae is a notch which marks the termination of the carotid groove for passage of the internal carotid artery.

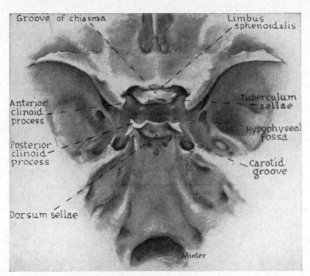

FIG. 7–23. A common type of sella turcica. (From *Head and Neck in Roentgen Diagnosis*, by Pendergrass, Schaeffer and Hodes, Charles C Thomas.)

The *carotid groove* begins at the medial side of the irregular foramen lacerum and ends medial to the anterior clinoid processes as described above. Occasionally there is a bony projection of this groove at its termination with the anterior clinoid process, producing the caroticoclinoid foramen.

The transverse distance between the anterior clinoid processes is considerably greater than the corresponding distance between the posterior clinoid processes, and occasionally the posterior clinoid processes project forward so that they are situated between them. On the lateral radiograph of the skull, this imparts to the sella an "overbridged" appearance, and it appears that the anterior and posterior clinoid processes are continuous with one another. Such continuity of bony substance does occur over the hypophyseal fossa but is rather rare.

Posterior Clinoid Processes. Occasionally the sphenoidal sinus extends into the posterior clinoid processes, giving them an aerated appearance. The superior petrosal process projects from the lateral border of the dorsum sellae, giving attachment to the petrosphenoidal ligament. The latter ligament is occasionally ossified, forming a foramen or canal (Dorello's canal) through which the inferior petrosal venous sinus and the abducens nerve (sixth cranial nerve) must pass before entering the cavernous venous sinus.

Normal Measurements of the Sella Turcica (Fig. 7–24). The antero-posterior dimension may be defined as the greatest distance between the anterior and posterior walls of the sella. A line is usually taken between a point below the tuberculum sellae and the anterior margin of the dorsum sellae. The depth is the greatest distance between the floor of the hypophyseal fossa and a line drawn between the tuberculum sellae and the top of the dorsum sellae. This latter line represents the position of the diaphragma sellae.

Camp,[1] in a study of 500 normal cases, stated that the minimal antero-posterior measurements were 5 mm. and the maximal 16 mm.; the average was 10.5 mm. The depth measurements were: minimal, 4 mm., maximal 12 mm.,

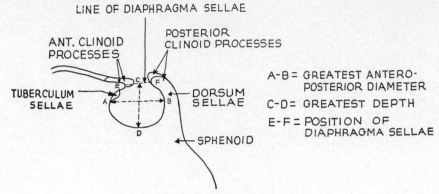

FIG. 7–24.   Method of measuring the sella turcica.

and average 8.1 mm. These correspond closely with those given by others. It is understood that these are the measurements when a 36-inch target-to-film distance is employed.

Other methods of measurement have been advocated, but have received lesser acceptance thus far.

ROUTINE RADIOGRAPHIC METHODS OF STUDY OF THE SELLA TURCICA

1. **Lateral Stereoscopic Projection of the Sella Turcica** (Fig. 6–26).   The technique employed is similar to that used for the lateral view of the skull as a whole, except that a small cone is applied and the central ray is directed over a point approximately midway between the anterior tubercle of the pinna and the outer canthus of the eye. Stereoscopic films are obtained.

2. **Towne's Projection of the Skull** (Fig. 6–25).   This view has already been described and should project the dorsum sellae and posterior clinoid processes into the foramen magnum. One can usually also identify the anterior clinoid processes.

3. **Postero-anterior View of the Skull** (Fig. 6–24).   In this projection the tuberculum sellae and the anterior clinoid processes are frequently identified, although detail is usually poor in view of the overlying skull structures.

4. **Body Section Radiographs.**   This method has not proved as useful here as in other parts of the anatomy, but may on occasion furnish corroborative information which has already been indicated by the other methods of investigation.

5. **Axial View of the Skull** (Fig. 6–27).   In this view the floor of the sella turcica and adjoining anatomic structures may be seen to good advantage.

REFERENCES

1. Camp, J.: Normal and Pathological Anatomy of the Sella Turcica as Revealed by Roentgenograms. Am. J. Roentgenol., *12:* 143–155, 1924.
2. Pendergrass, E. P., Hodes, P. J., Tondreau, R., and Marden, P.: The Tympanic Cavity and Auditory Ossicles—Roentgen Findings in Health and Disease. Am. J. Roentgenol., *76:* 327–342, 1956.
3. Pendergrass, E. P., Schaeffer, J. P., and Hodes, P. J.: *The Head and Neck in Roentgen Diagnosis.* 2nd Ed. Charles C Thomas, Springfield, Illinois, 1956.
4. Proetz, A. W.: The Displacement Method of Sinus Diagnosis and Treatment. Annals Publishing Company, St. Louis, 1931.

CHAPTER 8

The Radiographic
Study of the Brain

PNEUMOENCEPHALOGRAPHY AND VENTRICULOGRAPHY

APART FROM those regions which may normally contain calcium within the brain and adjoining structures (see Chap. 6), the brain itself is not normally radiopaque. Occasionally, an abnormality may contain excessive calcium and thus be manifest; a normally calcified structure may be displaced and thus give indirect evidence of abnormality; or there may be secondary changes in the cranial bones which give evidence of abnormality in the brain, vascular structures or meninges. For the most part, however, the brain must be investigated by the injection of a contrast medium into the various potential or real spaces surrounding and within the brain, or it must be studied indirectly by injecting contrast media into the arterial system leading to the brain, and examining the arteriograms and venograms so obtained.

The importance of these studies can hardly be emphasized sufficiently, since most neurosurgical procedures involving the brain require a radiographic study of the brain as a prerequisite. This examination, however, is a very specialized one, and requires considerable experience and intensive study, and is usually performed by the neurosurgeon and radiologist working together as a team.

Contrast Media Employed. Both positive and negative contrast media have been employed in the study of the potential and actual spaces within the brain. Thorotrast is the radiopaque medium that has been employed in very small quantities, but in view of its inherent radioactivity and irritative effects, it has never gained wide favor. The negative or radiolucent medium is the one most universally employed.

Among the negative contrast media, almost all available gases have been used at one time or another. Air (filtered through sterile cotton) is the most readily available and easily used, but has the disadvantage of being very slowly absorbed over a period of seven to eleven days, with considerable discomfort to the patient in the meantime. It has the advantage of permitting a 24-hour study, if such is desired, and there are some who insist that a complete study should encompass the 24-hour period. Many investigators, however, have come to prefer the more readily absorbed gases such as oxygen or helium, especially the former as it is more readily available.

319

The quantity of gas utilized is also variable. Some use very small quantities such as 15 to 20 cc. (Robertson[13]) and investigate the ventricles by tilting the patient in many planes and directions. Lindgren[10] has advocated the injection of small quantities of air (5 to 7 cc.) similarly without withdrawal of cerebrospinal fluid. By carefully positioning the patient's head (Fig. 8–1) a clearer visualization of the fourth ventricle, cerebral aqueduct, posterior fossa cisterns, and cisterna ambiens is obtained, after repeated small injections of air. Usually, however, practically all the cerebrospinal fluid is drained off, intermittently replacing it with the gas, utilizing 80 to 120 cc. during the course of the examination.

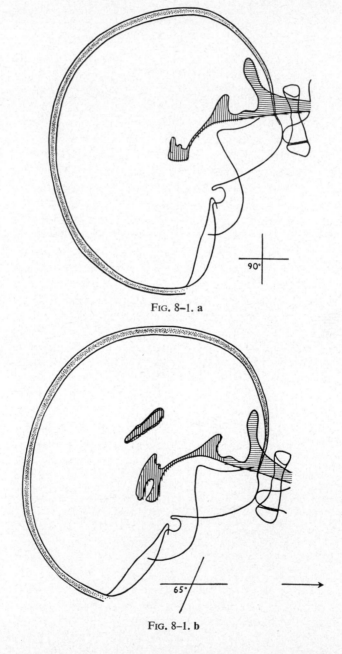

FIG. 8–1. a

FIG. 8–1. b

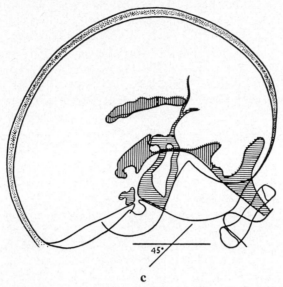

c

FIG. 8–1.   The relationship of posture to the distribution of gas in the cadaver. In **a** the flexion is 90 degrees, in **b** 65 degrees, in **c** 45 degrees. (From Robertson: *Pneumoencephalography*, Charles C Thomas.)

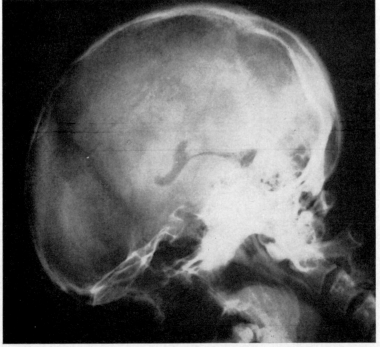

FIG. 8–1. **d,** Radiograph obtained by the Robertson-Lindgren technique (45 degree flexion).

Techniques of Investigation.   The contrast medium may be injected through the lumbar subarachnoid space, or directly into the ventricles through small trephine holes in the calvarium just behind the posterior horns of the lateral ventricles. The former method is called "pneumoencephalography" in contrast to the more direct surgical approach which is called "ventriculography." Ventriculograms must be employed in the presence of increased intracranial pressure to avoid a herniation of the medulla and cerebellum through the foramen magnum (pressure cone formation). The disadvantage of ventriculograms is that they fail to demonstrate the subarachnoid spaces surrounding the brain and the basal cisterns as satisfactorily as do the pneumoencephalograms, and the introduction of the trocar through the posterior cerebrum is not without danger of injury to the brain substance.

In either case, the procedure is accompanied by considerable discomfort to the patient, and cannot be used indiscriminately.

In children it is possible to employ a direct approach through the anterior fontanel if that is still open.

In accordance with techniques originally described by Laruelle[7] in 1933 and modified by E. Graeme Robertson,[13] Lindgren[10] and others, a spinal puncture is performed and a minimal amount of fluid is removed. A small quantity of gas (5 to 7 cc.) is first injected with the patient sitting in the erect position and the head flexed so that the acanthomeatal line is at 90 degrees with the horizontal. The patient's forehead is placed against the upright Bucky apparatus or grid casette. Additional films after further small injections are taken as the degree of flexion diminishes to 45 degrees and the gas passes from the fourth ventricle and cerebral aqueduct to the third ventricle. Often there is a clear visualization of the cisterna ambiens, and other basal cisterns. This technique is particularly valuable for visualization of the posterior fossa structures, without interference by gas shadows in other regions, as one can see by the accompanying illustration (Fig 8–1, **d**).

THE GROSS ANATOMY OF THE BRAIN AS RELATED TO RADIOLOGY

The Meninges.   The brain is completely invested by the meningeal membranes which are composed of three layers (Fig. 8–2): the dura mater, the arachnoid and the pia mater.

The cranial dura mater is at the same time the endosteal layer of the inner table of the calvarium, and its outer endosteal layer is everywhere adherent to the inner meningeal portion except where it separates to form venous sinuses

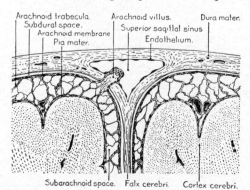

FIG. 8–2.   Schematic diagram of coronal section of meninges and cortex. (From Gray, *Anatomy of the Human Body*, Edited by C. M. Goss, courtesy of Lea & Febiger, Publishers.)

There are four projections of cranial dura mater which extend into the cavity of the skull: (1) the falx cerebri, which descends vertically in the longitudinal fissure between the two cerebral hemispheres; (2) the tentorium cerebelli, which arches over the cerebellum, and supports the occipital lobes of the brain; (3) the falx cerebelli, between the tentorium cerebelli and the occipital bone, which projects into the cerebellar notch; and (4) the diaphragma sellae, which roofs over the sella turcica.

Beneath the dura (and all of its projections), and between it and the arachnoid is the potential space known as the subdural cavity. This normally contains only a small amount of fluid.

The arachnoid is a thin membrane which does not dip into the sulci or fissures, with the exception of the longitudinal fissure.

The subarachnoid cavity or space lies between the arachnoid and the pia mater. There are numerous fine trabeculae between these two layers, producing intercommunicating channels in which the cerebrospinal fluid is contained. Since the pia mater is closely adherent to the brain whereas the arachnoid is not, the sulci and fissures contain greater quantities of gas during pneumoencephalography, and many can be differentiated.

At certain parts of the base of the brain the arachnoid is separated from the pia mater by wide spaces called subarachnoid cisterns. These will be described in greater detail subsequently.

In pneumoencephalography, the air is introduced into the subarachnoid space of the lumbar region and will circulate in this space almost exclusively. Frequently, however, it will enter the subdural space either overlying the brain, or beneath the tentorium cerebelli, and produce a tent-shaped appearance here. Occasionally, air will enter the subdural space exclusively, with virtually no visualization of the subarachnoid space. This variation has no abnormal significance, and upon repeating the examination a more satisfactory result is usually obtained. Subdural air overlying the brain may at times be confused with cerebral or cortical atrophy, unless the examiner is aware of this possibility.

Not infrequently after the introduction of air in the lumbar subarachnoid space, only the sulci surrounding the brain are visualized, and the ventricles are not. This appearance will be described more fully below.

Subdivisions of the Brain. The brain is divided into five principal parts (Figs. 8–3, 8–4): (1) the cerebrum, composed of two cerebral hemispheres, lying above a plane drawn between the internal occipital protuberance, the petrous ridges and the floor of the anterior cranial fossa; (2) the cerebellum, composed of two hemispheres and a small central portion called the vermis, lying in the posterior fossa; (3) the midbrain, which lies between the cerebral hemispheres above, and the hindbrain below; (4) the pons, lying beneath the fourth ventricle between the cerebral peduncles above and the medulla oblongata below; and (5) the medulla oblongata, which lies immediately above the spinal cord above the level of the foramen magnum.

The Convolutions of the Brain, Gyri, Sulci and Fissures, Lateral Aspect. The cerebral hemispheres have numerous folds following a rather definite pattern which are called gyri or convolutions, and these are separated from each other

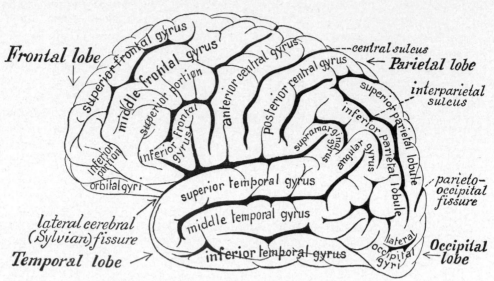

FIG. 8–3.   **a,** The subdivisions, major sulci and gyri of the lateral aspect of the brain. (From Sobotta and McMurrich, *Atlas and Textbook of Human Anatomy.*)

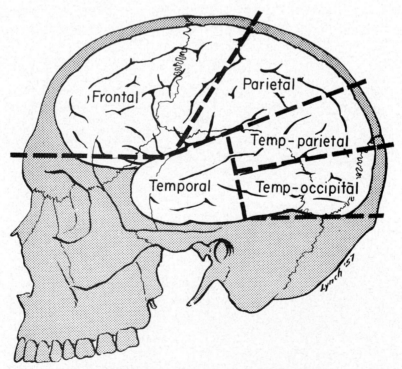

FIG. 8–3.   **b,** Diagram showing the position of the various subdivisions of the brain as considered clinically and radiologically (supratentorial).

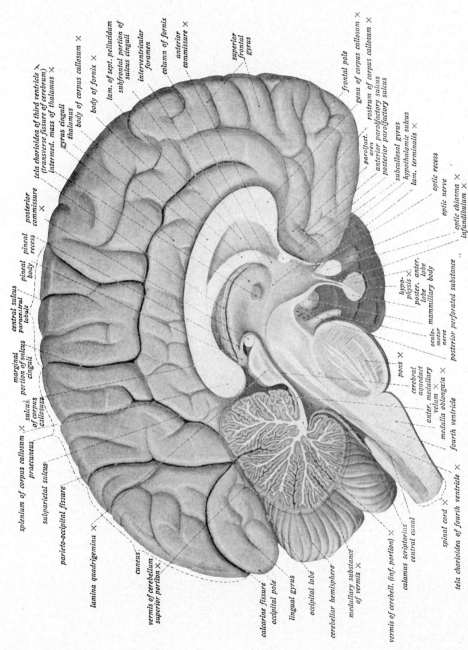

tela chorioidea of third ventricle ✕
(transverse fissure of cerebrum) ✕
intermed. mass of thalamus ✕
lam. of sept. pellucidum
subfrontal portion of
sulcus cinguli
interventricular
foramen
column of fornix
anterior
commissure ✕
superior
frontal
gyrus
gyrus cinguli
thalamus
body of corpus callosum ✕
body of fornix ✕

frontal pole
genu of corpus callosum ✕
rostrum of corpus callosum ✕
paralfact.
area
anterior parolfactory sulcus
posterior parolfactory sulcus
subcallosal gyrus
hypothalamic sulcus
lam. terminalis ✕
optic recess
optic nerve
optic chiasma ✕
infundibulum ✕

posterior
commissure
✕

pineal
recess

pineal
body

pineal
recess

central sulcus
paracentral
lobule

marginal
portion of sulcus
cinguli

sulcus
of corpus
callosum

hypo-
physis ✕
poster. anter.
lobe lobe
oculo-
mammillary body
oculo-
motor
nerve
posterior perforated substance

pons ✕
cerebral
aqueduct
anter. medullary
velum ✕
medulla oblongata ✕
fourth ventricle

splenium of corpus callosum ✕
praecuneus
subparietal sulcus
parieto-occipital fissure
lamina quadrigemina ✕
cuneus
vermis of cerebellum
superior portion ✕
calcarine fissure
occipital pole
lingual gyrus
occipital lobe
cerebellar hemisphere
medullary substance
of vermis ✕
vermis of cerebell. (inf. portion) ✕
calamus scriptorius
central canal
spinal cord ✕
tela chorioidea of fourth ventricle ✕

Fig. 8–4. MEDIAL SAGITTAL SECTION OF BRAIN: **a,** The subdivisions, major sulci and gyri. (From Sobotta and McMurrich, *Atlas and Textbook of Human Anatomy*.)

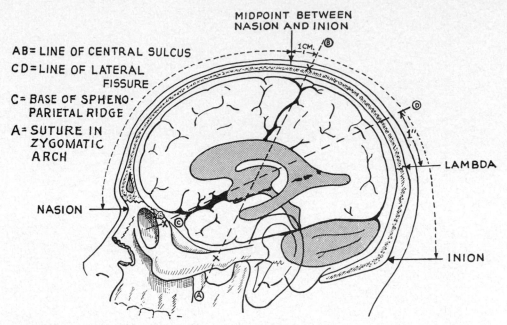

FIG. 8–4. MEDIAL SAGITTAL SECTION OF BRAIN: **b,** Relationship of the central sulcus and latera
fissure to the ventricles and skull.

by grooves called sulci, if they are shallow, and fissures when they are deep
(Figs. 8–3, 8–4). The fissures tend to separate the cerebral hemispheres into
various lobes. Thus, the lateral cerebral fissure separates the temporal lobe
below from the frontal lobe anteriorly and the parietal lobe superiorly, and the
central fissure separates the frontal lobe anteriorly from the parietal lobe
posteriorly. The central lobe, or island of Reil, lies deep within the lateral fissure, and is ordinarily not seen unless the latter structure is separated. The
demarcation of the occipital lobe from the parietal lobe is less clearly defined
by the lateral portion of the parieto-occipital fissure, and a line running from
this fissure to the preoccipital notch.

The right and left cerebral hemisphere are separated by the great longitudinal fissure, which is occupied by a projection of dura known as the falx
cerebri. In the depth of this fissure centrally is the corpus callosum, which
acts as a bridge connecting the two cerebral hemispheres. The falx is rigidly
fixed and virtually cannot be displaced except with considerable force.

The sulci over the lateral convexities of the cerebral hemispheres are difficult to identify on pneumoencephalograms.

In the frontal lobes are situated three major gyri, the superior, middle and
inferior, each separated by a corresponding sulcus.

The temporal lobes also possess three major gyri, the superior, middle and
inferior—and ordinarily these cannot be identified on the lateral pneumoencephalogram.

The parieto-occipital fissure and the calcarine fissure of the occipital lobe
are other division lines which may be identified, but other landmarks of the
occipital lobe are less constant.

The gyri of the cerebellar hemispheres are not recognizable as such unless a considerable measure of cerebellar atrophy exists.

The deduction of the presence of cerebral atrophy is based on an evaluation of the size and presence of these various sulci on the pneumoencephalogram, together with an estimation of ventricular enlargement. Assistance may also be obtained by studying Figure 8–4, **b,** in which the relationships of the ventricles and the central and lateral fissures to the skull are seen.

The Median Sagittal View of the Brain. A sagittal section of the brain shows the cerebral hemisphere above the cerebellum, which lies posteriorly and below the occipital lobe. The temporal lobe is seen together with the mid-brain, pons, medulla oblongata, corpus callosum and fornix, these latter structures being seen in cross section. The septum pellucidum is visible, interposed between the fornix and corpus callosum. The smooth medial surface of the thalamus is exposed, forming a portion of the lateral wall of the third ventricle.

In this section the third and fourth ventricles are opened in the sagittal plane and the cerebral aqueduct connecting their cavities, together with the foramen of Monro high on the wall of the third ventricle, are seen. The relationship of the pituitary body to the third ventricle and basal structures of the brain is well shown.

The Inferior Surface of the Brain (Fig. 8–5). This view of the brain shows the frontal lobes separated by the longitudinal fissure and anterior extremity of the corpus callosum. The olfactory tracts are embedded in the inferior aspect of the frontal lobes.

Posterior to the rostrum of the corpus callosum and centrally placed from before backward are situated (1) the optic chiasma, (2) the hypophysis, (3) the cerebral peduncles (enclosing the tuber cinereum, corpora mammillaria and posterior perforated substance), (4) the pons and (5) the medulla.

The temporal lobe and inferior surface of the cerebellum are seen and the various cranial nerves as they emerge from the brain substance are shown to good advantage.

The structures on the inferior aspect of the brain are identifiable on pneumoencephalograms in considerable part (Figs. 8–6, 8–14). The pons, medulla oblongata and cerebellum lie in close relationship to the fourth ventricle, the cisterna pontis, and the cisterna cerebellomedullaris, and are readily delineated by these air-containing structures.

Many of the other small structures are identified within the shadows of the basal cisterns, and these will be described in that connection below.

The Ventricular System (Fig. 8–6). The ventricles of the brain consist of a series of communicating cavities lined with ependymal epithelium. The ventricular system is divided into the two lateral ventricles, the third and the fourth ventricles. These ventricles are connected by small passageways—the interventricular foramina (Monro) connecting the two lateral ventricles with the third ventricle, and the cerebral aqueduct or aqueduct of Sylvius joining the third with the fourth ventricle.

THE LATERAL VENTRICLE (Fig. 8–6). The lateral ventricle consists of six parts: the anterior, posterior and temporal horns, and the body, which is arbitrarily divided into an anterior, middle and posterior third. The anterior horn, which is that portion anterior to the interventricular foramina, turns laterally at an angle of about 45 degrees around the head of the caudate nucleus and it terminates blindly in a pouch surrounded by the radiating fibers derived from the rostrum and genu of the corpus callosum (Fig. 8–7). When viewed from the anterior aspect, these anterior horns are separated by a wedge consisting of the genu of the corpus callosum, and more superiorly by the septum pellucidum. This latter structure widens anteriorly and is continuous with the anterior pillars of the fornix. At the junction of the anterior horn and body of the lateral ventricles, there is frequently a dip or indentation present so marked as to lead to a suspicion of a small tumor of the corpus callosum, but it is considered to be due to a condensation of fine nerve fibers.

The cavity of each lateral ventricle extends from the interventricular foramen to a point opposite the splenium of the corpus callosum. The outline of the lateral ventricle in transverse section is triangular with a roof, a floor and a medial wall. The roof and rostral boundary are formed by the corpus callosum. The floor from lateral to medial is formed by the caudate nucleus, the stria terminalis, the terminal vein, the thalamus, the choroid plexus and the lateral portion of the fornix. The medial wall is formed by the posterior portion of the septum pellucidum. The posterior third of the body of the lateral ventricle

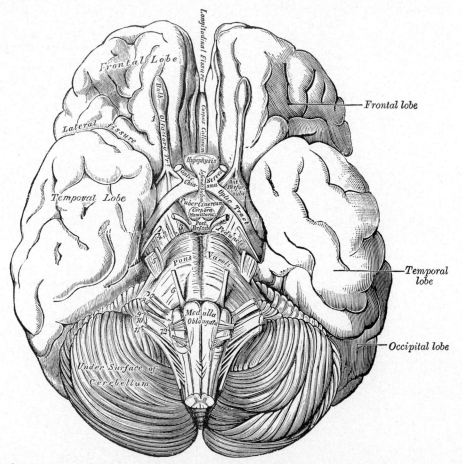

Fig. 8–5. View of the base of the brain. (From Gray, *Anatomy of the Human Body*, Edited by C. M. Goss, courtesy of Lea & Febiger.

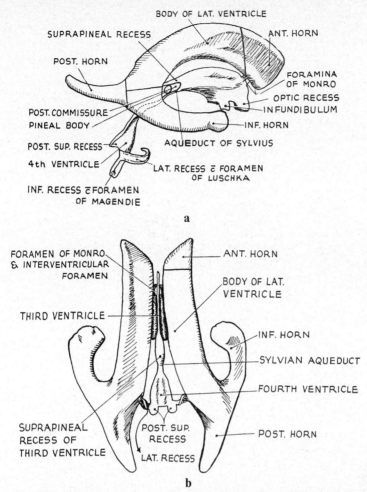

FIG. 8-6. VENTRICULAR SYSTEM OF THE BRAIN: a, Lateral projection; b, superior projection.

diverges from its junction with the middle third at an angle of approximately 35 degrees in a lateral direction and 60 degrees downward. The hippocampus is here added to the structures which form the floor of this portion of the body of the lateral ventricle (Fig. 8–7).

The occipital horn is the extension of the lateral ventricle into the occipital lobe. This is a variable structure and may not always appear.

The temporal horn courses downward and laterally and ends in a bulbous termination at a point about 2.5 cm. from the tip of the temporal lobe. In cross section it is a curved slit with the convexity dorsally placed, due to the swelling of the hippocampus. The roof is formed in great part by the inferior surface of the tapetum of the corpus callosum.

Near the junction of the body and the temporal horn, the glomus of the choroid plexus produces a defect in the gas shadow of each ventricle, and this may be augmented by the shadow of the hippocampus.

THE INTERVENTRICULAR FORAMINA (FORAMINA OF MONRO). The interventricular foramina (foramina of Monro) form a Y-shaped tubular structure connecting the paired lateral ventricles and the unpaired midline third ventricle.

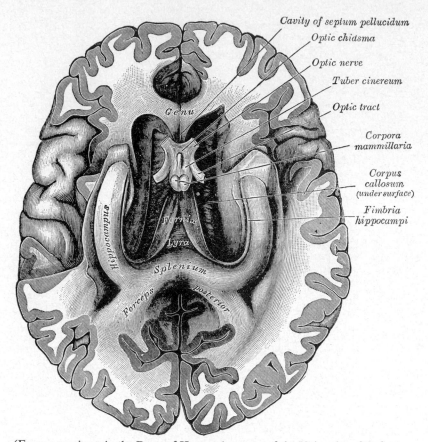

(From a specimen in the Dept. of Human Anatomy of the University of Oxford.

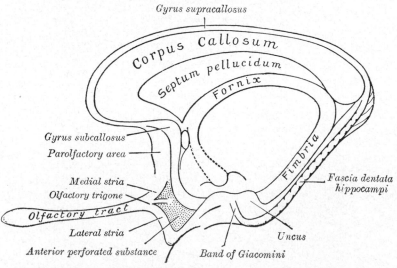

FIG. 8–7.   Relationship of the fornix and hippocampus to the ventricles. (From Gray, *Anatomy of the Human Body*, Edited by C. M. Goss, courtesy of Lea & Febiger.)

The lateral and posterior walls of each arm are formed by the anterior ends of the thalamus on which rest the choroid plexuses as they pass through these foramina from the roof of the third ventricle to the floor of the lateral ventricles. The anterior and medial walls are formed by the anterior pillars of the fornix.

THE THIRD VENTRICLE. The third ventricle is a midline cavity situated between the two thalami which in cross section is slitlike or lenticular in outline, and in sagittal section is trapezoid in shape. It is connected posteriorly with the fourth ventricle by the cerebral aqueduct. The anterior boundary is formed by the interventricular foramina, the anterior pillars of the fornix, and the anterior commissure and lamina terminalis. The floor is formed by the optic chiasma, infundibulum, tuber cinereum, corpora mammillaria, posterior perforate space, cerebral peduncles and tegmentum of the midbrain. The posterior boundary consists of the posterior commissure, pineal recess, pineal body and suprapineal recess. The posterior commissure can usually be identified just superior and posterior to the opening of the cerebral aqueduct. The roof is composed of a thin layer of epithelium stretching between the thalami. This latter is adherent to a layer of pia mater which is invaginated by the choroid plexuses of the third ventricle. Posteriorly, this invagination of the choroid produces a potentially weak covering, important as the site of occasional herniation. The lateral walls are formed by the medial surfaces of the thalami and hypothalamus. The middle commissure crosses the middle of the ventricle (also called the massa intermedia). The lowest portion represents the optic recess and infundibulum.

The width varies between 2 and 8 mm. and the length averages over 2 cm.

THE CEREBRAL AQUEDUCT. This narrow midline channel connects the third and fourth ventricles. It has an arched roof consisting of the quadrigeminal plate and posterior commissure, and a floor formed by the tegmentum of the midbrain. The cerebral peduncles lie anterior and slightly to either side. It measures about 1.5 cm. in length and 2 to 3 mm. in diameter.

THE FOURTH VENTRICLE. The fourth ventricle is a midline cavity which is diamond-shaped in the frontal projection and triangular in lateral cross section. It communicates superiorly with the third ventricle by means of the cerebra. aqueduct, and antero-inferiorly with the central canal of the medulla oblongatal Below in the midline and laterally in the lateral recesses it communicates with the cisterna magna (cerebellomedullaris) by the foramina of Magendie and Luschka respectively. The floor of this ventricle is made up of the ependymta covered surface of the pons and of the cephalic half of the medulla oblongaa.-Extending laterally and forward around the brain stem are the lateral recesses, at the extremities of which are located the foramina of Luschka, as described above.

The lateral boundaries of the fourth ventricle on each side from before backward are the superior, middle and inferior cerebellar peduncles. The roof of the fourth ventricle is composed of a tentlike structure called the medullary velum, which has an anterior and posterior segment and an apex (or fastigium) between. The peduncles of the cerebellum overlie this velum or covering. On the inner aspect of the posterior medullary velum is attached the choroid plexus of the fourth ventricle. Anterior to the plexus is the foramen of Magendie connecting the ventricle with the cisterna cerebellomedullaris.

The measurements of the fourth ventricle may be indicated as: 1.6 cm. (average) from the fastigium to the floor, and 4 cm. from the superior to the inferior angle.

The Subarachnoid Cisterns (Fig. 8–8). The important cisterns and their locations are:

CISTERNA CEREBELLOMEDULLARIS (CISTERNA MAGNA). This is the largest cistern, and is situated beneath the cerebellum and above the posterior surface of the medulla oblongata. It communicates with the fourth ventricle through the median aperture (foramen of Magendie), and the two lateral apertures (foramina of Luschka) which are the openings of the lateral superior recesses of the fourth ventricle.

CISTERNA PONTIS. The cisterna pontis is a large space situated on the ventral aspect of the pons. It is continuous anteriorly with the cisterna interpeduncularis and below with the subarachnoid cavity of the medulla spinalis. The pons may be readily delineated between the cisterna pontis and the floor of the fourth ventricle, having an average thickness of 2.8 cm. The basilar artery runs through the cisterna pontis and can frequently be identified on the pneumoencephalogram.

The measurement between the floor of the fourth ventricle and the dorsum sellae should not exceed 4 cm. (average 3.7 cm.). The cisterna pontis measures 5 to 12 mm. in its antero-posterior dimension.

CISTERNA BASALIS (CISTERNA CHIASMATICA AND INTERPEDUNCULARIS). The cisterna basalis consists of two parts—the cisterna chiasmatica, anterior to and between the optic chiasma, and the cisterna interpeduncularis, behind the chiasma. The chiasmatic portion of the basal cistern lies just above the hypophysis. Not infrequently the optic nerves, the oculomotor nerve and the infundibulum of the hypophysis may be clearly identified within this cistern. In the interpeduncular portion, the mammillary bodies, the oculomotor nerves and the posterior cerebral artery may occasionally be seen.

Occasionally, a third portion of the basal cistern is differentiated: a cisterna laminae terminalis, located above and anterior to the cisterna chiasmatica.

The basal cistern extends anteriorly upward over the knee of the corpus callosum, also forming the cisterna corpus callosi, which may frequently be identified on the antero-posterior and lateral pneumoencephalogram (Fig. 8–14).

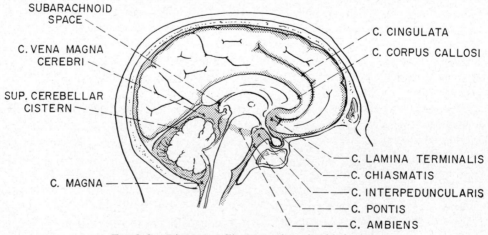

FIG. 8–8.   Diagram to illustrate subarachnoid cisterns.

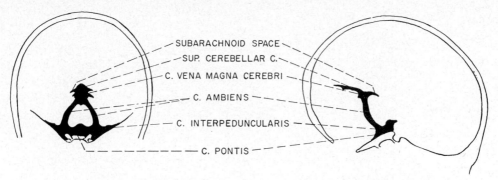

SUBARACHNOID SPACE
SUP. CEREBELLAR C.
C. VENA MAGNA CEREBRI
C. AMBIENS
C. INTERPEDUNCULARIS
C. PONTIS

FIG. 8–9. Cisterna ambiens in Towne's and lateral projections. (Modified from Robertson.)

CISTERNA AMBIENS (CISTERN OF THE GREAT CEREBRAL VEIN) (Fig. 8–9). This cistern occupies the interval between the quadrigeminal bodies and the splenium of the corpus callosum. It comes into relationship with the pineal body and the great cerebral vein of Galen. In the lateral roentgenogram this cistern is seen to consist of two parts—a dorsal portion, which is single and situated in the midline above the collicular plate, and a ventral portion, which is paired and situated laterally between the lateral aspects of the cerebral peduncles and the medial aspects of the hippocampal gyri. In the radiograph it is situated just ventral to the pineal body, and appears as a thin semilunar structure (Fig. 8–9).

CISTERNA OF THE LATERAL CEREBRAL FOSSA. This cistern is formed bilaterally in front of the temporal horns where the arachnoid bridges over the lateral fissure and the contained middle cerebral artery and its branches. This is not very frequently identified.

Cerebrospinal Fluid. It is probable that the cerebrospinal fluid is produced in the following regions (Fig. 8–10): (*a*) the choroid plexuses (1) of the ventricles, which produce most of the fluid; (*b*) the ependyma of the central canal of the spinal cord (7), lending a small current of fluid which tends to go cephalad; and (*c*) the perivascular linings of the blood vessels that enter and leave the brain in close proximity with the subarachnoid spaces.

The intraventricular fluid flows down the ventricles (2 to 5) to the fourth ventricle (6), and thereafter flows out of the fourth ventricle through the foramina of Magendie and Luschka into the subarachnoid space (8 to 13). There is probably no other communication between the intraventricular fluid and the subarachnoid fluid.

The fluid then distributes itself in the subarachnoid space underlying and covering the brain (8 to 13), and is ultimately absorbed by diffusion through the arachnoid villi (or granulations) into the great dural sinuses (14). There is also a small amount of absorption through the perineural lymphatics.

It is probable that the fluid in the subdural space is produced locally by its own mesothelial cells, but the exact relationship of this fluid to the cerebrospinal fluid is not known.

The Ventricles and Cisterns as They Appear on the Pneumoencephalogram (Figs. 8–11 and 8–13). The radiographic appearances of the ventricles and the cisterns of the brain follow closely the basic anatomy already described.

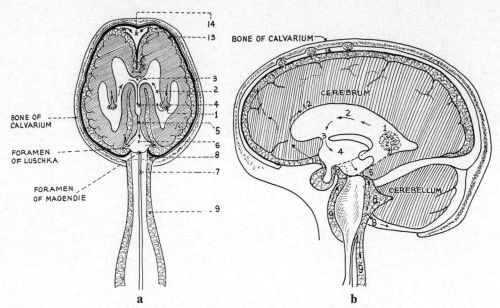

FIG. 8–10.   DIAGRAMS TO ILLUSTRATE THE CIRCULATION OF THE CEREBROSPINAL FLUID: **a,** Frontal projection; **b,** lateral projection. (See text for explanation.)

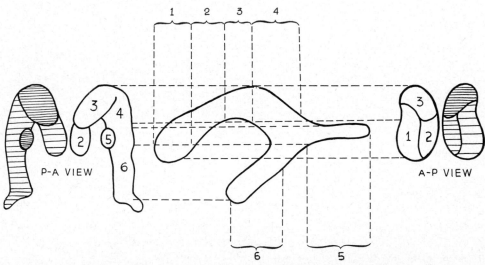

FIG. 8–11.   Lateral ventricle as seen in the antero-posterior and postero-anterior views in air contrast studies of the brain, with corresponding portions numbered. 1, Anterior horn; 2, 3 and 4, anterior, middle and posterior thirds of the body; 5, posterior horn; 6, temporal horn. (4 and 6 are not indicated on the A-P view but may be seen on the tracing in Fig. 8–15, **c.**). The anterior horn fills poorly on the P-A view, and the posterior horn poorly on the A-P view.

The lateral ventricles are arbitrarily divided into six parts as previously indicated, and this subdivision is of importance from the standpoint of varying degrees of radiographic density due to overlapping air shadows (Fig. 8–11). The slight divergence of the anterior horns, and the marked divergence of the posterior portion of the body (part 4) and temporal horns (part 6), produce the characteristic birdlike configuration in the frontal projections. The semilunar shaped slitlike appearance of the temporal horns is related to the indentation produced by the hippocampus and fornix. The perfect symmetry of the lateral ventricles in relation to the septum pellucidum is of the utmost importance in the exclusion of a space-occupying lesion which would tend to displace the ventricles and deform them in the frontal projections. If only one lateral ventricle should fill and it remain in normal position, a repeat examination is recommended since this may occur quite normally for undetermined causes.

In viewing the recumbent frontal projections, it must be remembered that the side that is uppermost will obtain the greatest quantity of air and hence demonstrate the greatest contrast.

In the lateral view of the lateral ventricles, the apparent "filling defects" produced by the caudate nucleus, calcar avis, and glomus of the choroid plexus are demonstrated in Figure 8–14, and must not be interpreted as abnormal. Occasionally, the roof of the lateral ventricle has a concave instead of a convex appearance, and in slight degrees this has no pathologic significance.

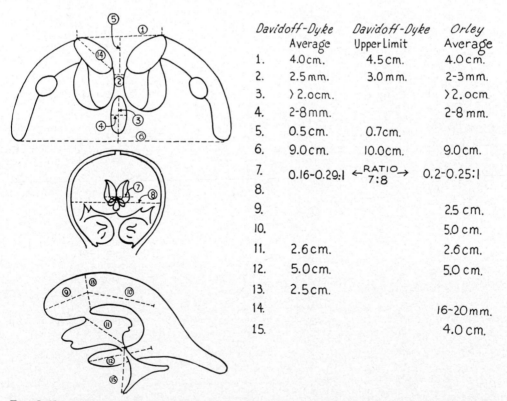

	Davidoff-Dyke Average	Davidoff-Dyke Upper Limit	Orley Average
1.	4.0 cm.	4.5 cm.	4.0 cm.
2.	2.5 mm.	3.0 mm.	2-3 mm.
3.	>2.0 cm.		>2.0 cm.
4.	2-8 mm.		2-8 mm.
5.	0.5 cm.	0.7 cm.	
6.	9.0 cm.	10.0 cm.	9.0 cm.
7.	0.16-0.29:1	←RATIO→ 7:8	0.2-0.25:1
8.			
9.			2.5 cm.
10.			5.0 cm.
11.	2.6 cm.		2.6 cm.
12.	5.0 cm.		5.0 cm.
13.	2.5 cm.		
14.			16-20 mm.
15.			4.0 cm.

FIG. 8–12. MEASUREMENTS OF VENTRICLES AS APPLIED TO PNEUMOENCEPHALOGRAPHY: a, Average measurements. (Modified from Orley: *Neuroradiology*, Charles C Thomas, Publisher.)

The slitlike midline appearance of the third ventricle is most important. In the frontal projection its size, position and contour are carefully noted and even slight deviations become of significance. In the lateral projection the shadow of the third ventricle is usually very faint when normal and slight abnormal encroachments could readily escape detection.

The cerebral aqueduct is about 1.5 cm. in length and 1 to 2 mm. in diameter. In its anterior half it is virtually horizontal but at about its midportion it curves sharply almost vertically downward, and produces a bent-knee appearance in the lateral view. The floor of the vertical segment of the cerebral aqueduct forms a continuous straight line with the floor of the fourth ventricle.

In the frontal projection, it forms a narrow 2 to 3 mm. wide strip inferior to the third ventricle, or superimposed upon the gas shadow of the hypothalamic portion of the third ventricle.

The fourth ventricle in the frontal projections is often obscured by the air in the ethmoid and sphenoid sinuses and the bones of the base of the skull. When seen, however, it presents a diamond-shaped appearance and occasion-

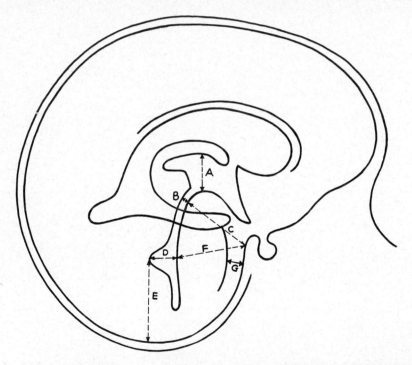

	MINIMUM	MAXIMUM	AVERAGE	ROBERTSON
A	1.10 cm.	1.60 cm.	1.42 cm.	1.3-1.9 cm.
B	0.10 cm.	0.20 cm.	0.15 cm.	0.1-0.2 cm.
C	3.0 cm.	3.9 cm.	3.44 cm.	3.0-3.7 cm.
D	1.0 cm.	1.9 cm.	1.46 cm.	1.1-2.1 cm.
E	3.0 cm.	4.0 cm.	3.26 cm.	————
F	3.3 cm.	4.0 cm.	3.61 cm.	3.1-4.3 cm.
G	0.5 cm.	1.2 cm.	0.82 cm.	0.5 cm.

FIG. 8–12. MEASUREMENTS OF VENTRICLES AS APPLIED TO PNEUMOENCEPHALOGRAPHY: b, Further measurements with an indication of range. (From Dyke and Davidoff: Am. J. Roentgenol., vol. 44, 1940; also Robertson, *Pneumoencephalography*, Charles C Thomas.)

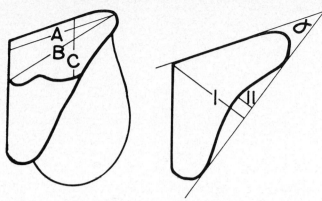

Fig. 8–13. Measurement of bodies and anterior horns of ventricles. *A* measures distance between septum pellucidum and supero-lateral angle above caudate nucleus. (Ruler placed parallel to and just below roof of ventricle.) *A* should measure less than 2 cm. Jirout's system of measurements is as follows: When the ventricles are dilated the dimension (I) and the angle alpha increase and the dimension (II) decreases. The dimension (I) is usually smaller than 1.5 to 1.6 cm. Angle alpha is 20 degrees to 35 degrees normally. (From Robertson: *Pneumoencephalography*, Charles C Thomas.)

ally the lateral recess is faintly delineated on either side as a thin 1.5 cm. streak which arches superiorly and has a small hook on its end. In the lateral projection, the fourth ventricle appears as an isosceles triangle with the floor parallel to the line of the dorsum sellae. This floor should not be more than 3.8 to 4 cm. from the dorsum sellae. The pons and cephalic half of the medulla oblongata separate the floor of the fourth ventricle from the cisterna pontis, with which it communicates indirectly. The roof of the fourth ventricle in the lateral projection has the angulated appearance previously described and delineates the cerebellar peduncles.

Occasionally a fluid level is visible in either (or both) the frontal and lateral projections at about the level of the fastigium.

The distance from the fastigium to the floor averages 1.46 cm. and from the superior to the caudal angles 4 cm.

The size and the shape of the lateral ventricles vary somewhat within normal limits. Accurate measurements have been carried out and can be found in various articles and texts (Fig. 8–13).[4]

The pneumoencephalographic appearance of the basal cisterns is very much as is illustrated in Figure 8–8. The cisterna magna is in the cerebellomedullary angle, and is separated on the lateral projection from the inferior portion of the cisterna pontis by the pons and superior portion of the medulla oblongata. Its superior margin is formed by the cerebellum, and it is continuous inferiorly with the spinal subarachnoid space. The cisterna pontis is readily seen between the dorsum sellae anteriorly and the pons posteriorly. This cistern as well as the other cisterns have already been described in conjunction with the anatomic exposition previously presented.

The Fissures and Sulci As They Appear on the Pneumoencephalogram. Normally, the width of a sulcus measures approximately 1 to 3 mm. Often there is a space produced by blood vessels crossing the subarachnoid space and these must be differentiated from sulci. These remain superficial in stereoscopy, in contrast with the perivascular subarachnoid spaces.

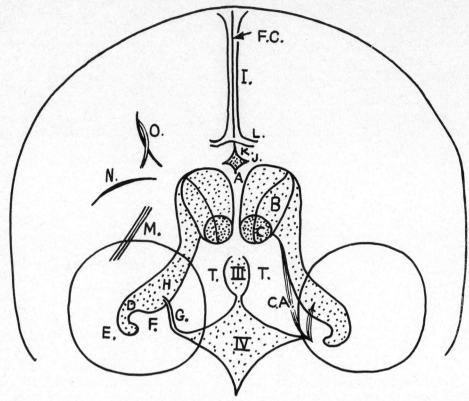

Fig. 8–14. DIAGRAM TO ILLUSTRATE THE VARIOUS ANATOMIC PARTS SEEN IN PNEUMOENCEPHAL OGRAPHY: **a,** Antero-posterior projection. *A,* Corpus callosum; *B,* caudate nucleus; *C,* choroid plexus; *D,* temporal horns; *E,* eminentia collateralis; *F,* fornix; *G,* lateral recess of fourth ventricle; *H,* foramen of Luschka; *I,* longitudinal fissure; *J,* callosal sulcus; *K,* cisterna corpus callosi; *L,* cingulate sulcus; *M,* air in depths of sylvian fissure; *N,* middle frontal sulcus; *O,* interparietal sulcus; *T–T,* thalamus; *C.A.,* cisterna ambiens; *F.C.,* falx cerebri.

The sulci of the median sagittal surface of the brain are more constantly identified than those overlying the lateral surface of the brain.

The callosal sulcus (Fig. 8–14) and the cisterna corpus callosi at the inferior margin of the falx cerebri form a diamond-shaped structure in the frontal projection. On the lateral view (Fig. 8–14, **b**) the callosal sulcus can be recognized near the roof of the lateral ventricles following the contour of the latter, particularly anteriorly.

Directly above the corpus callosum (about 1 or 1.5 cm.) on either side of the midline are the cingulate gyri whose course parallels the corpus callosum. The parolfactory area is of importance especially with regard to detection of sphenoid ridge meningiomas, and may be seen posterior and interior to the cingulate gyrus.

The parieto-occipital and calcarine fissures are readily identified behind th upturned margin of the cingulate sulcus.

The longitudinal cerebral fissure lies in the sagittal plane between the cerebral hemispheres, and frequently appears as a dense line in the center of the skull in the antero-posterior and postero-anterior views.

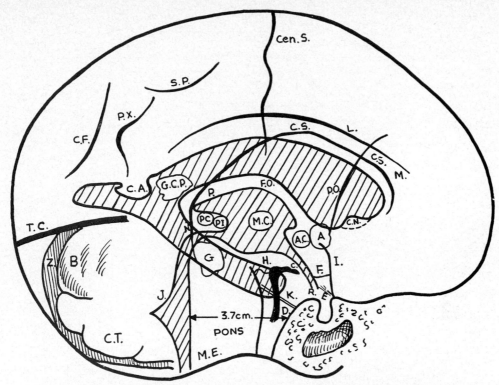

FIG. 8–14.   DIAGRAM TO ILLUSTRATE THE VARIOUS ANATOMIC PARTS SEEN IN PNEUMOENCEPHAL-OGRAPHY: **b,** Lateral projection. *A,* Lamina terminalis; *B,* cerebellar folia; *C,* posterior cerebral artery; *D,* basilar artery; *E,* optic chiasm; *F,* anterior communicating artery; *G,* colliculi; *H,* cerebral peduncles (mammillary bodies); *I,* tuber cinereum; *J,* superior medullary velum; *K,* oculomotor nerve; *L,* cingulate sulcus; *M,* cingulate gyrus; *N,* cisterna ambiens; *P,* pulvinar; *CN,* caudate nucleus; *FO,* fornix; *AC,* anterior commissure; *MC,* middle commissure; *PC,* posterior commissure, *CA,* calcar avis; *PI,* pineal; *R,* infundibulum; *CS,* callosal sulcus-cisterna corpus callosi; *PX,* parieto; occipital sulcus; *CF,* calcarine fissure; *SP,* subparietal sulcus; *PO,* parolfactory sulcus; *Cen. S.-*central sulcus (Rolando); *CT,* cerebellar tonsil; *TC,* tentorium cerebelli; *Z,* air outlining cerebellum; *GCP,* glomus of the choroid plexus.

On the lateral aspect of the brain, the central fissure can be identified as an S-shaped shadow centrally located over the cerebral hemispheres. The lateral fissure can occasionally be seen, which in turn permits the identification of the superior temporal sulcus.

The frontal lobe is divided into three major parallel convolutions, the superior, middle and inferior, all parallel with each other in the antero-posterior direction.

The convolutional pattern of the occipital lobe of the brain is extremely variable, making identification of structures very difficult or impossible in most instances.

Routine Views for Pneumoencephalograms and Ventriculograms.   The views employed are as follows:

1. Straight antero-posterior views:
   (*a*) Upright (Fig. 8–15)
   (*b*) Recumbent, with vertical x-ray beam (Fig. 8–16)
   (*c*) Recumbent, with horizontal x-ray beam (Fig. 8–17)

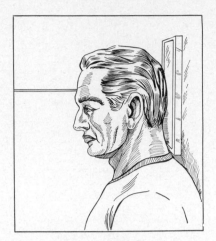

PATIENT. . . . . .ERECT
FILM . . . . .VERTICAL
PROJECTION. . . .ANT-POST SKULL
BEAM . . . . . . .HORIZONTAL

FIG. 8–15. ERECT ANTERO-POSTERIOR PNEUMOENCEPHALOGRAM: **a,** Method of positioning patient.

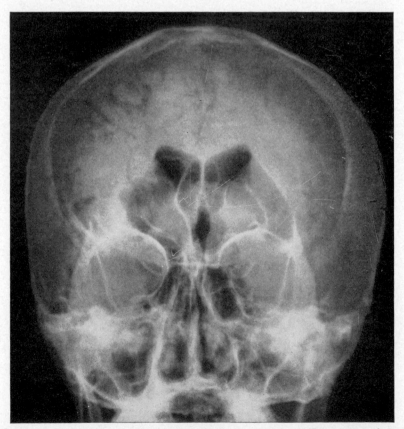

FIG .8 –15. ERECT ANTERO-POSTERIOR PNEUMOENCEPHALOGRAM: **b,** Pneumoencephalogram.

Points of Practical Interest with Reference to Figure 8–15:

1. This projection will vary somewhat depending upon the exact relationship of the central ray to the acantho-meatal line. When the acantho-meatal line is slightly above the horizontal plane, the petrous ridges are projected lower in relation to the orbits, and the temporal horns are more clearly shown. When the acantho-meatal line is slightly below the horizontal plane, there is less interference from the frontal sinuses as they are projected over the lateral ventricles; and one may at times see the fourth ventricle in frontal perspective also.

2. A head halter attached to a pulley mechanism anchored to the ceiling is helpful in maintaining the position of the head of the patient who is under the influence of considerable sedation. The head halter must, of course, not cast a shadow on the radiograph.

3. When maximum visualization of the posterior fossa structures is desired, this view is not applicable, and Towne's projection is preferable.

4. To make certain that the film is a perfectly straight one, so that deviation of the septum pellucidum to one side or the other may be measured, the examiner may note the relationship of the mastoid processes with the rami of the mandible. These must be perfectly symmetrical.

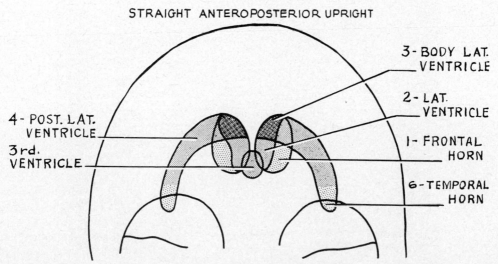

FIG. 8–15.   ERECT ANTERO-POSTERIOR PNEUMOENCEPHALOGRAM: c, Tracing of b.

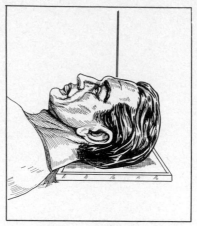

PATIENT......SUPINE
FILM.......HORIZONTAL
PROJECTION...ANT-POST. SKULL
BEAM.......VERTICAL

FIG. 8–16. RECUMBENT ANTERO-POSTERIOR PNEUMOENCEPHALOGRAM, X-RAY BEAM VERTICAL: **a.**
Method of positioning patient.

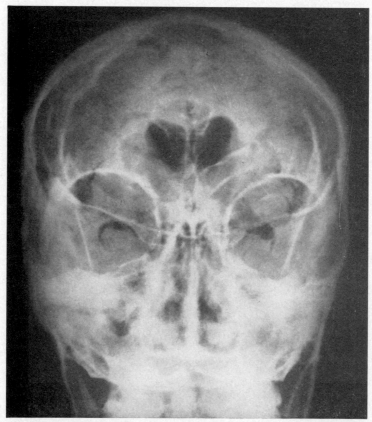

FIG. 8–16. RECUMBENT ANTERO-POSTERIOR PNEUMOENCEPHALOGRAM, X-RAY BEAM VERTICAL: **b.**
Pneumoencephalogram.

POINTS OF PRACTICAL INTEREST WITH REFERENCE TO FIGURE 8–16:
1. In this projection the air rises to the frontal horns and to the tips of the temporal horns, leaving the posterior portions of the lateral ventricles less distinctly visualized. The third and fourth ventricles, however, are indicated fairly clearly.
2. This view can usually be differentiated from postero-anterior projection by virtue of the marked magnification of the orbits.

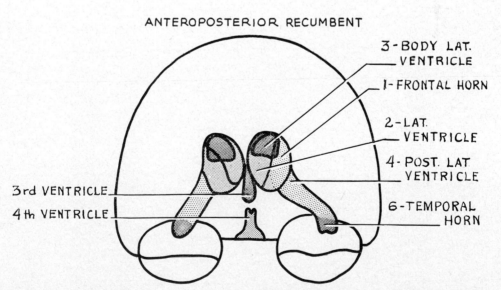

FIG. 8–16. RECUMBENT ANTERO-POSTERIOR PNEUMOENCEPHALOGRAM, X-RAY BEAM VERTICAL: c, Diagram of b. (Diagram does not show impression by hippocampus on temporal horns, or semilunar shape of latter.)

2. Both lateral views: upright and recumbent as above (Figs. 8–18 to 8–21)
3. Straight postero-anterior view, recumbent as above (Fig. 8–22)
4. Reversed Towne's position recumbent (Fig. 8–23)
5. Special views for studying the fourth ventricle (Fig. 8–24)

It is particularly important that these x-rays should be taken with the skull in a perfectly symmetrical position with regard to the film, whatever position is required. These are usually stereoscopic views, at least in part. Certain special positions may be taken as the occasion demands.

In every instance advantage is taken of the fact that air or oxygen is lighter ihan cerebrospinal fluid and will rise to the top. Thus, in addition to employtng a vertical x-ray beam in the antero-posterior, postero-anterior and lateral projections, it is possible to demonstrate that part of the ventricular system which is uppermost by employing a horizontal x-ray beam with the patient recumbent. Thus, selective filling of each part is obtained as desired. Upright films are not feasible when a general anesthetic is used.

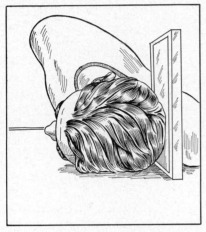

FIG. 8–17. RECUMBENT ANTERO-POSTERIOR TNEUMOENCEPHALOGRAM X-RAY BEAM HORIZON-PAL: **a,** Method of positioning patient; **b,** tracing of radiograph so obtained.

PATIENT.....RECUMBENT
FILM........VERTICAL
PROJECTION...ANT.-POST. SKULL
BEAM........HORIZONTAL

a

ANTEROPOSTERIOR, LAT. DECUBITUS

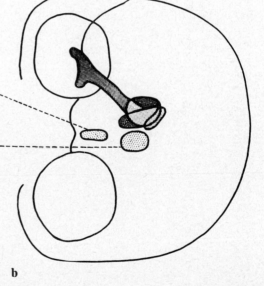

THIRD VENTRICLE

AIR TRAPPED IN
LOWERMOST
LATERAL VENTRICLE

b

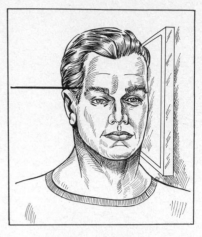

FIG. 8–18. ERECT LATERAL PNEUMOENCEPH-
ALOGRAM (BOTH LATERAL VIEWS ARE OBTAINED):
a, Method of positioning patient.

```
PATIENT.......ERECT
FILM ........VERTICAL
PROJECTION...LATERAL SKULL
BEAM .......HORIZONTAL
```

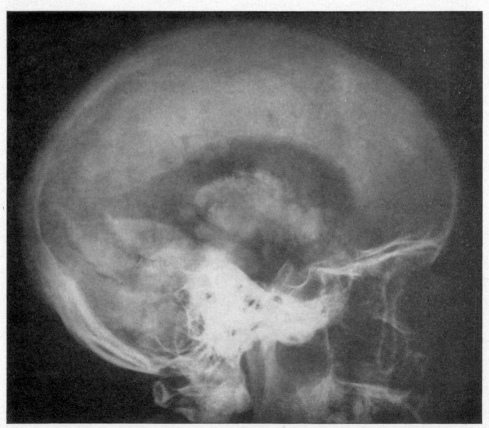

FIG. 8–18.   ERECT LATERAL PNEUMOENCEPHALOGRAM: **b**, Pneumoencephalogram.

POINTS OF PRACTICAL INTEREST WITH REFERENCE TO FIGURE 8–18:

1. The lateral ventricle which is closest to the film is shown in greatest detail, with the least magnification; yet both lateral ventricles may be seen adequately. In this respect the erect lateral is superior to the recumbent lateral, since in the latter, the air rises to the uppermost ventricle, and the ventricle which is closest to the film contains the least amount of contrast media, and may be poorly delineated.
2. The recumbent lateral studies will often give the better delineation of the temporal horns, particularly that temporal horn which is farthest from the film and uppermost.

STRAIGHT LATERAL ERECT

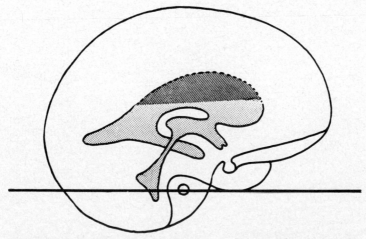

FIG. 8–18. ERECT LATERAL PNEUMOENCEPHALOGRAM: c, Tracing of b. (Subarachnoid space surrounding brain and cisterns is not illustrated.)

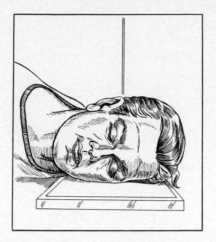

PATIENT..... RECUMBENT
FILM .... HORIZONTAL
PROJECTION..LATERAL SKULL
BEAM.......VERTICAL

FIG. 8–19. RECUMBENT LATERAL PNEUMOENCEPHALOGRAM (BOTH LATERAL VIEWS ARE OBTAINED):
a, Method of positioning patient.

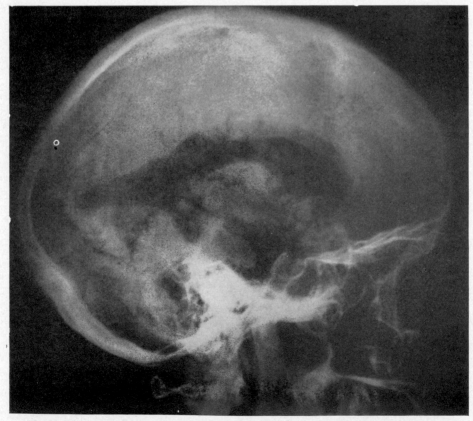

FIG. 8–19. RECUMBENT LATERAL PNEUMOENCEPHALOGRAM: b, Pneumoencephalogram.

Points of Practical Interest with Reference to Figure 8–19:

1. The position of the head is the same as in the case of the routine lateral skull. Extreme care, however, must be exercised to place the head so that its sagittal plane is perfectly parallel with the plane of the film. This will virtually superimpose the two lateral ventricles. The lateral ventricle which is uppermost will contain the greatest quantity of air, but it in turn will also be magnified to the greatest extent since it is farthest from the film. The third ventricle is ordinarily quite indistinctly visualized since it is a rather thin structure, from side to side.

2. No effort has been made in the tracing to indicate any of the air-containing structures except the ventricular system. For a discussion of these other air-containing structures see the text and diagrams.

STRAIGHT LATERAL RECUMBENT

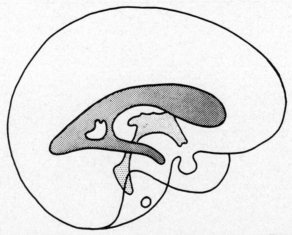

Fig. 8–19. RECUMBENT LATERAL PNEUMOENCEPHALOGRAM: c, Tracing of b.

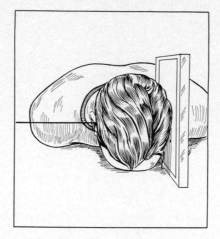

PATIENT......PRONE
FILM........VERTICAL
PROJECTION....LATERAL SKULL
BEAM........HORIZONTAL

a

LATERAL POSTERO-ANTERIOR DECUBITUS
(BROW DOWN)

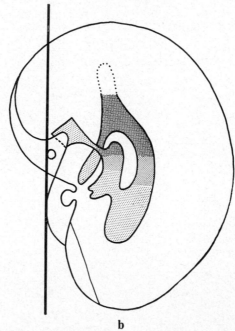

b

FIG. 8–20. RECUMBENT "DECUBITUS" LATERAL PNEUMOENCEPHALOGRAM WITH PATIENT PRONE (BROW DOWN): **a,** Method of positioning patient; **b,** tracing of radiograph so obtained.

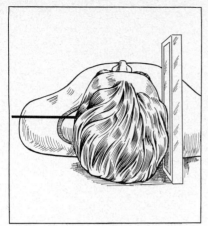

PATIENT.....SUPINE
FILM......VERTICAL
PROJECTION...LATERAL SKULL
BEAM.......HORIZONTAL

a

Fig. 8–21. RECUMBENT "DECUBITUS" LAT-
ERAL PNEUMOENCEPHALOGRAM WITH PATIENT
SUPINE: **a,** Method of positioning patient;
b, tracing of radiograph so obtained.

LATERAL ANTEROPOSTERIOR DECUBITUS
(BROW UP)

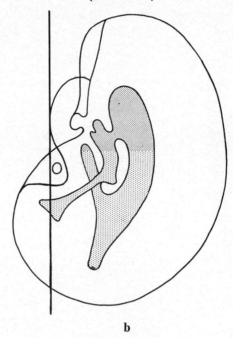

b

RECUMBENT POSTERO-ANTERIOR

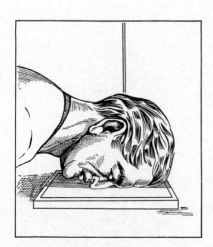

PATIENT.....PRONE
FILM........HORIZONTAL
PROJECTION...POST.–ANT. SKULL
BEAM........VERTICAL

a

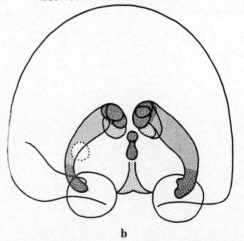

b

FIG. 8–22. RECUMBENT POSTERO-ANTERIOR PNEUMOENCEPHALOGRAM: **a,** Method of positioning
patient; **b,** tracing of radiograph so obtained.

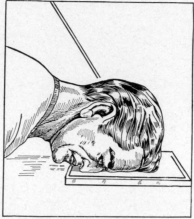

Fig. 8–23. RECUMBENT REVERSED TOWNE'S PROJECTION: **a,** Method of positioning patient.

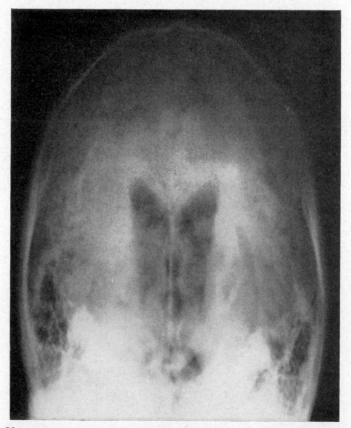

Fig. 8–23. RECUMBENT REVERSED TOWNE'S PROJECTION: **b,** Pneumoencephalogram.

POINTS OF PRACTICAL INTEREST WITH REFERENCE TO FIGURE 8–23:

1. Since the air rises to the uppermost portions of the ventricular system, this view has its chief application in visualization of the occipital horns, the posterior portions of the lateral ventricles, the posterior part of the third ventricle, and the fourth ventricle.
2. The true Towne position, with the patient supine and the central ray angled 35 degrees toward the feet, is most applicable to visualization of the temporal horns and the anterior sectors of the lateral ventricles.

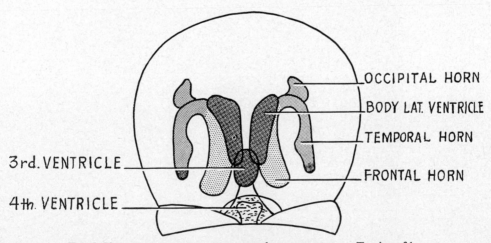

FIG. 8–23. RECUMBENT REVERSED TOWNE'S PROJECTION: c, Tracing of b.

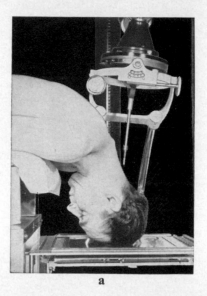

a

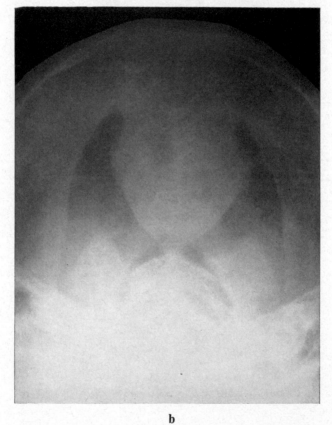

b

FIG. 8–24. SPECIAL PNEUMOENCEPHALOGRAPHIC METHODS FOR DEMONSTRATING FOURTH VENTRICLE FILLING. BASO-VERTICAL VIEW. **a,** Position of patient. **b,** Radiograph with vertical beam. (From Robertson: *Pneumoencephalography*, Charles C Thomas.)

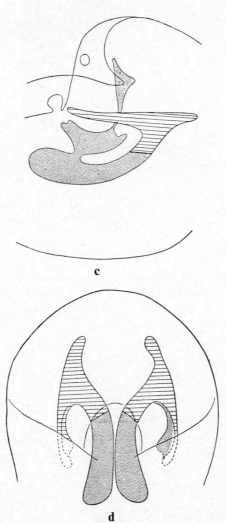

FIG. 8–24. SPECIAL PNEUMOENCEPHALOGRAPHIC METHODS FOR DEMONSTRATING FOURTH VENTRICLE FILLING. BASO-VERTICAL VIEW. c, Tracing of radiograph with beam horizontal. Air is trapped in the temporal and occipital horns and fourth ventricle particularly. d, Tracing of b. (From Robertson.)

THE RADIOGRAPHIC ANATOMY OF THE CIRCULATORY SYSTEM OF THE MENINGES AND BRAIN

The Blood Supply of the Meninges. The arterial supply of the dura mater is very extensive, the chief source being the middle meningeal arteries (Fig. 8–25) which anastomose from side to side. The dural supply of the anterior cranial fossa is derived from the middle meningeal artery and meningeal branches of the internal carotid and anterior and posterior ethmoidal arteries. That of the middle cranial fossa is supplied by the meningeal branches of the internal carotid artery. The dura of the posterior cranial fossa is supplied by the vertebral, occipital and ascending pharyngeal arteries, together with the middle meningeal.

The veins of the dura anastomose with the diploic veins. Many meningeal veins open directly into venous ampullae on either side of the superior sagittal sinus. Communication is established with the underlying cerebral veins, emissary and diploic veins.

The Arterial Supply of the Brain (Figs. 8–26, 8–27). The arterial supply of the brain is derived mainly from the internal carotid and vertebral arteries. The two vertebral arteries join to form the basilar artery which passes upward on the anterior surface of the brain stem. Just behind the dorsum sellae, it biturcates to form the posterior cerebral arteries.

The largest divisions of the internal carotid artery are the anterior and middle cerebral arteries. A branch goes posteriorly, anastomosing with the posterior cerebral artery to complete the circle arteriosus (of Willis), and another enters the inferior extremity of the choroid plexus of the lateral ventricle.

The major branches of the internal carotid artery (Fig. 8–27) are as follows: (1) the ophthalmic artery which passes through the optic foramen into the orbit; (2) the anterior choroidal artery, seen in about 59 per cent of angiograms, which is a small posterior branch near the division into the terminal branches. It supplies the choroid plexus of the lateral ventricle on the same side, the hippocampus, portions of the globus pallidus, and the posterior limb of the internal capsule. (3) The posterior communicating artery is seen in about 43 per cent of carotid angiograms and connects the middle and posterior cerebral artery on either side.

The anterior cerebral artery supplies the anteromesial brain surface. Its territory includes the whole of the medial aspect of the frontal and parietal lobes, as far back as the parieto-occipital fissure, and the subjacent white matter, knee and anterior four-fifths of the callosal body, the septum pellucidum, the anterior pillars of the fornix and part of the anterior commissure, part of the head of the caudate nucleus, the anterior part of the two outer segments of the lenticular nucleus, and the anterior half of the forelimb of the internal capsule.

The anterior cerebral artery is smaller than the middle cerebral and is joined to its mate of the opposite side by the anterior communicating artery. Both of these are seen in about 36 per cent of angiograms. Its first branch is the medial striate artery which runs backward into the anterior perforating substance to supply the head of the caudate nucleus and adjacent portions of the putamen and internal capsule. It gives off orbital and frontopolar arteries which supply the olfactory lobe, the gyrus rectus, and the medial portion of the orbital gyri. It then follows around the corpus callosum to be called the pericallosal artery, which anastomoses with the posterior cerebral artery in the vicinity of the splenium of the corpus callosum. The pericallosal artery has three branches—the anterior, intermediate and posterior medial; the anterior may appear to form a separate artery called the calloso-marginal artery which runs parallel to the pericallosal artery.

The middle cerebral artery supplies the outer aspect of the cerebral cortex, particularly the upper part of the posterior limb, and part of the anterior limb of the internal capsule, part of the head and the horizontal part of the caudate nucleus, and most of the lenticular nucleus. It supplies branches over the temporal lobe, the lateral part of the orbital surface of the frontal lobe, the parietal lobes and the angular gyrus.

The middle cerebral artery passes laterally into the lateral fissure where it divides into its cortical branches after curving out over the opercular margins of the lateral fissure, and spreads out over the convex surface of the brain. It gives off an ascending frontoparietal artery which supplies the lower frontoparietal region and in turn this latter artery branches to form the prerolandic, the rolandic and the anterior parietal arteries. The three terminal branches of the middle cerebral are somewhat variable and have been called the "group Sylvienne" by Egas Moniz. They cross superiorly, diagonally and posteriorly in the lateral (sylvian) fissure and are called the posterior parietal, the angular and the posterior temporal, respectively.

The vertebral artery (Fig. 8–26) gives off three branches before it unites with its fellow of the opposite side to form the basilar artery: the posterior spinal artery, the anterior spinal artery and the posterior inferior cerebellar, respectively. The basilar artery gives off the anterior inferior cerebellar artery, the superior cerebellar arteries, the internal auditory artery, pontine twigs and the posterior cerebral artery.

The posterior cerebral artery supplies the inferior surface of the occipital lobe, mesencephalon, basal ganglia, practically all of the thalamic and peduncular regions, and the geniculate bodies. It supplies almost the entire basilar surface of the temporal lobe also.

The posterior cerebral artery is seen in about 34 per cent of carotid angiograms, and all vertebral angiograms. This latter artery has two branches which arise from its proximal portion and supply the thalamus, lateral geniculate body, and posterior limb of the internal capsule (called the posterolateral and posteromedial branches respectively). The terminal branches of the posterior cerebral artery are: the anterior temporal, the middle or posterior temporal, the parieto-occipital and the calcarine arteries. These latter branches supply the medial and inferior aspects of the occipital lobe and the inferior portion of the temporal lobe.

The cerebellum is supplied by the posterior inferior cerebellar arteries, arising from the vertebral arteries, and the anterior superior and inferior cerebellar arteries arising from the basilar artery (Fig. 8–26). These are usually readily visualized on vertebral angiograms (Fig. 8–28).

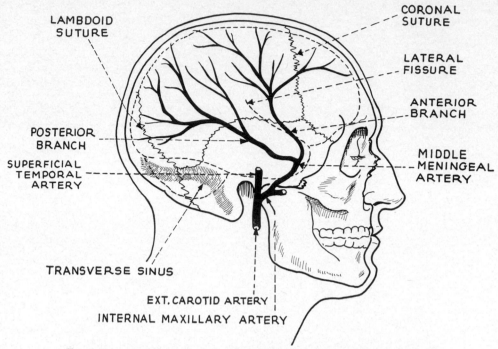

Fig. 8–25. **a.** Projection of middle meningeal artery in relation to the skull.

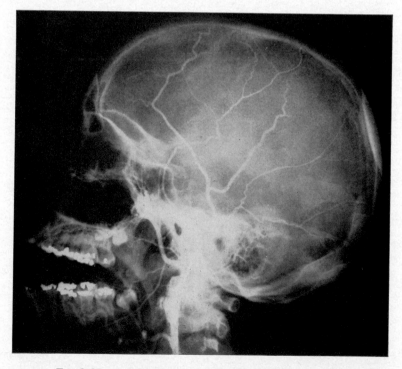

Fig. 8–25. **b,** Radiograph of external carotid arteriogram.

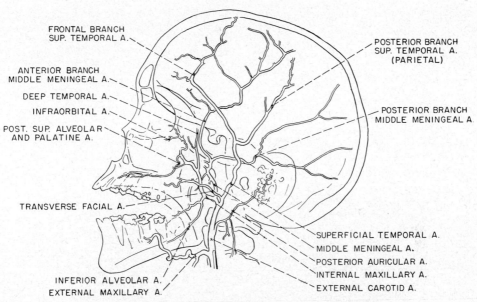

FRONTAL BRANCH
SUP. TEMPORAL A.

ANTERIOR BRANCH
MIDDLE MENINGEAL A.

DEEP TEMPORAL A.

INFRAORBITAL A.

POST. SUP. ALVEOLAR
AND PALATINE A.

TRANSVERSE FACIAL A.

INFERIOR ALVEOLAR A.
EXTERNAL MAXILLARY A.

POSTERIOR BRANCH
SUP. TEMPORAL A.
(PARIETAL)

POSTERIOR BRANCH
MIDDLE MENINGEAL A.

SUPERFICIAL TEMPORAL A.
MIDDLE MENINGEAL A.
POSTERIOR AURICULAR A.
INTERNAL MAXILLARY A.
EXTERNAL CAROTID A.

FIG. 8–25. **c,** Labeled tracing of external carotid arteriogram.

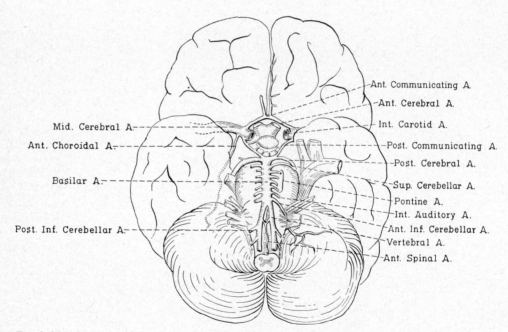

Mid. Cerebral A.

Ant. Choroidal A.

Basilar A.

Post. Inf. Cerebellar A.

Ant. Communicating A.

Ant. Cerebral A.

Int. Carotid A.

Post. Communicating A.

Post. Cerebral A.

Sup. Cerebellar A.

Pontine A.

Int. Auditory A.

Ant. Inf. Cerebellar A.

Vertebral A.

Ant. Spinal A.

Fig. 8–26.   Anatomy of the vertebral artery and branches in relationship with the base of the brain.

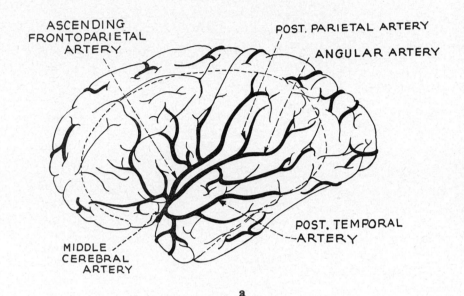

a

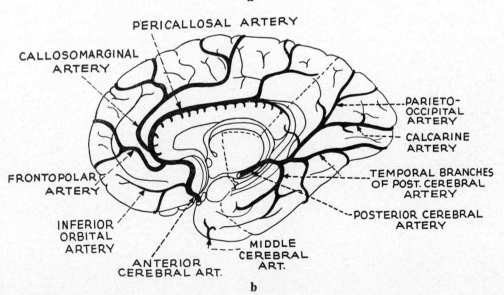

b

FIG. 8–27. CHIEF DIVISIONS OF THE INTERNAL CAROTID ARTERY. **a,** Lateral aspect; **b,** median sagittal aspect.

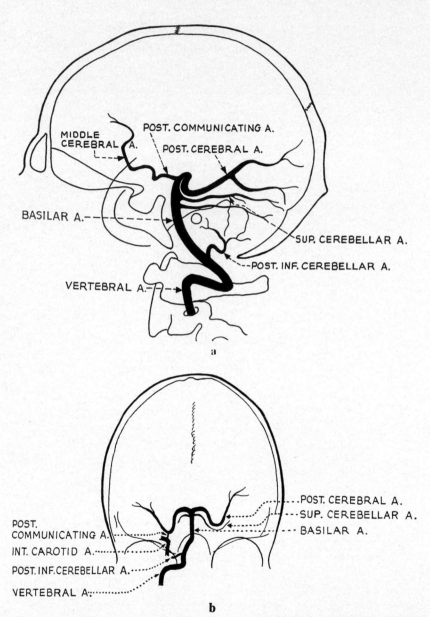

FIG. 8–28.   DIAGRAM OF VERTEBRAL ANGIOGRAMS: **a,** Lateral projection; **b,** Towne's projection.

Venous Drainage from the Brain[11, 12] (Fig. 8–29). The cerebral veins may be divided into three systems: (1) the external, or superficial veins; (2) the internal or deep veins; and (3) the dural sinuses. There are direct communicating chanuels between the superficial and the deep veins.

The superior cerebral veins (Fig. 8–29) have frontal, parietal and occipital components which empty into the superior longitudinal sinus. The middle cerebral vein, which empties into the cavernous sinus, communicates with the superior longitudinal sinus by means of the great anastomotic vein of Trolard, and with the transverse sinus by means of the posterior anastomotic vein of Labbe.

The deep cerebral veins first form among the choroidal and terminal veins which fuse in the region of the interventricular foramen to form the two internal cerebral veins. The striothalamic vein thus formed on each side meets the internal cerebral vein to form the so-called "venous angle"[11] (Fig. 8–29, **b**). Although somewhat variable, this marks the anatomic position of the interventricular foramen. The position of this angle has been plotted on localization graphs (Fig. 8–29, **c, d**) and by template[6] (Fig. 8–29, **e**). The shape of the venous angle is also important from the standpoint of localizing intracerebral space occupying lesions, but this is outside the scope of this text.

The internal cerebral veins join behind the pineal gland to form the great cerebral vein of Galen. This latter short but major channel also receives the basal veins of Rosenthal. The latter are formed by the union of three veins in the region of the anterior perforating substance, and wind backward around the cerebral peduncle. The vein of Galen empties into the straight sinus. The cerebellar veins drain into the transverse or straight sinus or into the internal cerebral veins, superior petrosal or occipital sinuses. The posterior portion of the inferior sagittal sinus and the vein of Galen outline the splenium of the corpus callosum. The vein of Galen has further importance in that it is a midline structure. If identified on a perfectly straight venogram, it can readily help determine a space-occupying lesion if displaced from the midline.

The dural sinuses (Fig. 8–30) are venous channels which drain the venous blood from the brain. They possess no valves but often fibrous septa project into their lumens and help maintain the rigidity of their walls. These sinuses are subdivided into two main groups: (1) *the postero-superior group*, which comprise the sagittal sinuses (superior and inferior), the straight sinus, two cransverse sinuses and the occipital sinus; and (2) *an antero-inferior group* tituated at the base of the skull. These comprise the cavernous sinuses, the intersavernous, the superior and inferior petrosal sinuses, and the basilar plexus. The first group is of greater importance in the study of radiographic anatomy.

The superior sagittal sinus occupies the convexity of the falx cerebri. It commences anteriorly where it receives a small vein from the nose through the foramen caecum, and passes directly backward to the internal occipital protuberance, where it turns to either the right or left side to end in the corresponding transverse sinus. The superior sagittal sinus receives blood from the venous lacunae in the dura mater on either side, the superior cerebral veins, and veins from the diploe and dura mater.

The inferior sagittal sinus is contained in the posterior half of the free margin of the falx cerebri. It passes backward to end in the straight sinus.

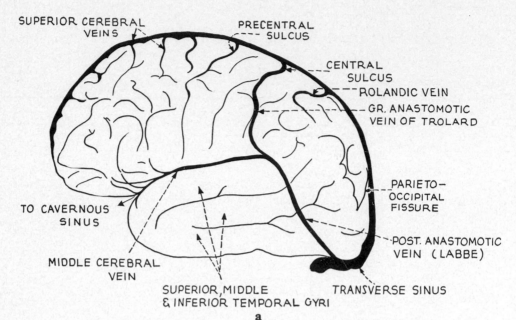

FIG. 8–29.   VENOUS DRAINAGE OF THE BRAIN: a, Superolateral aspect.

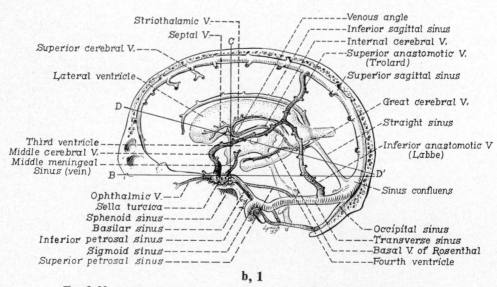

b, 1

FIG. 8–29. VENOUS DRAINAGE OF THE BRAIN: b, 1, Inner aspect, lateral view.

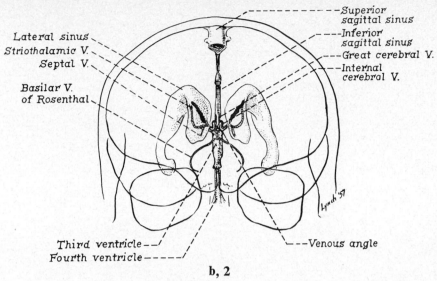

FIG. 8–29. VENOUS DRAINAGE OF THE BRAIN: **b, 2,** Inner aspect, frontal view.

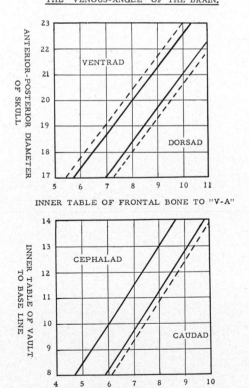

ORIENTATION CHART FOR FORAMEN OF MONRO OR
THE "VENOUS-ANGLE" OF THE BRAIN.

FIG. 8–29. **c,** Orientation chart for localizing the foramen of Monro or the "venous angle" of the brain. The normal range of variation of the "venous angle" in the ventrodorsad direction is represented by the broken lines; in the cephalocaudad direction the normal range of variation is shown by the anterior solid line and the posterior broken line. (From Mokrohisky, J. F., et al., in **Radiology,** vol. 67.)

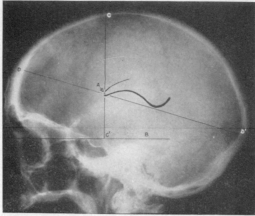

FIG. 8–29.   **d,** Method of orientation of the "venous angle." Base line, *B*, passes through the nasion and tuberculum sellae. Orientation in the cephalocaudad direction: measure *C–A* against *C–C"*. Orientation in the ventrodorsad direction: measure the longest anteroposterior diameter *D–D*. against *D–A*. (From Lin, Mokrohisky, Stauffer, and Scott: J. Neurosurg., vol. 12.)

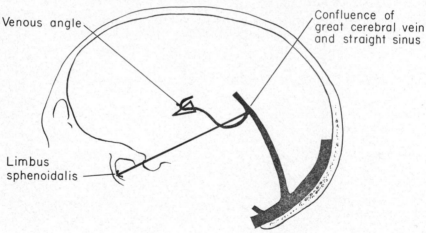

FIG. 8–29.   **e,** 1, Template method for demonstrating normal position of the venous angle: In a normal full-sized adult, the venous angle should fall within the triangle if the relations as shown are carried forward, to a straight line drawn as shown from the limbus sphenoidalis to the point of confluence of the great cerebral vein (of Galen) and the straight sinus.

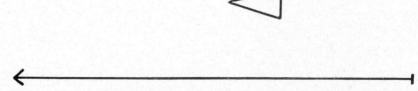

FIG. 8–29.   **e,** 2, Normal full-sized topogram (adult). Arrow from confluence of great cerebral vein and straight sinus to limbus sphenoidalis. The venous angle is inside the normal topogram. (From Laine et al.: Acta Radiologica, vol. 46.)

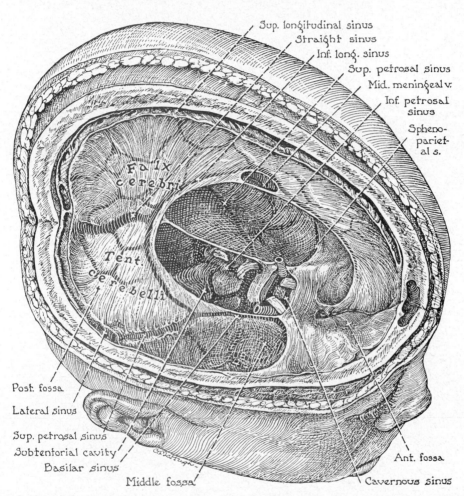

Sup. longitudinal sinus
Straight sinus
Inf. long. sinus
Sup. petrosal sinus
Mid. meningeal v.
Inf. petrosal sinus
Spheno-parietal s.

Falx cerebri

Tent. cerebelli

Post. fossa
Lateral sinus
Sup. petrosal sinus
Subtentorial cavity
Basilar sinus
Middle fossa
Ant. fossa
Cavernous sinus

FIG. 8–30.   Major dural sinuses surrounding the brain. (From Bailey, *Intracranial Tumors*, Charles C Thomas, Publisher.)

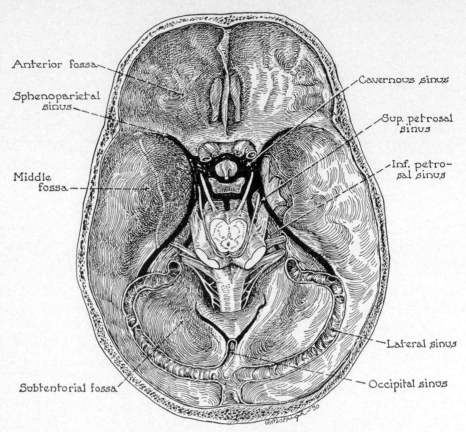

Anterior fossa

Sphenoparietal sinus

Middle fossa

Subtentorial fossa

Cavernous sinus

Sup. petrosal sinus

Inf. petrosal sinus

Lateral sinus

Occipital sinus

FIG. 8–30 (*continued*).   See preceding page for legend.

This sinus is directly related to the body of the corpus callosum, which lies immediately below it.

The straight sinus occupies the junction between the falx cerebri and tentorium cerebelli. It receives as major tributaries the inferior sagittal sinus and the great cerebral vein of Galen and also the superior cerebellar veins. It passes downward and backward to end in the opposite transverse sinus to that in which the superior sagittal sinus terminates.

The transverse sinuses commence at the internal occipital protuberance, as described above, and curve laterally and then downward and forward to end in the jugular foramen. They receive as branches the superior petrosal sinuses and emissary veins in their mastoid areas, together with some of the inferior cerebral and cerebellar veins.

The occipital sinus is usually single; it is situated in the attached margin of the falx cerebelli and passes backward from the foramen magnum to end in the confluence of the sinuses.

The antero-inferior group of sinuses at the base of the brain is less amenable to study. The sphenoparietal sinus is seen in the examination of angiography as it passes into the cavernous sinus; it is contained in the dura at the posterior margin of the anterior cranial fossa.

ANGIOGRAPHY OF THE BRAIN

Introduction. This examination entails the injection of radiopaque material into either the internal carotid or vertebral arteries. The method was intro, duced primarily to locate intracranial aneurysms, but more recently has received considerable prominence in the study of space-filling intracranial lesions- definite arterial patterns being established depending on the disorganization of the normal anatomy, and the nature of the pathologic condition. Hence, a knowledge of the normal arterial and venous patterns is important from this standpoint.[5]

Technique. The technique of examination will vary with the neurosurgeon's preference. Either the internal carotid or vertebral arteries may be exposed or they may be injected by the percutaneous method which requires great precision on the part of the operator. Another method for vertebral angiography, advocated by Egas Moniz, accomplished vertebral perfusion by retrograde flow after injection into the subclavian artery. The contrast material employed will show a considerable amount of variation. Diodrast may be used in concentrations of 35 per cent or Hypaque up to 50 per cent.

Thorotrast (25 per cent thorium dioxide) is highly opaque to x-rays and virtually nonirritating in the perivascular tissues, but it has long-life radioactivity and is concentrated in the reticuloendothelial system. It may be harmful in small quantities and hence is not used in many clinics except in arteriosclerotic individuals, old patients, or patients with a very poor prognosis. Tri-iodo-ethyl-stearate has been recommended abroad as an ideal contrast medium for this purpose, but its use at present is still experimental.

The following views are obtained routinely: (1) stereo-lateral, (2) an antero-posterior modified Towne's view with the central ray angled 12 degrees to the acanthomeatal line, and (3) similar projections in the capillary and venous phases as required. The antero-posterior projection is best when the supra-orbital ridge is projected over the superior margin of the petrous ridge. (4) Forty-five degree oblique views are helpful in some cases where overlapping sections of a blood vessel may obscure a small aneurysm.

Each injection consists of 8 cc. of contrast media injected rapidly. A total of 120 cc. must not be exceeded. Large amounts of contrast media should be used only in patients with good kidney function and over a sufficient interval of time to permit adequate excretion. Iodine sensitivity studies should be performed prior to the examination by the intravenous injection of a small amount of the contrast media.

The x-ray procedure varies in complexity depending upon the apparatus available. The ideal arrangement is the rapid cassette changer which enables serial films to be taken at $\frac{1}{2}$ second intervals for a period up to 7 seconds. If this is not available, it is possible to obtain good results by the manual method of changing cassettes; in the case of the internal carotid artery, the film obtained at the completion of the injection is usually adequate. In the case of the vertebral artery, the circulation is slower and the 1 second exposure after the injection is completed is preferable in the Towne's position (Fig. 8–28). The optimum time for venography is about 6 seconds after injection.

It should be emphasized that both the antero-posterior and lateral projections should be taken whenever possible, since only then can one consider the visualization complete in three dimensions (Fig. 8–31).

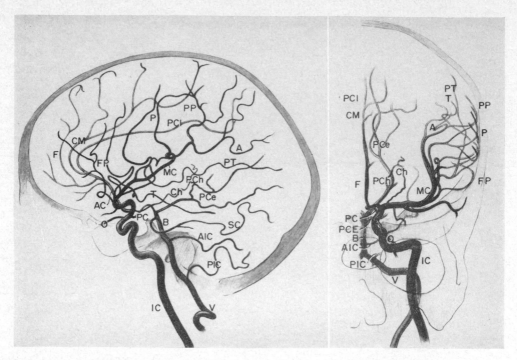

IC	–	Internal carotid	PT	–	Posterior temporal	V	–	Vertebral
O	–	Ophthalmic	PP	–	Posterior parietal	PIC	–	Posterior inferior cerebellar
PC	–	Posterior communicating	A	–	Angular	AIC	–	Anterior inferior cerebellar
Ch	–	Choroidal	AC	–	Anterior cerebral	B	–	Basilar
MC	–	Middle cerebral	F	–	Fronto-polar	S	–	Superior cerebellar
FP	–	Fronto-parietal	CM	–	Colloso-marginal	PCe	–	Posterior cerebellar
T	–	Temporal	PCI	–	Pericollosal	PCh	–	Posterior choroidal
P	–	Parietal					

a

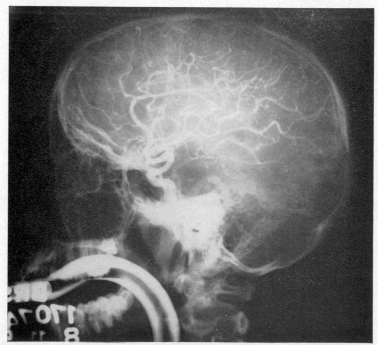

b

FIG. 8–31.   INTERNAL CAROTID ARTERIOGRAMS AND VENOGRAMS: **a,** Labeled diagram illustrating an idealized carotid and vertebral angiogram in the lateral and anteroposterior projections. **b,** Radiograph of an internal carotid arteriogram in the lateral projection.

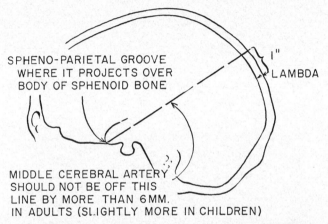

SPHENO-PARIETAL GROOVE
WHERE IT PROJECTS OVER
BODY OF SPHENOID BONE

1"

LAMBDA

MIDDLE CEREBRAL ARTERY
SHOULD NOT BE OFF THIS
LINE BY MORE THAN 6MM.
IN ADULTS (SLIGHTLY MORE IN CHILDREN)

Fig. 8–31. INTERNAL CAROTID ARTERIOGRAMS AND VENOGRAMS: **c**, 2, Diagram to illustrate the correct anatomic position of the middle cerebral artery from bony landmarks of the skull, *provided the lateral projection is a perfect one.* (Modified after Taveras.)

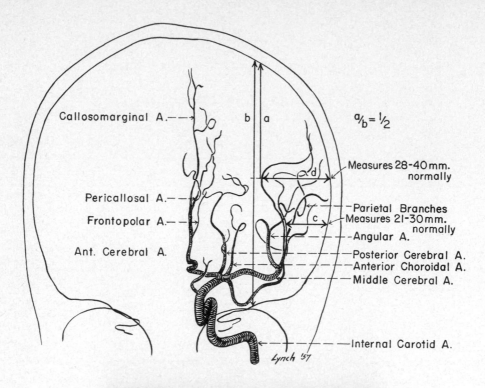

Callosomarginal A.

b | a

$a/b = 1/2$

Measures 28-40 mm. normally

d

Pericallosal A.

Parietal Branches
Measures 21-30 mm. normally

Frontopolar A.

c

Angular A.

Ant. Cerebral A.

Posterior Cerebral A.
Anterior Choroidal A.
Middle Cerebral A.

Internal Carotid A.

Lynch '57

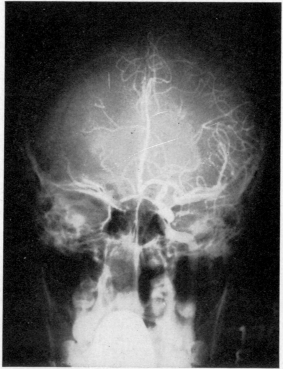

FIG. 8–31.　INTERNAL CAROTID ARTERIOGRAMS AND VENOGRAMS: **d,** Arteriogram diagram and radiograph, antero-posterior projection. (Measurements after Taveras.)

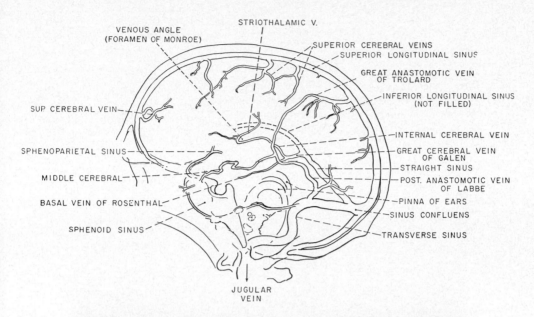

VENOUS ANGLE
(FORAMEN OF MONROE)

STRIOTHALAMIC V.

SUPERIOR CEREBRAL VEINS

SUPERIOR LONGITUDINAL SINUS

GREAT ANASTOMOTIC VEIN
OF TROLARD

INFERIOR LONGITUDINAL SINUS
(NOT FILLED)

SUP CEREBRAL VEIN

INTERNAL CEREBRAL VEIN

SPHENOPARIETAL SINUS

GREAT CEREBRAL VEIN
OF GALEN

STRAIGHT SINUS

MIDDLE CEREBRAL

POST. ANASTOMOTIC VEIN
OF LABBE

BASAL VEIN OF ROSENTHAL

PINNA OF EARS

SINUS CONFLUENS

SPHENOID SINUS

TRANSVERSE SINUS

JUGULAR
VEIN

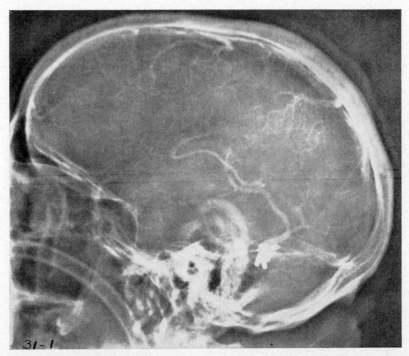

FIG. 8–31. INTERNAL CAROTID ARTERIOGRAMS AND VENOGRAMS: **e,** Venogram diagram and
representative radiograph.

Dural Sinus Venography.[12]   In an attempt to study the intracranial venous system more satisfactorily than in the end phase of an arterial injection, the following procedures have been done: (1) Direct injection through a catheter introduced into the anterior one third of the superior sagittal sinus; (2) retrograde injection through a catheter introduced into the basilar vein of the arm and passed upward to the superior bulb of the internal jugular vein; (3) direct measurement of venous pressure in the superior sagittal sinus.

1. The superior sagittal sinus venogram is performed by passing a catheter into the superior sagittal sinus through a small burr hole. Fifteen cc. of 35 per cent Diodrast or its equivalent is injected rapidly and the x-ray exposure made at the termination of the injection or serial films may be obtained. A slightly oblique Towne's view and a lateral view are obtained (Fig. 8–32). In the normal subject, the contrast media passes backward to the torcular Herophili and thence into the transverse sinuses and internal jugular veins (Fig. 8–32, **a**). The other dural sinuses ordinarily do not fill although occasionally a scalp or diploic vein or the orbital and facial veins anteriorly may be seen. Jugular compression, even if prolonged, never causes filling of the superior cerebral veins, but rather results in extensive filling of the vertebral and occipital plexuses of veins.

In about one half or more of the cases, only one of the transverse sinuses will fill, with apparently no particular predominance of one side or the other.

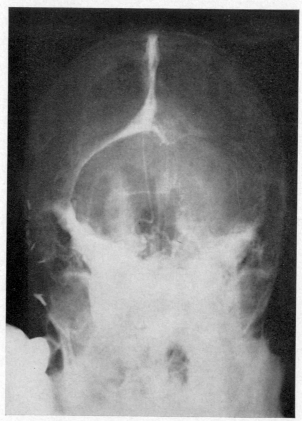

Fig. 8–32.   **a,** Normal superior sagittal sinus venogram.

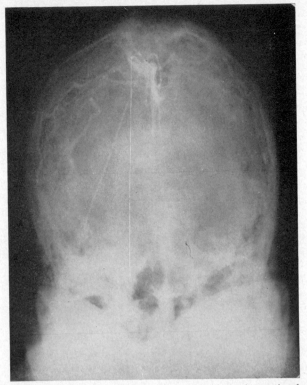

FIG. 8–32. **b,** Superior sagittal sinus venogram, Towne's view, obstruction by meningioma.

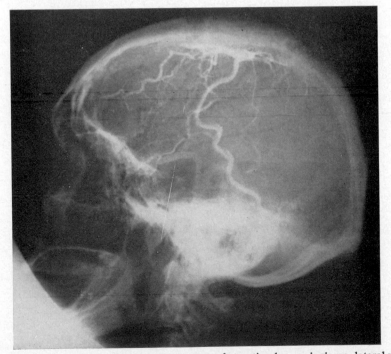

FIG. 8–32. **c,** Superior sagittal sinus venogram, obstruction by meningioma, lateral view.

Venous pressure in the superior sagittal sinus in the normal varies between 100 and 150 mm. of saline.

Abnormal patterns are obtained when the superior sagittal sinus or transverse sinus is invaded or obstructed (Fig. 8–32, **b, c**) by tumor or when either sinus is thrombosed.

2. Retrograde jugular venograms are performed by passing a cardiac catheter from the antecubital vein to the superior jugular bulb, applying compression or pressure on both jugular veins and injecting 25 cc. of 70 per cent Diodrast or its equivalent rapidly. A film or serial films are made in the lateral projection at the termination of the injection.

This results in filling of the superior and inferior petrosal sinuses and sometimes of the cavernous sinus and transverse sinus of the same side. The pterygoid and vertebral plexuses are apparently usually filled and occasionally the orbital and facial veins also.

THE UTILIZATION OF RADIOGRAPHS FOR LOCALIZATION OF INJECTION PROCEDURES IN RELATION TO THE BRAIN (CHEMOSURGICAL TECHNIQUES)

From time to time, neurosurgeons have developed injection procedures for certain areas of the brain. One that has been frequently used in the past has been the injection of the semilunar ganglion of the trigeminal nerve in treatment of the condition known as tic douloureux—a very painful condition affecting the trigeminal nerve. Radiographs are taken at the time of the needle insertion to assist the surgeon in making certain that the injection is in the immediate vicinity of the foramen ovale of the affected side.

The anesthesiologist occasionally calls upon the radiologist for somewhat similar assistance, depending upon the clinical requirements.

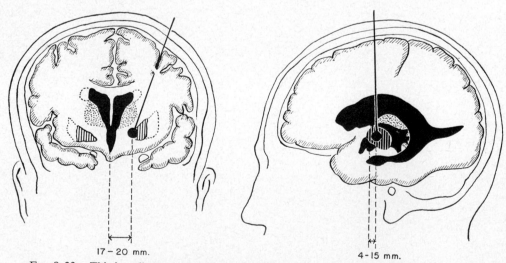

17 – 20 mm. 4 - 15 mm.

Fig. 8–33. This is a diagrammatic representation of chemopallidectomy. The cannula is placed into the brain through a small trephine opening. When it is properly localized, the small balloon at its tip is distended in either the globus pallidus or thalamus. The final lesion is made by injecting absolute alcohol into the cavity created by the balloon.

A more recent application of such studies is that of injecting the globus pallidus or the ventrolateral nucleus of the thalamus.[1] These basal ganglia are situated 4 to 15 mm. behind the foramen of Monro and 17 to 20 mm. lateral to the midpoint of the third ventricle (Fig. 8–33). Subject to the radiographic and physiologic confirmation of the correct placement of a cannula in this location, alcohol injections are carried out in selected patients with parkinsonism—a clinical condition characterized by a very marked tremor while at rest. This procedure is spoken of as chemopallidectomy.[1, 2, 3]

REFERENCES

1. Cooper, I. S.: Chemosurgery for Parkinsonism. Medical Science, 524–527, 1958.
2. Cooper, I. S., Bravo, G. J., Riklan, M., Davidson, N. W., and Gorek, E. A.: Geriatrics *13:* 127–147, 1958.
3. Cooper, I. S.: The Neurosurgical Alleviation of Parkinsonism. Charles C Thomas, Springfield, Ill., 1956.
4. Davidoff, L. M., and Dyke, C. G.: The Normal Encephalogram. 3rd edition. Lea & Febiger, Philadelphia, 1951.
5. Dyke, C. G., and Davidoff, L. M.: The Pneumo-encephalographic Appearance of Hemangioblastoma of the Cerebellum. Am. J. Roentgenol. *44:* 1–8, 1940.
6. Hodes, P., Campoy, P., Riggs, H., and Bly, P.: Cerebral Angiography: Fundamentals in Anatomy and Physiology. Am. J. Roentgenol., *70:* 61–82, 1953.
7. Laine, E., Delandsheer, J. M., Galibut, P., and Delandsheer, Arnott: Phlebography in Tumours of the Hemispheres and Central Gray Matter. Acta radiol., *46:* 203–213, 1956.
8. Laruelle, L.: Le Reparaje Ventriculaire. Rev. Neurol. *40:* 129, 1933.
9. Lin, P., Mokrohisky, J., Stauffer, H., and Scott, M.: The Importance of the Deep Cerebral Veins in Cerebral Angiography. J. Neurosurg., *12:* 256–277, 1955.
10. Lindgren, Erik: Radiologic Examination of the Brain and Spinal Cord. Acta radiol., Supplement 151, 1957.
11. Mokrohisky, J., Paul, R. E., Lin, P., and Stauffer, H.: The Diagnostic Importance of Normal Variants in Deep Cerebral Phlebography. Radiology, *67:* 34–47, 1956.
12. Ray, B. S., Dunbar, H. S., and Dotter, C. P.: Dural Sinus Venography. Radiology, *57:* 475–486, 1951.
13. Robertson, E. G.: Pneumoencephalography. Charles C Thomas, Springfield, Ill., 1957.

CHAPTER 9

The Vertebral Column
and Subarachnoid Space

THE VERTEBRAL COLUMN

THE VERTEBRAL COLUMN is composed of separate articulating segments called vertebrae. These are 33 in number and are distributed as follows: 7 cervical vertebrae, 12 thoracic, 5 lumbar, 5 sacral and 4 coccygeal.

Occasionally there is an extra vertebra in either the thoracic or lumbar spine regions, or there may be one less vertebra than normal, particularly in the lumbar spine. In the latter case, there may be an extra vertebra fused with the coccyx, either completely or partially.

At birth the vertebral column has only two curves with a figure-3 configuration (Fig. 9–1). It is a very asymmetrical 3 because the central angle is at the junction of the last lumbar and the first sacral segment, the so-called sacral-vertebral or lumbosacral angle. The cervical curvature begins to be formed two or three months after birth, when the child begins to lift its head significantly, and becomes further developed when he begins to sit upright, at seven to nine months of age. The lumbar curvature first appears at about one year of age, when walking is begun. The thoracic and sacral curves are the true primary curves of the spine. With advancing years the column loses its flexibility and resilience, and variable amounts of calcification occur at the junction of the vertebral bodies with the paraspinous ligaments. The fused sacrum and also the coccyx are hollowed out anteriorly, and this configuration of the sacrum is particularly important in the female when the pelvis is converted to a birth canal. A flattened sacrum encroaches upon the midpelvic dimension, usually making parturition more difficult.

CHANGES IN SPINAL CURVATURE WITH AGE

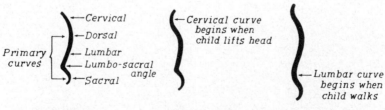

FIG. 9–1.   Changes in spinal curvature with age. (From Meschan, I., and Farrer-Meschan, R. M. F. Radiology, vol. 70, 1958.)

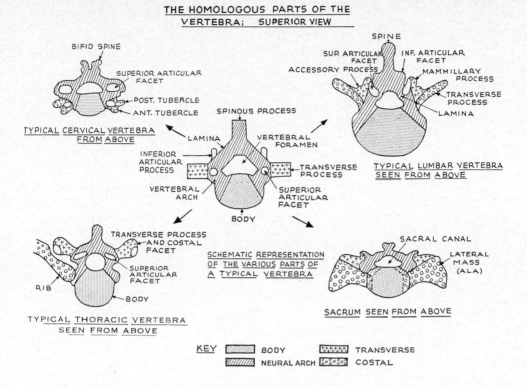

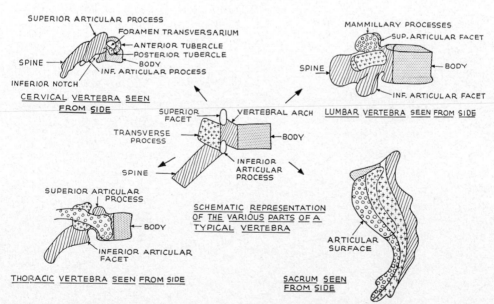

FIG. 9-2. Diagram of basic anatomy of the normal vertebral body and development of homologous parts in various portions of the spine. Superior and lateral views.

The coccyx is extremely variable in its configuration, making it virtually impossible to describe its normal contour. Its development follows no definite scheme.

The Anatomy of a Normal Vertebra.   A vertebra consists of the following parts (Fig. 9–2): (1) the body, (2) the transverse processes on each side, (3) the pedicles, (4) the laminae, (5) the superior articular processes, (6) the inferior articular processes, (7) the spinous process and (8) the partes interarticulares, situated between the two articular processes.

This basic anatomy is modified (Fig. 9–2) in certain parts of the spine to serve particular functions. In the cervical area, the vertebral bodies tend to be small, and the true transverse processes unite with the costal process laterally, enclosing the transverse foramen. The two processes together comprise the lateral mass, and are situated in a more anterior position than comparable portions of other vertebrae. In the thoracic spine, the costal process is separate from the transverse and participates in the formation of the head and neck of the rib with which it articulates. There are costal pits on both the body and transverse process for this articulation. In the lumbar and sacral spine, the costal and transverse processes are completely fused. The vertebral bodies become stouter and larger as one descends the spinal column. The costal elements tend to occupy the greater part of the lateral mass in the sacrum.

The Joints of the Vertebral Column.   In the adult spine, there are two major types of joints and a third ancillary system of joints: (1) the amphiarthrodial joint between vertebral bodies, the intermediate area being occupied by the intervertebral disk; (2) two diarthrodial joints which are true synovial joints between the articular processes of adjoining vertebrae; (3) diarthrodial joints in association with the costal facets of the thoracic spine; and (4) synovial joints (diarthroses) between the posterolateral margins of the lower five cervical bodies (joints of Luschka) (Fig. 9–3).[1] These latter joints are located anteromedially to the mixed nerve root and posteromedially to the vertebral artery, vein and sympathetics as these pass through the vertebral foramen (Fig. 9–4). On the anteroposterior projection of the cervical spine radiograph, the elements of the Luschka joints are formed by spur-like projections near the upper lateral margins of the lower five cervical vertebral bodies; and the corresponding under surfaces of the inferior margins of the vertebral bodies above. In oblique projections, the margins of these joints are seen close to the lower anterior portion of the intervertebral foramen.

The significance of disease in Luschka joints is based on the anatomic relationship of these joints to the neighboring structures—especially the mixed nerve roots, vessels, sympathetics and ligaments. There has been no observation of damage to the spinal cord resulting from disease in Luschka joints.

The true intervertebral joints (between the articular processes) are frequently called "apophyseal joints." There is an obliquity of these apophyseal joints, which will vary somewhat in different parts of the spine, and between individuals, but on the one side in the lumbar region they tend to be parallel, with their plane perpendicular to the corresponding sacro-iliac joint. The planes of the apophyseal joints of both sides tend to meet anteriorly at an angle of 60 to 90 degrees, whereas the planes of the two sacroiliac joints tend to approach one another posteriorly at a similar angle. The diarthrodial articulations be-

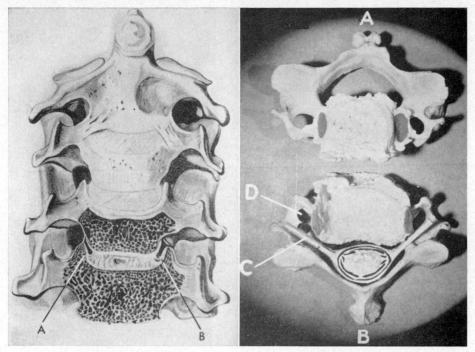

FIG. 9–3   FIG. 9–4

FIG. 9–3.   Reproduction from Lusckha's "Monograph," showing the joints (*A* and *B*) between the posterolateral aspects of the sectioned lower cervical vertebral bodies.

FIG. 9–4.   Photograph of the fifth (*A*) and sixth (*B*) cervical vertebrae showing Luschka joints in relationship to the mixed nerve roots and vertebral foramina. The joints are painted for contrast; the female segment is seen on *A* and the male part on *B*. It is apparent that Luschka joints are situated ventromedial to the nerves (*C*) which emerge through the intervertebral foramina and also medial to the vertebral vessels and sympathetics which pass through the vertebral foramina (*D*). (From Boreadis, A. G., and Gershon-Cohen, J., in Radiology, vol. 66, 1956.)

tween the last lumbar and first sacral segment (lumbosacral joints) are apophyseal joints like the rest, but their obliquity will differ on occasion from the others (Fig. 9–5). There are no apophyseal joints in the sacrum due to fusion of segments.

The Development of the Vertebral Column As a Whole.[9]   The primitive axial support of all vertebrates is the notochord. In humans, the notochord is only a transient structure except in the intervertebral disks where it persists as the nucleus pulposus (Fig. 9–6).

The axial skeleton differentiates from the mesenchyme, most of which occurs in serially arranged pairs of mesodermal segments, designated sclerotomes. The sclerotomes migrate to lie in paired segmental masses alongside the notochord. Each sclerotome differentiates into a caudal compact portion, and a cranial less dense half. At alternate segments there is an intersegmental artery between the less dense and a compact portion. The denser caudal part of each sclerotome mass then unites with the looser cranial half and thus forms the substance of the definitive vertebra. The intervertebral disk differentiates from the denser caudal region.

This so-called membranous vertebral column is succeeded at about the fourth week of fetal life by the cartilaginous vertebral column. Two cartilaginous centers appear on either side of the notochord and rapidly extend around it, thereby forming the bodies of the cartilaginous vertebrae (Figs. 9–6, 9–7). Second pairs of cartilaginous foci appear in the lateral parts of the vertebral arch and extend backward on either side of the neural tube to form the cartilaginous vertebral arch. Still different cartilaginous centers appear for each costal arch.

During the cartilaginous stage the notochord is progressively compressed into the central regions of the dense intervertebral disks. Eventually it disappears completely except as the nucleus pulposus of the intervertebral cartilage. The intersegmental artery persists as a narrow channeled anterior portal into the central portion of the vertebral body (Fig. 9–8). This appearance of the intersegmental artery produces an anterior notching of the vertebral bodies centrally, which may persist into adult life. Such persistence is probably without pathologic significance.

The anterior and posterior longitudinal spinal ligaments develop during the cartilaginous stage. In the ninth week of fetal life, anterior and posterior indentations into the cartilaginous body are produced by periosteal vessels, which form ventral and dorsal blood lakes (Fig. 9–9). These correspond with the arterial and venous supply to the vertebral bodies, as shown in the illustration.

There is considerable disagreement as to the exact changes which occur during the ossification stage. Ossification centers are said to form either dorsally and ventrally, or superiorly and inferiorly, in the vertebral body and are separated by cartilaginous septa, which soon disappear (Fig. 9–7). In either instance, the primary ossification center is hourglass shaped, and abnormalities in ossification will account for various unusual wedged appearances of the vertebral bodies. One can usually differentiate such wedging from traumatic or infectious wedging on the basis of the overdevelopment which is often discernible in contiguous vertebrae.

There are also separate ossification centers on each side which enter into the formation of the neural arch. Thus, for each vertebral segment there are three separate ossification centers.

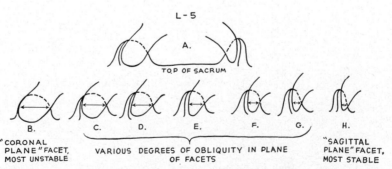

PATIENT WITH ASYMMETRICAL FACETS

L-5

A.

TOP OF SACRUM

B. C. D. E. F. G. H.

"CORONAL PLANE" FACET, MOST UNSTABLE   VARIOUS DEGREES OF OBLIQUITY IN PLANE OF FACETS   "SAGITTAL PLANE" FACET, MOST STABLE

FIG. 9–5. The plane of the lumbosacral facets in relation to stability. (Modified from Ferguson, A. B.: *Roentgen Diagnosis of Extremities and Spine*, Paul B. Hoeber, Inc.)

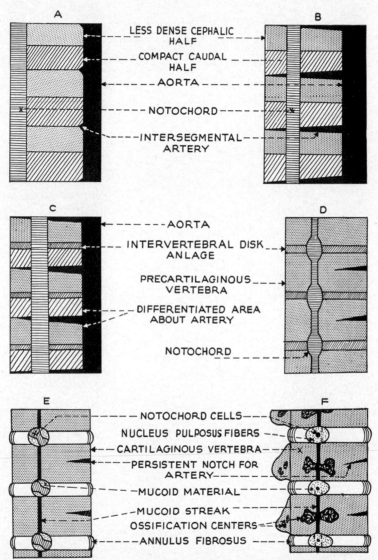

FIG. 9–6. Development of the vertebral column as a whole, demonstrating the membranous cartilaginous and early ossification stages. (After *The Intervertebral Disc*, by F. K. Bradford and C. Glenn Spurling.)

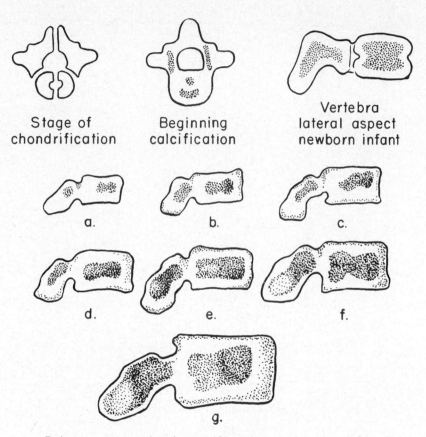

Stage of chondrification   Beginning calcification   Vertebra lateral aspect newborn infant

a.   b.   c.

d.   e.   f.

g.

Primary vertebral ossification centers from
sixth fetal week (a) to the neonatal period (g).

FIG. 9–7. **a,** Further diagram demonstrating the stage of chondrification, beginning calcification and gradual development of ossification in the vertebral body of the newborn.

AT BIRTH
VERTEBRAL BODY
AND NEURAL ARCH

2 YRS. OF AGE
LAMINAE FUSE POSTERIORLY
(STARTS IN LUMBAR AREA AND
ASCENDS, BUT SACRUM IS LAST)
(7 TO 10 YRS.)

BY 6-7 YRS. OLD
NEURAL ARCH UNITES WITH
VERTEBRAL BODY (EARLIEST
IN NECK, LAST IN SACRUM)

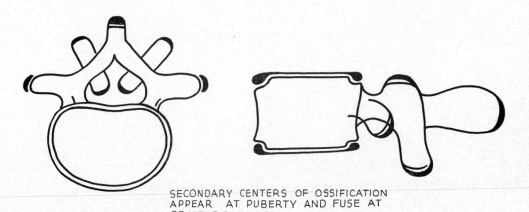

SECONDARY CENTERS OF OSSIFICATION
APPEAR AT PUBERTY AND FUSE AT
25 YEARS OF AGE

FIG. 9–7. **b,** Diagram to illustrate time of union of the laminae and the joining of the neural arches with the body. The secondary centers of ossification are also illustrated.

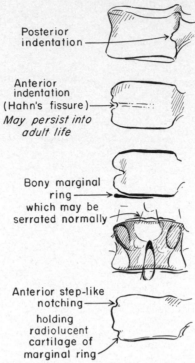

Posterior
indentation

Anterior
indentation
(Hahn's fissure)—
*May persist into
adult life*

Bony marginal
ring
which may be
serrated normally

Anterior step-like
notching
holding
radiolucent
cartilage of
marginal ring

FIG. 9–8.   The normal appearance of posterior and anterior indentations on vertebral bodies in relation to blood supply and venous drainage. The anterior steplike notching is a change in contour which is described in relation to the cartilaginous end plates of the vertebral body.

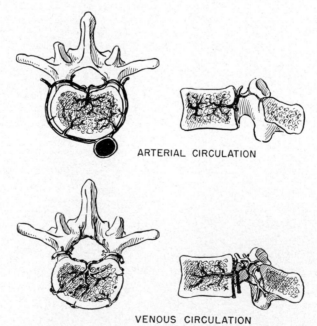

ARTERIAL CIRCULATION

VENOUS CIRCULATION

FIG. 9–9.   Diagrams illustrating the arterial and venous circulation of a vertebral body and its neural arch.

Aberrations in the further development of the neural arch are usually considered to represent defects in the development of the ossification rather than abnormalities in the centers *per se*. Figure 9–10 demonstrates the various areas of defective ossification which can occur in the formation of the neural arch.

At approximately the fifth to the sixth month of fetal life, the ossification center of the vertebral body has separated the cartilaginous body into two thick cartilaginous plates showing endochondral ossification toward the intervertebral disk side. Along the anterior and lateral periphery of the vertebral bodies, horseshoe-shaped cartilaginous plates appear, which represent cartilaginous ring apophyses (Fig. 9–7, **c**). Later these form the anlage of the bony ring apophysis which appears in adolescent life. These apophyses fit into notches in the superior and inferior portions of the vertebral bodies so that, prior to the ossification of the ring apophysis, the vertebral body has a notched appearance (Fig. 9–8). The rami of the lumbar neural arches unite during the first year of life, and similar changes follow in the neural arches of the thoracic and cervical regions. The tips of the transverse and spinous processes remain cartilaginous in the years before puberty. At about the sixteenth year, secondary centers appear at the tips of the transverse processes, the tips of the spinous processes, and at the upper and lower surfaces of the vertebral body (Fig. 9–7). These fuse with the rest of the vertebral body by age 25.

There are perhaps two other aberrations of development in relation to the vertebral body and the intervertebral disk which are noteworthy. Very often there is a posterior wedging of the fifth lumbar vertebra which persists even into adult life. Such posterior wedging is a relatively normal contour variation and has no pathologic significance. It is related to the junction of the lumbar curvature with the sacral curvature. Also the intervertebral disk between L_5 and S_1 may be narrowed throughout life. This likewise is related to the junction point between the lumbar and sacral curvature. *Narrowness of the interspace between L_5 and S_1, therefore, is without pathologic significance unless there are some other radiographic criteria, such as sclerosis of the end plates, irregularities of the end plates, or changes in the adjoining ligamentous structures.*

The *union of laminae* begins in the lumbar region soon after birth (Fig. 9–7, **b**), and spreading upward is completed in the cervical region early in the second year, but is deferred in the sacrum until the seventh to tenth years. After fusion of the laminae there is a gradual extension of the ossification process into the spinous processes.

The *bony union of the neural arch and the vertebral body* begins in the cervical area at the age of 3, and the process descends in the spine to reach the sacrum in the sixth or seventh year.

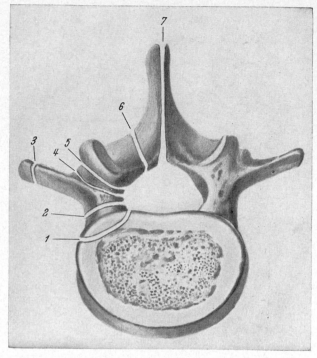

a

DEFECTS IN OSSIFICATION OF VERTEBRAE

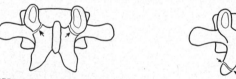

DEFECTS IN PARS INTERARTICULARIS

EXTRA-APOPHYSES

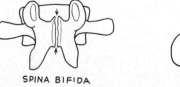

SPINA BIFIDA

b

FIG. 9–10.   **a,** Diagram illustrating the various areas for defective ossification in the neural arch and pedicles: *1,* Retrosomatic hiatus. *2,* Hiatus in the pedicle. *3,* Persistent epiphysis of the transverse process. *4* and *5,* Defects in the pars interarticularis. *6,* Retroisthmic hiatus. *7,* Bifid posterior spinous process. (From Köhler, Alban: *Borderlands of the Normal and Early Pathologic in Skeletal Roentgenology,* Grune & Stratton.)

b, Further tracings demonstrating defects in the pars interarticularis, spina bifida, and extra-apophyses as they may appear on various roentgenographic views.

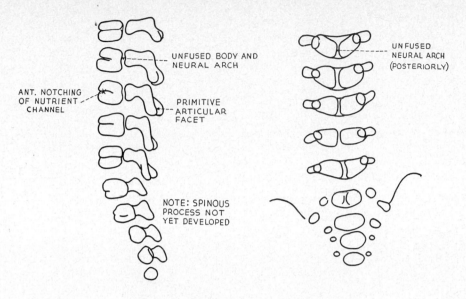

SPINAL COLUMN AT BIRTH

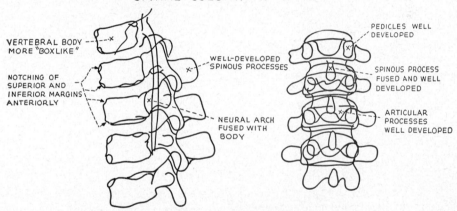

AGE 6 YEARS

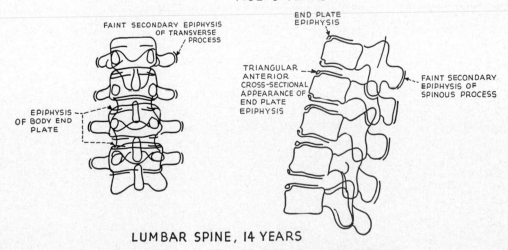

LUMBAR SPINE, 14 YEARS

FIG. 9–11. Spinal column at various stages of development.

DISTINGUISHING CHARACTERISTICS OF THE CERVICAL SPINE (Fig. 9–12)

The atlas and axis differ with regard to development from the rest of the vertebrae in that the ossification center for the body of C_1 separates from the rest of this vertebra, and unites with the body of C_2 to form the odontoid process. An epiphysis for the top of the odontoid process appears between the third and sixth years, and unites with the rest usually before 12 years of age. The spine of the atlas is represented by the tubercle on the posterior arch. (Spines are absent below the level of the third sacral segment.) The articular process of the atlas and the superior articular process of the axis are not truly homologous with the articular processes of the other vertebrae, and are virtually absent as such in these segments—the articular function in the atlas and superior articular process of the axis being taken over by a modification of the costal pits. The articular surfaces of C_1 and the upper articular surface of C_2 are thus more anteriorly situated than the other articulations in the cervical spine.

Occasionally occipitalization of the atlas will occur.[5, 6]

The alignment of C_1 with respect to the foramen magnum of the skull is illustrated in Figure 9–13, **a.** When a straight line is drawn along the front of the odontoid process, it meets the anterior margin of the foramen magnum, and a line drawn above the inner margin of the posterior arch of C_1 will meet the posterior margin of the foramen magnum. Lines drawn along the anterior margins and posterior margins of the vertebral bodies are practically parallel. A line connecting the anterior margins of the spinous processes forms a gentle continuous curvature, meeting the posterior margin of the foramen magnum. The curvature of the cervical spine virtually disappears when the neck is flexed, but these linear relationships persist, and a deviation becomes of definite significance.

Another mode of alignment of the cervical spine with respect to the skull is referred to as "Chamberlain's line" (Fig. 9–13, **a**): Normally, a line drawn from the hard palate to the inner table of the occipital bone will just fall above the odontoid process. An abnormality usually exists (basilar impression) if this is not found.

The undeflected contour of the line joining the posterior margins of the vertebral bodies is most important (Fig. 9–13, **a**). Deflections usually indicate small spurs which may encroach upon the spinal canal or intervertebral foramina.

The visualization of the odontoid process in the antero-posterior projection requires special techniques (Fig. 9–17). This is accomplished either by opening the mouth, by moving the mandible while the exposure is made (so that it does not obscure the upper cervical spine), or by body section radiography. Also, a short film-target distance is employed to distort the mandible out of clear view.

The symmetrical appearance of the odontoid with respect to the surrounding articulation is clearly demonstrated by the lines drawn as illustrated (Fig. 9–13).

The vertebral bodies below C_2 level are very regular and similar in appearances with the exception of C_5 which very frequently normally appears somewhat narrowed anteriorly. This variation of normal must not be misinterpreted.[10]

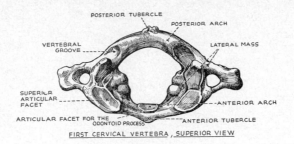

FIRST CERVICAL VERTEBRA, SUPERIOR VIEW

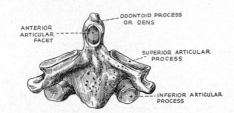

SECOND CERVICAL VERTEBRA, ANTERIOR VIEW

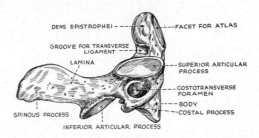

THE EPISTROPHEUS OR AXIS

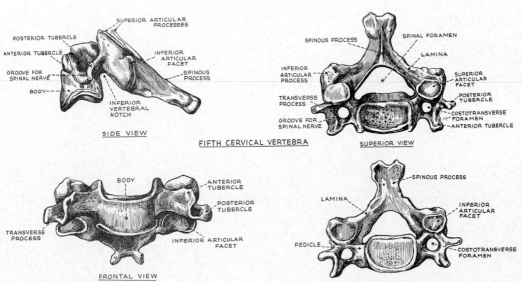

FIG. 9-12.   Distinguishing characteristics of cervical vertebrae.

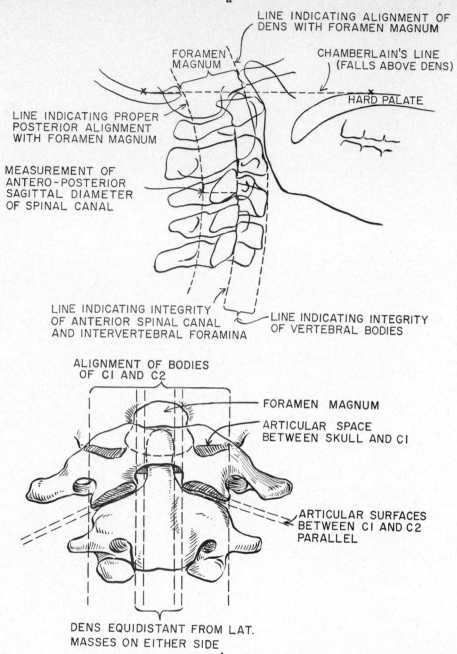

a

LINE INDICATING ALIGNMENT OF
DENS WITH FORAMEN MAGNUM

FORAMEN
MAGNUM

CHAMBERLAIN'S LINE
(FALLS ABOVE DENS)

HARD PALATE

LINE INDICATING PROPER
POSTERIOR ALIGNMENT
WITH FORAMEN MAGNUM

MEASUREMENT OF
ANTERO-POSTERIOR
SAGITTAL DIAMETER
OF SPINAL CANAL

LINE INDICATING INTEGRITY
OF ANTERIOR SPINAL CANAL
AND INTERVERTEBRAL FORAMINA

LINE INDICATING INTEGRITY
OF VERTEBRAL BODIES

ALIGNMENT OF BODIES
OF CI AND C2

FORAMEN MAGNUM

ARTICULAR SPACE
BETWEEN SKULL AND CI

ARTICULAR SURFACES
BETWEEN CI AND C2
PARALLEL

DENS EQUIDISTANT FROM LAT.
MASSES ON EITHER SIDE

b

FIG. 9–13. ALIGNMENT OF CERVICAL SEGMENTS WITH RESPECT TO EACH OTHER AND TO THE SKULL:
a, Lateral projection;   b, odontoid projection.

With the exception of C_1 and C_7, all of the vertebrae have somewhat bifid spinous processes. The transverse processes of C_7 may be considerably elongated, and its costal element may actually form a complete rib, in which case it is known as a cervical rib.

In the antero-posterior projection the lateral mass and the articular processes are projected over one another, and to separate the two one obtains the lateral projection, the articular processes being projected posteriorly (Fig. 9–14).

392

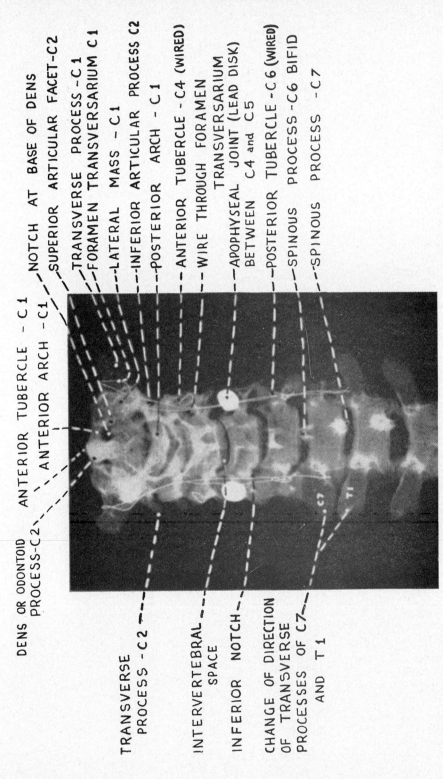

DENS OR ODONTOID PROCESS-C2

ANTERIOR TUBERCLE - C1

ANTERIOR ARCH - C1

NOTCH AT BASE OF DENS

SUPERIOR ARTICULAR FACET-C2

TRANSVERSE PROCESS - C1

FORAMEN TRANSVERSARIUM C1

LATERAL MASS - C1

INFERIOR ARTICULAR PROCESS C2

POSTERIOR ARCH - C1

ANTERIOR TUBERCLE - C4 (WIRED)

WIRE THROUGH FORAMEN TRANSVERSARIUM

APOPHYSEAL JOINT (LEAD DISK) BETWEEN C4 and C5

POSTERIOR TUBERCLE - C6 (WIRED)

SPINOUS PROCESS - C6 BIFID

SPINOUS PROCESS - C7

TRANSVERSE PROCESS - C2

INTERVERTEBRAL SPACE

INFERIOR NOTCH

CHANGE OF DIRECTION OF TRANSVERSE PROCESSES OF C7 AND T1

FIG. 9–14. RADIOGRAPHS, OF THE CERVICAL SPINE WITH CERTAIN ANATOMIC FEATURES INDICATED: a, Antero-posterior projection.

WIRES THROUGH
FORAMINA TRANSVERSARIA
ON BOTH SIDES
(COSTOTRANSVERSE FORAMINA)

PEDICLES

BODY - C 3

ANTERIOR TUBERCLES OF
TRANSVERSE PROCESSES
OF BOTH SIDES (WIRED)

TRANSVERSE PROCESSES
SUPERIMPOSED

POSTERIOR TUBERCLES
OF BOTH SIDES
(WIRED)

INFERIOR ARTICULAR FACET C7

SUPERIOR ARTICULAR FACET-T1

ODONTOID PROCESS - C 2

ANTERIOR TUBERCLE - C 1

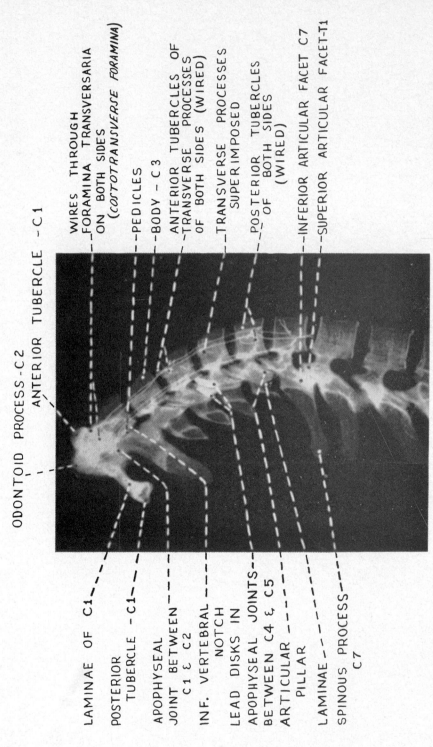

LAMINAE OF C1

POSTERIOR
TUBERCLE - C1

APOPHYSEAL
JOINT BETWEEN
C 1 & C 2

INF. VERTEBRAL
NOTCH

LEAD DISKS IN
APOPHYSEAL JOINTS
BETWEEN C4 & C5

ARTICULAR
PILLAR

LAMINAE

SPINOUS PROCESS
C7

FIG. 9-14. RADIOGRAPHS OF THE CERVICAL SPINE WITH CERTAIN ANATOMIC FEATURES INDICATED: **b,** Lateral projection.

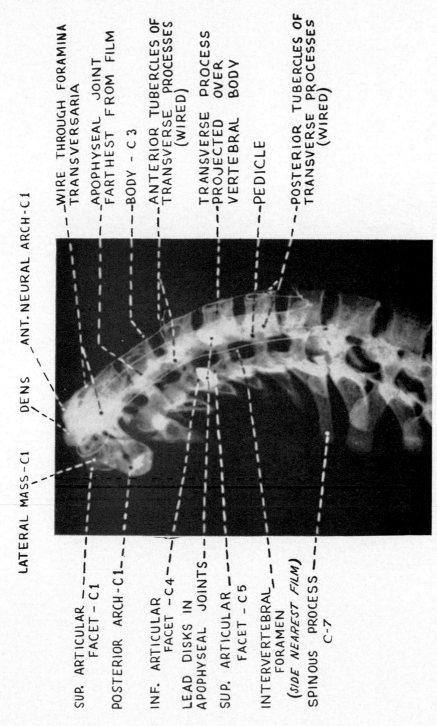

LATERAL MASS-C1

DENS

ANT. NEURAL ARCH-C1

WIRE THROUGH FORAMINA
TRANSVERSARIA

APOPHYSEAL JOINT
FARTHEST FROM FILM

BODY - C3

ANTERIOR TUBERCLES OF
TRANSVERSE PROCESSES
(WIRED)

TRANSVERSE PROCESS
PROJECTED OVER
VERTEBRAL BODY

PEDICLE

POSTERIOR TUBERCLES OF
TRANSVERSE PROCESSES
(WIRED)

SUP. ARTICULAR
FACET - C1

POSTERIOR ARCH-C1

INF. ARTICULAR
FACET -C4

LEAD DISKS IN
APOPHYSEAL JOINTS

SUP. ARTICULAR
FACET - C5

INTERVERTEBRAL
FORAMEN
(SIDE NEAREST FILM)

SPINOUS PROCESS -
C-7

FIG. 9–14. RADIOGRAPHS OF THE CERVICAL SPINE WITH CERTAIN ANATOMIC FEATURES INDICATED: **c**, Oblique projection.

The intervertebral foramina are best shown in the oblique projection (Fig. 9–19). These are ovoid in shape, and tend to diminish slightly in size between C_2 level and C_5, and then tend to increase slightly. Great variations in size are of definite significance from the standpoint of possible encroachment on nerve structures contained therein.

Some knowledge of the normal antero-posterior diameter of the bony cervical canal is of importance, since spur formation is common in this area, and these spurs may in turn be responsible for neurologic findings. In the measurement of the sagittal diameters of the cervical bony canal in 200 normal adults, Wolf *et al.*[12] concluded that a sagittal diameter of 10 mm. or less, due to posterior spurs, is likely to be associated with cord compression. Also a minimum sagittal diameter greater than 13 mm. suggests that simple spur formation could not be responsible for cord compression in this area. Other abnormalities are not of course excluded.

The average normal sagittal diameter of the spinal canal at the first cervical level is 22 mm.; at the second cervical level, 20 mm.; and at the levels between the third and seventh cervical, 17 mm., with a range in the latter instance of $+5$ mm

Encroachment upon the intervertebral foramina is visualized in the oblique views and is not measured by this expedient.

Changes with Growth and Development. The distinguishing characteristics of the atlas and axis as regards development have been described above. With regard to the other cervical vertebrae, at birth the laminae are united only by cartilage, and there is likewise no osseous union of the neural arch with the body (Fig. 9–11). This does not occur until the second or third year respectively. A faint cartilaginous line may persist until 6 or 7 years of age, and this may lead to confusion, particularly at the base of the odontoid process. Such cartilaginous lines may readily be confused with fractures.

The vertebral body does not take on its more definitive appearance until long after puberty, and particularly in the cervical region the anterior margins of the bodies tend to be slightly narrowed in comparison with the posterior margins. This configuration must not be misinterpreted as compression (Fig. 9–15). The only vertebral bodies that may persistently retain this infantile contour are C_5 and less frequently C_6. The secondary centers of ossification do not appear until puberty, and unite at about 25 years of age.

The change in curvature of the cervical spine with the changing posture of the growing individual has already been described.

ROUTINE RADIOGRAPHIC POSITIONS FOR STUDY OF THE CERVICAL SPINE

1. **Antero-posterior Views of the Cervical Spine** (Fig. 9–16). In this view, only the vertebrae below C_3 level are visualized unless the view is obtained with the mandible in motion. The lateral mass, consisting of the costal process, the transverse process and the costotransverse foramen, overlaps the articular process, and the anatomic parts are therefore difficult to distinguish. A mind's eye three-dimensional concept is most important to visualize these structures (Fig. 9–16).

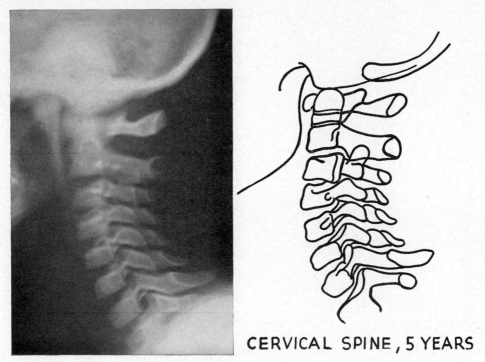

CERVICAL SPINE, 5 YEARS

FIG. 9–15. Radiograph and tracing of child's cervical spine to demonstrate irregularity and anterior narrowness of the vertebral bodies.

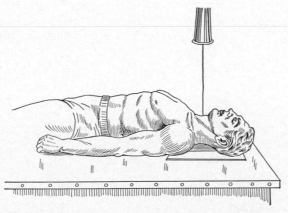

FIG. 9–16. ANTERO-POSTERIOR VIEW OF CERVICAL SPINE: **a,** Positioning of patient.

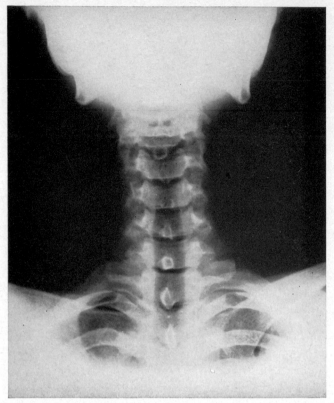

Fig. 9–16.   ANTERO-POSTERIOR VIEW OF CERVICAL SPINE: **b,** Radiograph.

POINTS OF PRACTICAL INTEREST WITH REFERENCE TO FIGURE 9–16:

1. The sagittal plane of the head is centered to the longitudinal axis of the table and the chin of the patient is extended sufficiently so that the lower edge of the anterior teeth of the patient is in the same perpendicular line as the tip of the mastoid processes.
2. The head should be immobilized by means of either sandbags or head clamps. These have been omitted in the drawings for the sake of clarity.
3. The central ray passes through the most prominent point of the thyroid cartilage. This ordinarily lies anterior to the fourth cervical segment.
4. Alternately, the central ray may be angled 15 or 20 degrees toward the head which gives one a somewhat clearer concept of the lower intervertebral spaces, and a better view for demonstration of possible cervical ribs.
5. Alternately also, the mandibular shadow may be blurred by utilizing regular, rhythmical motion of the lower jaw during the exposure. The head, of course, is rigidly immobilized to prevent movement of the cervical spine. When a view is obtained in this manner a concept of the upper two cervical segments may be obtained which otherwise is not possible in this projection, since these segments are invariably obscured by the shadow of the mandible (Fig. 9–16, d).

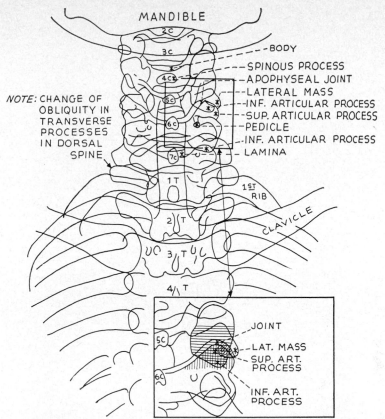

MANDIBLE

2C

3C ----BODY

----SPINOUS PROCESS

----APOPHYSEAL JOINT

4C ----LATERAL MASS

NOTE: CHANGE OF
OBLIQUITY IN
TRANSVERSE
PROCESSES
IN DORSAL
SPINE

5C ----INF. ARTICULAR PROCESS

----SUP. ARTICULAR PROCESS

6C ----PEDICLE

----INF. ARTICULAR PROCESS

7C ---- LAMINA

1 T

1ST
RIB

2 T

CLAVICLE

3 T

4 T

JOINT

5C LAT. MASS

SUP. ART.
PROCESS

6C

INF. ART.
PROCESS

FIG. 9–16. ANTERO-POSTERIOR VIEW OF CERVICAL SPINE: **c,** Labeled tracing of **b.**

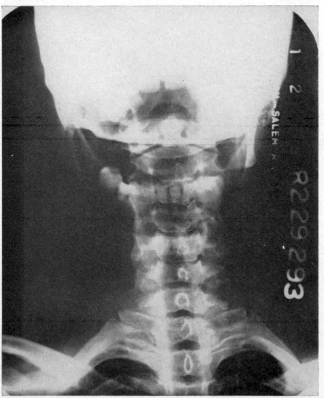

FIG. 9–16. **d,** Antero-posterior view of the cervical spine obtained with a rhythmic motion of the lower jaw during the exposure. This illustration virtually combines the anatomic features of Figures 9–16, **b** and 9–17, **b.** For anatomic detail, study these latter two illustrations.

399

2. **Antero-posterior View of the Upper Cervical Spine Through the Open Mouth or with the Mandible in Motion** (Fig. 9–17).   In this view, one must be careful to obtain the entire odontoid process. The base of the skull may obscure it in part. The relationship of the dens to its adjoining articulations has already been described (Fig. 9–13, **b**).

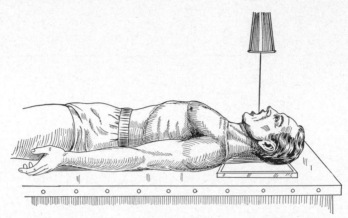

FIG. 9–17.   ANTERO-POSTERIOR VIEW OF UPPER CERVICAL SPINE WITH MOUTH OPEN PARTICULARLY TO SHOW ODONTOID PROCESS: **a,** Positioning of patient.

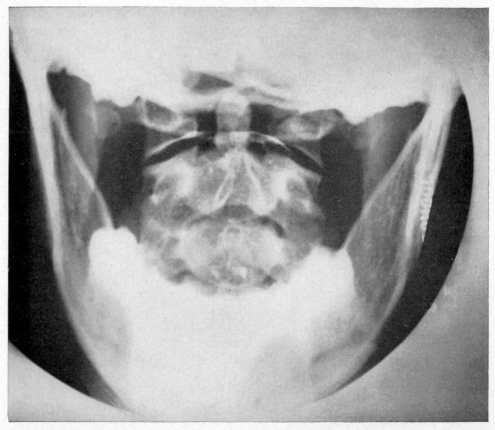

FIG. 9–17.   ANTERO-POSTERIOR VIEW OF UPPER CERVICAL SPINE WITH MOUTH OPEN PARTICULARLY TO SHOW ODONTOID PROCESS: **b,** Radiograph.

1. The mouth of the patient is opened as widely as possible and it may be kept in this position by a large cork or balsa wood block.
2. A line drawn between the lower margin of the anterior upper teeth to the tip of the mastoid process must be perpendicular to the film.
3. If the patient will softly say "Ah" during the exposure, the tongue will be more closely fixed to the floor of the mouth so that its shadow will not be projected over the atlas and axis.
4. Body section radiographs of the odontoid process and adjoining joints are frequently very helpful (Fig. 9–17, d).

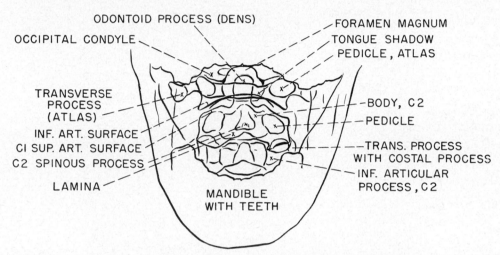

ODONTOID PROCESS (DENS)
OCCIPITAL CONDYLE
FORAMEN MAGNUM
TONGUE SHADOW
PEDICLE, ATLAS
TRANSVERSE PROCESS (ATLAS)
INF. ART. SURFACE
CI SUP. ART. SURFACE
C2 SPINOUS PROCESS
LAMINA
BODY, C2
PEDICLE
TRANS. PROCESS WITH COSTAL PROCESS
INF. ARTICULAR PROCESS, C2
MANDIBLE WITH TEETH

FIG. 9–17. ANTERO-POSTERIOR VIEW OF UPPER CERVICAL SPINE WITH MOUTH OPEN PARTICULARLY TO SHOW ODONTOID PROCESS: **c,** Labeled tracing of **b.**

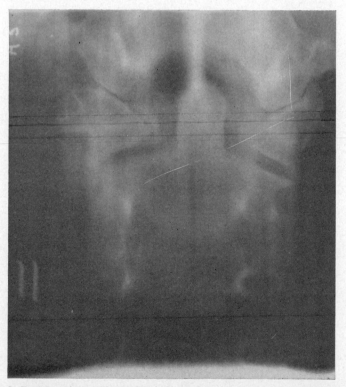

FIG. 9–17. **d,** Body section radiograph of the uppermost cervical segments showing in better detail the joint between the occipital condyles and the first cervical segment and also demonstrating more clearly the relationship of the foramen magnum and the projection of the odontoid process.

401

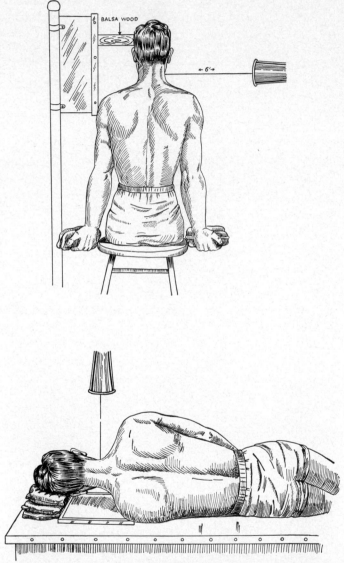

FIG. 9-18. LATERAL VIEW OF CERVICAL SPINE: **a,** Positioning of patient; erect (6 foot film-target distance) and recumbent views.

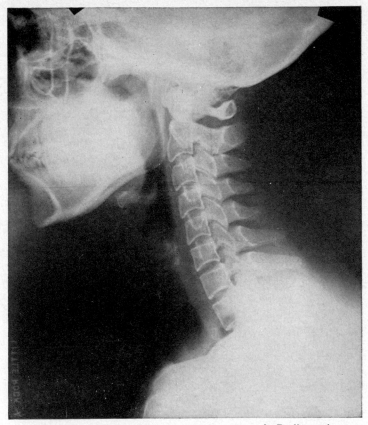

FIG. 9–18. LATERAL VIEW OF CERVICAL SPINE: **b,** Radiograph.

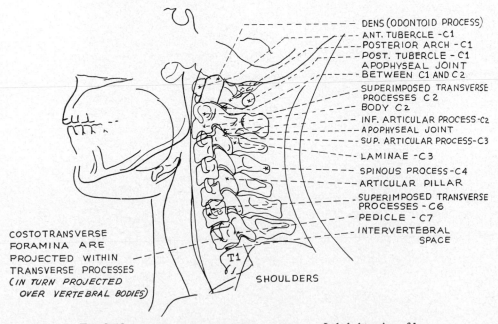

DENS (ODONTOID PROCESS)
ANT. TUBERCLE -C1
POSTERIOR ARCH -C1
POST. TUBERCLE - C1
APOPHYSEAL JOINT
BETWEEN C1 AND C2
SUPERIMPOSED TRANSVERSE PROCESSES C2
BODY C2
INF. ARTICULAR PROCESS-C2
APOPHYSEAL JOINT
SUP. ARTICULAR PROCESS-C3
LAMINAE -C3
SPINOUS PROCESS-C4
ARTICULAR PILLAR
SUPERIMPOSED TRANSVERSE PROCESSES - C6
PEDICLE - C7
INTERVERTEBRAL SPACE

COSTOTRANSVERSE FORAMINA ARE PROJECTED WITHIN TRANSVERSE PROCESSES (*IN TURN PROJECTED OVER VERTEBRAL BODIES*)

T1

SHOULDERS

FIG. 9–18. LATERAL VIEW OF CERVICAL SPINE: **c,** Labeled tracing of **b.**

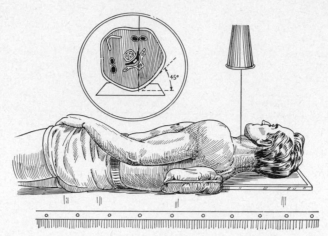

FIG. 9–19.   OBLIQUE VIEW OF CERVICAL SPINE: **a,** Positioning of patient.

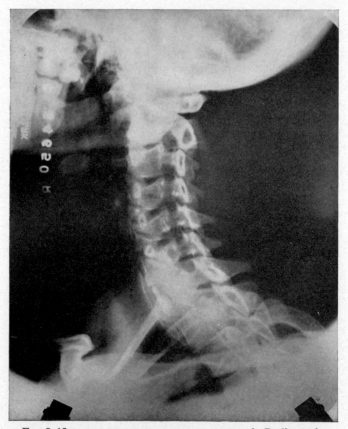

FIG. 9–19.   OBLIQUE VIEW OF CERVICAL SPINE: **b,** Radiograph.

Points of Practical Interest with Reference to Figure 9–19:
1. This view may be obtained in either the erect or recumbent position.
2. The entire body of the patient is rotated, and if the patient is supine, sandbags are placed beneath the shoulder and the buttocks to support the position of the patient at an angle of 45 degrees, with the table top. The sagittal axis of the head of the patient is perfectly straight with regard to the sagittal axis of the entire body.
3. The central ray is directed over the cervical spine at the level of the fourth cervical segment (at the level of the most prominent portion of the thyroid cartilage).
4. Alternately an additional angulation of the tube toward the head 15 degrees may be employed, with the patient in the same position as indicated herein.
5. It is best to employ a focal-film distance of at least 48 inches since the cervical spine is at such a great distance from the film in this projection.
6. Oblique studies of both sides are routinely obtained.
7. The intervertebral foramina which are farthest from the film are the ones which are shown most clearly.

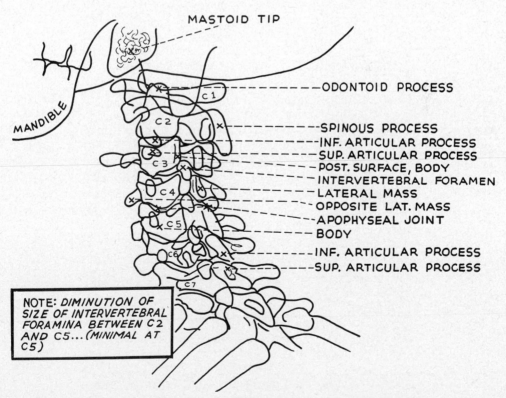

FIG. 9–19.   OBLIQUE VIEW OF CERVICAL SPINE: c, Labeled tracing of b.

3. **Lateral View of the Cervical Spine** (Fig. 9–18).   In order to obtain a good visualization of C_7, the patient sits up, and drops his shoulders as much as possible. Traction on the arms by means of heavy weights in the hands helps in lowering the shoulders. In order to obtain a true lateral projection, the patient's neck must be perfectly perpendicular to his shoulders, and also to the central ray. This places the cervical spine a considerable distance from the film. *Distortion and magnification are very considerable under these circumstances, unless a long film-target distance is employed* (6 ft.). Every effort is made to preserve the normal curvature of the cervical spine, but frequently this curvature will disappear in the event of muscular spasm. The normal alignment previously described is only slightly disturbed under these circumstances.

In this projection, the lateral mass is projected in part over the vertebral body, particularly in its costal element. The articular processes, however, are shown very clearly.

4. **Oblique View of the Cervical Spine** (Fig. 9–19).   In order to obtain comparable views of the intervertebral foramina, care must be taken to rotate the entire body 45 degrees, and not just the cervical spine. Actually, in this oblique projection, the head, neck and torso are in perfectly straight alignment. The anatomy so projected is shown in Figure 9–19.

DISTINGUISHING CHARACTERISTICS OF THE THORACIC OR DORSAL SPINE
(Fig. 9–20)

There are several distinguishing characteristics of the thoracic spine. The vertebral bodies of the upper eight segments articulate with two ribs on each side, and the lower four articulate only with the one rib with which they are numerically associated. There are also small costal facets on each transverse process of the upper ten thoracic vertebrae. The two different joints formed are called the costovertebral and costotransverse joints, respectively, with separate synovial cavities and joint capsules in each instance.

The superior and inferior surfaces of these bodies are ordinarily quite flat. Occasionally they appear defective centrally, with a notch appearing. These notches, when central and not too clearly defined, occur sufficiently frequently (in approximately 40 per cent of adult spines) to be considered without special significance, although Schmorl believed them to be due to defects in the end plates of the vertebra on a congenital basis (hence called "Schmorl's nodes"). However, when these nodes are excentric, or associated with an undulating appearance of the superior or inferior surfaces of the vertebral bodies, they may well be of definite pathologic significance.

The posterior surfaces of these vertebral bodies are slightly concave from side to side, producing a somewhat double contoured appearance on the radiograph.

There is a gradual increase in size from above downward in the vertebral supero-inferior dimensions, both anteriorly and posteriorly. The posterior dimension tends to be slightly greater than the anterior. Diminution in size of a vertebra in relation to the adjoining vertebral bodies, therefore, becomes of definite significance.

The twelfth thoracic vertebra differs from the others (Fig. 9–20) in that its transverse processes are each replaced by three tubercles, and its inferior apophyseal joint faces in a more lateral direction than do the joints above it.

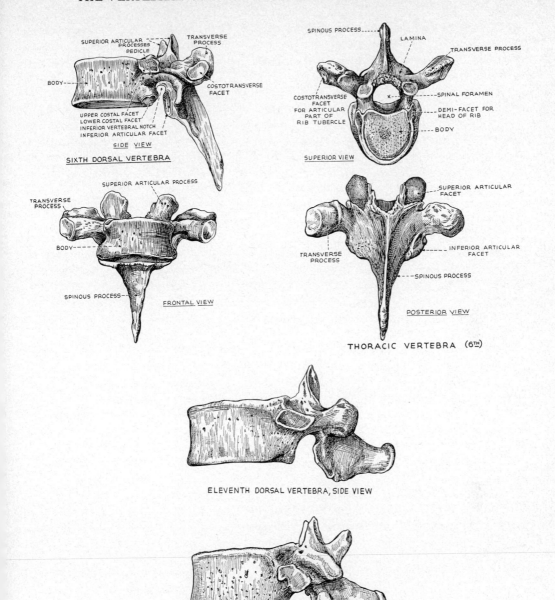

FIG. 9–20. Distinguishing characteristics of dorsal vertebrae.

The spinous processes are long and slender, being steepest in the middle of the thoracic spine (Fig. 9–25). These structures are to a very great extent obscured by the ribs which curve backward and overlie them. The laminae overlap one another (called imbrication), further obscuring detail. The intervertebral foramina are circular, and smaller than in the cervical or lumbar areas.

The paraspinal line (paravertebral soft tissue shadows), well delineated in frontal radiographs of the thoracic spine, must be differentiated from manifestations of disease.[2] A left paraspinal shadow delimited by the left pleura reflection is commonly visualized on films of the thoracic spine.[3] It roughly parallels the left margin of the vertebral column and the aorta and lies between these two structures (Fig. 9–21).

Above the level of the aortic arch the two pleural layers lie almost in contact anterior to the vertebral column, and because of the superposition of the tracheal air column the pleural air shadows are difficult to define radiographically. The right mediastinal shadow parallels the dorsal spine in corresponding fashion and lies between the dorsal spine and the right margin of the cardiac silhouette.

When there is a diffuse dilatation of the descending thoracic aorta, the left pleural reflection is pulled laterally, producing an apparent widening of the left paraspinal shadow, but at the same time this still maintains a relative symmetry in contour with the aorta.

Any bony changes may also alter the paraspinal shadow. Hypertrophic spurs on the lateral aspects of the vertebral bodies may reach a sufficient size to deflect the pleura on either or both sides. Inflammatory masses or neoplasms involving the vertebrae may likewise extend into the soft tissues and displace the pleura to the right or left at the affected levels.

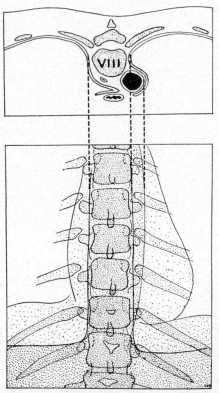

FIG. 9–21.   Upper: Cross section through the posterior mediastinum at the level of the eighth thoracic vertebra. Lower: Diagram taken from a roentgenogram depicting the posterior portions of the visceral and/or parietal pleura as lines along the vertebral column. Dotted lines indicate anatomical substrates of pleural lines and aortic lines in cross section. (From Lachman, E., in Anat. Rec., vol. 83, 1942.)

In the absence of demonstrable vertebral body disease and in the presence of an apparently normal aorta, other soft tissue abnormalities may be presumed to alter the paraspinal shadow. These may be related to tumors of nerve tissue origin, metastatic carcinoma, and other neoplasms, particularly those involving the mediastinum.

Changes with Growth and Development. As in the case of the cervical spine, at birth the laminae are not yet united, and the neural arch has not yet joined with the vertebral body. These small ossified segments therefore stand out clearly (see tracing of radiograph in Fig. 9–11). The laminae unite at about 1 year of age, when a more definitive appearance is obtained. The vertebral bodies do have a box-like appearance in this region, despite the lack of the secondary centers of ossification, unlike the cervical spine. The secondary centers of ossification appear at about puberty, the epiphyseal rings on the upper and lower margins of the vertebral body standing out most clearly. Occasionally, these do not appear homogeneously ossified, and this appearance must be differentiated from outright fragmentation, which is an indication of abnormality. The secondary centers unite at about 25 years of age (or somewhat sooner), at which time growth in height ceases completely.

ROUTINE RADIOGRAPHIC POSITIONS AND RADIOGRAPHIC ANATOMY OF THE THORACIC SPINE

1. **Antero-posterior View of the Thoracic Spine** (Fig. 9–22). In view of the primary curvature of the thoracic spine, some of the vertebral bodies are seen obliquely in the antero-posterior projection. The posterior and anterior margins of the vertebral body are projected separately, and will overlap the adjoining vertebral surface, producing a diminution in anatomic detail.

The transverse processes, though prominent, are obscured by the heads and necks of the ribs to a considerable degree.

The pedicles stand out prominently as ovoid structures, and their inner margins bear a rather definite relationship to one another. The distance between their inner margins is called the "interpedicular distance." This has been charted for a series of normal individuals by Elsberg and Dyke supplemented by Simril, Thurston, and also Schwarz (Figs. 9–23 and 9–24). Variations from their normal limits become of definite pathologic significance. It will be noted that the interpedicular distances diminish down to the fourth or fifth thoracic vertebra, and then gradually increase after a relatively stationary period. In view of the fact that the intervertebral foramina of the thoracic spine are smaller than those of the cervical or lumbar areas, a space-occupying lesion located in this area is apt to erode the pedicle along with the margins of the intervertebral foramina. This is manifest by a sudden and inordinate increase in the interpedicular distance on this projection.[11] Erosion of the pedicle will alter the normal ovoid contour of the pedicle as seen in frontal perspective, so that it will appear "semi-lunate" and concave medially.

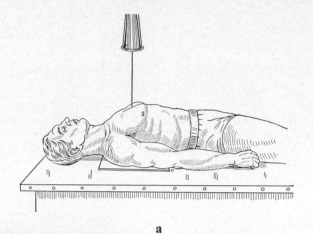

a

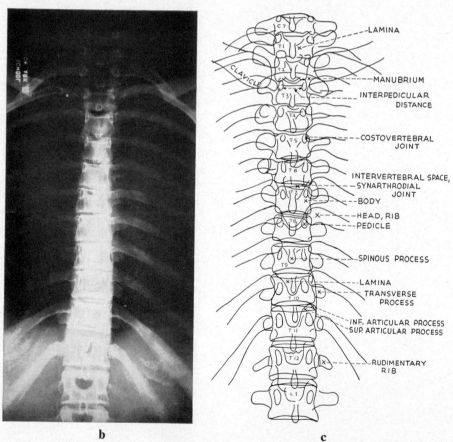

b   c

FIG. 9–22. ANTEROPOSTERIOR VIEW OF THE THORACIC SPINE: **a,** Positioning of patient; **b,** radiograph: **c,** labeled tracing of **b.**

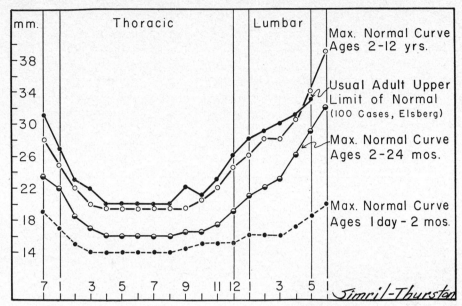

FIG. 9–23. Chart of interpedicular distances. (From Golden, *Diagnostic Roentgenology*, Thomas Nelson & Sons, Publishers.) (After Elsberg and Dyke.)

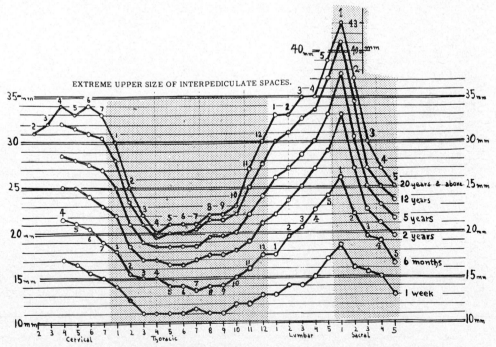

FIG. 9–24. Composite graph showing extreme upper measurements of interpediculate spaces in various age groups. (From Schwartz, G. S., in Am. J. Roentgenol., vol. 76, 1956.)

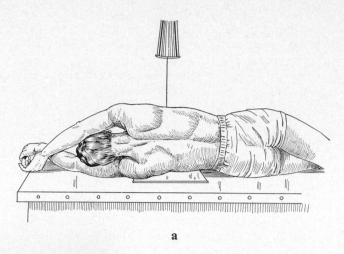

a

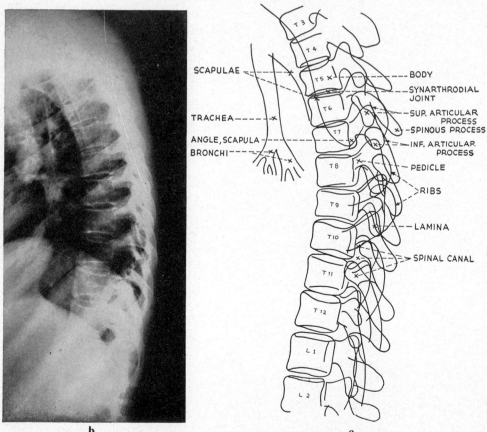

b   c

FIG. 9–25.   LATERAL VIEW OF THORACIC SPINE: **a,** Positioning of patient; **b,** radiograph; **c,** labeled
tracing of **b.**

2. **Lateral View of the Thoracic Spine** (Fig. 9–25).   The lateral projection gives an excellent perspective of the vertebral bodies and spinal canal. The various processes and synovial joints are obscured to a great extent by the overlapping laminae, spinous processes and ribs.

The gas shadows of the lung structures overlie the vertebral bodies of the thoracic spine, and frequently make the interpretation of minimal trabecular abnormality virtually impossible. In cases of doubt, body section radiographs are of considerable help.

It is not usually satisfactory to attempt to include the lower dorsal vertebrae with lumbar vertebrae on a single exposure, since separate techniques are required for maximum clarity.

The uppermost two or three vertebrae are usually not seen in the routine lateral radiograph, in view of the interference caused by the shoulder shadows. This portion of the spine is most difficult to radiograph. Ordinarily a routine study does not include this small section unless specifically requested or desired.

3. **Lateral (Slightly Oblique) View of the Upper Two Thoracic Segments** (Fig. 9–26).   The accompanying illustration demonstrates the manner in which this projection is used to obtain a clear view of these segments. The exposure factors must likewise be different from those for the remainder of the dorsal spine. Usually factors similar to those utilized in radiography of the lumbar spine are employed. The anatomic detail is somewhat distorted, but usually sufficiently clear.

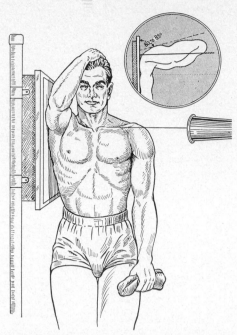

FIG. 9–26.   LATERAL (SLIGHTLY OBLIQUE) VIEW OF UPPER TWO THORACIC SEGMENTS: **a,** Positioning of patient—upright view. May also be taken in recumbent position.

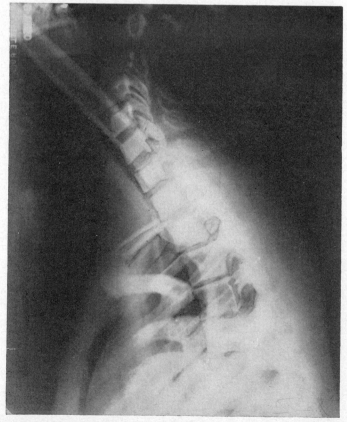

FIG. 9–26.   LATERAL (SLIGHTLY OBLIQUE) VIEW OF UPPER TWO THORACIC SEGMENTS: **b,** Radiograph (intensified).

POINTS OF PRACTICAL INTEREST WITH REFERENCE TO FIGURE 9–26:

1. The patient's midaxillary plane is placed against the midline of the film. The shoulder which is farthest from the film is depressed as much as possible with a heavy weight in the hand, whereas that which is closest to the film is rotated forward by placing the hand on the head and flexing the elbow. There may be a very slight rotation of the patient's body 5 to 10 degrees as shown.
2. The patient's axilla closest to the film is centered on the film and the central ray is directed perpendicular to the film at this central point.
3. The central ray is perpendicular to the film if the remote shoulder can be depressed adequately, but an angle of 15 degrees toward the feet may be employed when the shoulder cannot be well depressed.
4. A view of the uppermost two thoracic segments is not obtained on a routine lateral thoracic spine film, and when these two segments must be visualized some special means such as this must be employed.

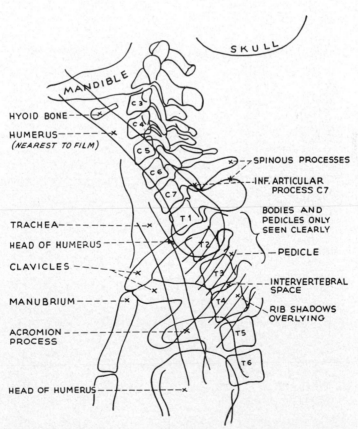

FIG. 9–26. LATERAL (SLIGHTLY OBLIQUE) VIEW OF UPPER TWO THORACIC SEGMENTS: **c,** Labeled tracing of **b.**

DISTINGUISHING CHARACTERISTICS OF THE LUMBAR SPINE (Fig. 9–27, a)

As previously indicated, the lumbar curvature is secondary to the erect posture of the human, and does not develop until the child learns to walk. Lumbar vertebrae differ from cervical and thoracic vertebrae in that they have no foramen in the transverse process and no facets for ribs. They are considerably larger than the other vertebrae.

The transition from the lower dorsal vertebrae to the lumbar is frequently very gradual, and the last ribs may have the appearance of transverse processes. Occasionally the last lumbar vertebra is fused in whole or in part with the sacrum, or the first sacral segment becomes a separate segment and has the appearance of the last lumbar. Its transverse processes may be partially or wholly fused with those of the sacrum, or an articulation in this location may exist.

Defects in the neural arch of the lower lumbar segments are particularly frequent (found in 5 to 10 per cent of the adult population), but these abnormalities are not within the scope of the present text.

In the lateral projection, there is a progressive increase in the width of the vertebral bodies or they remain the same in width, descending the spine, except in the case of the fifth lumbar which may vary somewhat. The *fifth lumbar interspace is usually narrower than adjoining interspaces, and this is without special significance when unaccompanied by other findings.* Otherwise the interspaces are equal in width, and variations are of special significance.

The posterior margins of the vertebral bodies ordinarily form a smooth curved line. Occasionally, the superior margin of the lower lumbar vertebra will fall out of this line. The author's method of drawing lines described in Figure 9–28 has proved of value in determining whether or not this alignment is normal. When these lines are drawn as described, it has been found in studying a large series of normal cases that they fall into certain definite categories and the anteriorly slipped vertebral body (spondylolisthesis) produces a definite variation in the arrangement of these lines.

Occasionally, it will appear that a margin is posteriorly displaced.[7] This may be due to the phenomenon of projection or to deformity in the posterior margin of the sacrum, but it is possible that a true posterior spondylolisthesis may exist, although the existence of this entity is doubted by some (Fig. 9–29).[7]

Ferguson (Fig. 9–30, **a**) has defined the lumbosacral angle as the angle formed between a horizontal line and the plane of the superior margin of the sacrum. This is an index of the angle between the lumbar and sacral spine, and when it exceeds 34 degrees, this author believes that an abnormality from the standpoint of stability exists.

Weight-bearing films in the lateral projection in flexion and extension may also be utilized to determine the stability at the lumbosacral junction as shown in Figure 9–30, **b.**

There are occasionally extra ossicles which form along the superior anterior margins of lumbar bodies. These are called "extra-apophyses" and have significance only in that they must be recognized as being different from fractures, and without pathologic significance (Fig. 9–10, **b**).

Fɪɢ. 9–27. Lumbar spine and sacrum: **a,** Distinguishing characteristics of the lumbar spine; **b,** sacrum (frontal and lateral projections).

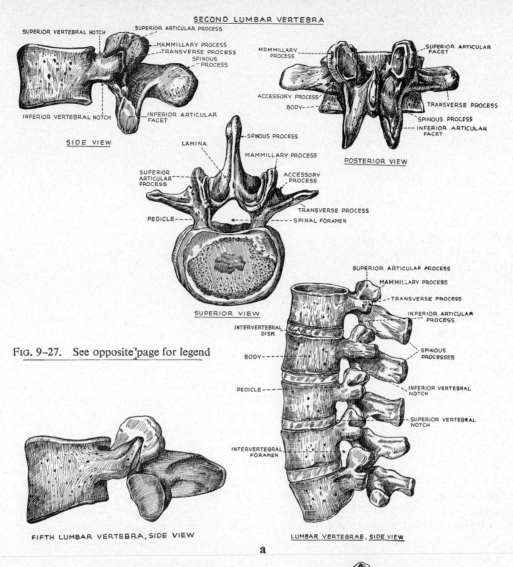

SECOND LUMBAR VERTEBRA

SUPERIOR VERTEBRAL NOTCH

SUPERIOR ARTICULAR PROCESS

MAMMILLARY PROCESS
TRANSVERSE PROCESS
SPINOUS PROCESS

INFERIOR VERTEBRAL NOTCH

INFERIOR ARTICULAR FACET

SIDE VIEW

MAMMILLARY PROCESS

SUPERIOR ARTICULAR FACET

ACCESSORY PROCESS
BODY

TRANSVERSE PROCESS
SPINOUS PROCESS
INFERIOR ARTICULAR FACET

POSTERIOR VIEW

SPINOUS PROCESS
LAMINA
MAMMILLARY PROCESS
SUPERIOR ARTICULAR PROCESS
ACCESSORY PROCESS
TRANSVERSE PROCESS
PEDICLE
SPINAL FORAMEN

SUPERIOR VIEW

FIG. 9-27. See opposite page for legend

SUPERIOR ARTICULAR PROCESS
MAMMILLARY PROCESS
TRANSVERSE PROCESS
INFERIOR ARTICULAR PROCESS

INTERVERTEBRAL DISK
BODY
SPINOUS PROCESSES
PEDICLE
INFERIOR VERTEBRAL NOTCH
SUPERIOR VERTEBRAL NOTCH
INTERVERTEBRAL FORAMEN

FIFTH LUMBAR VERTEBRA, SIDE VIEW

LUMBAR VERTEBRAE, SIDE VIEW

a

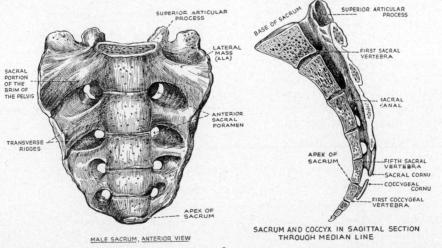

SUPERIOR ARTICULAR PROCESS

SACRAL PORTION OF THE BRIM OF THE PELVIS

LATERAL MASS (ALA)

ANTERIOR SACRAL FORAMEN

TRANSVERSE RIDGES

APEX OF SACRUM

MALE SACRUM, ANTERIOR VIEW

BASE OF SACRUM
SUPERIOR ARTICULAR PROCESS
FIRST SACRAL VERTEBRA
SACRAL CANAL

APEX OF SACRUM
FIFTH SACRAL VERTEBRA
SACRAL CORNU
COCCYGEAL CORNU
FIRST COCCYGEAL VERTEBRA

SACRUM AND COCCYX IN SAGITTAL SECTION THROUGH MEDIAN LINE

b

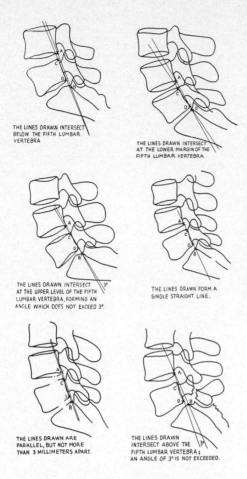

THE LINES DRAWN INTERSECT
BELOW THE FIFTH LUMBAR
VERTEBRA

THE LINES DRAWN INTERSECT
AT THE LOWER MARGIN OF THE
FIFTH LUMBAR VERTEBRA

THE LINES DRAWN INTERSECT
AT THE UPPER LEVEL OF THE FIFTH
LUMBAR VERTEBRA, FORMING AN
ANGLE WHICH DOES NOT EXCEED 3°.

THE LINES DRAWN FORM A
SINGLE STRAIGHT LINE.

THE LINES DRAWN ARE
PARALLEL, BUT NOT MORE
THAN 3 MILLIMETERS APART.

THE LINES DRAWN
INTERSECT ABOVE THE
FIFTH LUMBAR VERTEBRA;
AN ANGLE OF 3° IS NOT EXCEEDED.

FIG. 9–28. Lines to demonstrate various types of alignment in the lumbosacral lateral projection. A line AB is drawn between the posterior-inferior margin of L_4 and the posterior-superior margin of S_1. A second line CD is drawn between the posterior-superior and posterior-inferior margins of L_5. These two lines form the six definite normal configuration patterns as shown.

The presence of a defect in the pars interarticularis is not always associated with a "slipping" forward, but predisposes to such (called spondylolisthesis if slipping is present). (From Meschan, I: Radiology, vol. 47, 1945.)

SIGNS OF POSTERIOR DISPLACEMENT OF THE LUMBAR VERTEBRAE

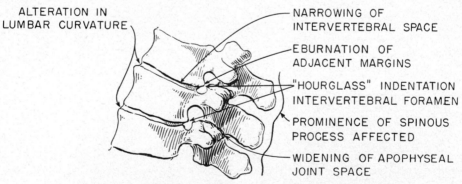

ALTERATION IN
LUMBAR CURVATURE

NARROWING OF
INTERVERTEBRAL SPACE

EBURNATION OF
ADJACENT MARGINS

"HOURGLASS" INDENTATION
INTERVERTEBRAL FORAMEN

PROMINENCE OF SPINOUS
PROCESS AFFECTED

WIDENING OF APOPHYSEAL
JOINT SPACE

OTHER CRITERIA:
ANTERIOR AND POSTERIOR MARGINS MUST BE DISPLACED
WITH REFERENCE TO UNDERLYING VERTEBRA

OTHER SIGNS OF DISC DEGENERATION MAY BE PRESENT

FIG. 9–29. Criteria for backward displacement of the lumbar vertebrae.

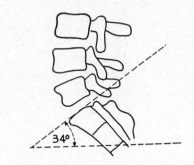

FERGUSON'S NORMAL LUMBOSACRAL
ANGLE

a

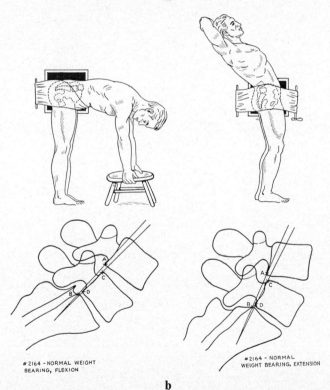

#2164 – NORMAL WEIGHT
BEARING, FLEXION

#2164 – NORMAL
WEIGHT BEARING, EXTENSION

b

FIG. 9–30. MEASUREMENT OF THE LUMBOSACRAL ANGLE: a, Ferguson's method of determining the normal lumbosacral angle in the lateral projection. b, Method of measuring stability at the lumbosacral angle by obtaining weight-bearing films in flexion and extension, and measuring the alignment of the fifth lumbar vertebra with respect to the fourth lumbar vertebra and the sacrum, as indicated in Figure 9–28. (From Meschan, I: Am. J. Roentgenol., vol. 53, 1945.)

The pars interarticularis (Fig. 9–31) is that slender, bony segment between the superior and inferior articular processes. Not infrequently (in about 5 per cent of population) it remains unossified, being formed by cartilage or fibrous tissue, and predisposes to the condition already described as spondylolisthesis.

The apophyseal joints of the lumbar area are more frequently affected in atrophic arthritic disease than are the higher portions of the spine, and it is indeed fortunate that they can be so clearly demonstrated. The obliquity of these joints will vary, and occasionally several oblique views must be obtained before definite abnormality can be excluded.

As previously indicated, the plane of the apophyseal joints is perpendicular to the plane of the sacroiliac joint on the same side, and it is the sacroiliac joint of the side that is *farthest* from the film (antero-posterior oblique) which is seen clearly, whereas the apophyseal joint of the side *closest* to the film is seen to best advantage.

Changes with Growth and Development in the Lumbosacral Spine. The development of the lumbar vertebrae parallels that of the thoracic vertebrae closely with minor differences. However, that of the sacral spine is different significantly.

In addition to the centers for the vertebral body and neural arches (Fig. 9–11) in the sacrum there are also centers for the costal processes present at birth. The costal parts fuse with the arches at the fifth year. The arch fuses with the body two or three years later, and the halves of the arches unite posteriorly between 7 and 10 years of age. The secondary centers of ossification which appear adjoining the wings of the sacrum on either side do not appear until 15 to 18 years of age and fuse in the early twenties. Before their appearance, the sacroiliac joints appear somewhat wider than one might expect, and this appearance must be considered normal.

The vertebral arches are incomplete below the third and fourth sacral segments and are wholly absent from the lower coccyx.

The coccyx is cartilaginous at birth and segments each ordinarily have only one primary center. They appear from above downward from birth to puberty, and fusion is very variable and usually occurs from below upward. The coccyx is one of the most variable bones in the human body, and interpretation of abnormality is frequently very difficult. The coccyx is more freely movable in the female and less likely to be fused with the sacrum, and the first segment of the coccyx more often than not fails to fuse with the second.

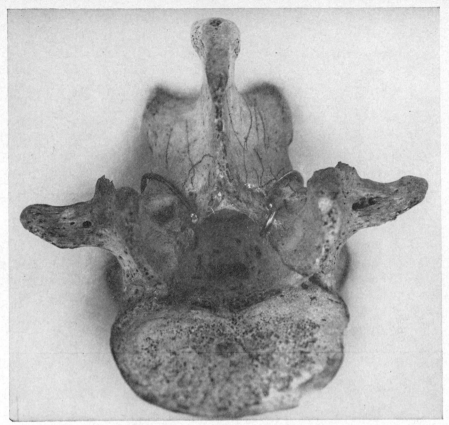

a

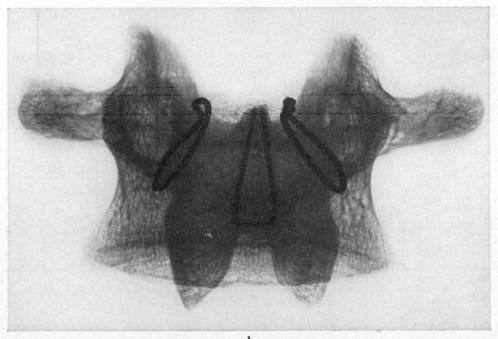

b

FIG. 9–31. VERTEBRAL BODY WITH WIRE DELINEATING THE PARS INTERARTICULARIS: a, Photograph; b, Radiograph in antero-posterior projection.

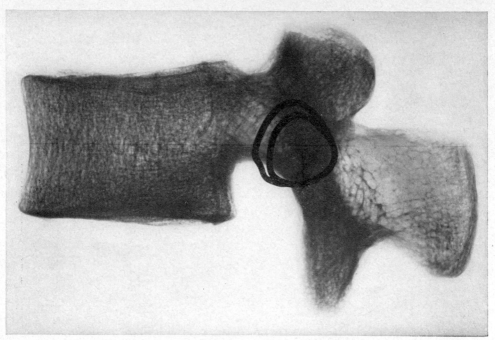

FIG. 9–31.   VERTEBRAL BODY WITH WIRE DELINEATING THE PARS INTERARTICULARIS: **c,** Radiograph in lateral projection.

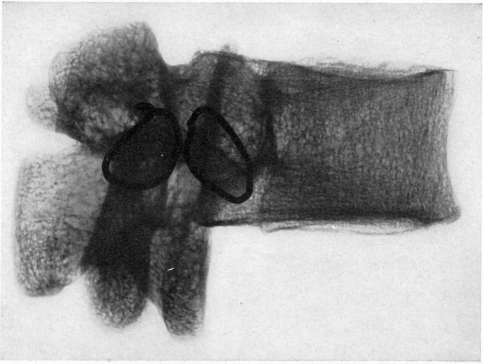

FIG. 9–31.   VERTEBRAL BODY WITH WIRE DELINEATING THE PARS INTERARTICULARIS: **d,** Radiograph in oblique projection.

ROUTINE RADIOGRAPHIC POSITIONS AND RADIOGRAPHIC ANATOMY

1. **Antero-posterior View of the Lumbosacral Spine** (Fig. 9–32).   The lumbar curvature will impose a degree of distortion and magnification on those lumbar vertebrae which are farthest from the film, and to diminish this effect the knees are flexed, which straightens the lumbar spine to some extent.

When interpreting the anatomy, it is possible to see through the vertebral body and delineate the laminae, spinous processes and articular processes. The transverse processes are irregular in appearance, and frequently asymmetrical.

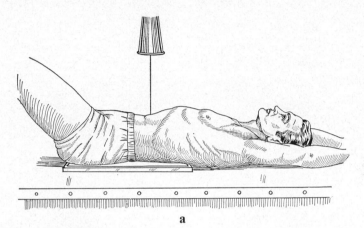

a

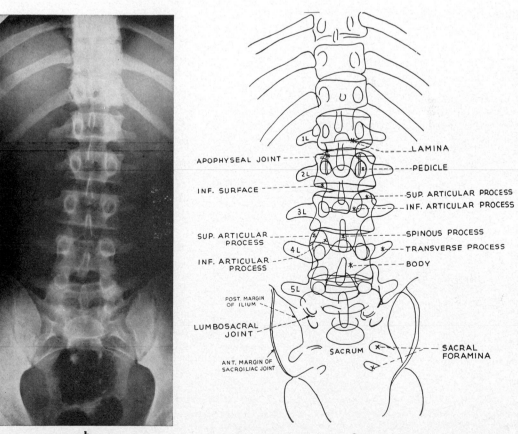

b   c

FIG. 9–32.   ANTERO-POSTERIOR VIEW OF LUMBOSACRAL SPINE: a, Positioning of patient; b, radiograph; c, labeled tracing of b.

2. **Lateral View of the Lumbosacral Spine** (Fig. 9–33). When a 36-inch film-target distance is employed the usual lumbar sag is quite permissible, in that it forms part of the arc of a circle with a 36-inch radius, and the vertebral surfaces are parallel to the rays from the target. However, if longer film-to-target distances are employed, it is best to eliminate the lumbar sag (with a balsa wood block), especially in women, so that an undistorted view of the lumbar spine can be obtained.

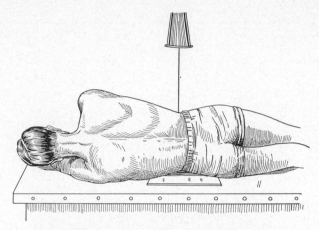

FIG. 9–33.   LATERAL VIEW OF THE LUMBOSACRAL SPINE: a, Positioning of patient.

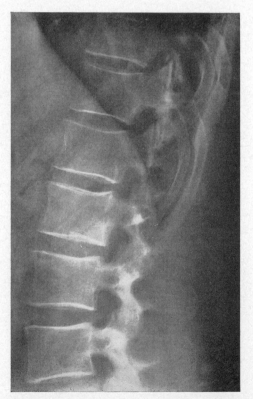

FIG. 9–33.   LATERAL VIEW OF THE LUMBOSACRAL SPINE: b, Radiograph (intensified).

This area requires special exposure factors to penetrate structures present, and the less dense structures such as the spinous processes frequently require a bright light source for visualization.

Occasionally the sacrum cannot be included satisfactorily in this study since exposure factors for some sacra are excessively high (Fig. 9–34).

3. **Oblique View of the Lumbosacral Spine** (Fig. 9–35). This view is obtained as shown. It has particular value in demonstrating the partes interarticulares and the apophyseal joints to best advantage. It has already been shown as a means of delineating the sacroiliac joints (Chap. 5).

CHARACTERISTIC FEATURES OF SACROCOCCYGEAL SEGMENT

The special radiographic anatomy of the sacrum and coccyx has already been dealt with (Chap. 5). The coccyx is ordinarily not seen to best advantage on the routine lateral view of the lumbosacral spine and special lateral views are therefore obtained (Fig. 9–34). The great normal variability of the coccyx makes interpretation of this structure extremely difficult, and indeed, usually impossible. In the antero-posterior projection gas and fecal material in the rectum and sigmoid colon add to the confusion. Special tilted views of the sacrum (Chap. 5) may be obtained as described to help overcome some of this difficulty.

The configuration of the anterior margin of the sacrum is of great importance obstetrically, in that a flat sacrum (one which has lost its concavity developmentally) diminishes the available space in the midpelvis (Chap. 17).

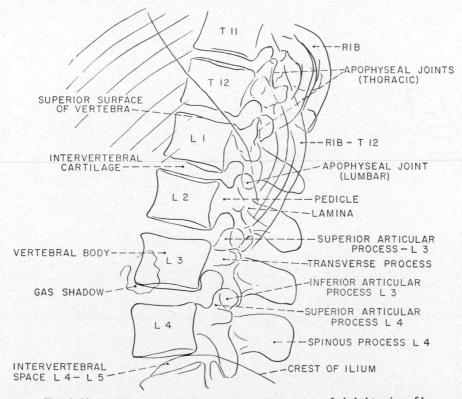

FIG. 9–33. LATERAL VIEW OF THE LUMBOSACRAL SPINE: c, Labeled tracing of b.

The secondary epiphyses projected in the sacroiliac joints (covering the auricular or alar surfaces of the sacrum) do not appear until 15 to 16 years, and until then the sacroiliac joints may have a somewhat "fuzzy" and widened appearance. This is a normal variation which one must learn to recognize.

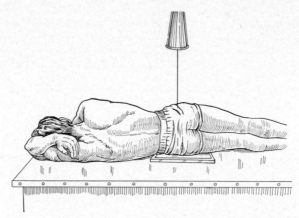

FIG. 9–34.   SPECIAL LATERAL VIEW OF SACRUM AND COCCYX: a, Positioning of patient.

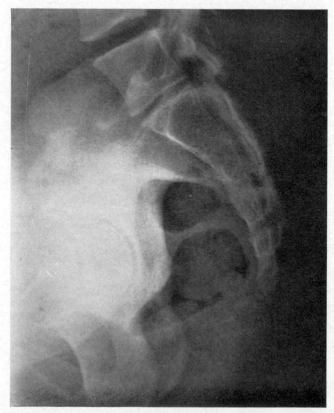

FIG. 9–34.   SPECIAL LATERAL VIEW OF SACRUM AND COCCYX: b, Radiograph.

1. The patient's hips and knees are flexed to a comfortable position to help immobilize the patient.
2. The coronal plane passing 3 inches posterior to the midaxillary line is adjusted to the longitudinal axis of the table.
3. It is usually desirable to place folded sheets or balsa wood blocks in the depression above the iliac crest to maintain the lower thoracic spine in a perfectly parallel relationship with the table top.
4. Although the film here is demonstrated immediately beneath the patient, a Potter-Bucky diaphragm is always employed.
5. If it is the coccyx which is the major interest, a somewhat lighter exposure technique would have to be employed and lesser detail with regard to the sacrum will then be obtained

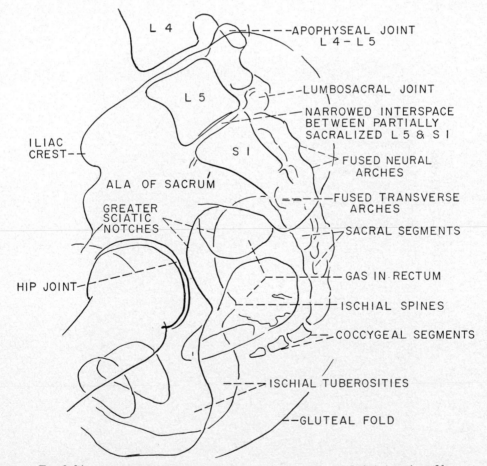

Fig. 9–34. special lateral view of sacrum and coccyx: c, Labeled tracing of b.

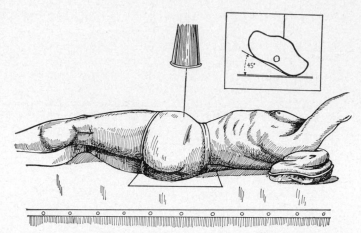

FIG. 9–35.   OBLIQUE VIEW OF LUMBOSACRAL SPINE: **a,** Positioning of patient.

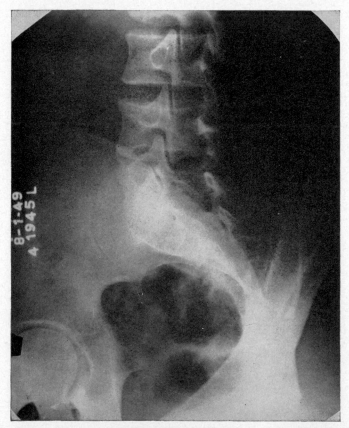

FIG. 9–35.   OBLIQUE VIEW OF LUMBOSACRAL SPINE: **b,** Radiograph.

POINTS OF PRACTICAL INTEREST WITH REFERENCE TO FIGURE 9–35:

1. The patient's body is placed obliquely with respect to the table top at an angle of 25 to 45 degrees. The coronal plane passing through the spinous processes is centered to the midline of the table.
2. If the lower lumbar apophyseal joints are of greatest interest the central ray passes through the level of the raised iliac crest. If the upper lumbar apophyseal joints are desired, the central ray passes through a point about 1 inch above the raised iliac crest.
3. The apophyseal joints closest to the film will be shown to best advantage, but occasionally it will require several attempts with varying degrees of angulation to obtain a clear view of all of the apophyseal joints. This may be necessary since the plane of the joint varies somewhat as one descends the lumbar spine (Fig. 9–5).
4. The sacroiliac joint which is farthest from the film will be opened up to best advantage. An angle of approximately 25 degrees is usually most satisfactory for the sacroiliac joint depiction.

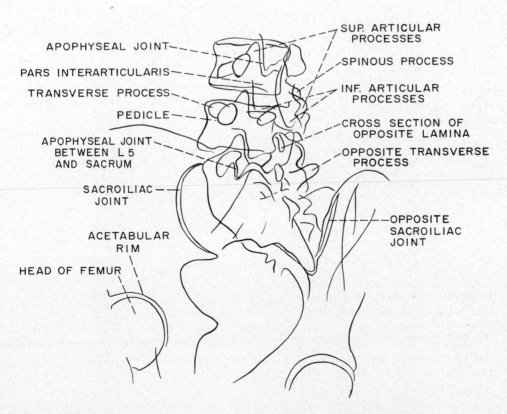

FIG. 9–35. OBLIQUE VIEW OF LUMBOSACRAL SPINE: c, Labeled tracing of b.

STRUCTURE OF THE INTERVERTEBRAL DISK (Fig. 9–36)

There is an intervertebral disk between each vertebral body between the second cervical and first sacral segments. Its development has already been described. This structure is considered here in considerable detail as it may

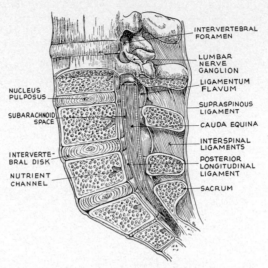

FIG. 9–36. Structure of intervertebral disk and its relationship to the subarachnoid space and adjoining ligamentous structures.

cause compression of the spinal cord when degenerated and posteriorly herniated.

The annulus fibrosus forms the major portion of the disk, and is composed of lamellated fibrocartilage intimately attached to the epiphyseal bony ring of the adjacent vertebral bodies. Its periphery is reinforced by the longitudinal ligaments.

The nucleus pulposus is the residuum of the notochord, and is composed of gelatinous matrix interspersed with fibers from the inner zone of the annulus fibrosus, with which it blends. It apparently functions to distribute the pressure evenly over the vertebral bodies.

There is a cartilaginous plate cemented to the adjoining surface of the vertebral body, which fuses with the epiphyseal ring of the body. There are vacuolated spaces in this calcified cartilage through which nutrition diffuses for maintenance of the intervertebral disk.

There are numerous places of congenital weakness in the intervertebral disks and cartilaginous end plates which are residua of small vascular channels which have disintegrated and become filled by cartilage as the individual grows and develops. These weaknesses in both the cartilaginous end plates and the disks permit the nucleus pulposus to protrude in one direction or another.

When this protrusion occurs into the adjoining vertebral bodies centrally, the phenomenon is referred to as a "Schmorl's node." When, however, the protrusion is posterior or lateral, a compression of a nerve structure may result. Thus, simple Schmorl's nodes of a central type are relatively frequent and asymptomatic. However, protrusion elsewhere may be of definite pathologic significance, producing clinical symptoms and signs.

THE VERTEBRAL CANAL AND SPINAL SUBARACHNOID SPACE

Radiographic Anatomy. The vertebral canal tends to be triangular in shape, and relatively large in the cervical and lumbar areas, and is small and ovoid in the thoracic area. It is bounded by the following structures: (1) Anteriorly lie the posterior longitudinal ligament, the posterior portions of the vertebral bodies and the posterior margins of the intervertebral disks. (2) Laterally are situated the pedicles of the vertebral bodies, the intervertebral foramina and the articulating facets. (3) Posteriorly lie the laminae, ligamenta flava and the spinous processes. The vertebral canal contains the following structures (Fig. 9–37): (*a*) Centrally, the spinal cord and its meninges are longitudinally placed.

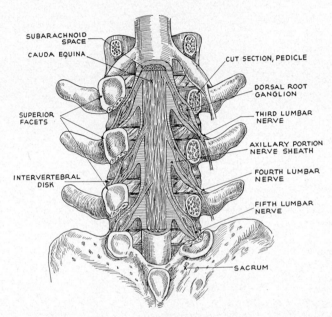

Fig. 9–37. Relationship of spinal nerve roots to axillary pouches of the subarachnoid space.

(*b*) The spinal nerves and vessels traverse the intervertebral foramina. (*c*) Between the inner margins of the vertebral canal and the meninges is the epidural space. This contains considerable fat, venous plexuses and nerves (supplying the meninges, intervertebral disks and ligaments). The fat is most abundant in the thoracic region. There is a small recurrent nerve from the spinal nerves adjoining the division of the latter into anterior and posterior rami which supplies the structures within the vertebral canal.

All of these structures are important in that their aberrations may cause encroachment on the vertebral canal; the site of involvement may be easily determined but the exact nature of anatomic and pathologic processes may remain obscure.

It will be recalled that the spinal cord lies loosely within its meninges and extends from the foramen magnum to the lower border of the first lumbar vertebra. It has two bulbous enlargements innervating the upper and lower extremities respectively, and below the lower enlargement, the cord narrows down to a cone-shaped structure, the conus medullaris, from which a slender filament, the filum terminale, extends downward to the first segment of the coccyx.

As in the case of the brain, the dura is normally closely applied to the arachnoid, with only a potential subdural space between. The dura ends in a cone-shaped cul-de-sac at a variable level, usually in the vicinity of the first or second sacral segment, but it may end somewhat higher. The space between the arachnoid and pia mater which invests the cord, the subarachnoid space, is bathed in spinal fluid, in direct communication with the ventricles of the brain and its surrounding spaces.

The spinal nerves arise at considerably higher levels than their corresponding intervertebral foramina. The cauda equina is formed by the spinal nerves which extend below the termination of the spinal cord at L_1 level, and these nerves lie free in the subarachnoid space except that just as they leave the vertebral canal they are invested for a short distance by the meningeal covering of the cord, called the nerve sheath. There is a small pouch on the inferior aspect of the nerve sheath near the point of exit called the axillary pouch, or subarachnoid pouch (Fig. 9–37). In the lumbar region, the nerve sheath curves under the vertebral pedicle to reach its exit, and thus has a relatively long extradural but intravertebral course, compared with other regions of the spine. The point of exit is below the inferior margin of the intervertebral disk, which is of considerable importance when an aberration of the disk exists, allowing pressure upon the nerve in this vulnerable location.

METHOD OF STUDY OF THE SPINAL SUBARACHNOID SPACE

Contrast Myelography. The contents of the vertebral canal are studied radiographically by introducing contrast media into either the subarachnoid space or epidural space. The subarachnoid space is the one more frequently used. The two major methods of study involve the use of either negative or positive contrast media in the subarachnoid space. Dardy (Ann. Surg., 1919) first advocated the use of air, and Sicard and Forestier (1922, 1926) introduced the use of iodized oil (Lipiodol, iodized poppy-seed oil). Various other media have been used. Oxygen has to a large extent replaced air as the negative contrast medium of choice, but has the disadvantage of demonstrating clearly only the lowermost lumbar subarachnoid space. Aqueous media like Thorotrast have been used, but they are irritating, and the removal of Thorotrast is very tedious. It has an inherent radioactivity and cannot be left in the vertebral canal. Skiodan is another aqueous contrast medium, but is irritating, and does not produce as satisfactory contrast as do the iodized oils.

The best results have been obtained with the oil-type media. Among these, pantopaque (ethyl-iodophenylundecylenate) (discovered in 1944) has been found to be most satisfactory. It is absorbed at the rate of about 1 cc. per year if left in the vertebral canal and may be slightly less irritating than Lipiodol. Ordinarily it is removed following the examination.

TECHNIQUE.   The technique of the examination is as follows: Three to 6 cc. of the iodized oil is injected into the lumbar subarachnoid space at the level of the third or fourth lumbar interspace. It is desirable to avoid the interspace where the pathologic condition is suspected, since the introduction of the needle at this level may introduce a small area of hemorrhage which may complicate interpretation of the findings. If Pantopaque is used, the needle may be left in place, and after the examination is complete, the Pantopaque is removed through the same needle. The oil is heavier than spinal fluid (except for light-weight Lipiodol which is not recommended) and sinks to the lowermost portion of the subarachnoid space where it delineates the caudal sac when the patient is almost erect (Fig. 9–38, c). By gradually tilting the patient to a position where his feet are elevated, the oil can be made to gravitate to upper portions of the spine as desired. Unfortunately, there is a tendency for the oil to break up into small globules when the lower segments of the dorsal spine are reached, and the examination of this area is frequently not very satisfactory. The oil may also be introduced into the cisterna magna and allowed to gravitate down the spine in similar fashion, and in this way the subarachnoid space of the cervical and upper dorsal areas is studied. These studies are always made fluoroscopically with spot films taken at intervals to demonstrate any areas desired or all areas sequentially. This can be done with the patient lying prone; oblique and lateral views are best obtained by Potter-Bucky diaphragm technique at the desired levels.

The width of the myelographic shadow varies considerably in accordance with the width of the vertebral canal. *If the width of the column is less than 16 mm., it is considered that the examination will not accurately reflect anatomic changes in the vertebral canal.*

Normal Radiographic Appearances. The usual appearance is illustrated in Figure 9–38. There is usually a straight column with small peaklike structures at regular intervals at the interspace levels. These are the axillary pouches of the inferior aspects of the nerve sheaths. Occasionally there is a slight undulating appearance with minimal indentations opposite the interspaces on both sides (Fig. 9–38) and anteriorly in the lateral view. When the indentations are accentuated, they are representative of abnormality.

The column in the thoracic region tends to be more narrow and cylindrical than the lumbar region, but again becomes wider in the cervical region.

The increased space between the posterior margin of the fifth lumbar vertebra and upper sacral segment from the anterior margin of the opaque column makes the lateral view difficult to interpret at these segmental levels, and it would be possible for a small abnormality to escape detection in the lateral projection alone. Fortunately, the antero-posterior projection is quite accurate at this site.

Occasionally the caudal sac will end opposite the fifth lumbar vertebra, and in these instances it is not possible to examine the fifth lumbar interspace area adequately.

There is a considerable variation of normal in the appearance of the terminal theca and the radicular extensions in this location. These are illustrated in Figure 9–39.

The abnormal configurations of the iodized oil column are out of the scope of this text, but suffice it to say that it is possible to distinguish between extradural defects, intradural and extramedullary defects, and intramedullary defects. By means of our knowledge of the frequency of certain pathologic entities in these specific locations, the aberration in anatomy in terms of pathology can be predicted with fair accuracy.

In cisternal myelography, a persistent globule of oil may occur between the two cerebellar tonsils and fail to descend. The column of iodized oil in the

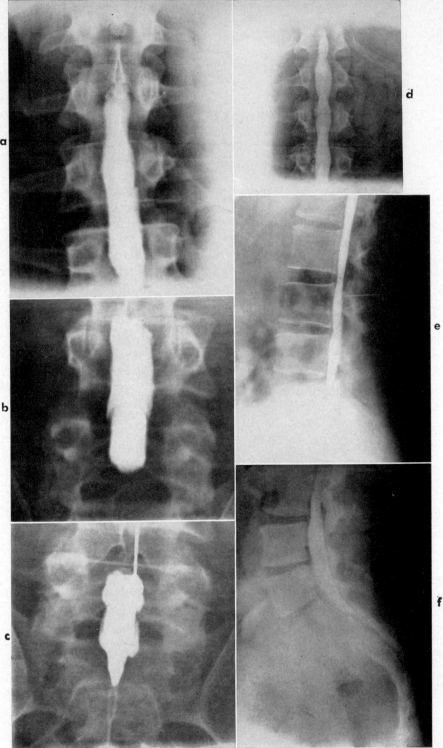

FIG. 9–38.

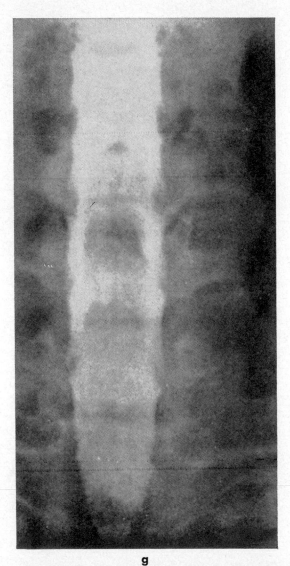

g

FIG. 9–38. LUMBAR AND CERVICAL MYELOGRAMS: **a** to **f**, Normal radiographic appearance of lumbar myelogram in antero-posterior and lateral projections. **a, b** and **c**, Antero-posterior spot film studies at upper lumbar, midlumbar and lumbosacral areas; **d**, antero-posterior spot film studies showing normal symmetrical indentations at interspace levels; **e**, lateral, upper lumbar myelogram; **f**, lateral lumbosacral area. **g**, Normal radiographic appearance of a cervical myelogram in the antero-posterior projection. (Cervical myelogram, courtesy of Bell and Douglas.)

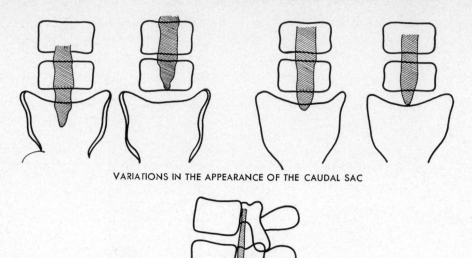

VARIATIONS IN THE APPEARANCE OF THE CAUDAL SAC

LATERAL PROJECTION

FIG. 9–39.   Variations in appearance of the terminal theca.

cervical spine is thinner (and hence more radiolucent) antero-posteriorly, and is relatively broader than the column elsewhere. The axillary nerve sheath peaks point at right angles to the spinal column, are more closely spaced, and the superior and inferior margins tend to be symmetrical. These differences may be explained anatomically by the shorter, more direct course of the cervical nerves.

Thoracic myelography normally is not very satisfactory, since the iodized oil column breaks up into small globules in the region of the thoracic curvature. However, if a definite point of obstruction is encountered, the passage of the globules is impeded, and they tend to coalesce, thus improving the diagnostic value of the procedure.

CERVICAL MYELOGRAPHY

Cervical Myelograms.   The lumbar puncture and the instillation of the oil are done in the usual manner, with the patient either lying on his side, or prone with a pillow under the abdomen to hyperextend the back. A short beveled 18- or 19-gauge needle is employed to reduce the incidence of subdural or epidural injection. In the absence of a complete block, 9 to 12 cc. of Pantopaque is employed. If a complete block has been demonstrated by a Queckenstedt test, only 2 to 3 cc. of contrast media need be employed to demonstrate the level of the block.

Following the appropriate examination of the lumbar and thoracic areas, the examiner's assistant assumes a position at the head of the table and takes

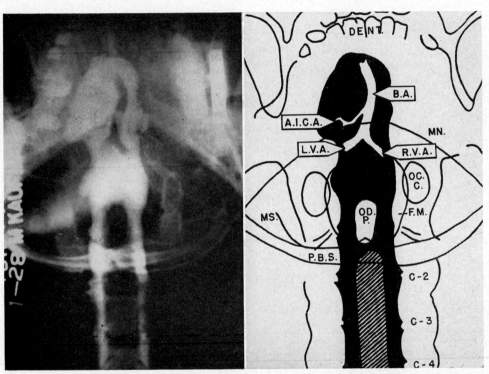

FIG. 9–40. **a,** Normal antero-posterior view of the foramen magnum and clivus myelogram.
(From Malis, L. I.; Radiology, Vol. 76, 1958.)

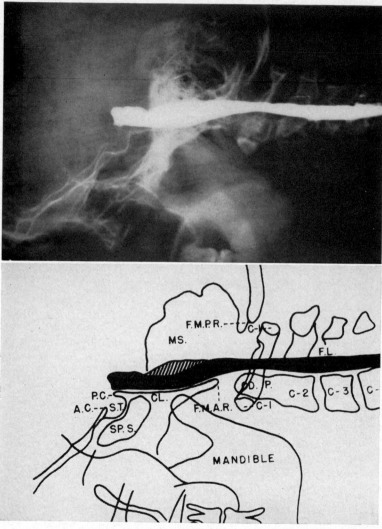

Fig. 9–40. **b,** Normal cross-table (horizontal beam) lateral view, in same position as Figure 9–40, **a.** B.A. basilar artery; A.I.C.A. ant. inferior cerebellar artery; L.V.A. left vertebral artery; R.V.A. right vertebral artery; Oc. C. occipital condyle; Od. P. odontoid process; MS. mastoids; F.M. foramen magnum; P.B.S. posterior base of skull; F.M.P.R. foramen magnum posterior rim; F.M.A.R. foramen magnum anterior rim; CL clivus; A.C. anterior clinoids; P.C. posterior clinoids; S.T. sella turcica; SP.S. sphenoid sinus; F.L. fluid level of Pantopaque. (From Malis, L. I.: Radiology, vol. 76, 1958.)

complete control of the patient's head. The patient is instructed to keep the head perfectly prone at all times and fully hyperextended unless otherwise moved by the examiner's assistant. With the patient's head fully hyperextended, the table is tilted to about 50 degrees, so that most of the oil trickles over the dorsal hump into the cervical region. The hyperextension of the head will keep the oil from going beyond the foramen magnum.

The table is then made level, with the patient's head still hyperextended. Under fluoroscopic control, with direction by the examiner, the assistant slowly flexes the patient's head until the oil column rises to C_2 level. The table may then be tilted slowly to about 10 to 15 degrees, which will ordinarily allow the oil to run in along the clivus. Under no circumstances is rotation of the head permitted.

Appropriate antero-posterior spot films and lateral horizontal beam studies are taken with the shoulder rest removed. The appearance of the normal cervical myelogram is illustrated in Figures 9–38 and 9–40. Figure 9–38 demonstrates the appearance of the mid- and lower cervical myelogram. Figure 9–40, **a** demonstrates the appearance high on the clivus, with the various parts labeled. The lateral projection is demonstrated in Figure 9–40, **b.**

Although intracranial Pantopaque is undesirable, it is probable that no serious sequelae result. With good technique and adequate cooperation from the patient, it is possible to examine the entire cervical subarachnoid space, including the entire area of the foramen magnum, and still recover all of the oil from the intracranial cavity. Following the procedure, the oil is removed from the lumbar needle as with lumbar myelograms.

REFERENCES

1. Boreadis, A. G., and Gershon-Cohen, J.: Luschka Joints of the Cervical Spine. Radiology, *66,* 181–187, 1956.
2. Dalton, C. J., and Schwartz, S. S.: Evaluation of the Paraspinal Line in Roentgen Examination of the Thorax. Radiology, *66:* 195–200, 1956.
3. Lachman, E.: A Comparison of the Posterior Boundaries of Lungs and Pleura as Demonstrated on the Cadaver and on the Roentgenogram of the Living. Anat. Rec., *83:* 521–541, 1942.
4. Malis, L. I.: Myelographic Examination of the Foramen Magnum. Radiology, *70:* 196–221, 1958.
5. McRae, D. L., and Barnum, A. S.: Occipitalization of the Atlas. Am. J. Roentgenol., *53:* 23–46, 1953.
6. McRae, D. L.: Bony Abnormalities in the Region of the Foramen Magnum: Correlation of the Anatomic and Neurologic Findings. Acta radiol., *40:* 335–354, 1953.
7. Melamed, A., and Ansfield, D. J.: Posterior Displacement of Lumbar Vertebrae. Am. J. Roentgenol., *58:* 307–328, 1947.
8. Meschan, I.: Spondylolisthesis. Am. J. Roentgenol., *53:* 230–243, 1945.
9. Meschan, I., and Farrer-Meschan, R. M. F.: Important Aspects in the Roentgen Study of the Normal Lumbosacral Spine. Radiology, *70:* 637–648, 1958.
10. Paul, L., and Moir, W.: Nonpathologic Variations in the Relationship of the Upper Cervical Vertebrae. Am. J. Roentgenol., *62:* 519–524, 1949.
11. Schwarz, G. S.: The Width of the Spinal Canal in the Growing Vertebra with Special Reference to the Sacrum. Am. J. Roentgenol., *76:* 476–481, 1956.
12. Wolf, B. S., Khilnani, M., and Malis, L.: Sagittal Diameter of Bony Cervical Spinal Canal and Its Significance. J. Mt. Sinai Hosp., *23:* 283–292, 1956.

CHAPTER 10

The Respiratory System

THE RESPIRATORY TRACT can be conveniently subdivided for discussion into: (1) the upper air passages, (2) the larynx, (3) the trachea and bronchi, (4) the lung parenchyma, (5) the vascular supply, venous drainage and lymphatics of the respiratory tract, (6) the lung hili and (7) the thoracic cage, pleura and diaphragm.

THE UPPER AIR PASSAGES

The upper air passages are usually amenable to direct and indirect inspection to such a great extent that radiography need not often be employed for further information. Nevertheless, considerable useful information can be obtained by fluoroscopic and radiographic methods, and hence a consideration of this subject is noteworthy.

Apart from the nasal air passages which have already been described, the upper air passages are referred to anatomically as the pharynx. This, in turn consists of three fundamental areas: (1) the nasopharynx, which extends from the nasal cavity anteriorly and the base of the skull superiorly to the tip of the uvula and margin of the soft palate below; (2) the oropharynx, which extends from the soft palate above to the epiglottis and its pharyngo-epiglottic folds, opposite the hyoid bone; and (3) the laryngeal pharynx, which extends from the hyoid bone above to the upper boundary of the esophagus below, opposite the sixth cervical vertebra (posterior to the larynx). The larynx itelf is considered separately.

The pharynx is approximately 12 cm. in length. It communicates with the nasal cavity, the oral cavity, the middle ear via the auditory (eustachian) tube, the esophagus and the trachea. The vital structures on either side of the pharynx are: the carotid arteries, the jugular veins, the ninth, tenth, eleventh and twelfth cranial nerves, the cervical sympathetic chain, important lymph nodal chains, and important fascial planes which may extend into the mediastinum.

The Nasopharynx (Fig. 10–1). The anterior boundary of the nasopharynx is formed by the choanae, with the vomer of the nasal septum between them. The posterior wall lies above the level of the anterior arch or tubercle of the atlas of the cervical spine, and usually contains considerable lymphatic tissue, which is continuous with a ring of lymphatic tissue around the circumference of the pharynx. The lymphatic tissue on the posterior wall of the nasopharynx comprises the adenoids of children, and tends to become atrophic in adults. As a result, the soft tissue width of the nasopharyngeal posterior wall is considerably greater in children than in adults, and tends to swell forward and downward toward the soft palate in the very young. The extent of this swelling is readily visualized on the lateral radiograph of the child's neck and furnishes an accurate means of evaluating the extent of adenoid hypertrophy. On the lateral wall is the pharyngeal recess or fossa of Rosenmüller, and below and in front of this are found the orifices of the auditive (eustachian) or auditory tubes. The elevated boundaries of the latter structure can usually be identified on the lateral radiograph of the neck.

The Oropharynx. The oropharynx is the common passageway of both the digestive tract (mouth to esophagus) and the respiratory tract (nasopharynx to larynx). It is bounded anteriorly by the posterior one third of the tongue which contains lymphoid follicles, and posteriorly by the soft tissue covering of the upper three cervical spine segments. The width of this soft tissue space is of considerable importance radiographically, particularly when compared with the width of the retrolaryngeal soft tissues. This relationship will be described in greater detail below (Fig. 10–2).

On each lateral wall of the oropharynx is the tonsillar fossa with its anterior and posterior pillars. Embedded between these pillars is the palatine or faucial tonsil.

The Laryngeal Pharynx (Fig. 10–3).   The laryngeal pharynx connects with the oropharynx above and the esophagus below. It is bounded posteriorly by

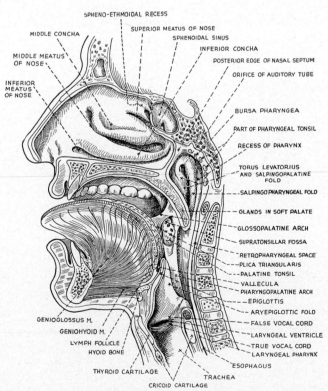

FIG. 10–1. Sagittal section of the head and neck to demonstrate the structure of the nasopharynx and larynx.

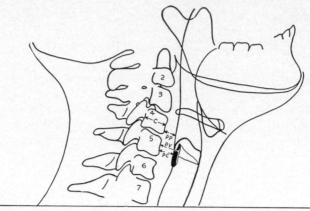

UPPER NORMAL LIMITS OF SOFT TISSUE SPACES OF NECK				
AGE	POSTPHARYNGEAL SOFT TISSUE		POSTLARYNGEAL SOFT TISSUE	
0-1	1.5c		2.c	
1-2	.5c		1.5c	POSTVENTRICULAR
2-3	.5c		1.2c	
3-6	.4c		1.2c	
6-14	.3c		1.2c	
ADULT	MALE .3c	FEMALE .3c	MALE .7c	FEMALE .6c	POSTCRICOID

PV = POSTVENTRICULAR SOFT TISSUE
PP = POSTPHARYNGEAL SOFT TISSUE   PC = POSTCRICOID SOFT TISSUE
C = ANTERO-POSTERIOR DIMENSION OF C-4 VERTEBRAL BODY AT ITS MIDDLE
(AFTER P. D. HAY: The Neck, In Ann. Roentgenology, N.Y., P.B. Hoeber, Publisher, 1930, Vol. 9.)

FIG. 10–2. Relative width of the posterior oropharynx to the soft tissues of the neck posterior to the larynx. (After P. D. Hay.)

GENERAL SCHEMATIC REPRESENTATION OF THE ROENTGEN ANATOMY OF THE LARYNX AND PHARYNX

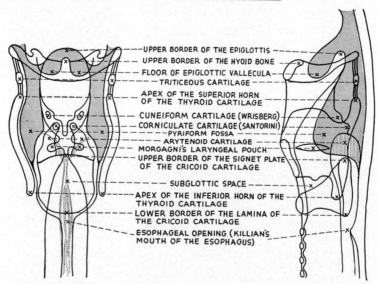

UPPER BORDER OF THE EPIGLOTTIS
UPPER BORDER OF THE HYOID BONE
FLOOR OF EPIGLOTTIC VALLECULA
TRITICEOUS CARTILAGE
APEX OF THE SUPERIOR HORN OF THE THYROID CARTILAGE
CUNEIFORM CARTILAGE (WRISBERG)
CORNICULATE CARTILAGE (SANTORINI)
PYRIFORM FOSSA
ARYTENOID CARTILAGE
MORGAGNI'S LARYNGEAL POUCH
UPPER BORDER OF THE SIGNET PLATE OF THE CRICOID CARTILAGE
SUBGLOTTIC SPACE
APEX OF THE INFERIOR HORN OF THE THYROID CARTILAGE
LOWER BORDER OF THE LAMINA OF THE CRICOID CARTILAGE
ESOPHAGEAL OPENING (KILLIAN'S MOUTH OF THE ESOPHAGUS)

FIG. 10–3. Geaner schematic representation of the roentgen anatomy of the larynx and pharynx.

the soft tissues overlying the fourth, fifth and sixth cervical vertebrae, and anteriorly by the posterior wall of the larynx. The posterior wall of the larynx contains the arytenoid cartilages and the lamina of the cricoid cartilage. The lateral walls of this area are attached to the thyroid cartilage and to the hyoid bone. The epiglottis is situated anteriorly and superiorly, in the median plane, with the aryepiglottic folds extending posteriorly and inferiorly from the epiglottis to the arytenoids. Beneath the level of these folds on either side are the pyriform sinuses. The valleculae are hollow pockets situated between the epiglottis and the dorsal aspect of the tongue just lateral to the median plane.

THE LARYNX

The cartilaginous framework is illustrated in Figure 10–4. This consists of three large single cartilages: the thyroid, cricoid and epiglottis; and three paired cartilages: the corniculate, the cuneiform and the arytenoids.

The thyroid cartilage is composed of two wings or laminae, and two superior and two inferior horns, or cornua. The superior margins of the two wings are convex and meet at the superior thyroid notch at an angle of 90 degrees in the male, and 120 degrees in the female, which explains the greater laryngea prominence in the male.

The cricoid cartilage attaches to and rests upon the first cartilaginous ring of the trachea, below the thyroid cartilage. It has the shape of a signet ring, being expanded posteriorly. This broad posterior aspect, or lamina, has a ridge centrally for attachment to the esophagus, an upper elliptical surface for attachment to the arytenoid cartilages, and inner impressions for attachment of the crico-arytenoid muscles. The inferior horns of the thyroid cartilage articulate with the lateral aspect of the cricoid ring.

The arytenoid cartilages are paired pyramidal cartilages surmounting the laminae of the cricoid posteriorly while the corniculate cartilages are mounted superiorly on the arytenoids. The cuneiform cartilages are embedded in the aryepiglottic folds.

The epiglottic cartilage is situated behind the root of the tongue above the thyroid cartilage, and behind the body of the hyoid bone. It lies in front and above the superior opening of the larynx and acts to deflect the swallowed bolus of food to either side into the pyriform fossae. The aryepiglottic folds act as a sphincter, preventing the food bolus from entering the larynx and trachea.

The thyroid, cricoid, and the greater part of the arytenoid cartilages are composed of hyaline cartilage which tends to calcify late in life and may be transformed into bone. The rest of the cartilages are composed for the most part of fibrocartilage, and do not calcify. The calcification may be irregular, and these open spaces must not be misinterpreted as erosion of the cartilage. Also, these areas of calcification must not be misinterpreted as foreign bodies in the esophagus or larynx. This distinction is readily made if one administers barium to the patient and the barium column is then seen to go behind the larynx.

The Cavity of the Larynx. The laryngeal aditus or superior laryngeal aperture or inlet is readily identified on the soft tissue films of the larynx (Fig. 10–5) as an opening which is bounded by the epiglottis in front, and the aryepi-

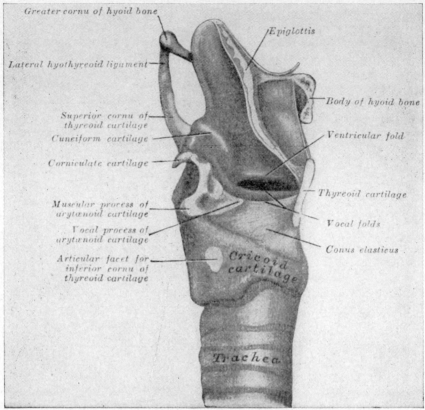

Fig. 10–4. Diagrammatic presentation of the cartilages and internal structure of the larynx. (From Gray, *Anatomy of the Human Body*, Edited by C. M. Goss, courtesy of Lea & Febiger, Publishers.)

glottic folds on each side. The pyriform recess or sinus is identified just outside the aditus on either side, between the aryepiglottic fold and the inner wall of the thyroid cartilage.

The vestibule or upper laryngeal compartment of the larynx extends from the laryngeal aditus to the ventricular folds (false vocal cords). The narrow opening between the ventricular folds is the vestibular slit.

The vestibule of the larynx as seen on the lateral radiograph of the neck is triangular in shape, with the base of the triangle formed by the ventricular folds, and arytenoid cartilages posteriorly. The anterior margin of this triangle is formed by the aryepiglottic folds, and the posterior by the epiglottis.

The middle laryngeal compartment is situated between the ventricular folds above and the vocal folds (true vocal cords) below. The ventricular folds are undermined on either side by a small lateral outpouching forming the laryngeal ventricle.

The "rima glottidis" is an elongated slitlike opening between the true vocal folds. This is the narrowest part of the laryngeal cavity.

The portion of the laryngeal cavity below the level of the vocal folds is the lower laryngeal compartment and is the inferior entrance to the glottis. It changes from a slit to a rounded cavity surrounded by the cricoid cartilage below, and is continuous with the trachea. This portion is a favorable site for the development of edema because of its loose connective tissue.

The sensory nerve supply of the larynx above the true vocal folds is carried by the superior laryngeal nerve and below the vocal folds by the recurrent laryngeal; the motor nerve supply (with the exception of the cricothyroid muscle) is carried by the recurrent laryngeal. The cricothyroid muscle is supplied by the superior laryngeal nerve.

The Normal Swallowing Act. The opaque mixture is projected from the mouth into the pharynx. The inferior constrictors of the pharynx contract, the thyroid cartilages and cords move upward, and the epiglottis moves slightly posteriorly. This closes off the laryngeal air passage. The pyriform sinuses and valleculae fill at this time, as the material passes into the hypopharynx. In the region of the cricopharyngeus muscle the barium column narrows, but becomes somewhat wider as it passes into the cervical esophagus. The aryepiglottic folds act as a sphincter, and the epiglottis divides the bolus into two equal streams which pass laterally into the pyriform sinuses. The epiglottis does not act as the sphincter or trap door. (A more detailed description of the swallowing act is presented on pages 593 and 594.)

The laryngeal structures return to their resting position after the bolus has passed into the esophagus.

Comparison of Width of the Retro-epilaryngeal Space with the Retrotracheal Space. Figure 10–2 presents the relationship of the soft tissues of the child and the adult in the specified regions at the levels of the fifth and sixth cervical vertebrae respectively. Roughly, up to the age of 1 year, the widths of these tissues equal one another and are approximately one and one half to two times the antero-posterior dimension of the fourth cervical vertebral body (C); however, in the adult, this ratio changes, so that the retropharyngeal space measured at C_5 level is about one third the width of the retrolaryngeal space, measured at C_6 level. Immediately below the middle compartment of the larynx, the retrolaryngeal space is considerably wider than the retrotracheal space, and this measurement is related to the junction with the esophagus.

RADIOGRAPHIC METHODS OF STUDY

The air passages are moderately well demonstrated by the fluoroscope and radiograph.

In addition to identifying the anatomic structures already described, the *fluoroscopic adjunct permits visualization of the movement of the vocal cords* in the antero-posterior projection, with phonation.

1. **Soft Tissue Lateral Film of the Neck (without and with Barium)** (Fig. 10–5). Visualization of the larynx is enhanced if the hypopharynx is distended with air by an expiratory effort with the mouth and nostrils closed. It is also helpful to extend the tongue. The technique is very similar to that employed for demonstration of the cervical spine, except that a "soft exposure" technique is employed. Barium may or may not be employed in the pharynx as desired.

The structures best visualized on the lateral film of the neck are: (1) the epiglottis; (2) the aryepiglottic folds; (3) the superior laryngeal compartment; (4) the ventricular and vocal folds, with the laryngeal ventricle between; (5) the thyroid, cricoid and arytenoid cartilages; (6) the retropharyngeal and laryngeal soft tissue spaces; (7) the trachea, thyroid, and surrounding soft tissue structures

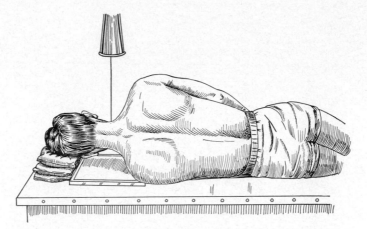

FIG. 10–5.   LATERAL SOFT TISSUE FILM OF NECK: **a,** Position drawing.

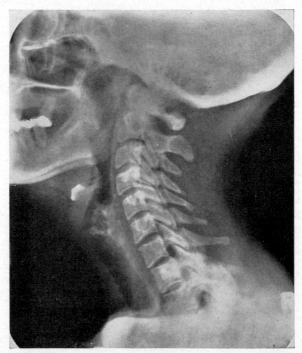

FIG. 10–5.   LATERAL SOFT TISSUE FILM OF NECK: **b,** Radiograph.

At the posterior margin of the laryngeal ventricle is a spherical shaped soft tissue mass produced by the arytenoids.

The pyriform sinuses and vallecula are best studied with the aid of barium in the pharynx.

2. **Antero-posterior Body Section Radiograph of the Larynx** (Fig. 10–6). If one obtains a section through the middle of the larynx in the coronal plane, the vestibule and the "zeppelin-shaped" laryngeal ventricle are clearly demonstrated, along with the true and false vocal cords. Ordinarily, such radiographs are obtained with the larynx at rest (Fig. 10–6, **a** and **b**); and during phonation 'Fig. 10–6, **c** and **d**).

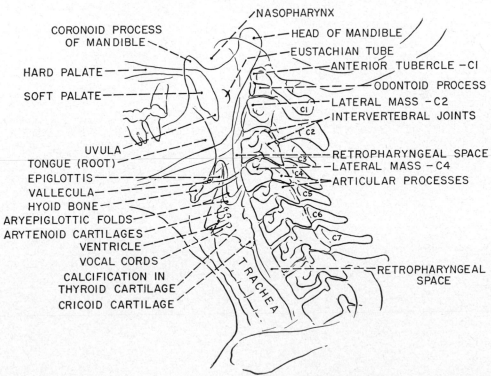

FIG. 10–5.   LATERAL SOFT TISSUE FILM OF NECK: **c,** Labeled tracing of **b.** (Diagrammatic for soft tissues only. For cervical spine structures see Figure 9–18.)

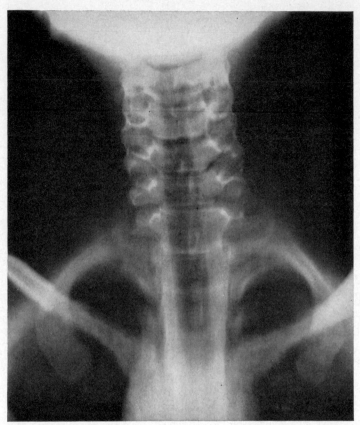

FIG. 10–6.   ANTERO-POSTERIOR BODY SECTION RADIOGRAPH OF LARYNX: **a,** Radiograph during rest.

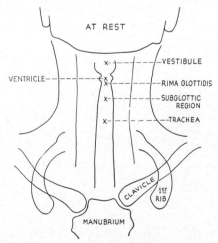

FIG. 10–6.   ANTERO-POSTERIOR BODY SECTION RADIOGRAPH OF LARYNX: **b,** Labeled tracing of **a.**

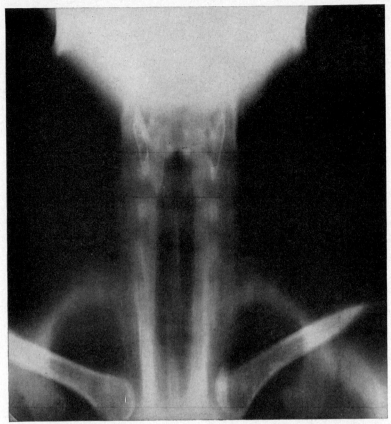

FIG. 10–6.   ANTERO-POSTERIOR BODY SECTION RADIOGRAPH OF LARYNX: **c,** Radiograph during phonation.

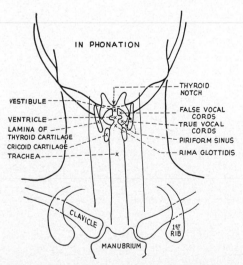

FIG. 10–6.   ANTERO-POSTERIOR BODY SECTION RADIOGRAPH OF LARYNX: **d,** Labeled tracing of **c.**

THE TRACHEA AND BRONCHI

The Trachea. The trachea consists of a framework of cartilaginous C-shaped rings which are connected posteriorly by a dense layer of connective tissue and muscle. The cartilages present marked irregularities, and they may be partially fused with adjoining cartilage rings. The carinal cartilage is formed by the fusion of tracheal and left bronchial cartilages, and the carina tracheae is a prominent ridge running antero-posteriorly across the bottom of the trachea between the origin of the bronchi. There is very little distinction between the epithelium lining the trachea and that lining the bronchi, and four types of cells are identified: (1) basal cells; (2) intermediate cells; (3) ciliated cells; and (4) goblet cells. The latter two types predominate.

The trachea begins at the level of the cricoid cartilage (sixth or seventh cervical vertebra). It extends downward through the neck, into the superior mediastinum, and ends at the upper border of the fifth to the eighth thoracic vertebra by bifurcating into the right and left bronchi. Bifurcation is lower in the adult than in the child (Fig. 10–7), usually at the level of the fourth costal cartilage in the child. The trachea moves upward upon swallowing, and downward in deep inspiration.

The trachea adheres to the midline, except toward its termination where it deviates slightly to the right. As it passes downward, it recedes from the surface, following the curvature of the vertebral column from which it is separated by the esophagus. In the infant, the trachea may be seen to deviate to the right as a normal occurrence (Fig. 10–8), and one must interpret tracheal shift in the infant with great caution. This is probably related to a relative redundancy of the trachea at this stage, and also to some irregularity in the position of the thymus. The trachea in the infant is roughly one third the length of the adult's, growing from approximately 4 cm. to a length in the adult of 12 cm.

Calcification of the tracheal rings may occur normally in the adult.

The Bronchi. The angle which the two bronchi make with the trachea varies according to the age of the individual (Kobler and V. Hovorka in Miller[2]) as follows:

AGE	RIGHT BRONCHUS	LEFT BRONCHUS
Newborn	10–35 degrees	30–65 degrees
Adult male	20 degrees	40 degrees
Adult female	19 degrees	51 degrees

From each main bronchus, lateral branches are given off. The dorsal branches are usually more slender than the ventral branches.

The right main bronchus is more nearly continuous with the trachea than is the left, but is shorter, and soon divides into two main branches—one above, and the other below the right pulmonary artery (Fig. 10–9): (1) the upper lobe bronchus (eparterial); (2) the continuation of the main stem (hyparterial).

The right upper lobe bronchus (Fig. 10–9) has three main branches: (1) the *apical* which divides in turn into an anterior and a posterior component; (2) the *posterior*, which supplies a pyramidal region along the axillary and posterior surface of the upper lobe; and (3) an *anterior* branch which supplies the anterior segment of the upper lobe.

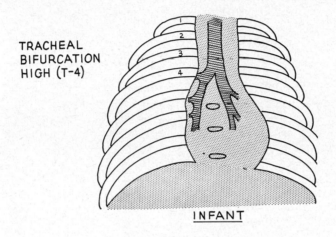

TRACHEAL
BIFURCATION
HIGH (T-4)

INFANT

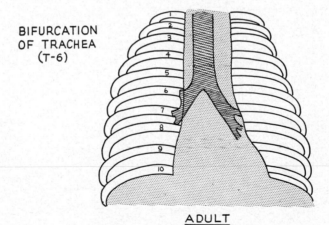

BIFURCATION
OF TRACHEA
(T-6)

ADULT

FIG. 10–7. Comparison of level of bifurcation of trachea in adult and child. (After Caffey, with permission of the publisher.)

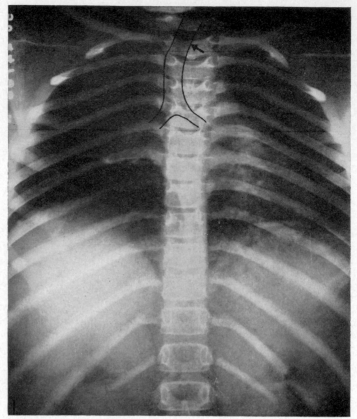

FIG. 10–8.   Radiograph (postero-anterior) of chest of infant to demonstrate slight normal deviation of trachea to the right, which occasionally occurs. This may result from a slight rotation of the infant's head, which may be very difficult to control, redundancy of the trachea, or slight thymic enlargement.

The right lower main stem thereafter subdivides into the *middle lobe bronchus* and the *lower lobe bronchus*.

The right middle lobe bronchus has two main branches: (1) a *medial* branch which supplies the sternocardiac region of the middle lobe; and (2) a *lateral* branch, which supplies the outer portion.

The *right lower lobe bronchus* has five main branches ordinarily: (1) the *superior branch*, which supplies the upper posterior and outer part of the apex of the lower lobe (this is sometimes an accessory lobe); (2) the *medial basal branch*, which arises directly from the inner side of the main stem, and supplies the inner side of the right lower lobe; (3) the *anterior basal branch*, which subdivides and supplies the anterior basal portion of the lower lobe; (4) the *posterior basal branch*, which supplies the posterior basal part of the right lower lobe; and (5) the *lateral basal branch*, which supplies the axillary portion of the basal part of the right lower lobe.

The absence of the middle lobe modifies the pattern of the bronchi in the left side. The left main bronchus is larger than the right but comes away from the trachea at a more acute angle. Opposite the inner end of the third anterior

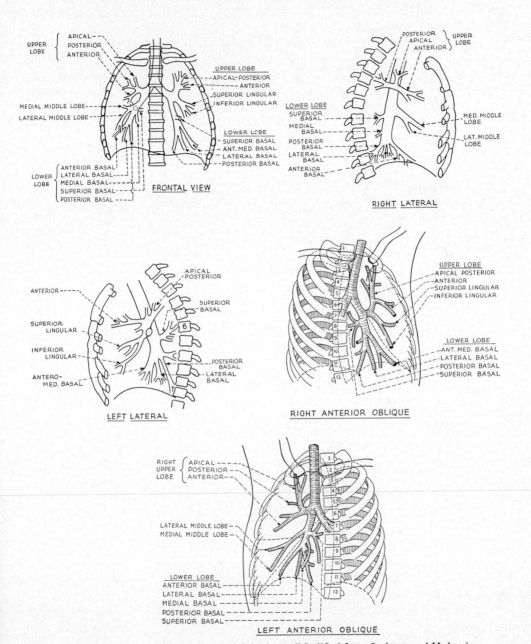

FIG. 10–9.   Bronchial distribution of the lung. (Modified from Jackson and Huber.)

interspace, it divides into an *upper lobe branch*, and a *lower lobe branch* which continues the line of the main stem. Above the curve of the bronchus, a shadow is seen with a free crescentic upper margin; this is the left pulmonary artery.

The *upper lobe bronchus* divides into an upper and a lower division, which almost immediately subdivide.

The *upper division* has two main branches: (1) the *apical-posterior branch*, which supplies the apical and posterior portions of the left upper lobe; and (2) an *anterior branch* which supplies the anterior portion of the apical area.

The *lower division* divides into two branches, similar to those of the right middle lobe but slightly different in direction: (1) a *superior branch*, and (2) an *inferior branch*, which supply the corresponding parts of the lingula portion of the left upper lobe.

The *left lower lobe bronchus* is almost identical with its counterpart on the right side with the one exception that the medial basal branch arises from the anterior basal branch rather than as a direct off-shoot from the left lower lobe bronchus. Otherwise, the superior, anterior basal, posterior basal and lateral basal branches are the same.

Bronchial Segments (Fig. 10–10).   The regions supplied by individual bronchi represent definite and separate bronchopulmonary segments of the lung which are combined according to a rather definite scheme into lobes. These are important to identify, and are fully illustrated in Figure 10–10.

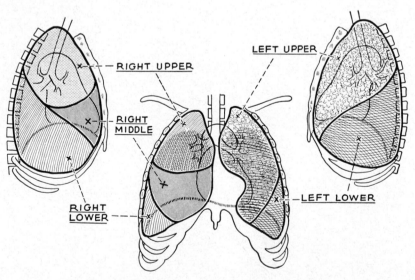

FIG. 10–10.   THE LUNG: a, Lobes and fissures.

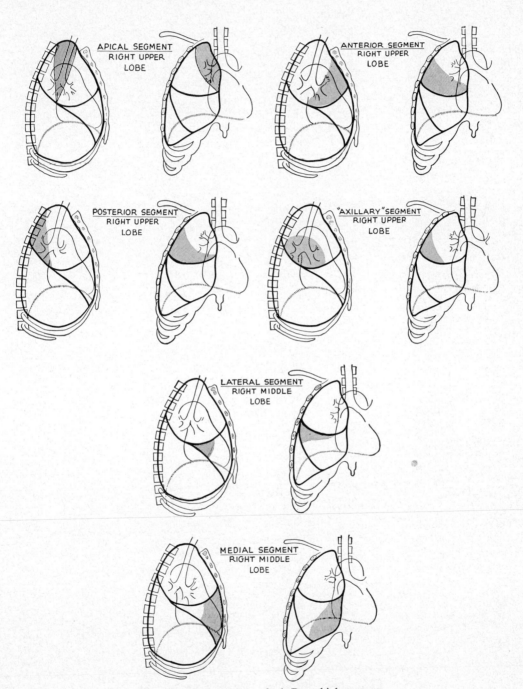

FIG. 10–10. THE LUNG: **b, 1,** Bronchial segments.

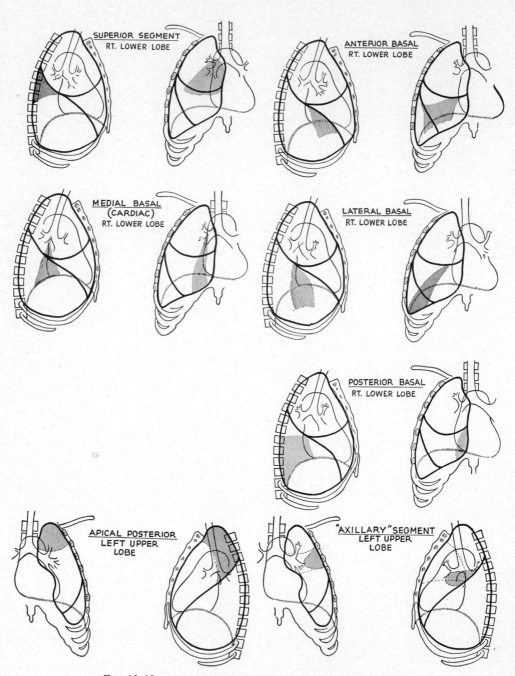

FIG. 10–10. THE LUNG: **b**, 2, Bronchial segments (*continued*).

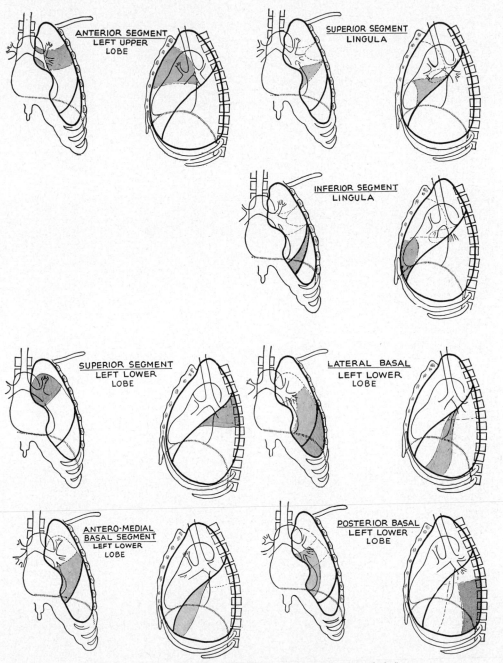

ANTERIOR SEGMENT
LEFT UPPER
LOBE

SUPERIOR SEGMENT
LINGULA

INFERIOR SEGMENT
LINGULA

SUPERIOR SEGMENT
LEFT LOWER
LOBE

LATERAL BASAL
LEFT LOWER
LOBE

ANTERO-MEDIAL
BASAL SEGMENT
LEFT LOWER
LOBE

POSTERIOR BASAL
LEFT LOWER
LOBE

Fig. 10–10.   the lung: **b**, 3, Bronchial segments (*concluded*).

THE LUNG PARENCHYMA; THE AIR SPACES

The Primary Lobule (Fig. 10–11). The bronchi continue to ramify until a point is reached where the walls no longer contain cartilage, forming the tubular bronchioli. Eventually the tubular character changes and there are small projections on all sides of the bronchiolus, known as alveolar ducts (Fig. 10–11). From the distal end of each alveolar duct, there are three to six spherical cavities called "atria." These atria, in turn, communicate with a variable number of larger and more irregular shaped cavities called "air sacs." Projecting from the wall of each air sac and atrium there are a number of smaller spaces called "pulmonary alveoli." This entire group of structures together with the accompanying blood vessels, lymph vessels and nerves form a primary lobule. The primary lobules are grouped into bronchial segments, in accordance with the pattern previously described.

The epithelium of the alveoli, like that of the bronchi and bronchioli, rests upon a network of reticulum, which is of some importance in connection with interstitial disease processes of the lungs.

The interchange of gases takes place in the alveoli, and the entire structure of the lungs is subservient to this end.

Fissures and Lobes of the Lungs (Fig. 10–10, **a**). The right lung is subdivided into three lobes, an upper, middle and lower, by two interlobar fissures. The major fissure separates the lower lobe on the one hand from the middle and upper lobes on the other. With minor differences to be described below, this fissure corresponds to the major fissure on the left side. The other fissure, or minor fissure, separates the upper from the middle lobe.

The left lung contains only a major fissure, and is subdivided into two lobes, an upper and a lower.

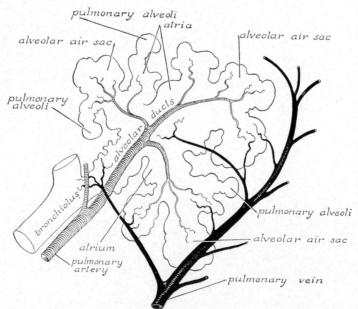

FIG. 10–11. Primary lobule of the lung. (Modified from Miller, *The Lung*, Charles C Thomas, Publishers.)

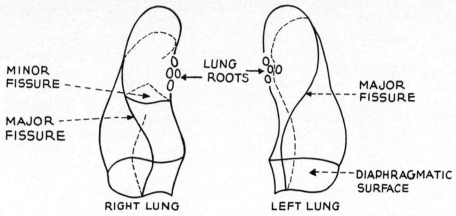

MINOR FISSURE

LUNG ROOTS

MAJOR FISSURE

MAJOR FISSURE

DIAPHRAGMATIC SURFACE

RIGHT LUNG   LEFT LUNG

FIG. 10–12.   Three-dimensional concept of interlobar fissures.

Each lobe of the lung is almost completely covered by visceral pleura, and each interlobar fissure is composed, therefore, of the visceral pleura of the two adjoining lobes which have extended down the fissure.

There is a considerable variation in the normal configuration and exact position of each fissure. From the radiologic point of view, the configuration of the entire surface of the interlobar fissure is of great importance. Each fissure must be visualized not as it is projected on to the surface of the thorax, but rather as a three-dimensional structure (Fig. 10–12).

Shape of the Interlobar Surfaces (Fig. 10–12).   The major fissure on the right side has the shape of an elongated and concave semi-ellipse. On the left side, it is rather crescentic. The major fissures reach to a variable distance from the hilus, and the minor (middle lobe) fissure is closed on the hilar surface.

There are pleural bridges uniting the various surfaces. There are also parenchymatous bridges uniting the various lobes with one another, particularly on the hilar and posterior aspects.

The right minor or middle lobe fissure is triangular, with the apex directed anteriorly. The base of the triangle is formed by the junction of the middle lobe fissure and the major fissure.

The upper par of the interlobar surface of the lower lobe looks anteriorly and somewhat laterally, while the lower part of this surface looks anteriorly and inward. This gives this surface a somewhat spiral appearance (resembling paropeller).

The minor (middle lobe) fissure on the right side is horizontal, at the level of the fourth costal cartilage.

The upper limit of the lower lobe posteriorly is at the vertebral end of the third rib or medial end of the spine of the scapula. The lower end is opposite the lateral part of the sixth costal cartilage.

The left upper lobe forms about one eighth of the diaphragmatic surface of the left lung in its anteromedian portion. On the right side, a rather large part of the middle lobe is in contact with the diaphragm (as much as one half).

The major fissure is steeper on the left side than on the right, forming an angle of about 60 degrees with the horizontal as against 50 degrees on the right side.

In addition to the spiral curvature of the major fissure, there is an upward convexity of the surface as well.

Radiographic Visualization of the Fissures. Ordinarily, the fissures are not visualized unless there is a considerable thickness of the fissure thrown into tangential view. Thus the interlobar fissure between the upper and middle lobes on the right is very frequently seen, since much of its surface is thrown into tangential projection in the postero-anterior projection. In the straight lateral projection, the major fissure may likewise be seen at least in part for the same reason. It is conceivable that if one were to try carefully to obtain a good surface tangential view of the various portions of the surface of any of the fissures it would be possible to demonstrate successively the various portions of the fissures.

Visualization of the fissures is very helpful from the standpoint of detection of disease, localizing the disease, and determining the nature of the disease present.

Segments of the Lungs (Fig. 10–10). While the segments of the lung do not have definite visceral pleural subdivisions as do the various lobes of the lungs, there is a certain amount of separability of these segments within the lung parenchyma. Each segment is supplied by a separate bronchial and arterial subdivision (see Fig. 10–16), and thus is a separable entity surgically.

ACCESSORY LOBES OF THE LUNGS

Inferior Accessory Lobe (Fig. 10–13). The segment of lung supplied by the medial basilar branch of the lower lobe bronchus on the right or the corre-

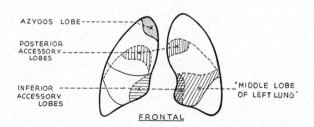

OCCASIONAL ACCESSORY LOBES OF LUNGS

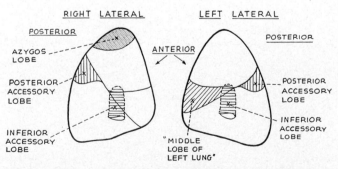

Fig. 10–13.   Diagrammatic presentation of accessory lobes of the lungs.

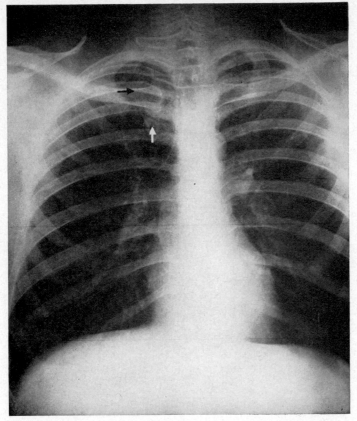

Fig. 10–14.   Radiograph of chest to show position and appearance of the azygos lobe.

sponding medial basilar branch of the anterior basilar branch of the left lower lobe bronchus may exist wholly or partially as a separate lobe. Schaffner found it in 45 per cent of 210 postmortem examinations, and radiologically it may be found in about 8 per cent of chest films (Twining). Fleischner has noted the variation in direction of the fissure of this lobe, and hence its variable appearance must be constantly borne in mind. It resembles closely at times an abnormally large pericardial fat pad in the right cardiophrenic angle, or any other abnormality which may be projected in this location.

Posterior Accessory Lobe.   The segment supplied by the superior branch of the lower lobe bronchus may not infrequently be an accessory lobe. It is probable, however, that it need not necessarily be a separate lobe even if it is shown sharply demarcated from the surrounding lung in disease, since the segmental distribution of the bronchi is discrete in any event.

Middle Lobe of Left Lung.   Although the lingular portion of the left upper lobe is separated from the rest of the upper lobe by a relatively avascular portion, and occasionally by an incomplete fissure, it is practically never a completely separate accessory lobe as in the case of the other lobes.

Accessory Azygos Lobe (Fig. 10–14).   Embryologically the azygos vein runs just lateral to the apex of the right upper lobe. As the apex grows upward, the azygos vein ordinarily glides medially so that it lies medial to the right lung apex.

If this gliding movement is interrupted, as the apex of the right upper lobe grows upward the azygos vein produces an indentation into the right upper lobe medially, carrying with it a fold of both visceral and parietal pleura. Thus, unlike the true fissures between lobes which consist of two layers of visceral pleura, this artificial fissure consists of four layers, two visceral and two parietal.

This false fissure appears radiologically as a thin line convex outward, always in the right upper lobe medially. It is usually thicker at its lower end, probably related to the fact that the azygos vein is situated in this location, and possibly to an associated fold of pleura. This thicker area must be carefully differentiated from any abnormality in the lung.

VASCULAR SUPPLY, VENOUS DRAINAGE AND LYMPHATICS OF THE RESPIRATORY TRACT

The Blood Vessels of the Lungs. PULMONARY ARTERY. The pulmonary artery (Fig. 10–15) follows closely the subdivisions of the bronchial tree. It arches over the right main-stem bronchus and lies dorsal and slightly lateral to the bronchus. The artery diminishes more rapidly in size than the bronchus it accompanies, and by the time it reaches the primary lobule, it is about one fourth or one fifth the size of the ductulus alveolaris. It finally ends in a capillary network which surrounds the alveolus. The pulmonary vein takes origin from the latter capillary network.

The common pulmonary artery divides into right and left pulmonary arteries. The right pulmonary artery passes under the aortic arch below the tracheal bifurcation, and crosses in front of the right bronchus between its upper lobe and lower division branches. It divides into three branches, two of which go to the upper lobe, and one supplies the middle and lower lobes. Each of the branches of these subdivisions follow the corresponding branches of the bronchial tree rather closely, with the artery lying along the upper side of the

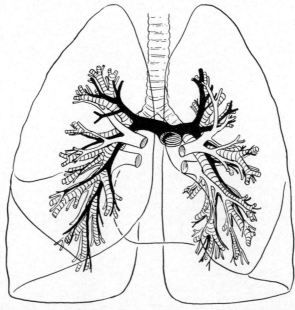

FIG. 10–15.   Pulmonary arteries and pulmonary veins shown in relation to the tracheo-bronchial tree.

bronchus most of the way. The left pulmonary artery is seen just below the aortic knob as it arches posteriorly into the left lung, and forms the crescentic shadow of the left hilus, above the downward curving left bronchus. It enters the hilus as three branches, and then subdivides into nine principal branches, five of which go to the upper lobe, and four to the lower lobe following corresponding bronchial branches.

CAPILLARIES. The network of capillaries is situated in the walls of the alveoli, and each capillary is common to two alveoli. The mesh of capillaries in the walls of the alveoli situated beneath the pleura is much coarser than that within the lung. The same holds true for the capillaries situated near the fibrous septa and larger blood vessels.

PULMONARY VEINS. Unlike the pulmonary artery which is virtually in the same sheath as the bronchus, the more peripheral pulmonary veins are situated far removed from the corresponding bronchus and are situated in the septa which unite several lobules. The pulmonary veins have four sources of origin: (1) the capillary network of the pleura, which is derived from the bronchial artery; (2) the capillary network of the alveoli; (3) the bronchopulmonary veins, which are situated on either side of the junction of two bronchi or bronchioli; and (4) the capillary network in the alveolar ducts, which gives origin to two venous radicles, one on either side of the duct.

The veins and arteries come closer together at about the fourth bronchial bifurcation and are more closely related, the veins lying anterior to and below the arteries. As they approach the hilum, they again become dissociated, the veins lying below and anterior to the arteries and diverging from them to enter the left atrium. The veins are not usually clearly distinguishable from the arteries in the usual radiograph (except perhaps in body-section radiographs).

BRONCHIAL ARTERY. The bronchial arteries vary in number and origin. Usually there are two for the left lung, and one for the right. They usually take origin from the descending limb of the upper thoracic aorta. They are embedded in the connective tissue which surrounds the bronchi. Usually there are two or three of these branches which accompany each of the larger bronchi or bronchioli, and each subdivision is accompanied by a corresponding subdivision of the bronchial artery. Anastomosing branches connect these arterial trunks. The bronchial arteries as a distinct set of vessels disappear at the appearance of the alveoli. The capillaries in the alveolar walls are derived from the pulmonary artery and not from the bronchial artery. The bronchial arteries terminate in a network of capillaries in the tunica propria of the muscular wall, and from this point onward, the pulmonary artery supplies the bronchial tree. (It is interesting to note that this point of transition from the bronchial to the pulmonary circulation is a favorite site for tubercle formation.)

BRONCHIAL VEINS. True bronchial veins are found only at the hilus of the lung. These arise from the first or first two dividing points of the bronchial tree, and receive branches from part of the pleura close to the hilus. These bronchial veins empty into the azygos, the hemiazygos, or one of the intercostal veins. Communications exist between the bronchial arteries and pulmonary veins via the capillaries, but Guillor (Miller) could not demonstrate such communication with the pulmonary artery directly. These vascular phenomena are of considerable importance from the standpoint of much of the circulatory pathology of the lungs.

The Lymphatics of the Lungs (Figs. 10–16, 10–17). The lung is provided with a great abundance of lymphatics, more than the liver, spleen or kidney (Miller). They may be divided grossly into a superficial and a deep set. The superficial lymphatics are situated in the pleura; the deep group are situated along the pulmonary artery, veins and bronchi, and form a dense network between the secondary lobules in the connective tissue septa. These two sets of lymphatics communicate with one another at the pleura and in the hilus. The pleural lymphatics are arranged in the form of irregular polyhedral rings, and have an unusually large diameter.

Lymphatics of the Bronchi. The larger bronchi have two sets of lymphatics which intercommunicate with one another, but the smaller bronchi have only a single plexus of lymphatics, which terminate at the alveolar ductules, where they join the lymphatics accompanying the pulmonary veins which form at this point.

There are no lymphatics in the walls of the air spaces distal to the alveolar ductules.

Lymphatics of the Pulmonary Artery. The larger branches of the pulmonary artery are accompanied by two lymph channels, one of which is situated between the artery and its accompanying bronchus. These intercommunicate freely by means of a rich plexus. The smaller arterial branches are accompanied by only single lymph channels. Communications between the periarterial and peribronchial lymphatics occur in many places but predominantly in the region of bifurcations, and at the distal end of the alveolar ductules.

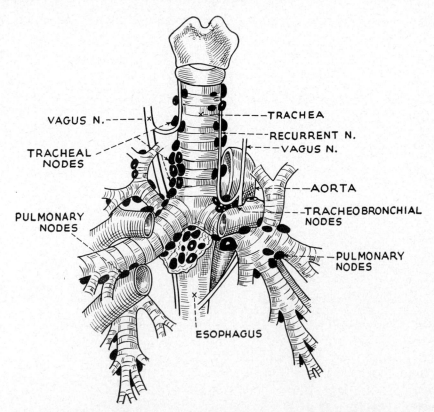

FIG. 10–16.   Lymph nodes of the tracheobronchial tree. (After Sukienikow.)

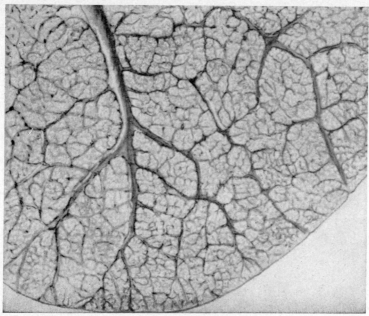

FIG. 10–17.   Drawing of lower surface of middle lobe showing lymphatic vessels outlining the lobules and acini of the lung parenchyma. (From E. W. Twining in *A Textbook of X-Ray Diagnosis,* H. K. Lewis & Co., Publishers.)

Lymphatics of the Pulmonary Veins.   As in the case of the arteries and bronchi, lymph channels accompany all of the veins, except in the region of the alveolar sacs.

There are no valves in the lung lymphatics except where the deep and superficial lymph systems meet.

Lymphatics of the Pleura.   There is only a single plexus of lymphatics in the pleura, arranged in polyhedral rings. There are smaller rings within these larger ones, with smaller lymph channels.

Direction of Lymph Flow.   The valves situated in the hilus, pleura, and at the junction of the deep and superficial systems permit flow in one direction only. *The flow in the peribronchial, periarterial and perivenous lymphatics is toward the interior of the lung,* or hilus.

The *valves situated just beneath the pleura permit flow of lymph only toward the pleura* and the *only communication between the superficial and the deep lymphatics is at this point.*

The valves situated in the pleura allow free circulation of the lymph within this space. The pleural lymphatics together with the lymphatics from the interior of the lung all enter the tracheobronchial lymph nodes.

In the presence of an obstructed lymph channel, a reversal of lymph flow can occur. These obstructed and distended lymphatics appear linear and stellate in relation to hilar lymph nodes.

Lymphoid Tissue.   Lymphoid tissue may occur in the form of lymph nodes, lymph follicles or small masses of lymphoid tissue. Lymph nodes in the normal lung are found associated with the larger divisions of the bronchi, and are situated at the places where branching takes place (Fig. 10–16). There is in old age a definite increase in the lymphoid tissue independent of that produced by disease, but dependent to a great extent on the amount of irritating particles inhaled (such as carbon). In the normal lung, lymph nodes are not present in the pleura.

The following groups of lymph nodes occur (Fig. 10–16): (1) the paratracheal group; (2) the tracheobronchial group, the right being more constant than the left, but those on the left are in close relation with the recurrent nerve (they are connected with the anterior and posterior mediastinal nodes, and also the inferior deep cervical nodes); (3) the bifurcation group which are likewise in communication with the posterior mediastinal nodes; (4) each group of bronchopulmonary nodes, lying in the hilus of the corresponding lung, in the angles between the branches of the bronchi; (5) the pulmonary groups, lying in the lung substance, usually in the angles of the branching bronchi up to the third branching. The nodes in the left upper lobe may lie in the anterior mediastinum in close relationship to the aorta and ductus arteriosus.

The hilar nodes receive lymph not only from the more peripheral lymphatics of the lung, but also from the pleura, by lymph channels which drain along the interlobar fissures and over the anterior and posterior lung surfaces toward the hilus. This accounts for the great frequency with which these fissures become visible in both pleural and pulmonary disease.

Lymphatic Pathways of the Mediastinum.   In the thorax, the thoracic duct receives tributaries from the intercostal and mediastinal tributaries, and communicates with the right bronchomediastinal trunk. The bronchomediastinal trunk receives the lymph from the right lung and empties via the right lymphatic duct into the beginning of the innominate vein. Near their terminations, both thoracic ducts lie close to the lower deep cervical lymph nodes.

THE LUNG HILI

The hilus of the lung (Fig. 10–18) is a wedge-shaped depressed area on the mediastinal surface of the lung above and behind the pericardial impression on the lung, within which the blood vessels, lymph vessels, nerves and bronchi enter and leave the lung. Bronchial lymph nodes are located among those structures. The hilus is surrounded by the reflection of the pleura from the surface of the lung on to the pulmonary root. The mediastinal surface of the lung presents the pericardial impression produced by structures in the posterior mediastinum, and the superior mediastinum in addition to the hili.

The term "root of the lung" is, strictly speaking, applied to a number of structures which enter and leave the lung on its mediastinal surface. It constitutes a pedicle which attaches the lung to the mediastinal wall of the pleural cavity. The large structures forming the pulmonary root are: (1) the two pulmonary veins, (2) the pulmonary artery, (3) the bronchus, (4) bronchial arteries and veins, (5) pulmonary nerves and (6) lymph vessels and some lymph nodes (bronchial).

In the case of the left lung, the major arteries, veins and branches are arranged in the form of a triangle, with the pulmonary veins forming the anterior and inferior apices of the triangle and the left pulmonary artery, the superior apex of the triangle; the bronchus is in the center of the triangle. The pulmonary artery lies higher in the left root than in the right, and crosses the bronchus on the left before it divides into its branches.

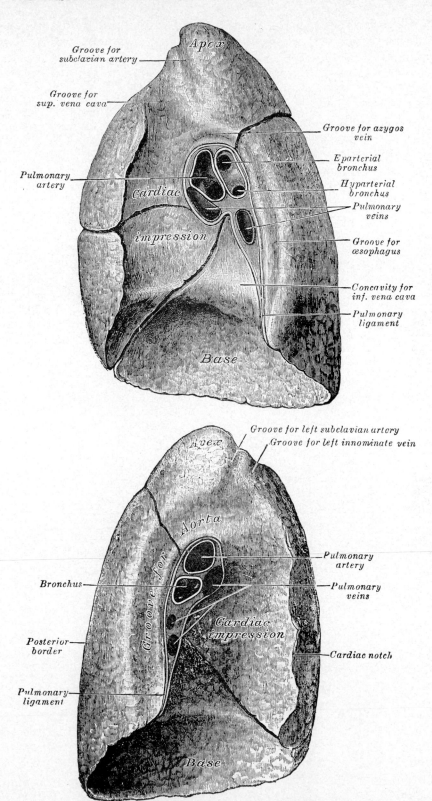

FIG. 10–18. Structures in the lung hili. (From Gray, *Anatomy of the Human Body,* by C. M Edited Goss, courtesy of Lea & Febiger, Publishers.)

These root structures can be moderately well distinguished on radiographs in the postero-anterior and oblique projections. By common usage, the terms "hilus" and "root" are used interchangeably.

THE THORACIC CAGE, PLEURA AND DIAPHRAGM

There are several important component parts of the thoracic cage, all of which may be visualized to some extent radiographically. These are: (1) the soft tissue structures of the thoracic wall, such as the skin, breasts and muscular tissues; (2) the bony structures of the thoracic cage, consisting chiefly of ribs, costal cartilage, sternum and thoracic spine; (3) the pleura, both visceral and parietal; and (4) the diaphragm.

SOFT TISSUE STRUCTURES OF THE THORACIC WALL

Skin and Subcutaneous Tissues. The skin and subcutaneous tissues of the thoracic cage cannot be entirely ignored in the consideration of the radiographic anatomy of the chest. Normally, these tegmental layers are seen only over the clavicle (see Chap. 4), and as outlining shadows of the thoracic cage; abnormally, shadows contained within the skin and subcutaneous tissues can produce very dense shadows which must be differentiated from pulmonary constituents. Free air in the skin and subcutaneous tissues also produce their individual

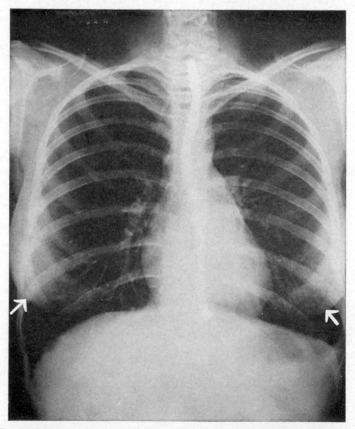

Fig. 10–19.   Projection of female breast shadows over the lung substance.

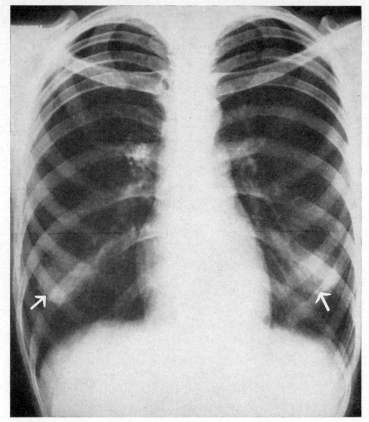

Fig. 10–20.   Radiograph showing areola and nipple shadows.

appearance. The fact that structures contained within the skin have radiographic significance must not be overlooked.

The Breasts (Figs. 10–19, 10–21).   The breasts are situated in the superficial fascia covering the anterior aspect of the thoracic cage, and in the female usually extend from the level of the second or third rib to the level of the sixth. The hemispherical shadow of the female breast is cast over that of the pectoralis major muscle, and together form a notable haziness which may obscure to a great extent the lung substance proper (Fig. 10–19). At the level of the fourth or fifth rib, the nipple, in turn, may cast an even denser shadow than that of the breast (Fig. 10–20), and has the appearance of a rather dense nodule. Occasionally the areola around the nipple may also be distinguished. Of course, the size and shape of the breasts vary considerably among both women and men, and will vary in the same woman according to the physiologic state of the breast.

The breast may be investigated radiographically in several ways: (1) soft tissue study tangential to the breast (Fig. 10–21); (2) study of the breast following injection of CO_2 into tissues around the breast (Fig. 10–22); and (3) by injection of opaque media into the lactiferous ducts (Fig. 10–23).

The main purpose of these studies is to demonstrate abnormal space-occupying lesions within the breast.

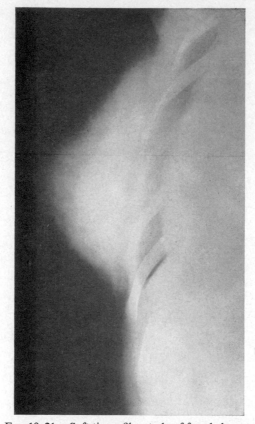

FIG. 10–21.   Soft tissue film study of female breast.

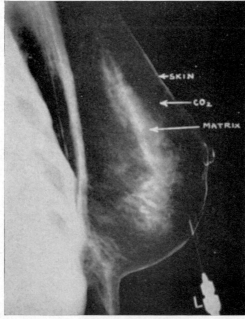

FIG. 10–22.   Study of breast following injection of soft tissues with air. (From N. F. Hicken et al., Am. J. Roentgenol., vol. 39, with permission of the author and publisher.)

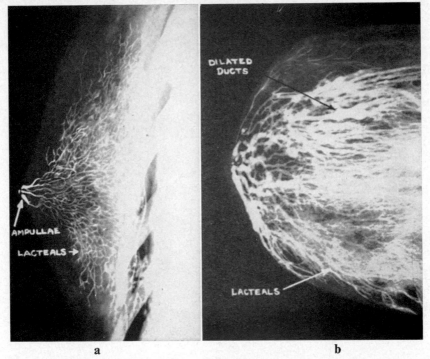

FIG. 10–23. RADIOGRAPHS OF BREAST AFTER INJECTION OF THE DUCTS WITH LIPIODOL: **a,** virginal breast; **b,** multiparous breast.

Muscular Tissues. The following muscles of the thoracic cage may produce a shadow upon the radiograph: (1) the pectoralis major and minor; (2) the sternocleidomastoid; (3) the serratus anterior; and (4) the intercostal muscles (may be seen on oblique views of the ribs and chest).

Their importance lies chiefly in the fact that they must be differentiated from abnormal shadows in the chest. By the injection of air, these muscle shadows can be delineated more clearly.

When it is desired to differentiate any of these soft tissue structures, it is well to mark or delineate the structures with wire, and compare a radiograph so obtained with one obtained without the delineation. This permits one at a glance to distinguish the cause of the shadow seen.

THE RIBS

Gross Anatomy Related to Radiographic Anatomy. The typical rib (Fig. 10–24) consists of a head, neck, tubercle, body or shaft, and costal cartilage. The body has an angle and a costal groove. The heads of the upper nine ribs articulate with two thoracic vertebrae—the one with which each rib is in numerical correspondence, and the one above. There are two articular facets for this purpose. The tenth, eleventh and twelfth ribs have only one articulation, and articulate with only one vertebral body.

Anatomic Features of Radiographic Significance.   The inferior aspect of the neck may have a notched appearance, and this notching must not be confused with the abnormal notching and undulation which occur more peripherally in association with dilated intercostal arteries (as in coarctation of the aorta).

The inferior margin of the rib where the costal groove is identified may have a somewhat irregular appearance, particularly at the angle of the rib. This irregularity at the angle is due to the fact that the bone is slightly thickened in this location.

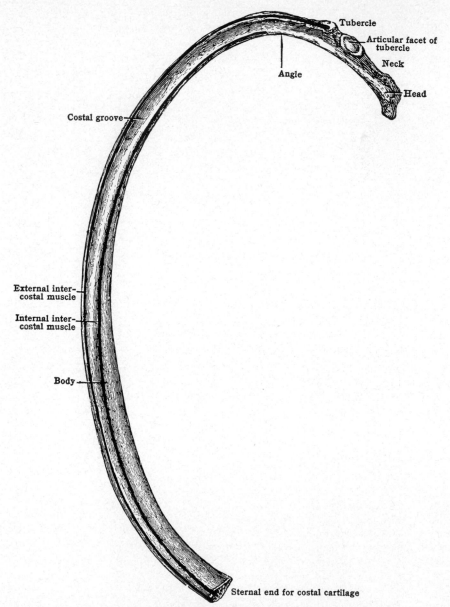

FIG. 10–24.   Anatomic drawing of a typical rib. (From R. J. Terry in Morris' *Human Anatomy*, Edited by Jackson, The Blakiston Co., Publishers.)

There is usually a slight widening of the rib as it joins the costal cartilage, and there is a ringlike shadow identified in this location (see Fig. 10–35). This slight flare of the ribs must not be confused with the abnormal rosary which occurs in vitamin D deficiency in children.

The overlying gas shadows over ribs are very disturbing at times, and make a study of bony detail extremely difficult. These gas shadows must not be confused with areas of true bone absorption or replacement.

The last rib may simulate a transverse process of the lumbar spine, but can be identified frequently by its articulation with the twelfth thoracic vertebra. This transition between the ribs and the transverse processes of the lumbar vertebrae is usually a gradual one, and is exemplified in the anatomic changes visible in the last three thoracic ribs.

Mode of Radiographic Examination of the Ribs.   Ribs may be studied in any of the routine radiographs of the chest. Ordinarily, however, for greatest accuracy, special studies of the ribs are desirable. These are obtained by placing the ribs in question in various degrees of obliquity (essentially the same as Fig. 10–27), centering over the area of maximum suspicion and obtaining movable grid films. Usually at least three such views are obtained. *It is not unusual to find that routine radiographs of the chest are inadequate for rib detail, and that the study is considerably better when done as a special procedure.*

THE STERNUM

Gross Anatomy and Correlated Radiographic Anatomy.   The sternum consists of the manubrium, body and xiphoid process. The body in youth consists of four segments. The manubrium ordinarily is united with the sternal body by a cartilaginous union only, until old age.

The manubrium has a suprasternal notch (Fig. 10–25), a clavicular articular surface on either side for articulation with the clavicle, and a rough portion just below the clavicular articulation where the cartilage of the first rib is implanted.

The angle between the body of the sternum and the manubrium is called the sternal angle, and the cartilage of the second rib joins the sternum at this point.

The body of the sternum is composed of four segments which fuse in adolescence, leaving a transverse ridge at each site of fusion. There are small protuberances on either side of the sternum at these junction lines, and the rib cartilages for the third, fourth and fifth ribs join the sternum at these protuberances.

The seventh rib cartilages join the sternum at the junction of the body and xiphoid process, and the sixth rib cartilages join the sternum slightly above this level.

The upper margin of the manubrium is at the level of the lower border of the body of the second thoracic vertebra; the sternal angle, with the upper border of the body of the fifth thoracic vertebra; and the xiphoid process, with the ninth thoracic vertebra.

With the exception of the manubrium, the sternum will ordinarily not be visualized on straight postero-anterior views of the chest, and requires special projections for the demonstration of its radiographic anatomy (Fig. 10–27).

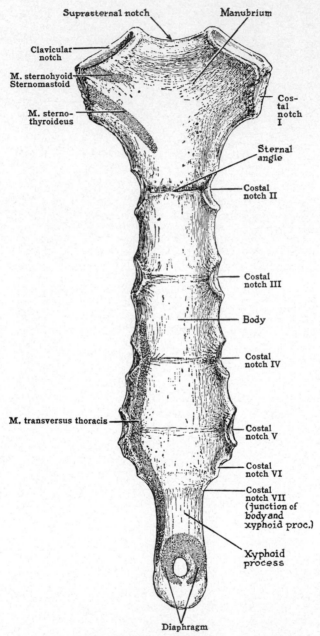

Fɪɢ. 10–25.   Gross anatomy of the sternum. (Adapted from Terry, R. J., in Morris' *Human Anatomy*, Edited by Jackson, The Blakiston Co., Publishers.)

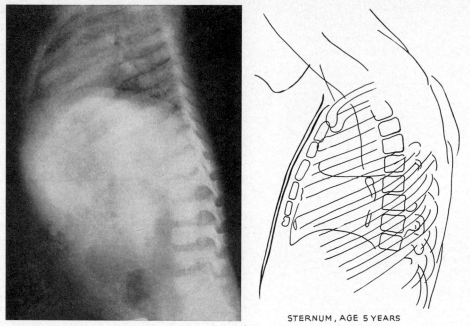

STERNUM, AGE 5 YEARS

Fig. 10–26.   Radiograph and tracing to show sternal segments.

Variations with Growth and Development (Fig. 10–26).   Ordinarily, there are one or two centers of ossification already present and ossified at birth for all segments of the sternum except the xiphoid process. The latter center of ossification usually does not appear until about 3 years of age.

The segments of the body of the sternum unite from below upward, so that the fourth and third segments unite first in childhood; the third unites with the second at puberty; the second with the first at about 21 years of age.

The body and the manubrium ordinarily do not unite until old age, and the body and xiphoid not until about 40 years of age.

These normal lines of fusion of the various segments must not be confused with fractures.

Modes of Radiographic Examination. 1. OBLIQUE VIEW OF THE STERNUM (Fig. 10–27).   Since the sternum overlies the heart and mediastinal structures, it must be projected away from these structures to be visualized radiographically. Either oblique projection may be employed as illustrated. In either case, the lung structures are projected over the sternum, so that bony texture is very difficult to evaluate accurately. Gross abnormalities are readily manifest, but minute changes in the sternum can escape detection.

The manner in which the film is obtained, and the associated anatomy are shown in Figure 10–27.

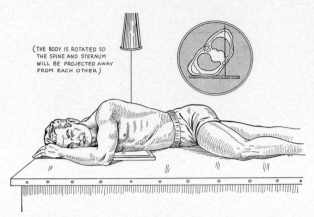

(THE BODY IS ROTATED SO THE SPINE AND STERNUM WILL BE PROJECTED AWAY FROM EACH OTHER.)

FIG. 10–27. OBLIQUE VIEW OF STERNUM AND STERNOCLAVICULAR JOINTS (ALSO RIBS): **a,** Position of patient similar in both.

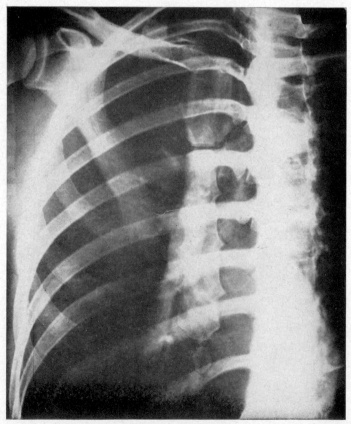

FIG. 10–27.   OBLIQUE VIEW OF STERNUM AND STERNOCLAVICULAR JOINTS (ALSO RIBS):   **b,** Radiograph of sternum.

POINTS OF PRACTICAL INTEREST WITH REFERENCE TO FIGURE 10–27, AND COMMENTS RELATING
    TO BODY-SECTION RADIOGRAPHY OF THE STERNUM:

1. Sometimes the sternum is difficult to visualize at best in this view with sufficient clarity.
   Under these circumstances, body-section radiography is recommended. The best technique
   for this is as follows:
   (a) A mobile cart is placed at right angles to the x-ray table, and the patient lies prone
       on the cart, with his chest overlapping the table, so that he is as nearly as possible
       perpendicular to the x-ray table.
   (b) *The long axis of the sternum is therefore in contact with the surface of the x-ray table
       but at right angles to the long axis of this table.*
   (c) The cassette is placed in the tray so that its long axis corresponds to that of the
       sternum.
   (d) The body-section study is thereafter made in the usual manner, and two or three
       "cuts" may be made.

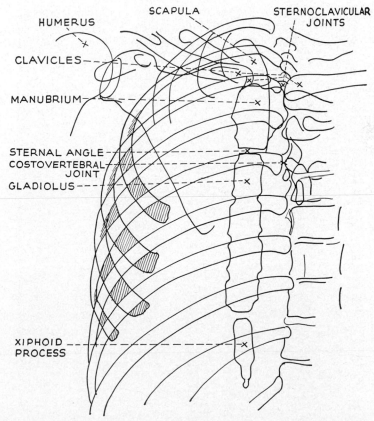

FIG. 10–27. OBLIQUE VIEW OF STERNUM AND STERNOCLAVICULAR JOINTS (ALSO RIBS): c, Labeled
tracing of b.

2. LATERAL VIEW OF THE STERNUM (Fig. 10–28). This view is particularly helpful since it shows the structure of the sternum in at least one perspective without the interference of overlying structures. This is only one perspective, however, and one cannot ordinarily obtain a clear anatomic concept from one projection alone. Moreover, in certain individuals, the sternum is somewhat depressed, and the ribs will overlie the sternum in considerable part. It is most difficult to obtain a clear idea of the structure of the sternum in such individuals.

This view is also valuable since it shows the relationship of the sternum to the underlying structures.

The method by which this view is obtained along with film and tracing are illustrated in Figure 10–28.

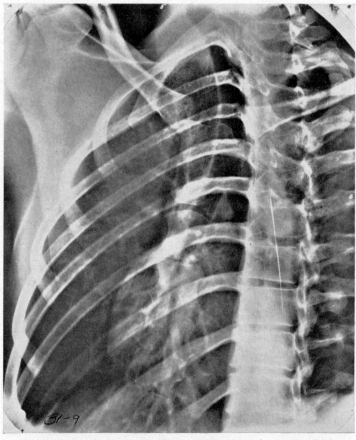

FIG. 10–27.   OBLIQUE VIEW OF STERNUM AND STERNOCLAVICULAR JOINTS (ALSO RIBS):   **d,** Radiograph of sternoclavicular joints.

3. BODY-SECTION RADIOGRAPHS OF THE STERNUM. Body-section radiographs must frequently be employed to obtain an unobstructed view of the sternum. A much more detailed visualization of the bony texture and structure can thus be obtained. Several sections are necessary, and one must use caution in interpretation since the entire sternum is not visualized at one level.

A study of the bony texture of the sternum is of particular interest and importance, since the sternal marrow is one of the important hematopoietic organs, and as such can be readily affected by diseases of the blood-forming apparatus, lymphoid structures, or any of the cellular components of the marrow.

Sternoclavicular Joints (Fig. 10–29). The sternoclavicular joint is a two-chambered synovial or diarthrodial joint with an articular disk between the two chambers. Each chamber is usually distinct and separate from the other, unless the articular disk happens to be unusually thin (as in the case of the temporomandibular joint).

These joints are usually demonstrated on oblique projections such as are employed for the sternum proper (Fig. 10–27), except that the tube is centered over the joint. *A comparison film of the opposite side is always obtained so that the two sternoclavicular joints can be compared in the same patient.*

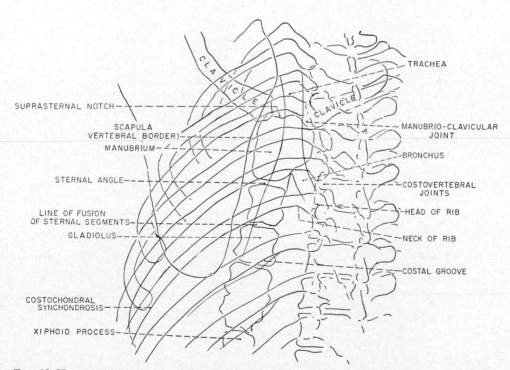

FIG. 10–27. OBLIQUE VIEW OF STERNUM AND STERNOCLAVICULAR JOINTS (ALSO RIBS): **e,** Labeled tracing of **d.**

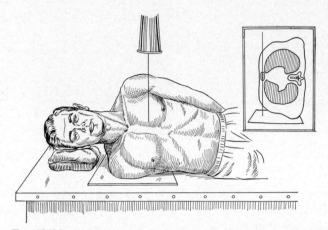

FIG. 10–28.   LATERAL VIEW OF STERNUM: **a,** Positioning of patient.

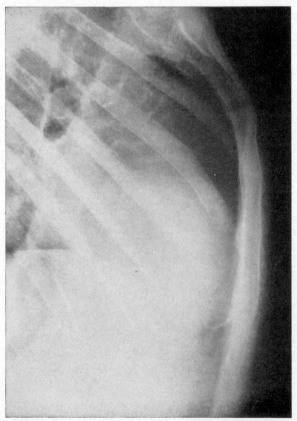

FIG. 10–28.   LATERAL VIEW OF STERNUM: **b,** Radiograph.

Points of Practical Interest With Reference to Figure 10–28:

1. This view of the sternum gives us maximum clarity of the sternum, but unfortunately has the following disadvantages:
   (a) When the sternum is depressed at all, it is concealed behind the costal cartilages and some lung in this projection. This is especially true of the condition called "pectus excavatum."
   (b) Abnormalities which do not affect the entire width of the sternum may be obscured by the unaffected portion. Body-section radiographs are helpful when this is suspected.
   (c) The various segments of the sternum must be recognized, and differentiated from other abnormalities which may be stimulated at the costo-sternal junctions.
2. The retrosternal mediastinal and pleural shadows should always be examined very carefully. This is also true of the shadows which are superficial to the sternum. The clue to abnormality is often found here where it may escape detection by inspection of the sternal shadow only.

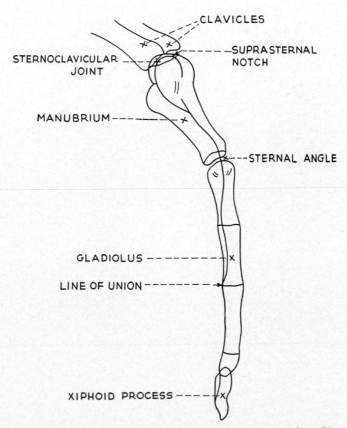

FIG. 10–28.   LATERAL VIEW OF STERNUM: c, Labeled tracing of b.

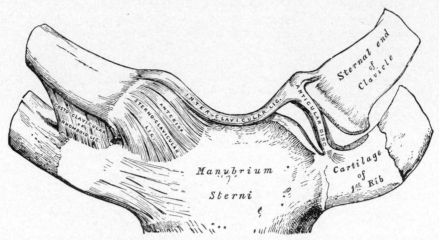

FIG. 10–29.   **a,** Gross anatomy of sternoclavicular joint. (From Gray, *Anatomy of the Human Body*, Edited by C. M. Goss, courtesy of Lea & Febiger.)

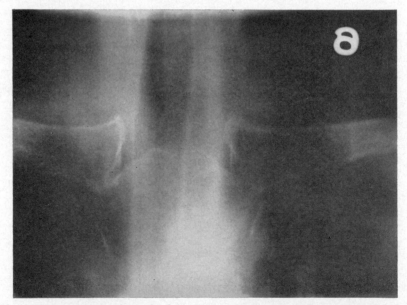

FIG. 10–29.   **b,** Body section radiograph of the sternoclavicular joints. This is obtained in the prone position, centering over the sternoclavicular joints.

THE PLEURA

Gross Anatomic Features as Applied to Radiographic Anatomy. The pleura lines the entire thoracic cavity, invests the entire lung, and invaginations of the pleura form the interlobar fissures. That portion which lines the thoracic cavity is called the parietal pleura, whereas that which invests the lung is spoken of as the visceral pleura. The interlobar fissures are formed by invagination into the lung of two closely approximated layers of visceral pleura.

The lines of pleural reflection do not accurately correspond on the two sides of the thorax. These lines of reflection also vary in different subjects depending upon body habitus.

The pleura is composed of a layer of endothelial cells resting on a membrane of connective tissue, within which are situated blood vessels, lymphatics and nerves.

There is a thin layer of serous fluid between the two opposing layers of pleura ordinarily, with a slow and steady filtration and absorption occurring normally. The visceral pleural blood supply is obtained from the bronchial arteries as previously indicated, whereas the parietal pleura is supplied by systemic arteries which are branches of the subclavian artery and thoracic aorta. Also, the reader is referred to the previous discussion of the lymphatics in connection with the lung. The superficial lymphatics drain the visceral pleura outward, and communicate by means of short tributaries with the deep lymphatics which drain in the opposite direction toward the lung hilus. The parietal lymphatics do not drain directly into the hilar lymph nodes but rather into the lymph trunks at the junction of the internal jugular and subclavian veins.

Ordinarily the pleura does not cast a significant radiographic shadow, except perhaps minimally in the costophrenic angles. When the pleural shadow can be identified, it is usually indicative of an abnormality.

There are usually small blebs or ruptured alveoli at the lung apices (Cunningham) which cast a shadow on the chest radiograph (Fig. 10–30). This may simulate pleural disease and must not be confused with an abnormal appearance of the pleura or lungs in this location.

Ordinarily, the costophrenic angles are very sharply delineated, and any significant degree of blunting is indicative of previous pleural disease; since these areas represent the most dependent portions of the pleura, disease is readily seen in these locations.

The cardiophrenic angles, however, vary considerably in appearance, and although the reflection of the pleura is normally sharp in this location also, a greater variability exists in the appearance of the pleural shadow here. An increased acuity of the appearance of this angle is of significance in detecting excessive fluid within the pericardial space, and thus an accurate conception of these angles must be constantly borne in mind.

THE DIAPHRAGM

Composition and Normal Attachments of the Diaphragm. The diaphragm consists of a peripheral muscular portion which completely surrounds a membranous aponeurotic membrane and arches over the abdominal contents, separating the abdomen from the chest. There is an extensive peripheral attachment to the xiphoid process, lower six costal cartilages, the ribs, the first three lumbar vertebrae on the right side, and the first two on the left side. With varying degrees of curvature, the fibers arch centrally and end in the central tendon. This latter tendon is more anterior than posterior, and thus is not truly central. It is incompletely divided into three lobes or leaflets. The middle one is anterior and intermediate in size, whereas the right lateral one is the largest and the left lateral the smallest. The crura of the diaphragm are two elongated musculotendinous bundles which arise on each side of the aorta, and are partly separated from the lumbar vertebrae by the upper lumbar arteries, but are firmly attached to the upper three vertebrae on the right and the upper two on the left. There is a tendency for the cupola of the diaphragm to descend with age (Fig. 10–31).

Normal Openings in the Diaphragm (Fig. 10–32). The diaphragm is pierced by numerous structures: the superior epigastric artery, the musculophrenic artery, the splanchnic nerves, and the sympathetic trunks behind; the aorta, azygos vein and thoracic duct, passing between the crura; the inferior vena cava, and small branches of the right phrenic nerve passing through the foramen venae cavae; and the esophageal opening, transmitting the esophagus and two vagus nerves.

Three-Dimensional Concept of the Diaphragm. The posterior attachment of the diaphragm is considerably lower than the anterior, and there is much lung

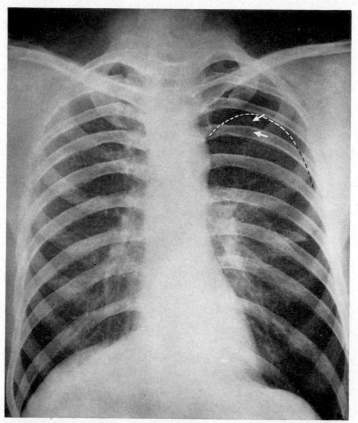

Fig. 10–30. Chest film to demonstrate small blebs or ruptured alveoli at lung apices: chest film of patient with spontaneous rupture into the pleural space of one of these blebs on the left. There are similar blebs in the right apex.

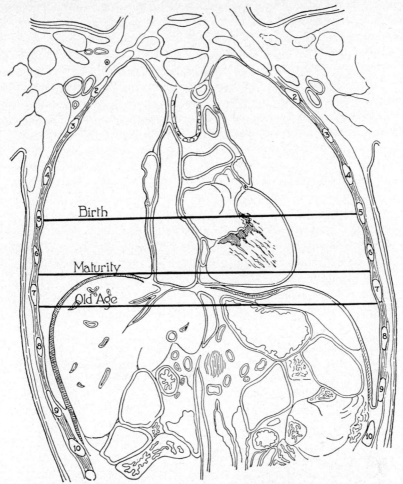

FIG. 10–31. Diaphragm at various ages. (From Scamon, in Meyers and McKinlay, *The Chest an the Heart*, Charles C Thomas, Publishers.)

substance and diaphragm which cannot be seen from the postero-anterior projection.

Moreover, much of the pleural space is likewise obscured from view by virtue of the attachments of the diaphragm. For that reason, it is important to attempt to visualize the structures behind it and obtain lateral and oblique projections frequently.

Occasionally, the diaphragm may have a slightly irregular appearance, and by projection, a structure which actually lies beneath the diaphragm will be projected above a portion of it. Every effort must be made to obviate such projection phenomena and understand them when they occur.

Tenting and Scalloping of the Diaphragm.   Occasionally, the contour of the diaphragm is broken into two or more arches, the outlines appearing as a scalloped margin (Fig. 10–33). This is usually due to an irregular contraction of the diaphragmatic musculature, and usually these irregularities become less evident in expiration.

Occasionally, several peaks are present on the diaphragmatic surface, which are likewise due to the rib attachments of the diaphragm. Occasionally, these are due to pleurodiaphragmatic adhesions which are abnormal, and the two processes must not be confused. This is spoken of as "tenting" of the diaphragm.

The Overlapping Shadows Due to Diaphragm, Liver and Heart Anteriorly (Fig. 10–36).   The anteromedian part of the diaphragmatic dome, the heart shadow, and the anterior margin of the liver overlap one another in the lateral projection, producing a triangular shadow which may be confused with an interlobar effusion or consolidation of the inferior portion of the right middle lobe. Care must be exercised not to make this error of interpretation.

Diaphragmatic Movements.   On quiet breathing, the range of motion of the diaphragm is about 1 to 2 cm. On deep breathing it will increase to 3 to 5 cm., or even somewhat more. There is usually an accompanying flare of the ribs upward and outward (Fig. 10–34). Occasionally, one half of the diaphragm will move somewhat more than the other, or in slightly different sequence, but marked differences in any area of the diaphragm or inequalities between the two sides are of definite pathologic significance.

The diaphragmatic position at rest is also of considerable importance, whether it be elevated or depressed, and localized elevations are likewise noteworthy, since they may be related to masses underlying the diaphragm.

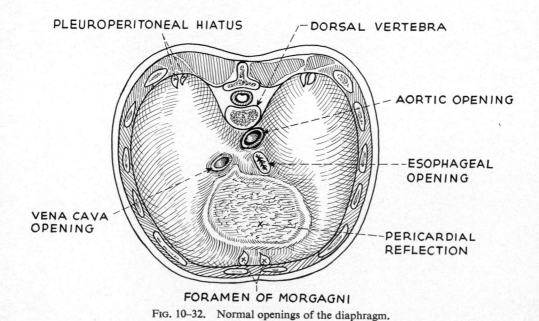

FIG. 10–32.   Normal openings of the diaphragm.

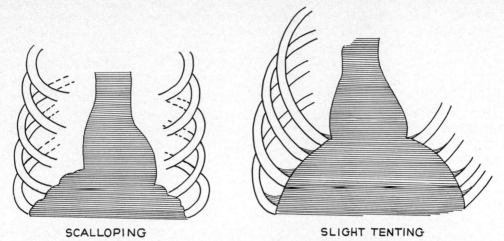

SCALLOPING   SLIGHT TENTING

FIG. 10–33. Diagrammatic illustration of tenting and scalloping of the diaphragm.

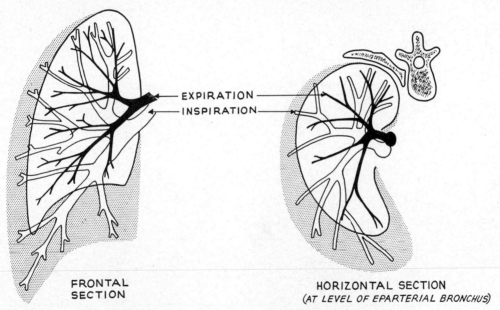

EXPIRATION
INSPIRATION

FRONTAL
SECTION

HORIZONTAL SECTION
(AT LEVEL OF EPARTERIAL BRONCHUS)

FIG. 10–34. Longitudinal and transverse sections through thorax, showing mode of expansion of lungs with respiration. (After Caffey, with permission of the publisher.)

ROUTINE POSITIONS IN THE RADIOGRAPHY OF THE CHEST

Chest Fluoroscopy. Fluoroscopy offers the first mode of examination of the chest. However, for consistent demonstration of fine detail, for avoidance of considerable magnification, and for the sake of permanent record and future comparison, radiography has no substitute.

A very useful routine to follow in fluoroscopy of the chest is as follows:

1. Notation of the position and contour of the trachea and larynx, in phonation and at rest.
2. Detection of the movement and symmetry of the two halves of the diaphragm.

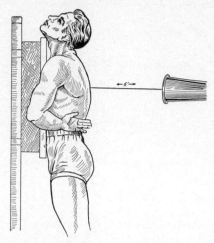

FIG. 10–35.   POSTERO-ANTERIOR VIEW OF CHEST: **a,** Positioning of patient.

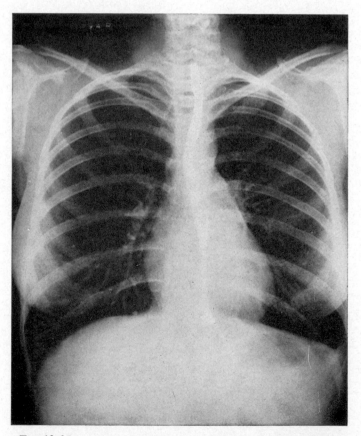

FIG. 10–35.   POSTERO-ANTERIOR VIEW OF CHEST: **b,** Radiograph.

3. Notation of the clarity of the costophrenic and cardiophrenic angles.
4. Examination of the lung fields, bilaterally, for notation of any differences in clarity of the two sides.
5. Examination of the lung apices, requesting the patient to move his scapula forward so as to improve the visibility of the lung apices.
6. Notation of the type of rib movement and flare with respiration.
7. Simultaneously, one must also study the heart and mediastinum, as well as the esophagus in its entirety.
   (These structures will be described subsequently.)

Fluoroscopy has the great advantage of offering the immediate opportunity of turning the patient in any degree of obliquity, or into the erect or recumbent positions. Spatial relationships as well as physiologic function are thus elucidated.

It has the disadvantage of requiring the exposure of the radiologist as well as the patient to considerably greater x-ray exposure than would be necessary by the film studies alone. Even though we may be well below presently considered tolerance levels for exposure to x-ray irradiation, any exposure must be regarded as potentially dangerous.

Postero-anterior View of the Chest (Fig. 10–35). This view is ordinarily obtained with a 6-foot film-target distance so that it can be utilized for study of

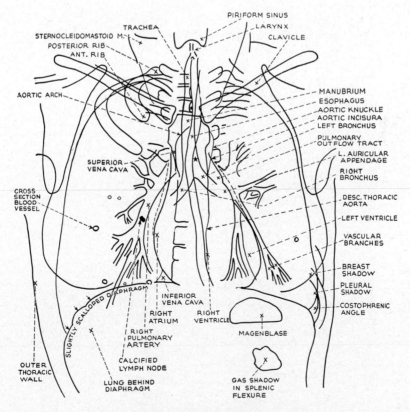

NOTE: ★ NORMAL DEFLECTION OF ESOPHAGUS

FIG. 10–35. POSTERO-ANTERIOR VIEW OF CHEST   c, Labeled tracing of b.

cardiac size and contour as well. The patient's shoulders are rotated forward, so that the scapulas are projected away from the lung fields, and the patient is asked to stop respiration after full inspiration and hold his breath for the film in inspiration, and similarly to stop respiration after forced exhalation for the film in expiration. Both of these studies have their definite indications. The film in inspiration will show the aerated lung to best advantage, and if there be any unaerated portions, they can be demonstrated by contrast. The film in expiration, on the other hand, will demonstrate any areas that are unusually well aerated. In either case, the mediastinum will normally remain stationary, but abnormally it will shift to one side or the other if unfixed by disease. The excursion of the diaphragm in the two phases of respiration may also be studied in this manner.

Films in both inspiration and expiration (exhalation) are particularly valuable in children, and it is our routine to attempt such films in all children under 8 years of age. Needless to say, it is not always possible to time the exposure in a child or infant exactly as one would desire it. The value of such a routine in children is as follows: (1) The history in relation to a child's chest abnormality is notoriously poor, since often the history is obtained from the parent who may be unaware of the fact that the child may have inhaled a foreign body. (2) The two frontal views of the chest, even though they may not be perfectly timed in relation to inspiration or expiration, usually supplement one another in any case

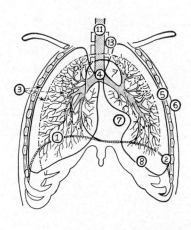

1. DIAPHRAGM
2. COSTOPHRENIC SINUSES
3. ZONES OF LUNG FIELDS
4. TRACHEA IN THORAX
   AND HILI
5. RIBS AND PLEURA
6. THORACIC WALL
7. HEART
8. UNDER DIAPHRAGM
9. HILI ON LATERAL VIEW
10. ANT. MEDIASTINUM
11. TRACHEA IN NECK
12. POST. MEDIASTINUM
13. VERTEBRA

Fig. 10–35.   d, A suggested routine to be followed in examining radiographs of the chest.

in an area of difficult diagnosis. Sometimes one of the films is faulty because of motion on the film or some other feature in the roentgen technique difficult to control in an infant or child. We are then particularly happy to have the two films for comparison.

Gross Subdivisions of the Lung Fields (Fig. 10–35, **d**). Arbitrarily one can subdivide the lung fields into three zones depending on the size of the vascular radicles. The vascular branches gradually assume a smaller caliber as one goes from the hilus to the lung periphery. The inner one-third zone contains the largest channels; the middle one-third zone contains vessels of intermediate size; whereas the peripheral one-third zone usually has vessels that are 1 mm. or less in diameter. This arbitrary subdivision permits one to attribute definite significance to shadows which are inordinately large in diameter or size, particularly in the middle and outer zones.

Lateral Views of the Chest (Fig. 10–36). When a lateral view of the one lung is desired, that side of the patient is placed closest to the film, and the arms are raised out of the projection as much as possible. A relatively close film-to-target distance (36 to 48 inches) is desired in this instance to "blur out" the lung which is farthest from the film.

The anatomic parts are illustrated in Figure 10–36. A detailed discussion of the anatomy will be deferred until after the entire thorax and its contents have been reviewed from the correlated gross anatomic standpoint.

Oblique Views of the Chest (Figs. 10–37, 10–38). These projections are obtained by rotating the thorax 45 degrees, with the side in question closest to the film. In postero-anterior oblique views the anterior aspect of the patient is closest to the film. On the other hand, in antero-posterior oblique views the posterior aspect of the patient is closest to the film.

The left postero-anterior oblique view (Fig. 10–37) (or right antero-posterior oblique) is ordinarily best for visualization of the trachea and its bifurcation. A portion of the left lung is obscured by the spine, but other portions of the left lung are seen in better detail. The right postero-anterior or (left antero-posterior) oblique (Fig. 10–38), on the other hand, gives the clearest visualization of the right retrocardiac space and right lung.

Antero-posterior View of the Chest (Fig. 10–39). This projection has the disadvantage of not permitting the scapulas to be projected out of the lung fields as readily as in the postero-anterior projection. The clavicle, however, is projected out of the subapical portion of the lung fields, and thus this view has this slight advantage. This projection is usually the only one possible in a very sick patient who cannot sit or stand up, and who cannot be rolled over onto his abdomen readily.

It will be noted that the rib structures appear different in this projection compared with the postero-anterior view.

Apical Lordotic View (Fig. 10–41). This projection is particularly useful for demonstration of the lung apices and subapical areas clearly. It also has its application in demonstrating the anterior mediastinum tangentially. Distortion of the lower chest areas is maximum in this view.

Lateral Decubitus Film Studies. By placing the patient on his one side or the other, utilizing a horizontal x-ray beam, one can obtain a postero-anterior projection. By gravity, the mediastinal structures will shift downward, and thus show the paramediastinal lung areas to better advantage (Fig. 10–40, **a, b, c**).

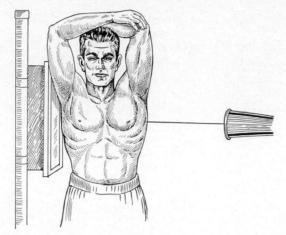

FIG. 10–36.   LATERAL VIEW OF CHEST: **a,** Positioning of patient.

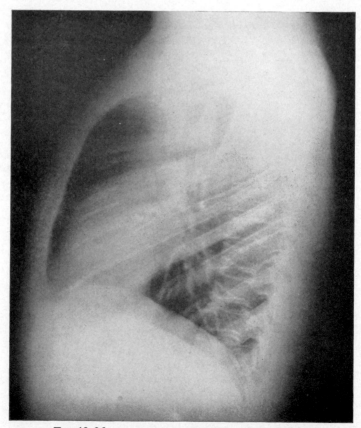

FIG. 10–36.   LATERAL VIEW OF CHEST: **b,** Radiograph.

If there be any free fluid in the chest, it will shift away from the side of the chest which is uppermost, and thus it is possible to obtain a clearer concept of a portion of lung or pleura which would otherwise be obscured. Also, this method offers an accurate means of estimating small amounts of free pleural fluid, which might otherwise escape detection.

Thus it is possible to detect amounts of fluid in excess of (but not less than) 100 cc. in this manner, whereas on other conventional views of the chest one cannot ordinarily detect fluid unless it exceeds about 300 cc. in volume.

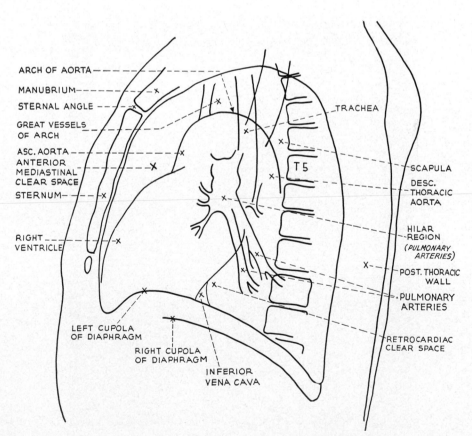

FIG. 10–36. LATERAL VIEW OF CHEST: c, Labeled tracing of b.

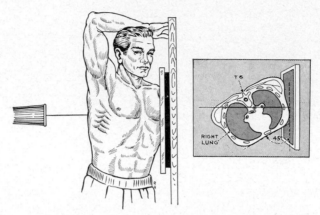

FIG. 10–37.   LEFT POSTERO-ANTERIOR OBLIQUE VIEW OF CHEST: **a,** Positioning of patient

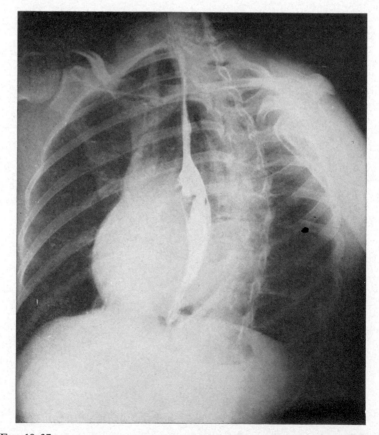

FIG. 10–37.   LEFT POSTERO-ANTERIOR OBLIQUE VIEW OF CHEST: **b,** Radiograph.

POINTS OF PRACTICAL INTEREST WITH REFERENCE TO FIGURE 10–37:

1. The 45 degree obliquity may be increased to 50 or 55 degrees on occasion, to obtain maximum clearance of the spine.
2. Ordinarily the left ventricle clears the spine, and the right ventricle forms a smooth uninterrupted convexity with the ascending portion of the arch of the aorta.
3. This view gives maximum clarity of the bifurcation of the trachea, the arch of the aorta and the posterior basilar portion of the left ventricle. Pulsations are ordinarily of maximum amplitude in this portion of the cardiac silhouette.
4. Although the right ventricle is seen very adequately in most instances in this view, the straight lateral is preferable, since the relationship of the right ventricle to the retrosternal space is more informative. Likewise, the left ventricle is more accurately evaluated in the straight lateral view by noting its relationship to the shadow of the inferior vena cava. It should not normally project more than 5 or 6 mm. beyond this shadow in the lateral projection.

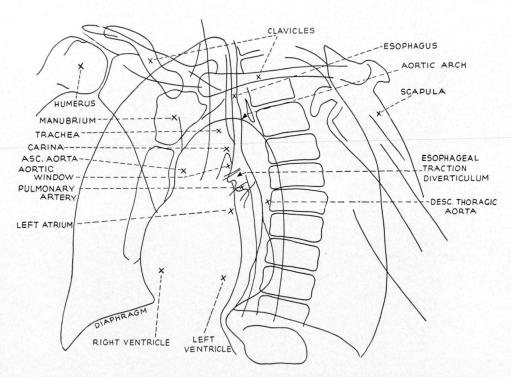

FIG. 10–37. LEFT POSTERO-ANTERIOR OBLIQUE VIEW OF CHEST: c, Labeled tracing of b.

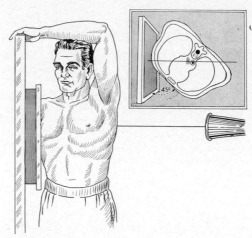

FIG. 10–38.   RIGHT POSTERO-ANTERIOR OBLIQUE VIEW OF CHEST: **a,** Positioning of patient.

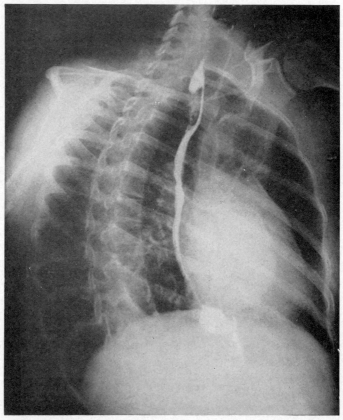

FIG. 10–38.   RIGHT POSTERO-ANTERIOR OBLIQUE VIEW OF CHEST: **b,** Radiograph. (The left atrium is enlarged slightly but is shown for demonstration of its indentation upon the esophagus. For a normal appearance see Figure 13–5.)

POINTS OF PRACTICAL INTEREST WITH REFERENCE TO FIGURE 10–38:

1. The patient's right shoulder is placed against the film and the body turned approximately 45 degrees from the film, resting the left arm in a convenient position, away from the body.
2. The central ray is directed just medial to the scapula nearest the x-ray tube at approximately the level of the sixth or seventh thoracic vertebra.
3. The patient is placed in proper position and then barium paste is administered. He is instructed to swallow and then take a deep breath and hold it while the x-ray exposure is made.
4. One demonstrates the maximum area of the right lung field in this view, but it is partially obscured by the shadow of the spinal column.
5. This view is most advantageous for demonstration of the left atrium and its possible enlargement, since any slight enlargement will cause a significant impression upon the esophagus as indicated.
6. This view is also of value for demonstration of the anterior apical portion of the left ventricle which is most significantly involved in anterior apical myocardial infarction, a rather common disease entity.

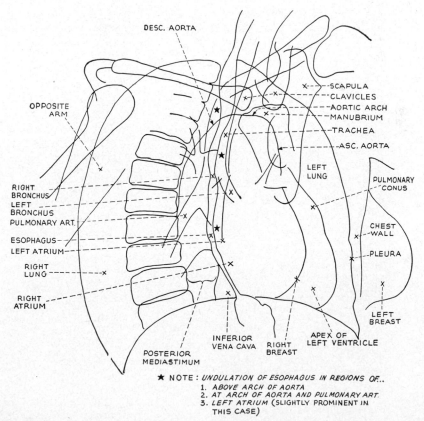

FIG. 10–38.   RIGHT POSTERO-ANTERIOR OBLIQUE VIEW OF CHEST: c, Labeled tracing of b.

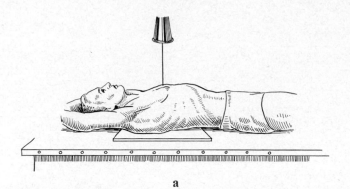

a

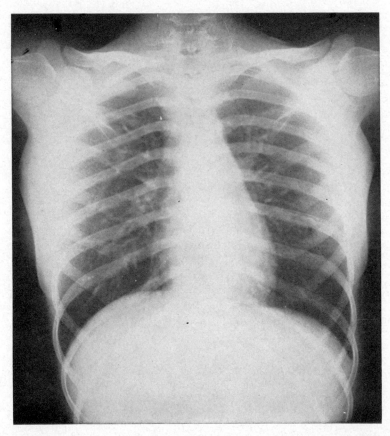

b

FIG. 10–39. ANTERO-POSTERIOR VIEW OF CHEST: **a,** Positioning of patient. **b,** Radiograph. The main differences between Figs. 10–35 and 10–39 are: (1) the projection of the clavicles; (2) the scapulas are projected over the lung fields in the antero-posterior view; (3) the superior mediastinal structures appear somewhat fuller in the antero-posterior view; (4) the obliquity of the ribs is different.

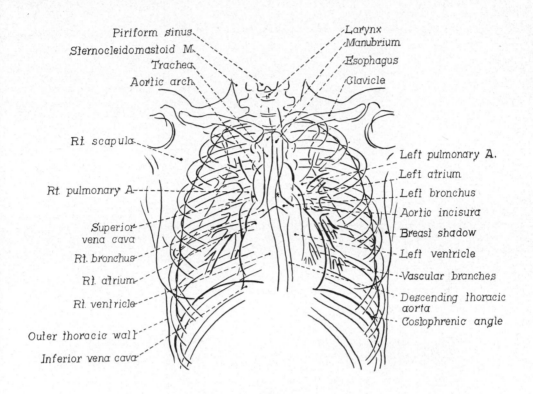

Note: ✳ Normal deflection of esophagus.

FIG. 10–39. ANTERO-POSTERIOR VIEW OF CHEST. **c,** Labeled tracing of **b.**

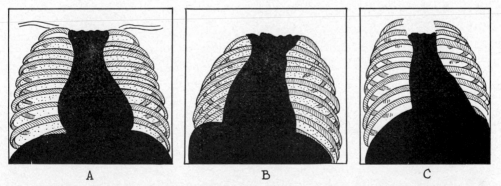

FIG. 10–40. DIAGRAM TO ILLUSTRATE CHANGES IN APPEARANCE OF MEDIASTINUM WITH POSITION OF PATIENT: **a,** Upright; **b,** lying on right side; **c,** lying on left side.

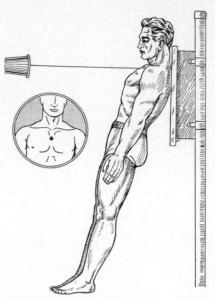

FIG. 10–41.   APICAL LORDOTIC VIEW OF CHEST: **a,** Positioning of patient.

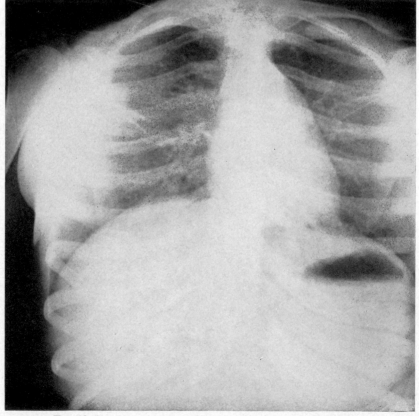

FIG. 10–41.   APICAL LORDOTIC VIEW OF CHEST: **b,** Radiograph.

Points of Practical Interest with Reference to Figure 10–41:

1. By standing the patient approximately 1 foot in front of the vertical cassette stand and then having him lean directly backward, a proper obliquity of the chest is obtained.
2. The top of the cassette is adjusted so that the upper border of the film is about 1 inch above the shoulders.
3. The central ray passes through the region of the manubrium. Occasionally a slight angle of 5 degrees toward the head may prove to be of advantage in demonstrating the apices more clearly.
4. This view gives one a very distorted view of the lung fields and mediastinum, but is of particular value in showing: (1) the apices more clearly; (2) the interlobar areas of the lungs; and (3) the region of the pulmonary sector of the cardiac shadow more clearly.

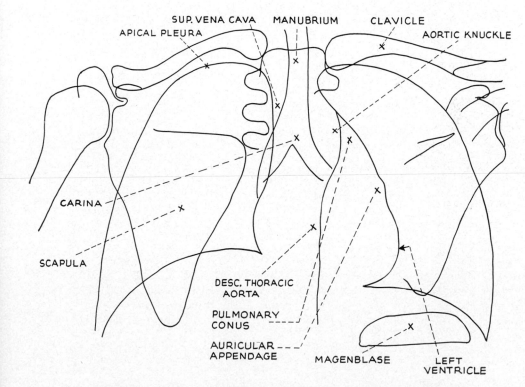

NOTE: *APICAL PORTION OF LUNG IS COMPLETELY CLEAR*

Fig. 10–41. apical lordotic view of chest: c, Labeled tracing of b.

BRONCHOGRAPHY

Methods. There are various methods and contrast media whereby the bronchi may be visualized. Most methods require the local anesthesia of the pharynx and larynx. Once that is accomplished, the simplest technique is to allow the contrast media to flow down over the back of the tongue with the tongue drawn forward, and the patient leaning forward. The patient is then rotated in various positions so as to distribute the contrast media in the various bronchial branches. It is usually difficult to obtain a satisfactory visualization of the upper lobe in this manner, but the lower lobe bronchi are ordinarily fairly well visualized. It is our preference to visualize the entire bronchial tree if possible, and hence the catheter technique illustrated in Figure 10–42 is recommended.

Another method is to puncture the trachea with a suitable needle and inject the contrast media directly. Occasionally this allows considerable leakage of air into the surrounding subcutaneous tissues, causing respiratory embarrassment to the patient; this is the main disadvantage of this method.

The most suitable technique which we have found for visualization of the entire bronchial tree requires the introduction of a catheter into the trachea after completely anesthetizing the throat, larynx, and upper trachea (Fig. 10–42). Small quantities of contrast media are then introduced into each major lung sector by positioning the patient as shown during the introduction of the media (Churchill's maneuvers) (see Fig. 10–42).

A simpler variant of this technique which will usually give satisfactory results is to inject 20 cc. of the media in position *B* (Fig. 10–42), and instruct the patient to inspire deeply immediately thereafter; then another 20 cc. is injected in position *G*, and the patient is similarly instructed to inspire deeply once again. Thereafter posteroanterior, stereoscopic erect films, both oblique projections, and a recumbent anteroposterior film are obtained in rapid sequence.

The ideal contrast agent has not as yet been developed for this purpose. Ideally, the agent should be nonirritating and nonsensitizing; it should be readily absorbed or expectorated so that it does not remain in the lungs for any significant period of time after the examination; if absorbed, it should not be toxic; if any of it remains even in microscopic quantities in the lung, it should not produce any irritant or granulomatous reactions within the lung. For many years the non-absorbable iodized oils such as Lipiodol or Iodochlorol were used, even though they beclouded the lung fields for years thereaf occasionally produced granulomas, and occasionally iodine sensitivity. In more recent times, Dionosil, either aqueous or in oil suspension, has been favored by us, although this, too, is not ideal. The aqueous Dionosil is very irritating and requires a general anesthetic, which in turn makes film-making more difficult, and the procedure more time-consuming, expensive, and hazardous.

Fig. 10–42. Technique of bronchography. In positions *A*, *B*, *C*, *G* and *H* the patient is rocked backward and forward, still maintaining the general position as indicated in the diagram. In positions *D* and *I*, the patient is rolled slightly from side to side, likewise still maintaining the general position as indicated in the diagram. This rocking or rolling motion is efficacious in obtaining a better distribution of the iodized oil medium in the bronchi.

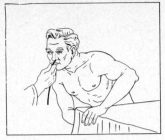

Ⓐ INTRATRACHEAL CATHETER INSERTED

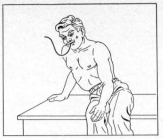

Ⓑ 5cc. INJECTED

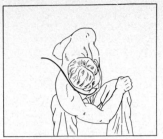

Ⓒ 3cc. INJECTED

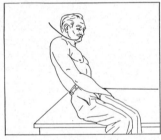

Ⓓ 4cc. INJECTED

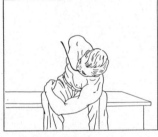

Ⓔ A-P RECUMBENT

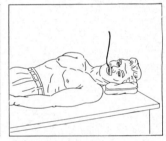

Ⓕ RIGHT LATERAL RECUMBENT

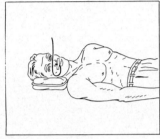

Ⓖ 4cc. INJECTED

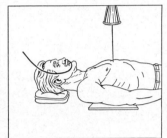

Ⓗ 3cc. INJECTED

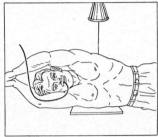

Ⓘ 4cc. INJECTED

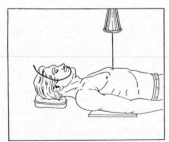

Ⓙ A-P RECUMBENT

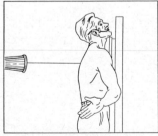

Ⓚ P-A ERECT

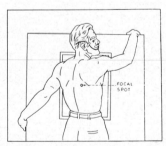

Ⓛ LEFT ANT. OBLIQUE

TECHNIQUE OF

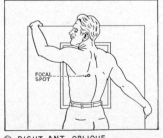

Ⓜ RIGHT ANT. OBLIQUE

BRONCHOGRAPHY

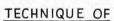

Dionosil in oil suspension leaves the lungs in about four days, but mild pneumonitis, granulomas, and other manifestations of irritation can result. A combination of Lipiodol and sulfanilamide (Visciodol) has been shown to leave the lung rapidly, but high sulfanilamide levels result.[3]

More recently, some experiments with 50 per cent colloidal barium in saline plus a 2 per cent methylcarboxycellulose mixture would appear to offer some promise[4] but experience with this latter medium is still too limited.

Our own preference at this time is Dionosil in oil suspension, although admittedly this is not as yet ideal in either contrast or benignity of reaction.

The following film studies are obtained after the injection of the contrast media:

1. Antero-posterior recumbent and lateral views of the side first injected, immediately after injection, and before the second side is injected (Fig. 10–43, **a** and **b** or **e**);

2. An antero-posterior view of the chest after both sides are injected.

3. An erect postero-anterior view of the chest (after both sides are injected) (Fig. 10–43 **d**);

4. Both oblique views after both sides are injected (stereoscopic views may be obtained if desired) (Fig. 10–43, **c** and **f**).

The above study may be combined with fluoroscopy, if a good spot-film apparatus is available which will give detail as good as the conventional studies. One advantage of the fluoroscopic examination is that it permits visualization of the filling as it occurs, so that the examiner knows immediately whether or not further filling is required. Moreover, a concept of the physiologic function of the bronchial tree is also thereby acquired. Balanced against this great advantage, however, is the fact that spot films are seldom as satisfactory in minute detail as are conventional long distance and small focal spot-film studies. The examiner must therefore adapt the technique to his requirements.

Ordinarily, both sides of the lung are injected at the same examination if the patient's respiratory capacity will permit. In many patients, injection of only one side at a single sitting is possible.

The radiographic anatomy of the bronchi and their distribution have been illustrated in previous diagrams (see Fig. 10–9).

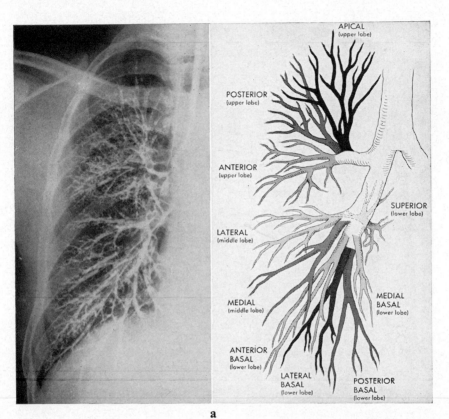

a

FIG. 10–43. THE NORMAL HUMAN BRONCHIAL TREE. a, Postero-anterior projection, right, (From Lehman, J. S., and Crellin, J. A.: Medical Radiography and Photography, vol. 31, 1955.)

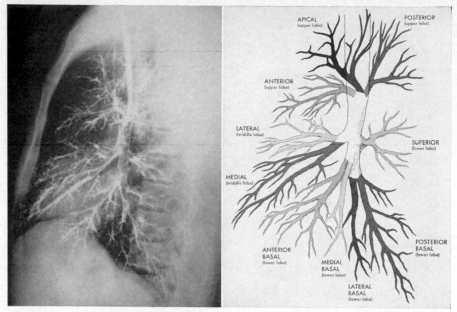

b

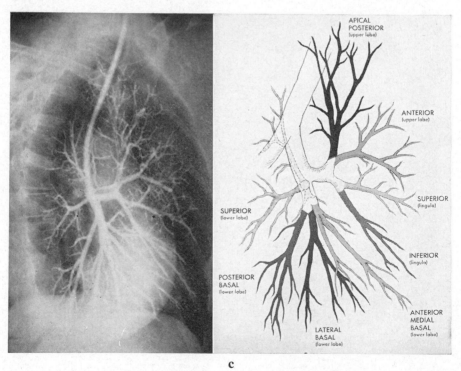

c

FIG. 10–43. THE NORMAL HUMAN BRONCHIAL TREE. **b,** Right lateral projection. **c,** Right anterior oblique projection. (From Lehman, J. S., and Crellin, J. A.: Medical Radiography and Photography, vol. 31, 1955.)

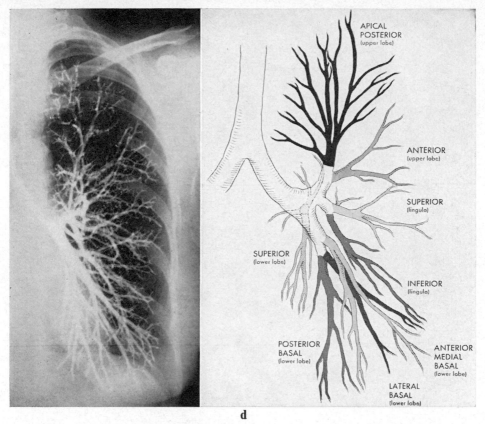

d

FIG. 10–43. THE NORMAL HUMAN BRONCHIAL TREE. d, Left postero-anterior projection. (From Lehman, J. S., and Crellin, J. A.: Medical Radiography and Photography, vol. 31, 1955.)

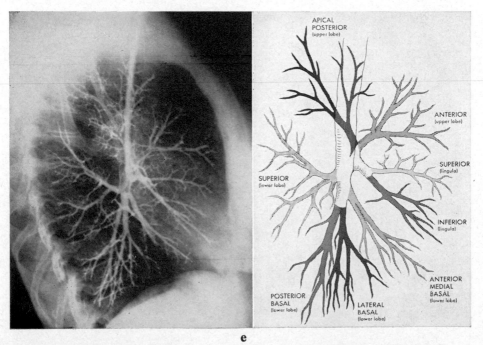

e

FIG. 10–43. THE NORMAL HUMAN BRONCHIAL TREE. e, Left lateral projection.

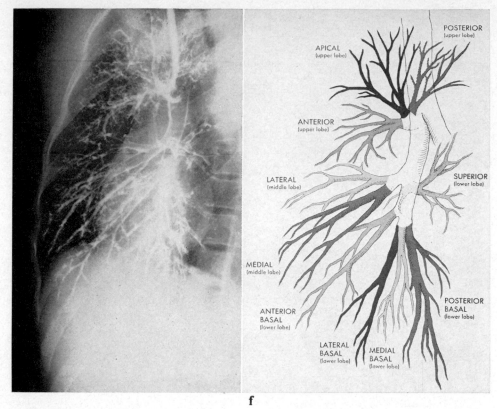

f

Fig. 10–43. THE NORMAL HUMAN BRONCHIAL TREE. f, Left anterior oblique projection. (From Lehman, J. S., and Crellin, J. A.: Medical Radiography and Photography, vol. 31, 1955.)

REFERENCES

1. Hicken, N. F., Best, R. R., Hunt, H., and Harris, T. T.: The Roentgen Visualization and Diagnosis of Breast Lesions by Contrast Media, Am. J. Roentgenol., *39:* 321–343, 1938.
2. Miller, W. S.: The Lung. 2nd Ed., Charles C Thomas, Springfield, Illinois, 1950.
3. Johnson, P. M., and Irwin, G. L.: Personal communication.
4. Nelson, S. W., Molnar, W., and Christofordis, A.: The Use of Barium and Bismuth Suspensions in Bronchography. Abstract, Meeting of Radiological Society of North America, 1958.

CHAPTER 11

The Mediastinum

THE MEDIASTINUM (EXCLUDING HEART AND AORTA)

Basic Anatomy. The pericardium and its contents comprise the middle compartment of the mediastinum, and the other structures of the mediastinum are related to this major compartment (Fig. 11–1). Thus the anterior mediastinum is situated between the pericardium and the sternum, and the posterior mediastinum between the posterior aspect of the pericardium and the spine. Anatomically, the superior mediastinum is also differentiated, being that portion which lies superior to a line drawn between the fourth dorsal vertebra and the sternal angle at the junction of the manubrium and body of the sternum.

The organs of the mediastinum are partially enveloped by the parietal pleura of each thoracic cage and, strictly speaking, the mediastinum lies between two pleural sacs.

The structures of the *superior mediastinum* are in direct continuity with those of the posterior mediastinum and consist of: (1) the aortic arch and its major branches; (2) the innominate veins and part of the superior vena cava; (3) the trachea, esophagus and thoracic duct; (4) the thymus; and (5) nerves, principally the vagi, phrenic and left recurrent nerves.

In addition to the heart and pericardium, the *middle mediastinum* lodges the phrenic nerves, the accompanying blood vessels, and important lymph nodes adjoining the trachea and bronchi.

The *anterior mediastinum* contains portions of the two pleural sacs which approach each other posterior to the sternum. There are also fibro-areolar tissue, lymph structures, and branches of the internal mammary artery within the anterior mediastinum.

The *posterior mediastinum* contains a prolongation of many of the structures of the superior mediastinum as previously described. In addition, it also contains the azygos and hemiazygos veins and the thoracic duct.

Ordinarily, the mediastinum is quite mobile, changing its position readily with positional changes and volume changes in each thoracic cage. Also, the mediastinum changes its shape in inspiration and expiration (Fig. 11–2). The mediastinum will vary in size and configuration with body build, being long and thin in the asthenic individual, but short and stocky in the sthenic person. The mediastinum also changes as the individual grows, as is illustrated in Figure 11–2.

There are several so-called weak spots of the mediastinum, where protrusion may more readily occur from one side of the chest to the other (Nitsch, Maier).

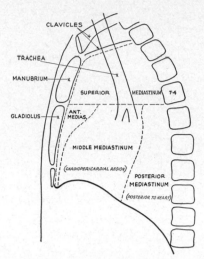

FIG. 11–1. Compartments of the mediastinum.

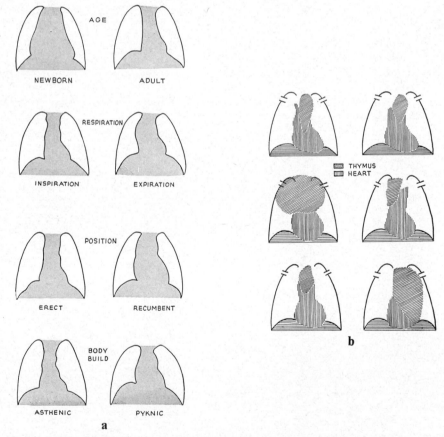

FIG. 11–2. **a,** Normal factors causing variation in the supracardiac shadow and cardiac contour.
b, Variations in size and position of supracardiac thymic shadow in the infant.

There is one situated anteriorly in the region of the shrunken thymus gland. Another weak spot exists where the esophagus and aorta are slightly separated in the lower posterior mediastinum; herniation of lung almost invariably occurs from right to left in this situation. The third is situated in the upper posterior mediastinum where the two pleural surfaces are almost in complete contact (between T_3 and T_5 and the esophagus in this area).

Radiologic Examination of the Mediastinum. The reader is referred to the remarks regarding fluoroscopy of the chest in Chapter 10.

Fluoroscopy is the first phase of any mediastinal investigation, since it is very difficult otherwise to study these many overlapping structures.

Movement of the anatomic part with deglutition helps establish its continuity with the larynx and trachea. The exact relations of the heart, aorta and pericardium may be studied by virtue of their pulsations. Film studies are then made in those positions which demonstrate the desired anatomy to best advantage. If fluoroscopy and routine film studies fail to complete the diagnosis, a contrast medium is introduced into those structures which permit investigation in this manner, and by a process of elimination, the remaining structures are studied. Thus it is possible to introduce barium sulfate into the esophagus, iodized contrast media into the heart and major blood vessels, iodized oil into the trachea, and occasionally air or carbon dioxide into the pericardial sac (when it contains excessive fluid). A systematic study of the anatomic structures of the chest may clarify disease processes in the mediastinum.

The relationships of structures in the mediastinum are illustrated in Figure 11–3.

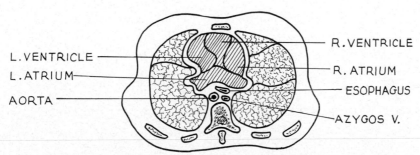

L.VENTRICLE
L.ATRIUM
AORTA
R.VENTRICLE
R.ATRIUM
ESOPHAGUS
AZYGOS V.

FIG. 11–3. Cross section of chest and heart showing antero-posterior relationships of cardiac chambers and retrocardiac structures.

THE CARDIOVASCULAR SYSTEM

BASIC ANATOMY OF THE CARDIOVASCULAR SYSTEM

Introduction. The heart, its major blood vessels, and the blood contained within these structures are all of the same order of density, and hence any studies of the heart without contrast media in the blood must necessarily be contour studies.

These studies therefore presuppose a knowledge of the normal positions of the various cardiac chambers, so that they can be placed in proper position for study; they also are based upon a knowledge of the normal contours of these chambers when in these various degrees of obliquity.

The Heart. The heart is enclosed within the pericardium, and normally there is only a thin layer of fluid between the inner layer of pericardium and the epicardium of the heart. The heart is obliquely situated in the chest so that about one third of it is situated on the right and about two thirds on the left of the median plane (Fig. 11–4).

The heart contains four chambers—two atria and two ventricles. The atria are separated from the ventricles by the coronary sulcus. The groove which separates the two atria is barely visible on the posterior surface, and is hidden from view on the anterior surface by the pulmonary artery and the aorta There are two grooves which separate the ventricles—the anterior longitudinal sulcus near the left border of the heart, and the posterior longitudinal sulcus, on the diaphragmatic surface of the heart. The base of the heart is the upper posterior and right aspect of the heart, while the apex is the rather pointed portion of the heart which extends inferiorly and to the left.

The right atrium is slightly larger than the left, and forms the upper right margin of the heart (Fig. 11–4, **a**). It has a principal cavity, and a smaller anterior pouch called the auricle. The superior and inferior venae cavae open into the right atrium as does also the coronary sinus. These channels return the blood from the upper and lower parts of the body, and the heart musculature respectively.

Situated in the lower part of the septum between the right and left atria is the fossa ovalis, an oval depression which corresponds with the foramen ovale of the fetus.

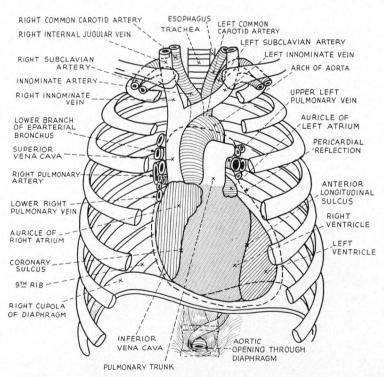

FIG. 11–4. PROJECTIONS OF THE HEART IN THE THORACIC CAGE WITH LUNG AND RIB STRUCTURES REMOVED: **a,** Frontal projection.

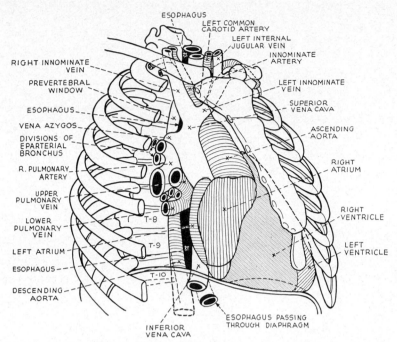

FIG. 11–4. PROJECTIONS OF THE HEART IN THE THORACIC CAGE WITH LUNG AND RIB STRUCTURES REMOVED: **b,** Right anterior oblique projection.

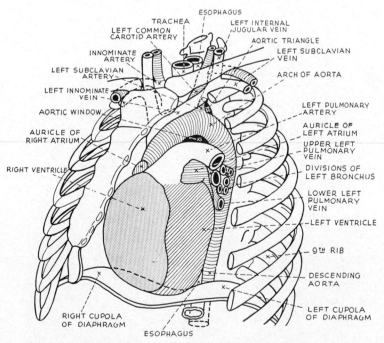

FIG. 11–4. PROJECTIONS OF THE HEART IN THE THORACIC CAGE WITH LUNG AND RIB STRUCTURES REMOVED: **c,** Left anterior oblique projection.

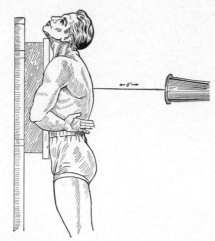

Fig. 11–5. CARDIAC ESOPHAGRAMS: **a,** Postero-anterior projection: **(i)** Position of patient.

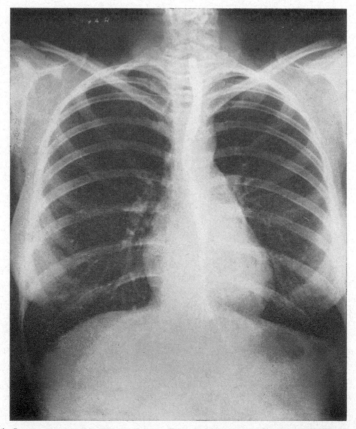

Fig. 11–5. CARDIAC ESOPHAGRAMS: **a,** Postero-anterior projection: **(ii)** Radiograph.

POINTS OF PRACTICAL INTEREST WITH REFERENCE TO FIGURE 11–5, **a**:

1. The exact course of the esophagus in this projection is noteworthy. At the base of the neck there is a slight deflection toward the left so that the esophageal projection falls behind the left sternoclavicular joint in a perfectly centered film. Thereafter it courses to the right at the level of the transverse portion of the arch of the aorta. From this position, there is a slight gradual deflection toward the left so that the diaphragm is penetrated to the left of the midline. An enlargement in any of the contiguous structures will alter this course perceptibly.

2. It is also important to trace the aortic shadow as it courses to the left of the middle, with its left margin ordinarily separate and distinct from the paraspinous shadow. This is a straight line normally below the level of the arch of the aorta; abnormally, it becomes convex, or S shaped with elongation of the aorta.

3. The position of the "left" ventricular apex with reference to the left hemidiaphragm is important. This portion of the cardiac silhouette is not always due to the left ventricle, but may be related to the right ventricle, particularly in congenital heart disease.

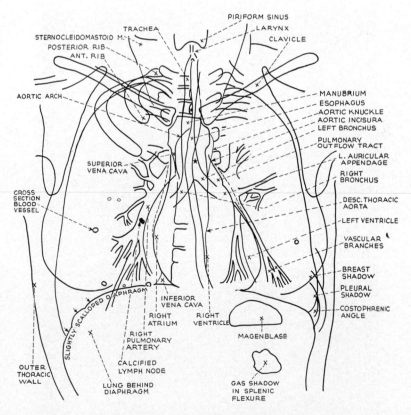

NOTE: ★ NORMAL DEFLECTION OF ESOPHAGUS

FIG. 11–5. CARDIAC ESOPHAGRAMS: **a,** Postero-anterior projection: **(iii)** Labeled tracing of **a (ii).**

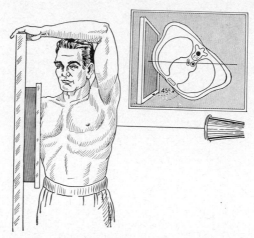

FIG. 11–5. CARDIAC ESOPHAGRAMS: **b,** Right anterior oblique projection. (There is a minima enlargement of the left atrium in this case, purposely chosen to show its position.) **(i)** Position of patient.

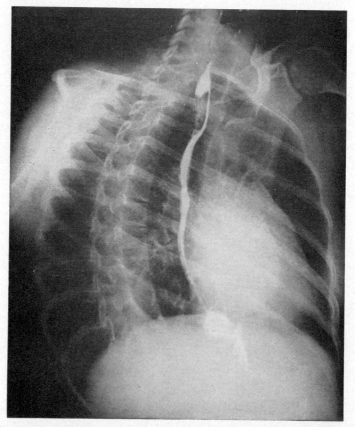

FIG. 11–5. CARDIAC ESOPHAGRAMS: **b,** Right anterior oblique projection: **(ii)** Radiograph.

POINTS OF PRACTICAL INTEREST WITH REFERENCE TO FIGURE 11–5, **b**:

1. The relative convexity of the pulmonary sector is noteworthy. This area becomes concave in many (but not all) cases of pulmonic or infundibular stenosis; or increased in prominence with dilatation of the pulmonary artery.
2. When the heart enlarges diffusely, the esophagus is often displaced posteriorly—but this type of displacement is not sharply localized to the region of the left atrium. For this reason, the region of the left atrium as it impinges on the esophagus must be known accurately by the student. Once this can be established, the differential diagnosis becomes more delimited.
3. Air shadows in the esophagus may produce some confusion in interpretation. These are frequent and normal, except possibly when excessive.

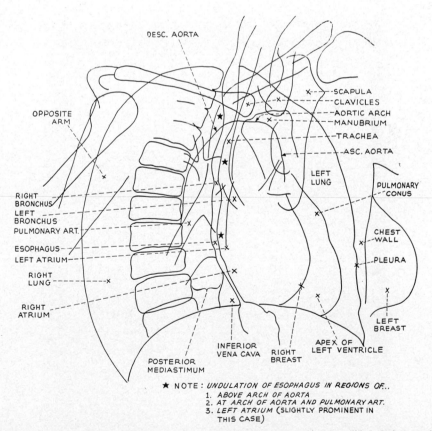

FIG. 11–5. CARDIAC ESOPHAGRAMS: **b,** Right anterior oblique projection: **(iii)** Labeled tracing or **b (ii).**

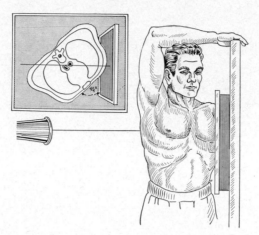

Fig. 11–5. Cardiac esophagrams: **c,** Left anterior oblique projection: **(i)** Position of patient.

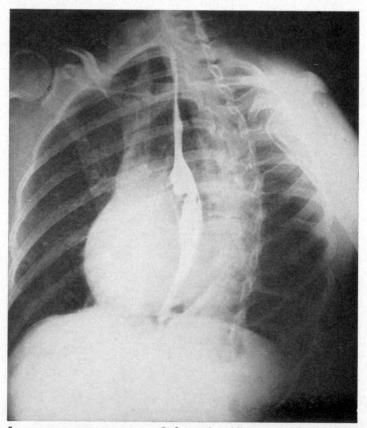

Fig. 11–5. Cardiac esophagrams: **c,** Left anterior oblique projection: **(ii)** Radiograph.

POINTS OF PRACTICAL INTEREST WITH REFERENCE TO FIGURE 11–5, c:

1. The student should learn to identify the following anatomic areas on the cardiac silhouette particularly, in this view: right and left ventricle; arch of aorta; left atrium; and the position of the aortic and mitral valves. The relative prominence of each of these areas should be noted.
2. The trachea and its bifurcation can be clearly identified in this projection. Position and contour description will help detect such abnormalities as narrowness, deflection, compression and filling defects.

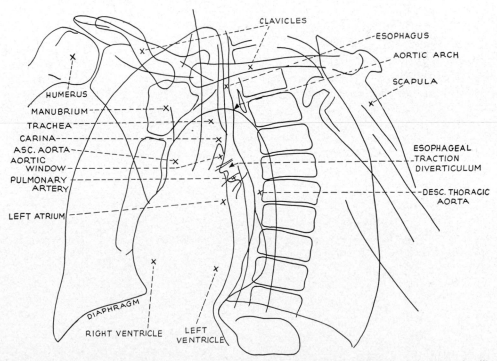

FIG. 11–5. CARDIAC ESOPHAGRAMS: c, Left anterior oblique projection. (iii) Labeled tracing of c (ii).

The left atrium, like the right, contains a principal cavity and an auricle. There are four pulmonary veins which open into the upper part of the posterior surface of the left atrium. The left atrium forms the greater part of the posterior surface of the heart, and the base of the heart. It is in close proximity with the esophagus in this sector, and any enlargement of the left atrium must necessarily displace the esophagus posteriorly, and usually to the right (Figs. 10–38 and 11–5, **b**).

The right ventricle forms the larger part of the anterior (or sternocostal) surface of the heart, and it also forms a small portion of the diaphragmatic surface. Its upper and left portion forms a conical pouch called the conus arteriosus or pulmonary conus. The wall of the right ventricle is thinner than that of the left, bearing a ratio of about 1 to 3 to the latter. The opening of the pulmonary artery is situated at the uppermost part of the conus arteriosus, above and to the left of the right atrioventricular opening.

The left ventricle forms much of the left cardiac border below the coronary sulcus, and a considerable part of the diaphragmatic surface of the heart. The left atrioventricular orifice is below and to the left of the orifice connecting with the aorta.

There are four series of valves regulating blood flow between the chambers of the heart and great vessels, situated between left atrium and left ventricle (mitral valves), left ventricle and aorta (aortic valves), right atrium and right ventricle (tricuspid valves), and right ventricle and pulmonary artery (pulmonary valves). There are three cusps to each of the above valves, with the exception of the mitral valve, which has two only. The tricuspid and mitral valves are attached by means of narrow bands (chordae tendineae) to the papillary muscles of the ventricular walls. (The position of the cardiac valves with respect to the chest and heart is indicated in Fig. 11–6.)

The Cardiac Cycle. The heart normally pulsates regularly by contraction at a rate of approximately 60 to 80 times per minute. Its wave of contraction is known as systole, and its period of rest as diastole. The atrial systole normally precedes the ventricular. When the ventricles contract, the bicuspid and tricuspid valves close, preventing the regress of the blood from the ventricles back to the atria, and as the pressure rises, the pulmonic and aortic valves open and allow the flow of the blood into the pulmonary artery and the aorta. When the ventricular contraction ceases, these latter valves close. During the period of rest, the blood from the systemic and pulmonary veins flows into the atria.

Fluoroscopically, the pulsations in the various portions of the heart vary somewhat in their appearance and sequence, the contractions being most forceful in the region of the left ventricular apex posteriorly (best seen in the left anterior oblique projection). The sequence and character of the pulsations, as well as the rhythmicity, require close study, since variations from the normal pattern are of considerable significance.

The Aorta. The aorta begins at the upper part of the left ventricle, where it is about 3 to 3.5 cm. in diameter, and arches upward, posteriorly and to the left over the root of the left lung. This portion is known as the aortic arch, and hence consists of an ascending, transverse and descending portion. It then descends within the thorax, posteriorly at first on the left side of the vertebral

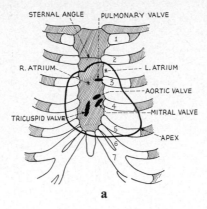

PROJECTION OF CARDIAC VALVES IN ROUTINE POSITIONS IN RADIOGRAPHY

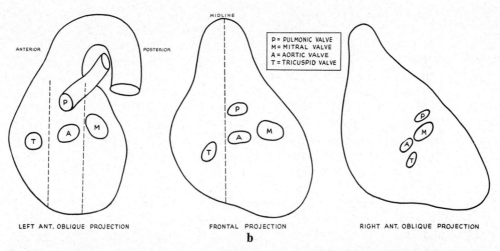

Fig. 11–6. POSITION OF CARDIAC VALVES WITH RESPECT TO: **a**, the chest, and **b**, the heart, in the frontal plane, left anterior oblique, and right anterior oblique projections.

column, gradually coming closer to the midline, and thereafter passes into the abdomen through the aortic hiatus in the diaphragm. It divides into the right and left common iliac arteries at the level of the fourth lumbar vertebra.

The ascending aorta measures about 5 cm. in length. It commences at the base of the left ventricle at a level with the lower border of the third costal cartilage, and passes upward and to the right as high as the upper border of the second right costal cartilage. The ascending aorta is enclosed within a sheath of pericardium common to it and the pulmonary artery. It is covered at its commencement by the pulmonary artery and right auricle. At its right side lies the right atrium and superior vena cava. The pulmonary artery passes upward to lie at the left side of the ascending aorta, and runs parallel to it for a short distance.

The arch of the aorta commences behind the second right sternocostal articulation and passes upward, backward and to the left in front of the trachea, after which it turns and descends to become the descending aorta at the lower border of the fourth thoracic vertebra.

The relations of the aortic arch are of considerable importance. Anteriorly it is related to the remains of the thymus gland, the pleura and lungs. Behind and to the right lies the trachea. The innominate, left common carotid and left subclavian arteries are branches from the convexity of the arch. Four nerves pass downward on the left side of the arch: the left phrenic, the lower of the superior cardiac branches of the left vagus, the superior cardiac branch of the left sympathetic, and the left vagus. On the right side are the deep portions of the cardiac plexus, the left recurrent nerve, the esophagus and the thoracic duct.

An embryonic channel, the ductus arteriosus, may persist into adult life and connect the left pulmonary artery and the aorta.

The descending aorta (thoracic aorta) is contained in the posterior mediastinum. In its course through the thorax it passes from the left side of the vertebral column, becoming more medial in its descent, and finally lies in front of the vertebral column at the level of the diaphragm. It is related anteriorly to the root of the left lung, pericardium, esophagus and diaphragm. It lies immediately in front of the vertebral column. On its right side lie the azygos vein and thoracic duct and on the left are situated the left pleura and lung. It ends at the lower border of the twelfth thoracic vertebra to pierce the diaphragm and become continuous with the abdominal aorta.

The Pulmonary Artery.   The pulmonary artery is a short, wide artery about 5 cm. in length extending from the conus arteriosus upward and backward, passing in front of and then to the left of the ascending aorta. Under the aortic arch it divides into right and left branches.

The entire artery is contained within the pericardium. On either side of its origin is the auricle of the corresponding side, and a coronary artery.

The right branch of the pulmonary artery is longer than the left, and passes horizontally to the right under the ascending aorta and superior vena cava, and in front of the right bronchus, to the root of the right lung where it divides into two branches. These follow the course of the right main stem bronchus rather closely as previously indicated (Chap. 10).

The left branch of the pulmonary artery passes horizontally in front of the descending aorta and left bronchus to the root of the left lung, where it likewise divides into two main branches, one for each lobe of the lung. It is connected with the distal concavity of the arch of the aorta by the ligamentum arteriosum. On the left of the latter structure is the left recurrent nerve. The further branches of the left pulmonary artery have been previously described in connection with the blood supply of the lungs (see Chap. 10).

VARIOUS FACTORS INFLUENCING CARDIAC CONTOUR (see Fig. 11–2)

Constitutional Features.   The general contour of the chest cavity is closely related to the contours of the organs contained therein. Thus, it has been demonstrated in anatomic sections that the outline of the circumference of the heart is in close relationship to the form of the circumference of the chest. In a circular chest, the cardiac contour tends to be circular also; in an ovoid chest, it tends to be ovoid.

If one arbitrarily divides the population into three groups, the asthenic or the long, slender type, the pyknic or the short, stocky type, and the athletic or muscular, well-proportioned group, one finds the following cardiac contours:

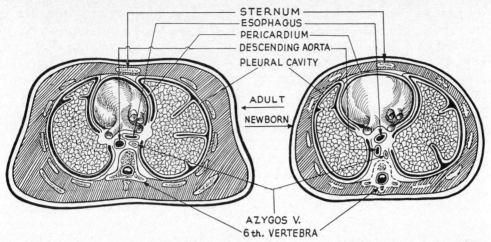

STERNUM
ESOPHAGUS
PERICARDIUM
DESCENDING AORTA
PLEURAL CAVITY

ADULT

NEWBORN

AZYGOS V.
6th. VERTEBRA

FIG. 11–7. Differences in infantile and adult posterior mediastinal relationships. (Modified after Caffey.)

In the asthenic variety, the mediastinum as a whole is long and narrow, the diaphragm is low, and the cardiac silhouette tends to be long, narrow, and rather straight up and down. Only the pulmonic shadow tends to be prominent. Extreme types of this group are called "pendulous hearts," which indeed is most descriptive.

In the pyknic individual, the mediastinal shadow as a whole tends to be short and wide. The diaphragm is high, and the convexity of all the cardiac contours is marked. The heart appears diminished in height, and somewhat boot-shaped, and is pushed upward and transversely by the high diaphragm. This type is indicated as horizontal or transverse.

In the athletic and sthenic individual, heart size tends to be at the upper limits of normal, and cardiac contour approaches the median group type.

Age. Age is an important factor which conditions the relative size and shape of the heart and contiguous mediastinal structures. In younger individuals the cardiac shadow tends to be more globular, and to reveal less differentiation than in the adult. In the newborn, the transverse diameter is very long in comparison with the diameter of the chest. The right side of the heart is larger than the left, and the atria and auricular appendages are large in comparison with the ventricles. The right border of the heart is therefore curved and the aortic knob cannot be differentiated.

During the last half of the first year, the long axis of the heart tends to rotate and descend slightly in the thorax, and the thymic shadow begins to regress. A rather definitive cardiac shadow is established between the sixth and the eighth year, but there is a relative prominence of the pulmonary artery (and conus) on the left in the frontal projection which persists in a variable degree throughout adolescence, and does not completely disappear until the early twenties.

As age progresses (Fig. 11–2), there is a gradual diminution of the size of the base of the heart, and a tendency to increasing prominence of the aortic knob and superior vena cava shadows. The cardiac and retrocardiac structures change their relationships slightly, as shown in Figure 11–7. When arteriosclerosis of the aorta is present, there is usually an elongation and tendency to redundancy of the entire thoracic aorta, but particularly the aortic arch.

Cardiac Cycle.   The size and shape of the cardiac silhouette will vary in accordance with systole and diastole. Differences in the greatest transverse diameter of 1.0 to 1.5 cm. can be detected from one extreme phase to the other in some individuals. This difference tends to be greater with contraction rates below sixty per minute.

For a most accurate assay, the cardiac configuration and size must be studied in identical phases of the cardiac cycle; when such accuracy is lacking, due allowance must be made for this variable factor.

Body Position.   There are quite definite changes in the cardiovascular silhouette in the different positions of the body. The change from the erect to the recumbent position causes a broadening of the cardiac silhouette, particularly at its base. The area of the cardiac shadow increases in proportion to increase in diameter and the broad diameter. These changes are probably secondary to the changes in position of the sternum, ribs and diaphragm.

In the lateral prone position, the mediastinal structures tend to shift with gravity toward the lowermost side. The lower leaf of the diaphragm ascends and increases its respiratory excursions, while the uppermost leaf descends. The mediastinal shadow tends to return to the midline on deep inspiration against the forces of gravity. This movement with deep inspiration is greatest in asthenic individuals.

Respiration.   During ordinary quiet or tidal respiration, no significant changes in the cardiac silhouette are noted. However, with forced inspiration, there will be changes produced depending upon whether we are dealing with a predominantly costal or diaphragmatic type of breathing. In the diaphragmatic type, there is a slight caudal shift of the heart which one does not ordinarily observe in the costal type of forced inspiration. There is a tendency for the left heart border to move medially, and the left contour is less curved. The vascular basilar shadows are elongated. The retrosternal and retrocardiac shadows are increased in radiolucency.

In forced expiration, there is a rise of the cardiac shadow together with some displacement to the left. The cardiac base appears wider and shortened, and the retrosternal and retrocardiac shadows are diminished in radiolucency. When one performs the Valsalva experiment by closing the glottis at the end of full inspiration and forcing expiration, there is a slow decrease in the size of the entire cardiac silhouette, probably related to the increased intrathoracic pressure. There is also a slowing of the heart rate in some, while in others the rate increases.

BASIC METHODS OF CARDIAC STUDY RADIOLOGICALLY

Role of Radiologic Examination of Heart.   It is important first to consider the part that the radiographic examination plays in the total clinical examination of the heart. Our basic physical diagnostic armamentarium consists of *inspection* to determine normal and abnormal pulsations, vascular distention and cyanosis; *percussion* to determine mediastinal size; *palpation* to verify further facts noted above as well as the detection of palpable thrills; and *auscultation* for study of cardiac and mediastinal sounds.

The radiographic examination of the heart gives more accurate data regarding cardiac size, contour and pulsations than any of the above methods, *but it can never be a substitute for auscultation, for the determination of palpable thrills, and for the detection of cyanosis.*

Thus the cardiac roentgenologic examination is a very useful adjunct in the total examination but it must not be regarded as independent of all other means of study.

First we will consider the basic methods of radiographic study of the heart, and subsequently (Chap. 12) we shall describe several specialized studies of the heart and major blood vessels in carefully chosen cases.

Fluoroscopy. The fluoroscopic examination of the heart always forms an integral part of the fluoroscopic examination of the chest as a whole. The two are inseparable, but for the sake of anatomic clarity the chest examination has been described in Chapter 10 and the cardiac study will be described here.

The fluoroscopic examination of the heart precedes the film studies—and indeed the appropriate film studies to be obtained depend in great measure upon fluoroscopic findings.

1. After the previously described study of the respiratory apparatus is completed, the heart and mediastinal structures are studied in the *frontal projection.* The pulsations along the left cardiac border are investigated and the radiologist proceeds around the periphery of the mediastinum, studying carefully the pulsations of the pulmonary arteries, aorta and right atrium. The cardiac position is carefully noted, both in inspiration and expiration, and changes with respiration detected as described previously.

2. The patient is thereafter turned in the *right anterior oblique position* and once again the cardiac contour and pulsations are carefully noted. The pulsations in the region of the apex of the left ventricle are particularly important since this area is prone to suffer from vascular disease. The pulmonary conus is observed and this projection forms the most accurate concept regarding this vessel. The anterior margin of the ascending aorta is then studied and thereafter the posterior mediastinal space. Normally this space is clear since it is occupied by structures of lesser opacity, such as the esophagus, aorta and veins. The prominence of the left atrium with respect to the posterior mediastinum is particularly noteworthy.

3. The patient is then turned in the *left anterior oblique position.* In this position the posterior basilar portion of the left ventricle is best studied. The pulsations here are usually of greater amplitude than elsewhere. Some concept regarding left ventricular size is obtained from the fact that in 45 degree obliquity the left ventricle normally clears the spine. The anterior margin of the heart in this projection is formed by the right ventricle. Indeed this position and the lateral view afford the best means of assaying right ventricular contour. A fairly straight line is formed between the anterior margin of the right ventricle and the ascending aorta in this projection. Any unusual convexities either in the right ventricle or the ascending aorta become of pathologic significance. Thereafter in this projection the arch of the aorta is carefully followed. This position affords the most accurate means of seeing the aortic arch in its entirety. Beneath the arch of the aorta, between it and the left pulmonary artery there is normally found a clear area known as the "aortic window." The integrity of this space is noteworthy, since any enlargement of a contiguous structure will cause its obliteration.

4. By carefully restricting the size of the fluoroscopic field, the cardiac shadow is thereafter studied in all positions for any areas of calcification. Care must be exercised to determine that the calcification is projected within the heart in every view, since calcified mediastinal lymph nodes can give rise to considerable confusion.

The heart normally does not contain calcification but the following cardio-pericardial structures may abnormally contain calcium: the pericardium, the coronary vessels, the myocardium, the endocardium, the papillary muscles, the cardiac valves, and the rings at the bases of the cardiac valves. These pathologic entities are outside the scope of the present text, but the method of study is briefly described, since fluoroscopy in this connection should be a routine procedure in every examination. Among these entities, calcified valves deserve particular note because of their greater frequency.

The cardiac valves in the living person are farther to the right and nearer to the midline than one might expect from anatomic textbooks which are based upon cadaver studies. It should be stated, moreover, that since calcified valves are themselves pathologic, and frequently associated with cardiac hypertrophy and dilatation, a study of cardiac valves in such subjects can hardly reflect upon or be compared with normal studies on human cadavers.

The positions of the valves with respect to the heart in the frontal plane are indicated in Figure 11–6. In the right anterior oblique view the mitral and aortic valves are projected so very close to one another (Fig. 11–6, **b**) that they cannot be readily differentiated. However, in the left anterior oblique projection (Fig. 11–6, **b**), the mitral valve appears in the dorsal one third of the cardiac shadow, while the aortic valve area is likely to be found in the middle segment. In the frontal view (Fig. 11–6, **a**), they are near the midline, or just to the left of it, at about the middle or within the lower one third of the mass of the cardiac shadow.

Fluoroscopic visualization requires full dark adaptation of the eyes, as well as a small fluoroscopic field. Calcified valves may be differentiated by their characteristic "dance" which is synchronous with the cardiac pulsations. Their motion is jerky and steplike.[9]

The demonstration on roentgenograms requires a very small focal spot, extremely rapid exposure, and coning down over the valve area in the proper degree of obliquity as determined fluoroscopically.

5. Barium sulfate paste is thereafter administered orally and the relationship of the esophagus and heart and mediastinum is carefully studied in the frontal, oblique and lateral projections. Since the esophagus is so closely applied to the descending aorta on the one hand and the posterior cardiac structure on the other, changes in the course of the esophagus become of considerable value in the int$_e$rpretation of cardiovascular structures.

6.   may then be lowered into a recumbent position and a study of the mediastinum repeated as described above in the frontal and oblique projections, noting carefully the changes previously described as occurring with change in body position.

The Esophagram.   Esophagrams are radiographs of the chest, with barium delineating the esophagus, obtained in the frontal, oblique and lateral projections as desired, after study in similar positions during fluoroscopy.

The optimum positions for examination of the heart and aorta are: (1) the postero-anterior view (Fig. 11–5, **a**) of the chest with barium in the esophagus employing a 6-foot film-to-target distance; (2) the right anterior oblique (Fig. 11–5, **b**) with esophagram; and (3) the left anterior oblique (Fig. 11–5, **c**) with barium in the esophagus.

Occasionally, where it is not feasible to obtain the above views, the left posterior oblique view is obtained instead of the right anterior oblique, and the right posterior oblique instead of the left anterior oblique. (4) An antero-posterior recumbent study (Fig. 11–8) is obtained for comparison with the erect antero-posterior film (at identical distances) in cases where shift of fluid in the pericardium can possibly be demonstrated.

1. THE 6-FOOT POSTERO-ANTERIOR VIEW OF THE HEART WITH BARIUM IN THE ESOPHAGUS. The various parts demonstrated in silhouette along the right margin of the central mediastinal shadow are as follows (Fig. 11–5, **a**): the inferior vena cava, in the right cardiophrenic angle; the right atrium, forming the major portion of the right cardiac shadow; the ascending portion of the arch of the aorta; and the superior vena cava, extending above and to the right of the latter. The anatomic parts contributing to the left side of the shadow are as follows (from above downward): the aortic knob, which forms a knuckle-like shadow superiorly; the aortic incisura, which is the notch between the aortic knob and the pulmonary artery below it; the left auricular appendage may protrude very slightly below the pulmonary artery; and the large sweeping convex shadow below this, which extends down to the diaphragm, is the border of the left ventricle. There is frequently a less dense shadow in the vicinity of the left ventricular apex, due to the pericardial fat pad, which has a triangular appearance and should not enter into the computation of the cardiac size.

The esophagus after it descends into the thorax lies in close proximity with the aorta. It has various impressions upon it, and the uppermost indentation is that produced by the arch of the aorta, which displaces the esophagus to the right and posteriorly. Normally, in this projection, the esophagus descends straight downward, and any deviation becomes of significance from the standpoint of cardiac chamber enlargement. A study of the esophagus in this view is therefore of value in detection of such abnormalities as rightsided aorta, left atrial enlargement and abnormalities of the descending thoracic aorta.

This 6-foot film of the heart is also called a "teleroentgenogram" and is obtained for evaluation of cardiac size and contour in the postero-anterior projection. Actually, this is usually the routine chest film obtained in most clinics. As indicated in Chapter 1, distortion and magnification are two major problems in radiography which to a great extent can be obviated if a long film-to-target distance is utilized. The degree of magnification and distortion will vary in accordance with the relative distances of the anatomic part, and the tube target from the film. A 6-foot film-to-target distance has been found to be practicable, and for all ordinary adult chests the magnification is no greater than 5 to 10 per cent. Since this study is usually combined with a study of the lung fields, an extremely short exposure is employed, about one tenth to one twentieth of a second (or even less). A short exposure of this type will usually portray the heart in some phase between systole and diastole, and hence allowance must be made for such differences as may occur in the various phases of the cardiac

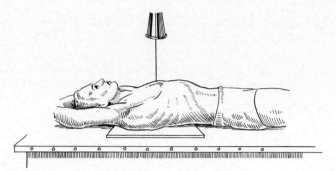

FIG. 11–8. ANTERO-POSTERIOR RECUMBENT STUDY OF CHEST: **a,** Positioning of patient.

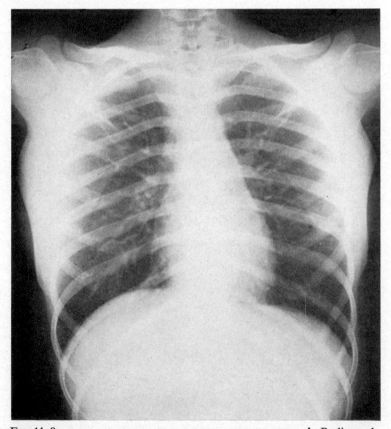

FIG. 11–8. ANTERO-POSTERIOR RECUMBENT STUDY OF CHEST: **b,** Radiograph.

POINTS OF PRACTICAL INTEREST WITH REFERENCE TO FIGURE 11–8:

1. Although it is difficult to obtain a view of the upper lung fields in this projection because of the shadows of the scapulae, considerable improvement will result if the patient crosses his arms above his head, thus rotating the scapulae outward.
2. The clavicles, on the other hand, are projected above the lung apices sufficiently so that this area of the lungs may be more clearly shown.
3. The analysis of the cardiac silhouette is not as favorable in this projection in the adult, because of the straightening of the left margin, and broadening of the base.

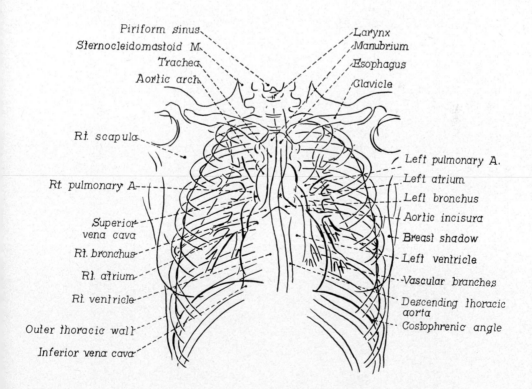

Note: ✳ Normal deflection of esophagus.

FIG. 11–8.   ANTERO-POSTERIOR RECUMBENT STUDY OF CHEST: c, Labeled tracing of b.

cycle, which may be 1 cm. or more. The cardiac size will also vary somewhat in the different phases of respiration, being smallest in deep sustained inspiration.

The pericardium, which invests the entire heart and is attached to the diaphragm below and the base of the major vessels above, ordinarily does not cast a shadow of its own, and is normally not distinguishable.

2. THE RIGHT ANTERIOR OBLIQUE VIEW WITH ESOPHAGRAM. In this position the patient is rotated so that his right side is in contact with the cassette, and he is rotated away from the cassette approximately 45 degrees (Fig. 11–5, **b**). The esophagus occupies the space between the descending aorta and the posterior margin of the cardiac shadow, and there is a slight undulation of the esophagus produced by the impression of certain structures upon it. We depend upon the esophagus to delineate most accurately the retrocardiac structures. The uppermost impression upon the esophagus after it enters the thorax is that produced by the arch of the aorta, as it displaces the esophagus to the right and posteriorly. Just below this indentation, there is frequently another slight posterior impression produced by the left atrium. This impression is virtually absent normally, and an impression beyond a minimal degree (such as is illustrated in Fig. 11–5, **b**) is indicative of left atrial enlargement, a most significant finding. The right atrium forms the lowermost slight convexity in the cardiac outline posteriorly in this projection.

The retrocardiac space is ordinarily fairly considerable, and when encroached upon is likewise an indication of abnormality.

The descending thoracic aorta overlaps the anterior margin of the thoracic spine in its descent, and it is significant that the esophagus descends in practically the same sheath as the aorta. Elongation and tortuosity of the aorta will therefore have a definite bearing on the appearance of the esophagus.

The trachea and left bronchus can be identified as a straight air shadow above the shadow of the left atrium, and just above the left atrium, the pulmonary artery can usually be seen as a circular opaque shadow (seen end on).

Between the left atrial impression and that of the aorta, there is frequently a lesser impression produced by the bronchial bifurcation.

The anterior border of this central mediastinal shadow permits delineation of the following structures: the ascending portion of the arch of the aorta is seen superiorly; there is usually a small notch between this shadow and that of the pulmonary conus which has a slight anterior convexity; below this shadow is that of the left ventricle or right ventricle depending upon the degree of rotation of the patient. This view forms a valuable one for visualization of the anterior apical area of the left ventricle (frequently involved by infarction) and the main pulmonary artery (frequently involved in congenital heart disease).

3. THE LEFT ANTERIOR OBLIQUE VIEW WITH BARIUM IN THE ESOPHAGUS. In this position, the patient is rotated 45 degrees with the left anterior shoulder against the cassette (Fig. 11–5, **c**). When sufficiently rotated, the left ventricle just barely clears the anterior margin of the thoracic spine. This is the posterior basilar portion of the left ventricle. Above this lies the left atrium. The arch of the aorta is seen in its entirety. The anterior margin of the silhouette is formed inferiorly by the right ventricle (this is the only view in which the right ventricle is adequately and definitely seen), and above this by the right atrium. The tracheal bifurcation is seen very clearly in this projection. The left pulmonary artery is seen in the clear space above the left atrium, and that portion beneath the arch of the aorta is known as the "aortic window."

The aortic triangle is frequently identified above the arch of the aorta, bounded by the arch of the aorta below, the dorsal spine posteriorly, and the left subclavian artery anteriorly. The latter can be faintly identified as branching from the aortic arch.

In this projection, the esophagus is normally not diverted from a relatively straight course. Deviations, if they can be described, are of pathologic significance.

4. THE ANTERO-POSTERIOR RECUMBENT STUDY OF THE CARDIOPERICARDIAL SHADOW (Fig. 11–8). There is a normal configuration change of the cardiopericardial shadow as a result of the change in posture from the erect to the recumbent position. This has been previously described and is due to the upward shift of the diaphragm. In the presence of fluid in the pericardial space in excess of about 300 cc., this configuration change becomes most marked as a result of the shift of the pericardial fluid from the lower portion of the space to the base of the heart. This produces a marked widening of the base of the heart.

These recumbent studies are also sometimes necessary in the event that the patient cannot stand erect.

In any case the film-target distance should be carefully stated so that adjustment can be made for distortion and magnification. (Method of determination of magnification will be described in conjunction with pelvicephalometry in Chap. 17.)

5. THE LATERAL VIEW OF THE CHEST WITH BARIUM IN THE ESOPHAGUS (Fig. 11–9). The lateral view of the chest with barium in the esophagus is a valuable adjunct in the study of the heart particularly in the following circumstances:

(1) It allows one another perspective for study of the relationship of the esophagus to the left atrium. The course of the esophagus is normally straight. Indentation in the region of the left atrium is usually an indication of enlargement of this chamber.

(2) The right ventricle is seen in silhouette anteriorly, and when enlarged encroaches upon the anterior mediastinal clear space. The right ventricle in this perspective usually forms a smooth convexity anteriorly from its junction with the aorta, gradually meeting the anterior chest wall in the vicinity of the xiphoid process of the sternum inferiorly. Its junction with the chest wall above this level is usually an indication of chamber enlargement. This is particularly of value in congenital heart disease.

(3) The pulmonary arteries form an ovoid structure identifiable below the arch of the aorta. These can be evaluated for size, and differentiated from other mediastinal structures which may on occasion be enlarged, such as mediastinal lymph nodes.

(4) The ascending portion of the aorta and arch of the aorta can be fully evaluated as to size and contour.

(5) The relationship of the left ventricle posteriorly projected to the shadow of the inferior vena cava shadow is of importance in evaluating the size of the left ventricle. Ordinarily the shadow of the inferior vena cava is seen about 5 to 8 mm. behind that of the adjoining left ventricular shadow. With enlargement of the latter chamber, particularly in association with mitral insufficiency, the left ventricle protrudes beyond these confines posteriorly. Such enlargement of the left ventricle is not apt to occur with relatively pure mitral stenosis.

(6) In attempting differentiation of diffuse cardiac enlargement from peri-cardial effusion, a careful study of the pulsations of the heart *posteriorly* in this projection may be very helpful. This may be more accurately ascertained with the aid of kymograms. With pericardial effusion, pulsations in this area are usually completely lacking, whereas with diffuse cardiac enlargement some degree of pulsation is usually manifest here.

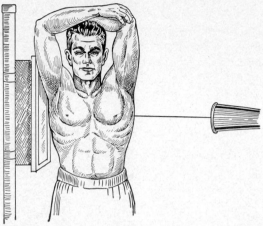

FIG. 11–9.   THE LATERAL VIEW OF THE CHEST WITH BARIUM IN THE ESOPHAGUS.   **a,** Position of patient

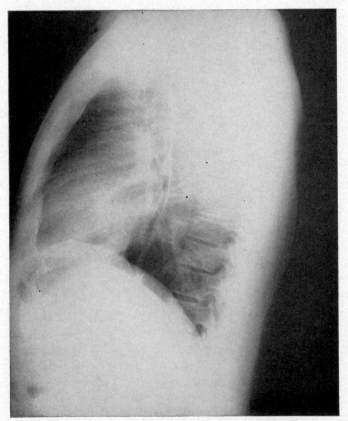

FIG. 11–9.   LATERAL VIEW OF THE CHEST: **b,** Radiograph.

POINTS OF PRACTICAL INTEREST WITH REFERENCE TO FIGURE 11–9:

1. The following areas are of particular interest and value for identification:
    (*a*) The relationship of the right ventricle to the posterior margin of the sternum. With enlargement of the right ventricle, its shadow "rises" higher on the sternum.
    (*b*) The degree of clarity of the anterior mediastinal clear space.
    (*c*) The relationship of the left ventricle posteriorly to the shadow of the inferior vena cava. This will allow early and accurate detection of enlargement of the left ventricle.
    (*d*) The relationship of the esophagus to the left atrium.
    (*e*) The relative prominence of the pulmonary arteries. This requires considerable experience, but is very valuable from the standpoint of detecting abnormalities of lymph node origin, or tumor masses.

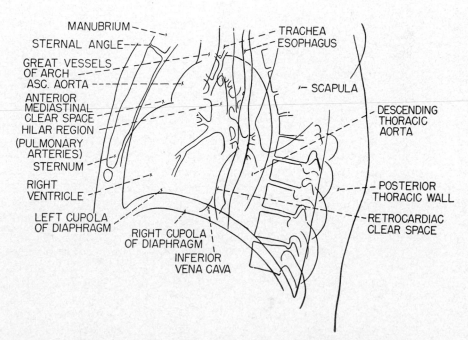

FIG. 11–9. LATERAL VIEW OF THE CHEST: c, Labeled tracing of b.

Cardiac Mensuration.   Mensuration of the heart is an effort to correlate various cardiac measurements, which can be obtained from radiographs, with cardiac weight and size, since, pathologically, *increase in cardiac weight or size is the most consistent indication of cardiac disease.* Such correlation between the radiographs and the actual specimen are inaccurate at best, but it is impossible for the physician to obtain more accurate data regarding cardiac size in life by any other means.[1]

1. THE DEFINITION OF THE "NORMAL" SIZED HEART.   It can be assumed that the majority of a large population is normal, and the problem of determining the "normal" sized heart on a radiograph becomes one of correlating various cardiac measurements with any other bodily factors which will allow a high statistical correlation in the majority of the population. This is statistically called a "high correlation coefficient." It is thus possible to determine the number of chances in a hundred which the individual case has of being within normal limits. In the individual case, this statistical approach may cause inaccuracy, but in the consideration of a large group it is a satisfactory means of assay. *We must be cognizant of the fact that the boundary between the normal and the abnormal is an arbitrary one, based upon statistical correlation alone.*

2. CRITERIA FOR RADIOLOGIC ESTIMATION OF CARDIAC SIZE.[2,5]   Many bodily factors and arithmetical constants have been correlated with various cardiac measurements.

The cardiac radiographic measurements may be obtained in one of several ways: (1) direct measurement on teleroentgenograms; (2) direct measurement on teleroentgenographic kymograms, which allows one to measure the heart in a definite phase of the cardiac cycle; and (3) orthoroentgenographic measurement. In this last method the cardiac contour is traced on a special fluoroscopic screen, in which the central ray of the fluoroscopic x-ray tube is focused on each point of the heart boundary in a definite phase of the cardiac cycle and respiration. Each method has its own arithmetical constants and charts which are not interchangeable. The teleroentgenographic method in which the measurements are obtained on a 6-foot chest film is the simplest to apply, the most universally used, and sufficiently accurate. The cardiac image is magnified to the order of 5 per cent.

The most frequent and useful cardiac measurements obtained from the teleroentgenogram are (Fig. 11–10):

Transverse Diameter.   This is the sum of the maximum projections of the right and left borders of the heart from the midline (TR plus TL).

Long Diameter.   This is the distance between the small notch on the right border of the heart between the right atrium and the superior vena cava and the left ventricular apex (L).

Broad Diameter.   This is the greatest diameter of the cardiac shadow perpendicular to the long diameter (B). Occasionally, it is necessary to extend the right cardiac margin interiorly in its natural curvature to delineate the lower margin of this diameter.

Aortic Arch Diameter.   This is the sum of the maximum extensions to the right and to the left of the aortic shadow from the midline as projected above the base of the heart (AR plus AL). When the esophagus is also delineated, the maximum extension to the left of the aortic shadow from the lateral margin of

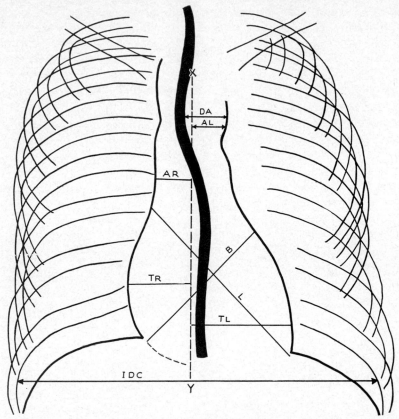

FIG. 11–10.   Diagram of teleroentgenograms of heart showing most frequent and useful cardiac measurements obtained therefrom: *TR*, Maximum projection of the right cardiac border from the midline; *TL*, maximum projection of the left cardiac border from the midline; *TR* plns *TL*, the greatest transverse diameter of the heart; *L*, the long diameter of the heart which extends from the junction of the cardiac silhouette and vascular pedicle on the right to the apex on the left' omitting consideration of the fat pad frequently seen in this location; *B*, the broad diameter of the heart, which is the greatest diameter of the cardiac shadow perpendicular to the long diameter. It may be necessary to extend the lower right heart border in its natural curve; *XY*, the midline in a perfectly straight P-A projection (falls over spinous processes of dorsal spine); *AR*, the maximum extension to the right of the vascular pedicle from the midline. (Note: The vascular pedicle shadow usually includes superior vena cava as well as aorta.) *AL*, the maximum extension to the left of the vascular pedicle from the midline; *AR* plus *AL*, the aortic arch diameter; *DA*, the measurement of the descending aorta which represents the distance from the left margin of the esophagus to the outermost left margin of the aortic knob; *IDC*, the greatest internal diameter of the chest.

the esophagus is a measure of the diameter of the descending limb of the arch of the aorta. Normally, this measurement may vary between 1.8 and 3.8 cm.; a measurement greater than 4 cm. is most certainly abnormal. These measurements have no correction for magnification, and do not take into account the 3 mm. thickness of tissue between the lumen of the esophagus and the aorta.

   Frontal Cardiac Area.   This may be determined with a fair degree of accuracy in accordance with the formula:

$$A = \pi/4\ L \times B$$

where A is the frontal area, and L and B are the long and broad diameters respectively. The frontal area of the heart gives one a reasonably accurate concept of cardiac size, and most correlation schemes use this as their basis.

The bodily factors which are most frequently employed for correlation are body height, weight, surface area, age and sex. Weight is a better criterion than height but fails in the presence of obesity. Height is therefore a valuable criterion to compensate for this failure. Height groups are also found to be better criteria than age groups in children.

The correlation coefficient of body surface area with cardiac frontal area has been found to be as high as 0.84 to 0.92 (1.0 being perfect). Since the surface area equals $0.425 \text{ W} \times 0.725 \text{ H} \times 71.84$ (where W and H are the weight and height respectively), there is a sufficiently high correlation between surface area and the product of height and weight to use the latter as a substitute for surface area.

Another bodily factor which has been employed is the area of the chest correlated with cardiac frontal area.[7]

The greatest internal diameter of the chest has a poor correlation with cardiac frontal area.

Eyster and Hodges[3,4] devised a very intricate mathematical formula for this correlation; although it is slightly more accurate than the less complicated correlations, the cumbersome nature of this formula has made it less popular.

The age factor will be considered subsequently.

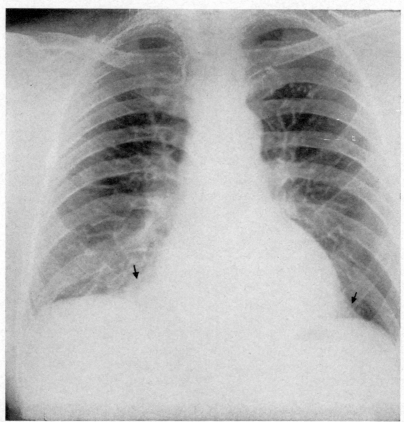

FIG. 11–11.   Pericardial fat pads. These are distinguished from the cardiac margins in both the right and left cardiophrenic angles.

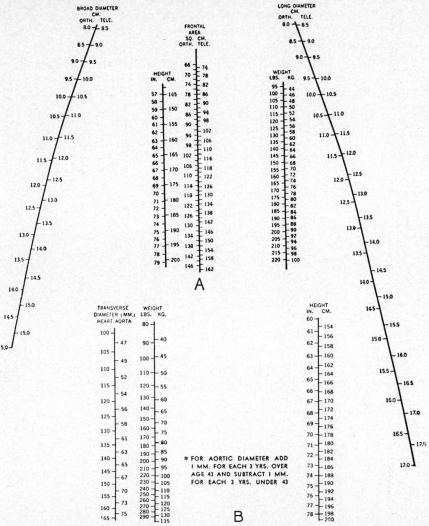

FIG. 11–12. **A,** Nomogram showing the frontal area of the heart predicted from height and weight, and actual area obtained from the measured long and broad diameters (for both ortho-diagrams and teleroentgenograms). Values exceeding 10 per cent above predicted values are abnormal. (Ungerleider and Gubner, in American Heart Journal, vol. 24.) **B,** Nomogram showing the predicted transverse diameter from height and weight, and diameter of the aorta. For the aortic diameter add 1 mm. for each three years over age 43 and subtract 1 mm. for each three years under 43.

3. MEANS OF APPLYING THE ABOVE CRITERIA.   The procedure for evaluating cardiac size radiographically is carried out as follows:

(*a*) A 6-foot target-to-film distance view of the chest is obtained with the patient erect, well centered, and respiration suspended in ordinary inspiration. In a well-centered film, the clavicles are symmetrical with respect to the spine which falls behind the cardiac shadow.

(*b*) The right and left cardiac borders are delineated and distinguished from extrapericardial fat pads in both the right and left cardiophrenic angles (Fig. 11–11).

(*c*) A line XY (Fig. 11–10) is drawn which bisects the thoracic spine and thorax (lies over the spinous processes).

(*d*) The maximum perpendicular projections of the right and left cardiac borders from the midline are drawn (TR and TL). This is the "greatest transverse diameter" of the heart. Ordinarily this measurement is less than one half the greatest internal diameter of the thorax. However, it is more accurate to correlate TR plus TL with body height and weight. A nomogram has been prepared[10] (Fig. 11–12) from which the predicted transverse diameter of the heart is obtained from heights ranging from 56 to 80 inches, and weights ranging from 95 to 300 pounds. (This same nomogram contains the predicted diameter of the aorta also.) A transverse diameter more than 10 per cent above the predicted value should be regarded as abnormal, and the heart is most certainly enlarged if the value is over 15 per cent in excess of the predicted transverse diameter.

(*e*) The long diameter, L, is then drawn and measured.

(*f*) The broad diameter, B, is drawn perpendicular to L and measured.

(*g*) The frontal area[5] may be computed by multiplying the product of L times B by $\pi/4$; or more simply from the nomogram prepared by the above authors (Fig. 11–12).

(*h*) The predicted frontal area for the given height and weight is also obtained from this nomogram, and the actual frontal area should not exceed the predicted value by more than 10 per cent to be within normal limits.

(*i*) The transverse diameter of the aorta is obtained by drawing lines AR and AL as described above. From the nomogram (Fig. 11–12) the predicted aortic diameter is obtained but an age correction must be applied: 1 mm. is added for each three years over the age of 43 years, and subtracted for each three years under 43 years.

(*j*) If the esophagus has been delineated with barium paste, the right border of the descending arch of the aorta is indicated by the aortic indentation of the esophagus, and the diameter of the aorta at this level is determined directly, 2 mm. being subtracted for the wall of the esophagus.

(*k*) As much as possible, each cardiac chamber is examined for enlargement and for this purpose the oblique as well as the frontal esophagrams are necessary:

(i) LEFT VENTRICLE. This chamber in frontal projection normally falls within the left midclavicular line; in the left anterior oblique view with 60 degree or more rotation, it should clear the spinal column. The student should also acquire a mind's eye impression of the normal convexity on the left.

(ii) RIGHT VENTRICLE. The right cardiac margin is 5 cm. or less from the midline. The left pulmonary artery segment must not be unduly prominent or straightened. In the left anterior oblique projection, the outer anterior border of the right ventricle forms a continuous straight line with the ascending aorta. In the right anterior oblique, the pulmonary conus segment is straight or only slightly convex anteriorly.

(iii) LEFT ATRIUM. In the frontal esophagram, the esophagus in its retrocardiac portion is straight and not displaced to the right. The cardiac waist above the left ventricle is not unduly full or convex to the left. In the right anterior oblique projection, there is no significant displacement posteriorly of the esophagus by the left atrium—and the esophagus proceeds downward in a smooth curve paralleling the anterior margin of the thoracic spine. In the left anterior oblique view, the infrabronchial space is clear, and the aortic window clearly identified.

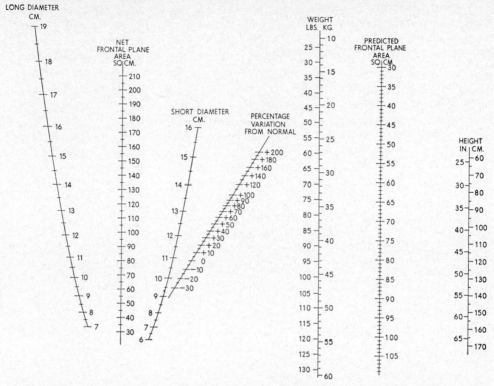

FIG. 11-13.   Nomograms showing the frontal area of the hearts from 6-foot chest films in children between the ages of 3 and 16 years inclusive. (From R. R. Meyer, Radiology, vol. 53, 1949.) The long and short diameters are obtained as previously described and the net frontal plane area is obtained from the nomogram portion reading "net frontal plane area." Next, the predicted frontal plane area is obtained from the nomogram by placing a straight edge between the appropriate body weight and height. When the ruler is placed so that it connects the values for "net" and "predicted rontal plane area," the "percentage variation from normal" is read off the sloping center scale at the point intersected by the ruler.

(iv) RIGHT ATRIUM.   The right heart border should not extend more than 5 cm. to the right of the midline in the frontal projection.

(v) AORTA.   In the frontal projection, there is no convexity to the right of the vascular pedicle at the base of the heart. The aortic knob falls 1 to 2 cm. below the clavicles, and the measurement of the descending limb of the arch of the aorta does not exceed 3.8 cm., or 4 cm. in markedly sthenic individuals. In the left anterior oblique projection, the anterior margin of the ascending limb of the arch of the aorta forms a smooth continuous convexity with the anterior border of the right ventricle. The aortic window is well preserved.

(vi) MAIN PULMONARY ARTERY.   The pulmonary artery is best visualized in the right anterior oblique projection, and normally is not visualized in the other projections to good advantage. It forms a continuous straight line, or a curve very slightly convex anteriorly above the left ventricular margin when the patient is rotated 45 degrees. Abnormality of the conus is also best reflected in this segment—but may also be demonstrated by secondary enlargement or distortion—or increased pulsations of the pulmonary arteries.

4. CARDIAC MENSURATION IN CHILDREN.   The Ungerleider nomograms are utilized only for adults between 56 and 80 inches in height, and 95 to 300 pounds in weight.

Similar nomograms for children between the ages of 3 and 16 years (Fig. 11–13) have been prepared by Meyer.[6] The frontal area of the heart in these children is calculated by multiplying the product of the long and broad diameters by 0.68, and the predicted frontal area is obtained from the nomogram. The two values are readily compared.

The wide variability in the newborn heart makes the evaluation at this time impossible with any degree of accuracy. Studies must be made serially to furnish any significant information. Rapid changes in size and contour are of particular importance. Caffey favors the cardiothoracic ratio determined from teleroentgenograms in erect frontal plane views of the heart. During the first year of life, the greatest transverse diameter of the heart is approximately 55 per cent of the thoracic width and may be as high as 70 per cent at birth, and 58 per cent by the second month of life. It gradually diminishes to 53 per cent by the end of the first year (Bakwin and Bakwin). Between the first and sixth years of age the ratio tends to diminish further to between 40 and 50 per cent.

REFERENCES

1. Bardeen, C. R.: Determination of Size of Heart by Means of X-Rays. Am. J. Anat., *23:* 423–485 1918.
2. Daley, R. M., Ungerleider, H. C., and Gubner, R.: Evaluation of Heart Size Measurements., Am. J. Roentgenol., *48:* 551, 1942 (abstract).
3. Eyster, J. A. E.: Determination of Cardiac Hypertrophy by Roentgen Ray Methods. Arch. Int. Med., *41:* 667–682, 1948.
4. Hodges, P. C., and Eyster, J. A. E.: Estimation of Transverse Cardiac Diameter in Man. Arch. Int. Med., *37:* 707–714, 1926.
5. Hodges, P. C., and Eyster, J. A. E.: Estimation of Cardiac Area in Man. Am. J. Roentgenol., *12:* 252–265, 1924.
6. Meyer, R. R.: A Method for Measuring Children's Hearts. Radiology, *53:* 363–370, 1949.
7. Newcomer, E., and Newcomer, N.: Heart Measurements. Radiology, *27:* 521–532, 1936.
8. Roesler, H.: Measurement of Cardiovascular System. In Golden, Ross: Diagnostic Roentgenology. Thomas Nelson and Sons, New York, 1941, p. 209.
9. Roesler, H.: Clinical Roentgenology of the Cardiovascular System. Charles C Thomas, Springfield, Ill., 1943, p. 269.
10. Ungerleider, H. E., and Gubner, R.: Evaluation of Heart Size Measurements. Am. Heart J., *24:* 494–510, 1942.

CHAPTER 12

Special Studies of the Heart and Major Blood Vessels

SPECIAL STUDIES OF THE HEART IN VIVO

NEWER advances in surgery of the heart and of the peripheral vascular system have necessitated that diagnostic studies in relation to heart disease depict abnormalities with great accuracy. Special techniques in cardiac radiology, and the greater collaborative efforts of radiologist, cardiologist and physiologist, have helped greatly in the achievement of this aim.

The most important of these special cardio-radiologic techniques are: (1) venous angiocardiography; (2) selective angiocardiography; (3) aortography; (4) peripheral arteriography and venography.

Lymphangiography is still highly experimental and has not achieved wide acceptance.

However, before delving into these special contrast studies, a few comments in relation to orthodiagraphy and kymography are in order.

Orthodiagraphy. An orthodiagram is an outline drawing of the heart made on a celluloid cover or transparent paper placed over the fluoroscopic screen while moving the screeen and x-ray tube independently, so that only the central ray is employed to record every point on the cardiac border. Since only the central ray is employed, the complete absence of divergent beams eliminates the element of magnification. Also, it is possible to plot the points in a given phase of the cardiac cycle, and in a given respiratory phase also, eliminating these variables as well. It is very time-consuming and requires specially constructed independently moving fluoroscopic screen and x-ray tube; the advantages gained are not usually sufficiently great to warrant the performance of this procedure.

Magnification of Teleroentgenograms and the Fallacy of Comparison of Orthodiagrams with Teleroentgenograms. In the method of orthodiagraphy the central ray is employed in a designated phase of respiration and cardiac cycle. Teleroentgenography, on the other hand, is a 6-foot projection of the heart in suspended inspiration in no definite phase of the cardiac cycle. Even at 6 feet a certain amount of magnification (approximately 5 per cent) is inevitable, depending upon the distance of the heart from the film on the one hand, and the distance of the heart from the tube-target on the other. Differences of cardiac measurements in systole and diastole will impose an additional 5 to 10 per cent variation. Differences produced by body habitus and phase of respiration, as well as body position, impose additional corrections to be remembered.

The complexity of this comparison can be seen immediately, and it is readily apparent that no actual constant arithmetical factor can be given between ortho-diagraphy and teleroentgenography. Reference to the Ungerleider and Gubner charts (Chap. 11) discloses that the two methods are considered separately.

Kymography[4] (Fig. 12–1).   The conventional multiple-slit kymograph consists of a sheet of lead in which multiple parallel slits about 1 mm. wide have been cut about 1 cm. apart. This is placed over a cassette, and the lead sheet is made to move the distance between the slits (1 cm.) during three to five cardiac systoles. As the slits descend, an outline of the pulsations of each portion of the cardiac outline is obtained. The peaks represent diastole, and the valleys systole. The configuration of the contractions can be studied, and abnormalities in pulsations recorded for future reference and comparison. However, respiratory changes, the changes in contour with the rotary movement of the heart, and the neutralization effects of one chamber on another all make this method of recording pulsations rather inaccurate. A more accurate method has been advocated[4] which employs the current in a photoelectric cell as the recording medium of the pulsation. The cardiac pulsations at a given point will interrupt

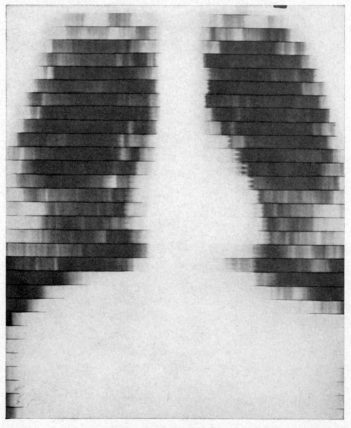

Fig. 12–1.   Postero-anterior kymogram.

the passage of a fine x-ray beam through the chest at this point, and this variation in the intensity of the x-ray beam after it has passed through the body is recorded by means of a photoelectric cell. Records can be obtained which are indicative of abnormality at given points in the cardiac outline, but here, too, the torsion of the heart with pulsations and the respiratory effect will modify the curve obtained, and thus produce inaccuracies.

Application of Special Contrast Studies to a Study of the Heart and Major Blood Vessels (Venous Angiocardiograms).   In 1938, Robb and Steinberg[12, 13] described a method for visualization of the cardiac chambers and major blood vessels leading from the heart, by means of the rapid injection of a relatively large quantity (50 cc.) of double concentration (70 per cent) Diodrast into a vein of the arm or leg. This method of examination was called "cardioangiography."

Originally, their method required timing the films in accordance with the major and lesser circulation times which were obtained prior to the Diodrast injection. More recently, apparatus has been devised which permits obtaining films at very rapid intervals, up to 12 per second. This allows the production of sequential films for twelve or more seconds after the injection depending on the "program selection." With the aid of such apparatus, it is unnecessary to time the exposures with great accuracy, so long as a sufficient number of exposures is obtained while the dye is passing through the right side of the heart, and then the left side of the heart and aorta.

It is essential in this method of examination that a large bulk of the dye (up to 50 cc.) be injected very rapidly (in two seconds or less), so that the concentration of the dye in the blood will be sufficiently high to produce a good contrast not only in the right side of the heart, but also in the left. For this reason a special syringe with a large bore and a large bore needle (12 gauge) must be employed. It is sometimes advisable in children to expose a vein in the ankle and insert the needle under direct visualization. Special automatic pressure injectors have also been devised for this purpose. At best, the concentration of the dye in the left side of the heart under normal conditions allows only a moderate intensification and visualization of the anatomy.

In normal individuals, the superior vena cava and the right atrium are visualized in one to one and one-half seconds; the right ventricle and pulmonary arteries in three to five seconds (Fig. 12–2); and the left atrium, left ventricle and aorta in six to ten seconds following the beginning of the injection period.

On the right side (Fig. 12–2, **a**), the following structures can be identified: the superior vena cava and its tributaries (which may be referred to as the inflow tract), the right atrial and ventricular cavities and walls; the auricular appendage; the tricuspid valve; the trabeculae; the ventricular septum; the pulmonic valve and the pulmonary artery with its subdivisions.

On the left side (Fig. 12–2, **b**), the following components may be seen: the pulmonary veins; the left atrial and ventricular cavities and walls; the auricular appendage; the aortic valve and the entire thoracic aorta with its main branches.

For most purposes, this examination yields most information in the right posterior oblique view (Fig. 12–2, **c** and **d**); however, diagrams of films obtained in the antero-posterior (Fig. 12–2, **a** and **b**), left posterior oblique (Fig. 12–2, **e** and

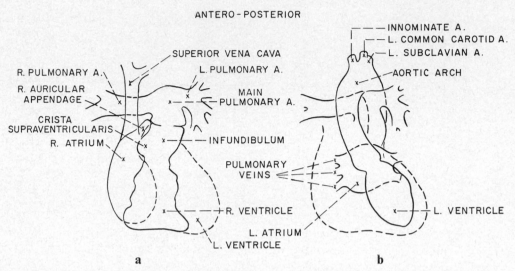

FIG. 12–2. MAJOR STRUCTURES VISUALIZED IN VENOUS ANGIOCARDIOGRAMS IN THE ANTERO-POSTERIOR
           PROJECTION: **a,** lesser circulation phase; **b,** greater circulation phase.

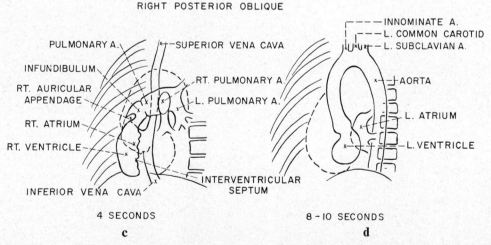

FIG. 12–2. MAJOR STRUCTURES VISUALIZED IN VENOUS ANGIOCARDIOGRAMS IN THE RIGHT POSTERIOR
           OBLIQUE PROJECTION: **c,** lesser circulation phase; **d,** greater circulation phase.

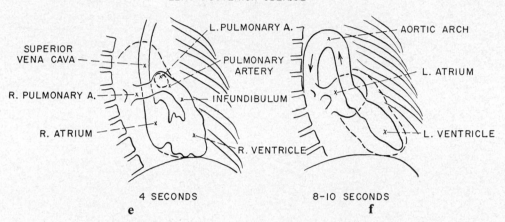

FIG. 12–2.   MAJOR STRUCTURES VISUALIZED IN VENOUS ANGIOCARDIOGRAMS IN THE LEFT POSTERIOR OBLIQUE PROJECTION: e, lesser circulation phase; f, greater circulation phase.

FIG. 12–2.   MAJOR STRUCTURES VISUALIZED IN VENOUS ANGIOCARDIOGRAMS IN THE RIGHT LATERAL PROJECTION: g, lesser circulation phase; h, greater circulation phase.

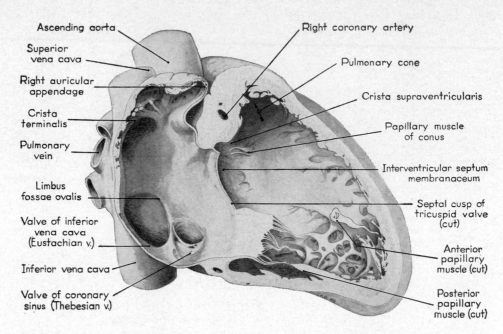

FIG. 12–3. **a,** Right side of the heart opened in a plane approximately parallel to the septa, to show the interior of the right atrium and the right ventricle. A segment of the septal leaflet of the tricuspid valve has been cut away to expose more fully the region of the membranous portion of the interventricular septum. (From Gould: *Pathology of the Heart*, Charles C Thomas, 1953.)

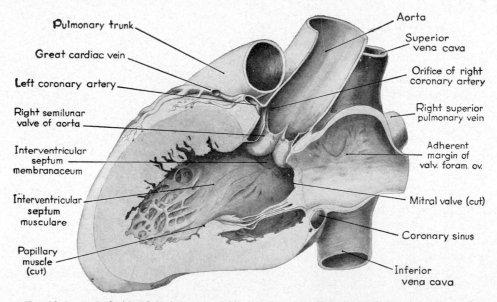

FIG. 12–3. **b,** Left side of the heart opened in a plane approximately parallel to the septa, to show the interior of the left atrium and left ventricle. A segment of the anterior leaflet of the mitral valve has been cut away to expose more fully the region of the membranous portion of the interventricular septum and the aortic orifice. (From Gould: *Pathology of the Heart*, Charles C Thomas, 1953.)

f) and lateral views (Fig. 12–2, **g** and **h**) are also included to demonstrate the anatomic arrangements of the shadows in these other positions as well. The antero-posterior and right lateral projections are ideal for visualization of the main stem of the pulmonary artery, and for the blood vessels in the hilus of the lung.

Ordinarily, the *superior vena cava* (Fig. 12–4, 12–5) begins in front of the second right costal cartilage and passes directly downward, forming the right border of the supracardiac shadow, to end in the right atrium at the level of the third interspace. It lies to the right of the ascending aorta midway between the sternum and the spine. It curves gently backward at the level of the pulmonary artery and then forward again to enter the right atrium.

The *right atrium* is oval in shape and lies at the level of the ninth and tenth thoracic vertebrae, resting partially upon the diaphragm. It lies directly behind and slightly above the inflow tract of the right ventricle. It is separated from the right ventricle by the coronary sulcus. In all of the views it is slightly lower in position than the left atrium. In the antero-posterior projection, it lies obliquely behind and to the right of the right ventricle, forming the lower right cardiac margin.

The *right ventricle* is roughly a triangular cavity having a horizontal inflow tract which extends from the tricuspid valve to the apex of the chamber, and a vertical outflow tract going from the apex to the pulmonary orifice. It ends in the pulmonary infundibulum. It lies on the anterior aspect of the heart, and overlaps the shadow of the left ventricle in the antero-posterior projection, but lies to the right of the midline for the most part. It is best seen in the oblique projections, particularly the right posterior oblique, in which case both the inflow and outflow tracts are clearly visualized, and also the lateral view. The interventricular septum may also be identified in these projections. The bulbous dilatation seen superiorly is the pulmonary infundibulum. The pulmonic valves can be frequently identified. The wall of the right ventricle ordinarily measures about 2 to 3 mm. and its thickness can be readily determined.

The *pulmonary artery* appears as a short broad tube which begins behind the interspace between the third and fourth left costal cartilages. It curves slightly upward and backward toward the spine, passing under the arch of the aorta, and bifurcates in front of the body of the seventh thoracic vertebra into its right and left branches. The pulmonary sinuses lie just above the pulmonic valve, and are visible in all projections except the antero-posterior. The pulmonary artery is seen best in the straight lateral projection, since it passes almost directly posteriorly. The right and left main branches of the pulmonary artery are seen in all projections, but best in the oblique views, in which cases they are seen in cross section or their side view is demonstrated as they pass obliquely backward in the chest. The left main branch arches slightly upward and then posteriorly and downward to divide at the left hilus into its superior and inferior divisions. The right main branch arches downward, posteriorly and transversely to end at the right hilus by dividing into its two major divisions.

The *pulmonary veins* may be seen converging toward both sides of the superior pole of the left atrium.

The *left atrium* (Fig. 12–4, **i**, **j**) is clearly demarcated from the shadow of the left ventricle in the left posterior oblique view. It is situated posteriorly, slightly superiorly, and somewhat to the right of the left ventricle, and this chamber overlaps the projection of the left ventricle in every view except the left posterior oblique. In this oblique view, it overlaps the shadow of the descending thoracic aorta. The region of the mitral valve can usually be delineated.

The *left ventricle* is inferior and to the left of the left atrium, and also extends anterior to the left atrium. Usually, the left ventricular wall can be moderately well measured as being 7 to 10 mm. in thickness. The interventricular septum can usually be distinguished as it extends obliquely to the right and anteriorly from below upward. Usually the shadows of the left atrium and left ventricle overlap one another in all but the left posterior oblique view, in an ovoid area which, therefore, appears highly intensified. The aortic valves can usually be distinguished in both oblique projections and in the left lateral view, and the aortic sinus is distinguishable as a bulbous area above the aortic valves.

The *arch of the aorta* is demonstrable as it first extends anteriorly and upward, and then arches posteriorly and to the left. It descends down the left

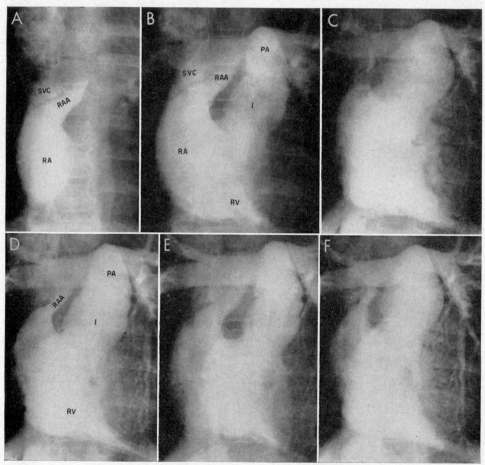

Fig. 12–4.   REPRESENTATIVE ANGIOCARDIOGRAMS.   *A–F*, Lesser circulation phase, frontal projection. Right auricular appendage lies directly to the right of the infundibulum and the right ventricle and lower part of the pulmonary artery which, consequently, in lateral projection, are overlapped by the appendage. AO, aorta; I, infundibulum; IVC, inferior vena cava; LA, left atrium; LV, left ventricle, PA, pulmonary artery; RA, right atrium; RAA, right auricular appendage; RV, right ventricle; SV, sinus venosus; SVC, superior vena cava. (From Kjellberg et al.: *Diagnosis of Congenital Heart Disease,* Year Book Publishers.)

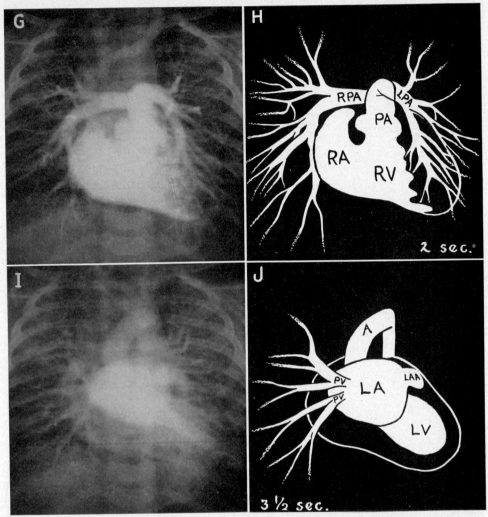

FIG. 12–4. *G* and *H*, Normal frontal angiocardiograms of a 4½ month old infant. At 2 seconds, most of the opaque material has traversed the superior vena cava and left innominate vein, which are still faintly seen. The right atrium, right ventricle, and pulmonary arteries are well filled. Just above the infundibulum of the right ventricle, localized lateral bulges in the pulmonary artery wall identify the sinuses of the pulmonary valve and clearly define the end of the pulmonary conus. Attention is directed to the arborization and tapering of the peripheral pulmonary arterial vessels. Their pattern contrasts sharply with that of the pulmonary veins, which are well seen at 3½ seconds (*I, J*). At this time, the left atrium is in full diastole, and the left ventricle has begun to opacify the aorta. (From Abrams and Kaplan: *Angiocardiographic Interpretation in Congenital Heart Disease*, Charles C Thomas.)

side of the thoracic spine and in the posterior mediastinal space as a tubular structure approximately 3.5 cm. in diameter. The wall thickness of the aorta is usually in the order of 3 mm.

The *innominate, left common carotid and left subclavian arteries* can occasionally be distinguished as they branch from the arch of the aorta, along its anterior aspect.

The *aortic triangle* is likewise delineated. It is bounded anteriorly by the left subclavian artery, posteriorly by the spine, and inferiorly by the arch of the aorta.

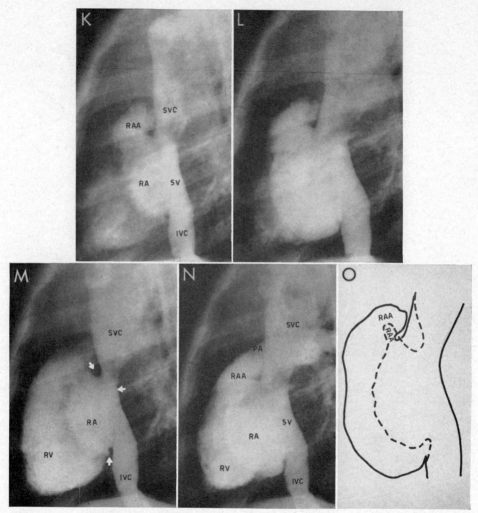

Fig. 12–4. REPRESENTATIVE VENOUS ANGIOCARDIOGRAMS. *K–O*, Lesser circulation phase, lateral projection. During atrial systole, the atrioventricular border is shifted dorsally, while the dorsal wall of the atrium remains in the same position. The crista terminalis presses into the lumen like a membrane (*M*, lower arrow). Sphincter mechanism of the venae cavae is clearly visible. *O*, collective picture of appearance of atrium in late diastole (solid line) and late systole (broken line). (From Kjellberg et al.: *Diagnosis of Congenital Heart Disease*, Year Book Publishers.)

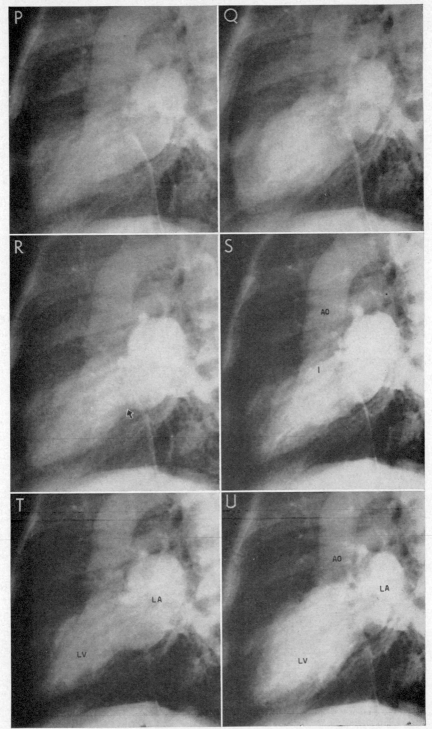

FIG. 12–4.   REPRESENTATIVE VENOUS ANGIOCARDIOGRAMS.   *P–U*, Greater circulation phase, lateral view. Conditions during filling and contraction in left atrium and ventricle. Arrow in *R* points to atrioventricular plane. (From Kjellberg, et al.: *Diagnosis of Congenital Heart Disease*. Year Book Publishers.)

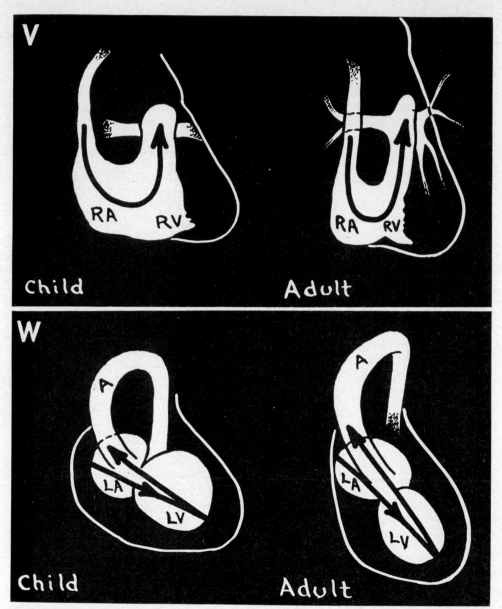

Fig. 12–4. *V*, Semidiagrammatic tracings of the normal right heart as seen in representative frontal angiocardiograms of children and adults. Note the more horizontal relationships of the cardiac chambers in the child, and the much tighter "U"-shaped curve of the right heart in the adult. This difference reflects the change from a relatively transverse position of the heart in infancy and childhood to a more vertical position in adult life, and parallels the changing configuration of the thoracic cage.

Fig. 12–4. *W*, Semidiagrammatic tracings from angiocardiograms of the normal left heart and aorta in children and adults. Frontal projection. The axes of both the inflow and outflow tracts of the left ventricle lie in a more horizontal position in infants and children than in adults. This reflects the transverse position of the heart and the relatively greater horizontal diameter of the chest in the early years. (From Abrams and Kaplan: *Angiocardiographic Interpretation in Congenital Heart Disease*, Charles C Thomas.)

CATHETERIZATION OF THE HEART

Cardiac Catheterization.[6, 11]   In view of the great technical advances made by cardiac surgeons in relation to open heart surgery and repair of defects, the roentgen examination of the heart and its inflow and outflow tracts has become much more exacting. The surgeon must know the answers to many questions, such as: the size and extent of a defect or stenosis; the degree of over-riding of the aorta; and the appearance of the pulmonary arteries, veins and systemic arteries.

In recent years, the technique of cardiac catheterization has been increasingly applied and developed in this direction. By passing a catheter into the right heart and thereafter sequentially into the pulmonary artery one is afforded the following opportunities: Blood samples may be obtained from any of these areas or all of them and gas analysis performed on these samples to determine the site of shunt formation. The volume of blood shunting may be calculated. Pulmonary blood flow may be readily calculated. Pressures in the various chambers are recorded and evaluated in relation to the dynamics of the cardiac circulation. If the catheter takes an abnormal route, a defect may be recognized directly, for example a patent interatrial septum. At the end of these procedures, one may selectively inject into any region a quantity of opaque media under sufficient pressure to visualize carefully a given area without too much interference from adjoining areas. This latter technique is called "selective angiocardiography," in contrast to the previously described venous angiocardiography.

Selective Angiocardiography.   There are several different types of catheters used for this purpose—the modified Cournand, the Lehman, the Rüsch and the Rodriguez-Alvarez—each with its own advocates. A mechanical pressure device for the injection must be employed to give one a satisfactory jet of contrast media within one half to one second. There are a number of these available commercially, varying in complexity and cost from several hundred dollars to several thousand. Injection directly into the right ventricle is by far the most common procedure, and the injection is followed by serial films taken as rapidly as 12 per second (simultaneously in two planes), or by cineradiographs for cinema depiction. Care must be exercised in accurate localization of the catheter tip, lest the injection be made into a coronary vein.

The projection planes most frequently employed are the straight frontal (anteroposterior), right posterior oblique and lateral.

The Rodriguez-Alvarez and Lehman catheters are thin-walled, and permit a greater volume of injection per unit time. Although 70 per cent Urokon has a faster flow rate than 90 per cent Hypaque warmed to 55 degrees Centigrade (because of lesser viscosity), the reaction rate is greater with the former media. Either medium is ordinarily used in quantities of 0.5 to 0.7 cc. per kilogram of body weight, with a pressure of injection of at least 6 kilograms per square centimeter.

In cineradiography, there is still considerable disagreement as to which film emulsion is best for all purposes. Eastman K Linograph and Shellburst are of fine grain and contrast but somewhat slower than Cineflure which, however, has a somewhat larger grain size.*

---

* Personal communication from John A. Campbell and Eugene Klatte.

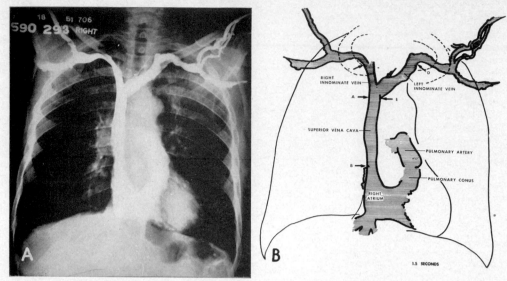

FIG. 12–5.   The superior vena cava and innominate veins as visualized by venous angiocardiography.
(From Roberts, Dotter, and Steinberg: Am. J. Roentgenol., vol. 66, 1951.)

Thoracic Aortography.   In this procedure, a catheter is threaded directly into a major artery by open exposure of the artery, or by threading a catheter through a percutaneous needle. Again, a pressure type injector must be employed and the injection accomplished within two seconds for pulse rates of 60 per minute. The injection rate must be more rapid with faster pulse rates. Injection directly into the left atrium for demonstration of an atrial septal defect must be very rapid (½ to one second). In the latter circumstance, oblique projections, rather than frontal and lateral, are preferred. Fifteen to 20 cc. of 50 per cent Urokon or Diodrast or its equivalent are used.

Direct injections into the renal, hepatic or other arteries are also possible by this technique, especially if a special type of catheter with a curved tip is employed.

The main dangers are irritation, spasm, or even thrombosis of an adjoining more peripheral artery such as the carotid, and the sequelae which may follow loss of blood supply to a vital part.

The retrograde injection directly into the base of the aorta proximal to the aortic valvular cusps has permitted visualization of the coronary arteries.[10,17] It is probable that this technique or some variant of it will assume increasing significance in the near future (Figs. 12–6, 12–7).

Selective Arteriography.   Selective injection into an artery can be accomplished either by direct percutaneous puncture (as in the case of carotid arteriography, Chapter 8), or by catheterization techniques. Ten to 20 cc. of opaque media are required as with selective angiocardiography, and serial films are best if the area to be covered is not too large. If, however, the area to be covered is greater than 14 inches square, simpler rapid film changing devices must be employed. There are several such available employing films up to 70 cm. in length and permitting as many as four films in rapid sequence. Another expedi-

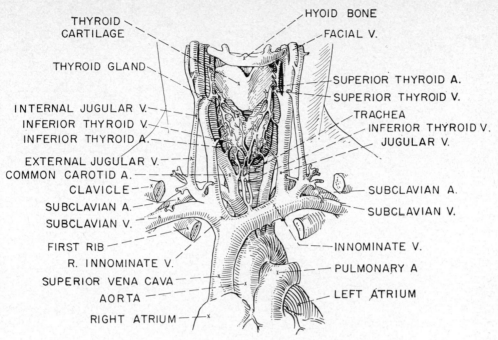

THYROID CARTILAGE

THYROID GLAND

INTERNAL JUGULAR V.
INFERIOR THYROID V.
INFERIOR THYROID A.

EXTERNAL JUGULAR V.
COMMON CAROTID A.
CLAVICLE
SUBCLAVIAN A.
SUBCLAVIAN V.

FIRST RIB
R. INNOMINATE V.
SUPERIOR VENA CAVA
AORTA
RIGHT ATRIUM

HYOID BONE
FACIAL V.

SUPERIOR THYROID A.
SUPERIOR THYROID V.
TRACHEA
INFERIOR THYROID V.
JUGULAR V.

SUBCLAVIAN A.
SUBCLAVIAN V.

INNOMINATE V.
PULMONARY A
LEFT ATRIUM

FIG. 12–6. **a,** Diagram of major circulation in the neck.

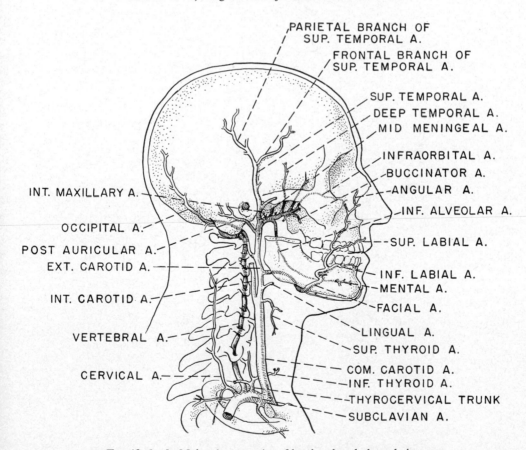

PARIETAL BRANCH OF
SUP. TEMPORAL A.
FRONTAL BRANCH OF
SUP. TEMPORAL A.

SUP. TEMPORAL A.
DEEP TEMPORAL A.
MID MENINGEAL A.

INFRAORBITAL A.
BUCCINATOR A.
ANGULAR A.
INF. ALVEOLAR A.

INT. MAXILLARY A.

OCCIPITAL A.

POST AURICULAR A.
EXT. CAROTID A.

INT. CAROTID A.

VERTEBRAL A.

CERVICAL A.

SUP. LABIAL A.

INF. LABIAL A.
MENTAL A.
FACIAL A.

LINGUAL A.
SUP. THYROID A.
COM. CAROTID A.
INF. THYROID A.
THYROCERVICAL TRUNK
SUBCLAVIAN A.

FIG. 12–6. **b,** Major deep arteries of head and neck, lateral view.

555

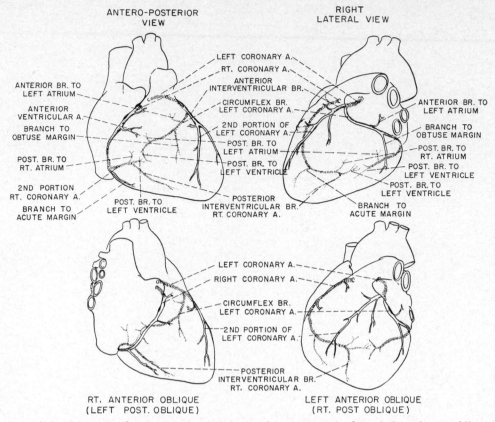

ANTERO-POSTERIOR
VIEW

RIGHT
LATERAL VIEW

LEFT CORONARY A.
RT. CORONARY A.
ANTERIOR
INTERVENTRICULAR BR.

ANTERIOR BR. TO
LEFT ATRIUM

ANTERIOR
VENTRICULAR A.

BRANCH TO
OBTUSE MARGIN

POST. BR. TO
RT. ATRIUM

2ND PORTION
RT. CORONARY A.

BRANCH TO
ACUTE MARGIN

CIRCUMFLEX BR.
LEFT CORONARY A.

2ND PORTION OF
LEFT CORONARY A.

POST. BR. TO
LEFT ATRIUM

POST. BR. TO
LEFT VENTRICLE

POST. BR. TO
LEFT VENTRICLE

POSTERIOR
INTERVENTRICULAR BR.
RT. CORONARY A.

ANTERIOR BR. TO
LEFT ATRIUM

BRANCH TO
OBTUSE MARGIN

POST. BR. TO
RT. ATRIUM

POST. BR. TO
LEFT VENTRICLE

POST. BR. TO
LEFT VENTRICLE

BRANCH TO
ACUTE MARGIN

LEFT CORONARY A.
RIGHT CORONARY A.

CIRCUMFLEX BR.
LEFT CORONARY A.

2ND PORTION OF
LEFT CORONARY A.

POSTERIOR
INTERVENTRICULAR BR.
RT. CORONARY A.

RT. ANTERIOR OBLIQUE
(LEFT POST. OBLIQUE)

LEFT ANTERIOR OBLIQUE
(RT. POST OBLIQUE)

Fig. 12–7. Diagram of coronary circulation as might be seen in frontal, lateral and oblique projections. (Modified from Guglielmo and Guttadauro: Acta Radiol., Supp. 97, 1952.)

ent is to cover the tube orifice with a narrow slit and move the tube over the area to be covered during the exposure. A third method is to use a sufficient tube-film distance to give one coverage of an entire 70 cm. film (or 36 inch cassette), utilize a two-second exposure, and a plastic filter so adjusted as to give one a diagnostic film coverage of both the thicker and thinner parts of the body simultaneously.

Figure 12–8 and Figure 12–9 are included for reference in relation to such special procedures.

Abdominal Aortography. The abdominal aorta may be injected either by catheterization or direct needle puncture at the level of the twelfth thoracic vertebra. For the latter purpose, a 15 to 20 cm., 18 or 20 gauge needle may be inserted directly into the aorta. Approximately 12 to 20 cc. of 70 per cent Diodrast or its equivalent in Hypaque, Urokon or Renografin are injected rapidly at a rate of 2 to 4 cc. per second and serial films obtained if possible (see previous section on selective arteriography). Otherwise the moving tube technique or the plastic bolus and long exposure technique are employed as previously described.

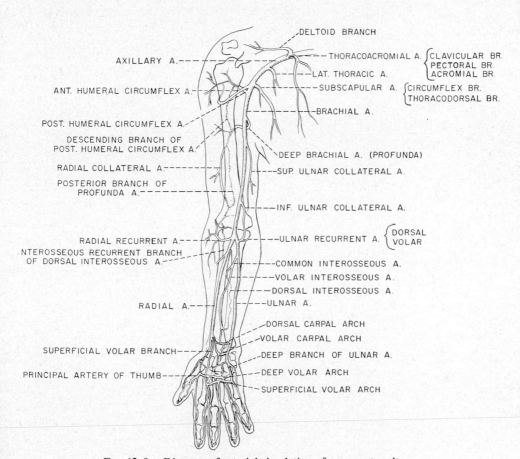

FIG. 12–8. Diagram of arterial circulation of upper extremity.

In the low thoracic or high abdominal aortogram, one may obtain a visualization of the entire aortic circulation or any branch or segment thereof. The accompanying illustrations show the anatomy which may be visualized (Fig. 12–10), and special visualizations of branches of the abdominal aorta may also be obtained (Fig. 12–11).

The method of aortography is useful also for visualization of the placenta in the pregnant uterus. Since there is a puddling of dye in the sinusoidal circulation of the placenta this can be readily visualized (Fig. 12–11, **b**), and abnormal implantation of the placenta thereby determined.

One of the areas of greatest usefulness is in the demonstration of renal architecture (Fig. 12–11, **f**). This technique has permitted accuracy of diagnosis of a wide variety of pathologic conditions of the kidney, such as neoplasms, anomalies, aneurysms, and causes of renal hypertension.

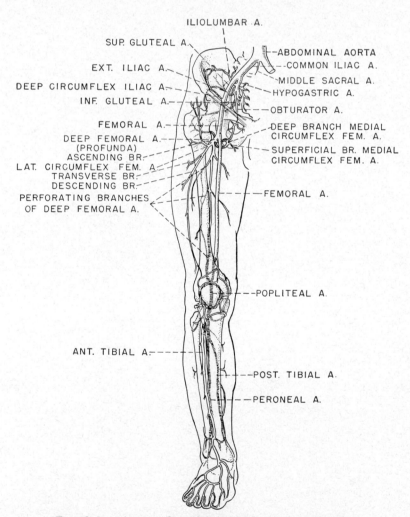

FIG. 12–9. Diagram of arterial circulation of lower extremity.

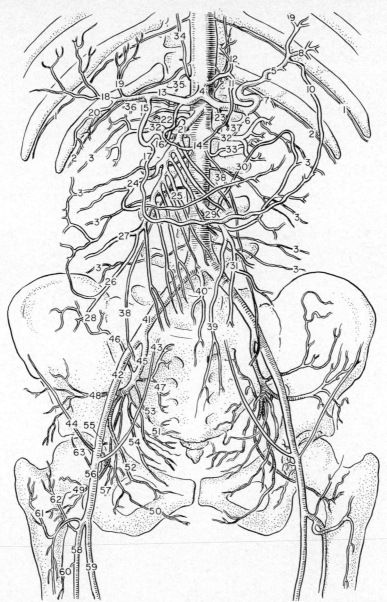

FIG. 12–10. THE ARTERIES OF ABDOMEN, PELVIS AND THIGH. (Modified from Muller, R. F., and Figley, M. M., Am. J. Roentgenol., vol. 77, 1957.) 1, Intercostal artery; 2, subcostal artery; 3, lumbar arteries; 4, celiac axis; 5, splenic artery; 6, dorsal pancreatic; 7, great pancreatic artery; 8, terminal branches to spleen; 9, short gastric branches; 10, left gastroepiploic; 11, left gastric artery; 12, esophageal branches; 13, common hepatic; 14, right gastric artery; 15, gastroduodenal artery; 16, anterior superior pancreaticoduodenal; 17, right gastroepiploic; 18, right hepatic artery; 19, left hepatic artery; 20, cystic artery; 21, superior mesenteric; 22, inferior pancreaticoduodenal; 23, inferior pancreatic; 24, middle colic artery; 25, intestinal branches; 26, ileocolic; 27, right colic; 28, appendiceal; 29, inferior mesenteric; 30, left colic; 31, sigmoid; 32, renal artery; 33, accessory renal; 34, inferior phrenic; 35, superior suprarenal; 36, middle suprarenal; 37, inferior suprarenal; 38, internal spermatic (or ovarian); 39, superior hemorrhoidal; 40, middle sacral; 41, common iliac; 42, external iliac; 43, inferior epigastric; 44, deep circumflex iliac; 45, hypogastric; 46, iliolumbar; 47, lateral sacral; 48, superior gluteal; 49, inferior gluteal; 50, internal pudendal; 51, middle hemorrhoidal; 52, obturator; 53, uterine; 54, vesical; 55, superficial epigastric; 56, common femoral; 57, superficial external pudendal; 58, deep femoral (profunda); 59, superficial femoral; 60, perforating muscular branches; 61, lateral femoral circumflex; 62, medial femoral circumflex; 63, superficial circumflex iliac.

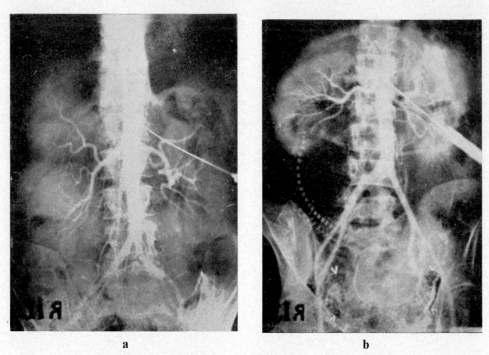

a   b

Fig. 12–11. AORTOGRAMS: a, Representative aortogram. b, An aortogram for placentography showing a placenta previa. The sinusoidal placental circulation produces a laking of opaque material in the region of the placenta. Usually a film taken at approximately six or eight seconds following the beginning of the injection period is most satisfactory for this purpose. (From *Manual of Roentgenographic Technique*, L. R. Sante, Edward Bros., Inc., Publishers.)

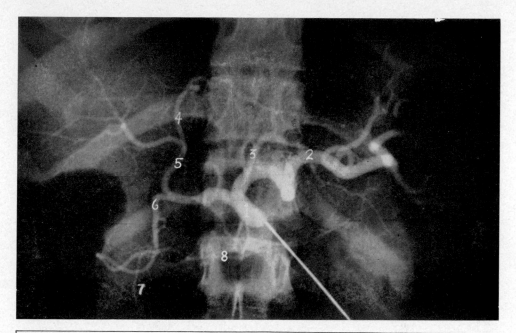

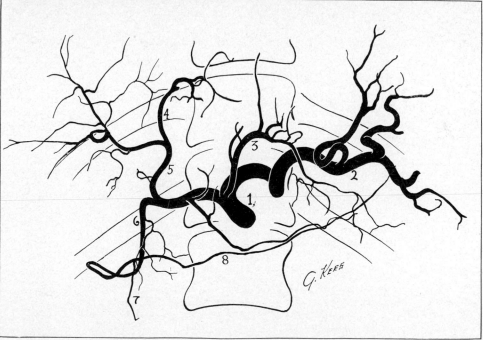

FIG. 12–11. AORTOGRAMS: c, Radiograph and tracing of the celiac artery an its major branches by the method of aortoraphy. (Through the courtesy of Drs. Parke G. Smith, Arthur T. Evans, Benjamin Felson, and Edward C. Elsey, Cincinnati General Hospital and Christ Hospital, Cincinnati, Ohio.) *1*, Celiac artery; *2*, splenic artery; *3*, left gastric artery; *4*, right gastric artery; *5*, hepatic artery; *6*, gastroduodenal artery; *7*, superior pancreaticoduodeal artery; *8*, right gastroepiploic artery.

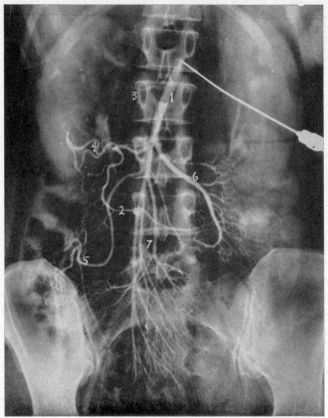

FIG. 12–11. AORTOGRAMS: d (i), Radiograph of the superior mesenteric artery and its branches. (Through the courtesy of Drs. Parke G. Smith, Arthur T. Evans, Benjamin Felson, and Edward C. Elsey, Cincinnati General Hospital and Christ Hospital, Cincinnati, Ohio.) *1*, Superior mesenteric artery; *2*, middle colic artery; *3*, pancreaticoduodenal inferior artery; *4*, right colic artery; *5*, ilio-colic artery; *6*, jejunal artery; *7*, ilial artery.

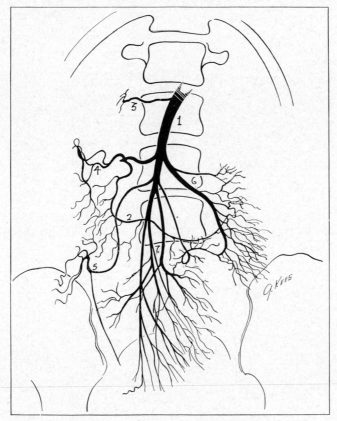

FIG. 12–11. AORTOGRAMS: **d (ii)**, Tracing of d **(i)**.

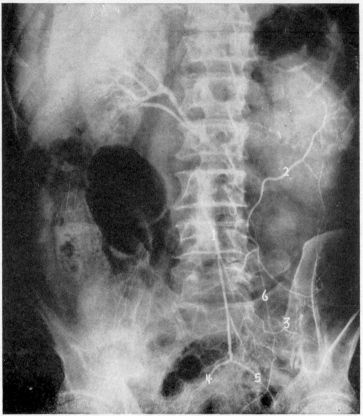

Fig. 12–11. AORTOGRAMS: e (i), Radiograph of the inferior mesenteric artery by the method of aortography. (Through the courtesy of Drs. Parke G. Smith, Arthur T. Evans, Benjamin Felson, and Edward C. Elsey, Cincinnati General Hospital and Christ Hospital, Cincinnati, Ohio.) *1*, Inferior mesenteric artery; *2*, left colic artery; *3*, sigmoidal artery; *4*, right hemorrhoidal artery; *5*, left hemorrhoidal artery. In addition, *6* demonstrates the left spermatic artery.

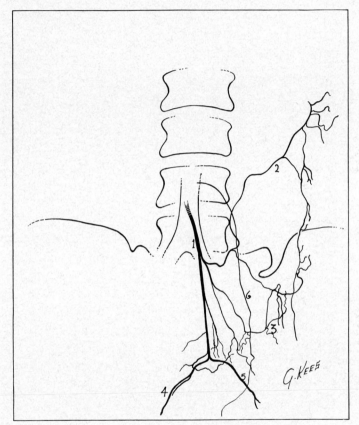

Fɪɢ. 12–11. ᴀᴏʀᴛᴏɢʀᴀᴍs: e (ii), Tracing of e (i).

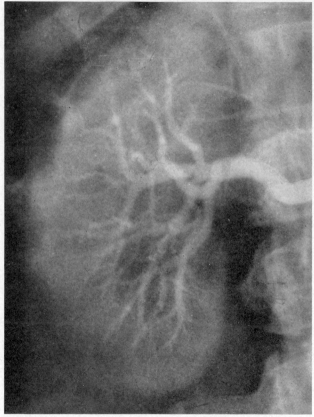

Fig. 12–11.   AORTOGRAMS: **f (i),** Radiograph of the normal renal circulation as demonstrated by the method of aortography. (Through the courtesy of Drs. Parke G. Smith, Arthur T. Evans, Benjamin Felson, and Edward C. Elsey, Cincinnati General Hospital and Christ Hospital, Cincinnati, Ohio)

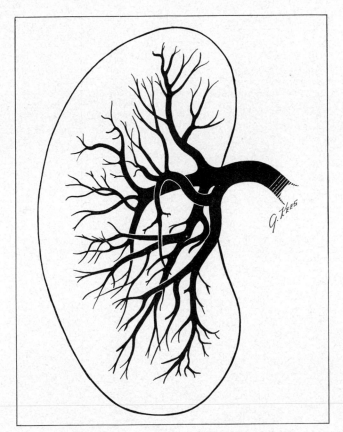

FIG. 12–11.   AORTOGRAMS: **f (ii)**, Tracing of **f (i)**.

UTILIZATION OF CONTRAST MATERIAL FOR DEMONSTRATION OF THE CORONARY CIRCULATION AT AUTOPSY

The demonstration of coronary artery circulation at autopsy by means of dissection alone has its limitations in that only the relatively large branches can be so studied. Injections of the coronary arteries by radiopaque material were carried out by Gross,[9] but the method has been improved considerably by Schlesinger.[14] Schlesinger employed a tinted radiopaque mass mixture of lead acetate solution and disodium phosphate in agar-agar under carefully controlled conditions of temperature and pressure, injecting the coronary arteries with this substance, and then allowing the substance to solidify in the arteries (Fig. 12–12). Then by a special technique of incising the heart, he was able to spread the heart out so that the major branches could be identified according to a very regular pattern first described by Spalteholtz. A roentgenogram and a labeled tracing of the heart obtained in this manner are shown in Figure 12–13. (There is a small area of coronary sclerosis in the left coronary artery in this particular specimen, but it is a good illustration of this application of radiographic anatomy to a study of the dead rather than the living.)

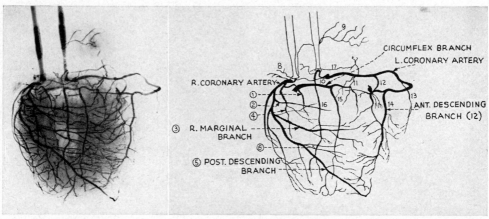

FIG. 12–12.   Radiograph and tracing of the coronary circulation at autopsy according to Schlesinger's method, prior to incising the heart.

Right Coronary Artery	*Left Coronary Artery*
1. A. adiposa dextra	*10.* A. adiposa sinistra
2. R. ventriculi dextri anterior	*11.* A. septi ventriculorum
3. R. marginis acuti	*12.* R. collateralis descendens anterior primus
4. R. ventriculi dextri posterior	*13.* R. collateralis descendens anterior secundus
5. R. sulci longitudinalis posterioris	*14.* R. ventriculi sinistri anterior
6. R. ventriculi sinistri posterior	*15.* R. marginis obtusi
7. R. ventriculi sinistri accessorius	*16.* R. ventriculi sinistri posterior
8. R. atrialis dexter anterior	*17.* R. atrialis sinister anterior C. R. auricularis
9. R. atrialis sinister posterior	*18.* R. atrialis sinister posterior

A = artery
R = ramus (branch)

(Photographs supplied through the courtesy of Lieutenant-Colonel H. C. Harrell, M. C., Chief, Radiological Service, Army and Navy General Hospital, Hot Springs, Arkansas.)

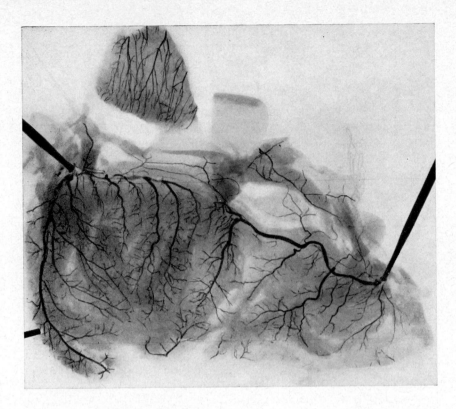

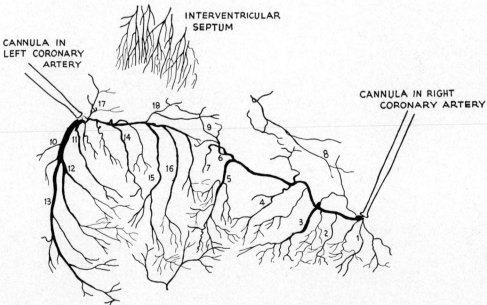

FIG. 12–13. Radiograph and tracing of injected heart after incision according to the method described by Spalteholtz and modified by Schlesinger. For anatomic correlation refer to Figure 12–12.

PHLEBOGRAPHY OF THE LOWER EXTREMITY[15]

Technique. Numerous slight variations in technique are described, but there is general agreement that the contrast medium shoud be injected into one of the superficial veins of the foot or ankle. The contrast media in common use in this country are 35 to 50 per cent solutions of either Diodrast or Neo-iopax or an equivalent organic iodide such as Hypaque or Renografin.

In the method utilized by Epstein, Wasch and Loewe[7] in their investigation of the normal phlebogram, 20 cc. of the media was injected within sixty seconds into any available vein on the dorsum of the foot or over either malleolus with a hypodermic needle. Two and sometimes three exposures were made using the Potter-Bucky diaphragm, each exposure being made as rapidly as possible as follows:

1. First exposure: leg slightly in inversion. Exposure made immediately upon completion of the injection centering just below the knee.
2. Second exposure centering just above the knee.
3. Third exposure, centering just below the groin.

They also studied some of the patients in the lateral projection as well.

Patients may also be injected in this manner with 30 mm. mercury pressure around the calf in an effort to visualize the deep system of veins, since this pressure will occlude the superficial veins, but not the deep. We have found this method of considerable value particularly since the deep veins are of greater interest clinically.

An alternative technique for demonstration of competency of femoral vein valves is to catheterize the saphenous vein in the groin, pass the catheter to the femoral vein, and introduce 15 to 20 cc. of the dye rapidly *with the patient erect*. Films are obtained immediately of the thigh and leg, and thereafter at one minute intervals for four minutes. (Direct percutaneous puncture of the femoral vein in the groin may be employed in lieu of the catheterization method described.)

If the femoral valves are competent, the passage of the dye will be stopped almost entirely at the first set of valves approximately 8 to 10 cm. from the inguinal ligament. A very small amount of dye may escape down to the second set of valves, but no farther. This method may be referred to as the "gravity method" of phlebography.[3,13] Another indication of abnormality is a visualization of an unusual number of the veins which communicate with the femoral vein in the thigh. Normally the dye should virtually disappear in less than one minute. Persistence for two minutes or longer is an indication of venous stasis and poor venous circulation.

Normal Anatomy (Fig. 12–14, **a** and **b**). The superficial veins form a continuous network around the leg and the thigh. The lesser saphenous vein (Fig. 12–15) begins behind the lateral malleolus, courses along the posterior surface of the Achilles tendon, and passes upward to enter the popliteal vein in the groove between the two heads of the gastrocnemius muscle. It anastomoses freely with the greater saphenous vein which arises in front of the medial malleolus and courses upward on the medial aspect of the tibia, making a slight curve at the medial tibial and femoral condyles. It then extends upward on the medial and anterior aspect of the thigh to enter the femoral vein in the fossa ovalis. Numerous branches are received throughout its course and it communicates freely with the deeper veins (Fig. 12–16).

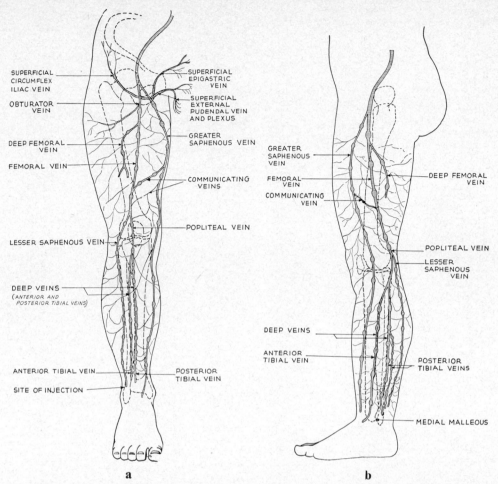

FIG. 12–14. Diagram of the anatomy of conventional venograms of the leg: **a,** Antero-posterior projection; **b,** lateral projection.

There are a variable number of valves in both of these veins, with the greater number usually in the long saphenous. Although anatomically it is said there may be eight to twenty valves in the long saphenous and six to twelve in the lesser, usually there is a considerably smaller number identifiable radiographically (four or five).

The deep leg veins are usually paired veins (Fig. 12–17), and accompany the anterior and posterior tibial and peroneal arteries. They communicate with each other freely and also with the superficial veins. They contain numerous valves.

The anterior tibial veins arise from the dorsum of the foot and lie in the anterior compartment of the leg, in front of the interosseous membrane. The posterior tibial veins arise from the plantar veins, and the peroneal veins arise from the dorsal surface of the calcaneus. These latter two veins are situated in the posterior compartment behind the interosseous membrane. The peroneal vein enters the posterior tibial below the knee.

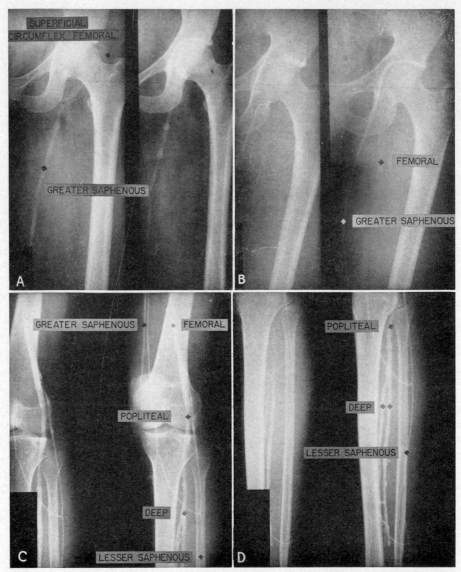

Fɪɢ. 12–15. Representative conventional venograms of the lower extremity demonstrating primarily the lesser and greater saphenous veins and several deeper veins of leg and thigh. (Courtesy of Dr. E. C. Baker, Youngstown, Ohio.)

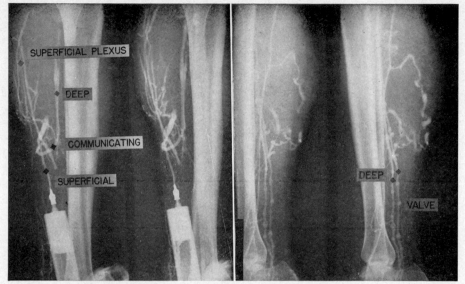

FIG. 12–16   FIG. 12–17

FIG. 12–16.   Venograms of leg demonstrating the communicating veins joining superficial and deep veins. (Courtesy of Dr. E. C. Baker, Youngstown, Ohio.)

FIG. 12–17.   Venograms of deep veins of leg, showing their paired nature. (Courtesy of Dr. E. C. Baker, Youngstown, Ohio.)

The popliteal vein is formed by the junction of the anterior and posterior tibial veins (Fig. 12–15, **d**), and this vein is very subject to slight variations.

The femoral vein (Fig. 12–18) and its tributaries comprise the deep veins of the thigh. It accompanies the femoral artery, and terminates as it enters the pelvis as the external iliac vein. The femoral veins are said to contain two bicuspid valves, but usually it is possible to see three or four valves in the femoral vein radiographically.

The deep femoral vein has numerous tributaries, and since these are not often seen radiographically in the usual examination, they need no further consideration in this test.

The great variability and the superposition of veins make the radiographic interpretation of venograms very difficult. Only those veins will fill which happen to be patent at the time of examination and it is most unusual to obtain a complete filling of all of the major veins in a single examination. Indeed, excessive filling of smaller tributaries is an indication of abnormality.

In the interpretation of these studies, it is well to repeat them on several separate occasions by the routine method of injection of a vein in the foot so that the constancy of a given finding will add weight to its reliability.

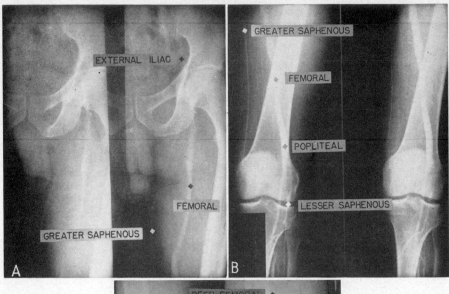

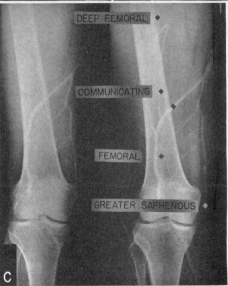

FIG. 12–18. Venograms demonstrating the external iliac vein, the femoral vein, and its major tributaries. (Courtesy of Dr. E. C. Baker, Youngstown, Ohio.)

PERCUTANEOUS SPLENOPORTAL VENOGRAPHY[5, 8]

Two methods are available for visualizing the portal circulation: (1) the direct approach through an abdominal incision; and (2) the percutaneous approach by splenic puncture. The latter technique provides fairly complete coverage of the portal venous system, and provides valuable information for the surgeon prior to a direct portacaval or splenorenal shunt in treatment of bleeding esophageal varices.

The procedure is performed under general anesthesia, with a rapid film changer preferably. A 16 gauge needle is inserted in the mid-axillary line of the ninth or tenth intercostal space. The patient is maintained in apnea as the spleen is approached, to prevent laceration of the spleen. The needle is advanced about

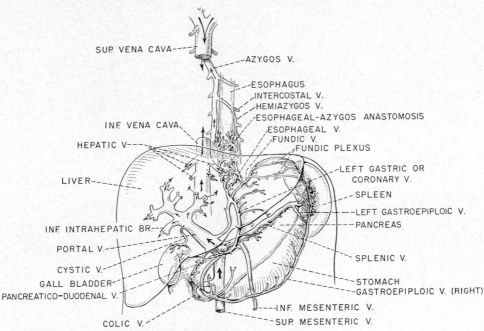

FIG. 12–19. Anatomic diagram of the portal circulation and relationship to esophageal veins and azygos venous systems.

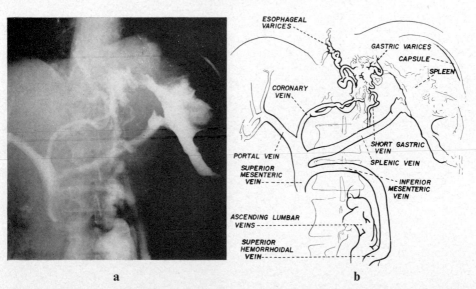

a   b

FIG. 12–20. **a**, Roentgenogram at 12 seconds demonstrates coronary vein, gastric and esophageal varices. The anastomosis between the inferior mesenteric vein and superior hemorrhoid plexus is demonstrated. The latter is also seen to drain into the vertebral venous plexus. **b**, Tracing of **a**. (From Evans, J. A., and O'Sullivan, W. D: Am. J. Roentgenol., vol. 77; 1957.)

2 or 3 cm. into the splenic pulp, and 50 cc. of 70 per cent Urokon or similar contrast substance are forcefully injected in 5 or 6 seconds. Exposure rates of one per second for about 12 to 15 seconds are adequate. The patient is maintained in apnea during the injection and exposure.

It is apparently customary to find 50 to 100 cc. of blood in the peritoneal cavity when the abdomen is opened, although occasionally the blood loss may be greater. In occasional cases, splenectomy is necessitated. Under no circumstances should the procedure be done except prior to surgery for performance of a shunt. Its main purpose is to demonstrate patency of the various major vessels of the portal circulation, to save the surgeon hours of search for a nonexistent or thrombosed vein which he is hoping to utilize in the anastomosis.

The basic anatomy of the area is illustrated in Figure 12–19. Typical splenoportograms are shown in Figure 12–20.

THE VERTEBRAL AND AZYGOS VENOUS SYSTEMS

The vertebral veins form a large accessory drainage area which is taking on increasing importance in diagnostic radiology. At the base of the brain, these anastomose freely with the cranial veins and sinuses; in the neck with the

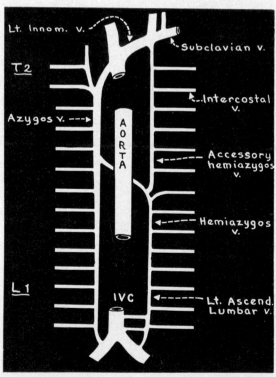

FIG. 12–21.　Diagrammatic representation of the azygos venous system. The segmental lumbar veins are joined to each other by a longitudinal vessel, the ascending lumbar vein. The right ascending lumbar vein, as it enters the thorax, becomes the azygos vein, and the left ascending lumbar vein is continuous with the hemiazygos vein. The hemiazygos vein crosses in front of the vertebral column at the level of T8 or T9 to join the azygos vein. The accessory hemiazygos vein is continuous with the hemiazygos, receives the upper thoracic veins on the left, and joins the left superior intercostal vein above. (From Abrams, H. L.: Radiology, vol. 69, 1957.)

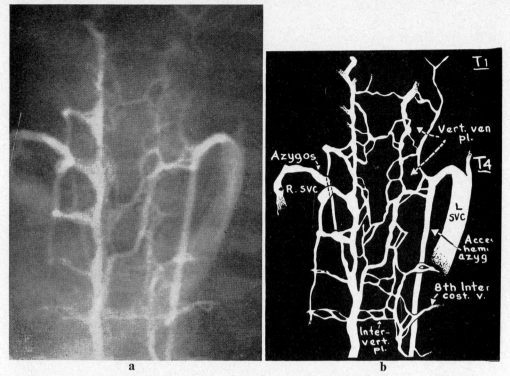

a   b

FIG. 12–22.   The vertebral veins at the upper thoracic level. The vertebral venous plexuses are opacified following the injection of the opaque medium into the left saphenous vein. The primitive paired arrangement of both the azygos and the superior vena cava is preserved, the accessory hemiazygos emptying into the left superior vena cava, and the azygos into the right superior vena cava. The medial portions of the intercostal veins are opacified. R.SVC, Right superior vena cava. L.SVC, Left superior vena cava. Access. hemiazyg, Accessory hemiazygos vein. (From Abrams, H. L., Radiology, vol. 69, 1957.)

deep cervical veins; in the thorax and abdomen with the intercostal and lumbar veins; and in the pelvis with the large venous plexuses anterior to the sacrum. The sacral and lumbar veins communicate directly with the inferior caval system, the lumbar and intercostal veins with the azygos system, and the azygos system with the superior vena cava and its branches (Fig. 12–21). A representative radiographic appearance of these veins at the upper thoracic level is shown in Figure 12–22.[2]

One application clinically of this knowledge is in vertebral trans-skeletal phlebography, where 20 cc. of 70 per cent Diodrast or its equivalent are injected rapidly into the spinous process of either the lumbar or the thoracic vertebrae and antero-posterior and lateral films are made immediately thereafter.[1]

OSSEOUS PHLEBOGRAPHY[16]

The osseous venous system and the deep veins that drain it can be demonstrated by the injection of 10 to 20 cc. of 50 per cent Hypaque into the appropriate bone (#15 bone marrow needle under general anesthesia). Injections in this manner are carried out not only into spinous processes, but into tumorous areas, the pelvic girdle and the sternum.

REFERENCES

1. Abrams, H. L.: The Vertebral and Azygos Venous Systems, and Some Variations in Systemic Venous Return. Radiology, *69:* 508–526, 1957.
2. Albala, M. M., Barrick, C. W., and Jenkinson, E. L.: Vertebral Trans-Skeletal Phlebography. Radiology, *67:* 229–232, 1956.
3. Bauer, G.: Roentgenological and Clinical Study of Sequels of Thrombosis. Acta chir. scandinav. (Supp. 61), *86:* 1, 1942.
4. Boone, B. R., Chamberlain, W. E., Gilbeck, F. G., and Henny, G. C.: Interpreting the Electro-kymogram of Heart and Great Vessel Motion. Am. Heart J., *34:* 560–681, 1947.
5. Brewer, A. J., and Hallenbeck, J. A.: Roentgenologic Findings in Splenic Portography. Am. J. Roentgenol., *77:* 324–331, 1957.
6. Cournand, A., Baldwin, J. S., and Himmelstein, A.: Cardiac Catheterization in Congenital Heart Disease. The Commonwealth Fund, New York, 1949.
7. Epstein, B. S., Wasch, M. G., Lowe, L. L.: An Evaluation of Phlebography of the Lower Extremity. Am. J. Roentgenol. *60:* 650–657, 1948.
8. Evans, J., and O'Sullivan, W. D.: Percutaneous Splenoportal Venography. Am. J. Roentgenol., *77:* 312–323, 1957.
9. Gross, L.: The Blood Supply of the Heart. Paul B. Hoeber, New York, 1921.
10. Guglielmo, L. D., and Guttadauro, M.: A Roentgenologic Study of the Coronary Arteries in the Living. Acta radiol., Supp. 97, 1952.
11. Kjellberg, S. R., Mannheimer, E., Rudhe, U., and Jonsson, B.: Diagnosis of Congenital Heart Disease, Year Book Publishers, Inc., Chicago, 1955.
12. Robb, G. P. and Steinberg, I.: Practical Method of Visualization of Chambers of the Heart, the Pulmonary Circulation, and the Great Blood Vessels in Man. J. Clin. Invest. *17:* 507, 1938; Am. J. Roentgenol., *41:* 1–17, 1939.
13. Roberts, D., Dotter, Charles, and Steinberg, I.: The Superior Vena Cava and Innominate Veins. Am. J. Roentgenol., *66:* 341–352, 1951.
14. Schlesinger, M. J.: An Injection Plus Dissection Study of Coronary Artery Occlusions and Anastomoses. Am. Heart J., *15:* 528, 1938.
15. Starkloff, Gene B., Bricker, Eugene M., McDonald, James J., and Litzow, Louis T.: Proximal Femoral Venography. Ann. Surg., *131:* 413–417, 1947.
16. Steinbach, H. L., Jergesen, F., Gilfillan, R. S., and Petrakis, H. L.: Osseous Phlebography. Surg., Gynec. & Obst., *104:* 215–226, 1957.
17. Thal, A. P., Lester, R. G., Richards, L. S. and Murray, M. J.: Coronary Arteriography of the Heart. Surg., Gynec. & Obst., *105:* 451–464, 1957.

CHAPTER 13

The Upper
Alimentary Tract

PRINCIPLES INVOLVED IN STUDY OF THE ALIMENTARY TRACT

THE WALLS of the alimentary tract are intermediate in radiographic density, and hence require some type of contrast material for detection by means of the x-ray. Normally, there is a variable amount of gas in the stomach and colon which permits a relatively gross and inadequate visualization of these structures. In the normal adult, gas in the small intestine is considered abnormal and the introduction of contrast material into the small intestine is therefore essential.

Although negative contrast is employed in the visualization of the gastrointestinal tract, it is usually supplementary to the more significant positive contrast with radiopaque media.

Since the physiology and function of the gastrointestinal tract are readily altered by so many factors such as hypotonicity or hypertonicity, alkalinity, acidity, proteins, fats, carbohydrates, amino acids, and any slight mechanical irritation, it is essential for any opaque contrast medium to be physiologically inert.

The most commonly used medium thus employed in present-day radiography of the gastrointestinal tract is barium sulfate in water suspension, although bismuth salts, radioactive Umbrathor and barium sulfate in isotonic saline, "buttermilk" or other commercial suspensions are also employed by some, or used on special occasions. In certain patients, where obstruction by barium mixtures may occur, organic soluble iodides are utilized by intubation techniques. In infants or other patients where aspiration is a potential danger small quantities of iodized oil are helpful, at least until it is certain that aspiration is not taking place. Iodized oil is a poor contrast agent beyond the esophagus because it distorts the normal physiologic pattern.

On certain occasions, there is advantage gained by so-called double contrast in which, following the introduction of the barium suspension, gas is introduced. The gas and barium suspension are thus mixed and are advantageous in outlining polyps and small tumors. The gas employed may be air, carbon dioxide, or a mixture of both, as when ginger ale or carbonated water is introduced into the stomach.

The actual radiologic methods include: (1) fluoroscopy, (2) spot-film radiography, (3) routine radiography in certain positions; any or all of the usual erect, recumbent, supine, prone, lateral or oblique positions are employed.

There are two major principles involved in the radiologic anatomy of the gastrointestinal tract:

1. We are examining a dynamic, moving, functioning system of organs. They are not static. Their structure must at all times be considered along with their function, and the two aspects are inseparable.

2. When the lumen of a hollow organ is filled with contrast substance, we can visualize the inner lining with accuracy, but the wall of the organ outside the innermost lining is studied only indirectly as it affects the lumen or the mucosa. It is conceivable that considerable abnormality may exist outside the lumen within the wall of the organ, which may not be reflected in the mucosal pattern.

THE MOUTH AND OROPHARYNX

The mouth and oropharynx are so readily examined by direct inspection and palpation that it is not usual to employ the radiograph except for demonstration of hidden structures.

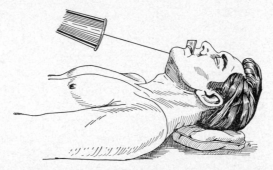

Fig. 13–1.   OCCLUSAL TYPE DENTAL FILM OF FLOOR OF MOUTH: a, Positioning of patient.

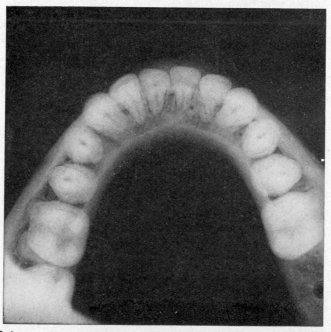

Fig. 13–1.   OCCLUSAL TYPE DENTAL FILM OF FLOOR OF MOUTH: b, Radiograph.

In a direct lateral view (Fig. 10–5), the air within the mouth and pharynx permits a contrast visualization of the tongue surface, the hard and soft palate, and the nasopharynx and oropharynx.

Special views of the salivary glands may be obtained after the injection of iodized oil into the ducts. Soft tissue studies of the floor of the mouth or the cheek are also feasible.

Brief mention of the radiography of the teeth has already been made (see Chap. 6), and no further consideration of the teeth is contemplated at this time.

Soft Tissue Study of the Mouth and Pharynx by Lateral Projection. The method by which this film is obtained is illustrated in Figure 10–5. The projection is identical with that employed for a lateral view of the cervical spine, except that technical factors are varied slightly to emphasize the soft tissues rather than the skeletal structure.

The structures which are demonstrated in profile are: the tongue and floor of the mouth; the hard and soft palate and uvula; the vallecula at the base of the tongue, and the pyriform sinuses on either side; the nasopharynx above the palate, with turbinates, and eustachian orifice; the lymphoid structures in hei nasopharynx; and the epiglottis. The laryngeal structures seen in this protjecton have been previously described (Chap. 10).

The width of the soft tissues projected under the sphenoid is considerably narrower in the adult than in the child, owing to the markedly enlarged lymphoid apparatus in the child. This view affords a ready means of investigating these lymphoid and adenoid structures (Chap. 10).

The width of the retro-oropharyngeal soft tissues in the child is also considerably greater than it is in the adult, when these structures are compared with the retrolaryngeal soft tissues, between the larynx and the cervical spine. Thus in the newborn and infant, the ratio of the retro-oropharyngeal soft tissues to the retrolaryngeal soft tissues is approximately 1 to 1, while in the adult it is usually in the order of 1 to 3. These measurements are of particular value in the detection of space-occupying lesions such as inflammations and tumors

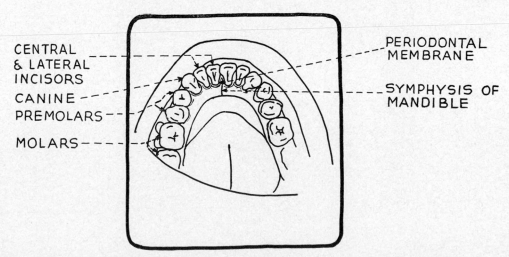

FIG. 13–1. OCCLUSAL TYPE DENTAL FILM OF FLOOR OF MOUTH: c, Labeled tracing of b.

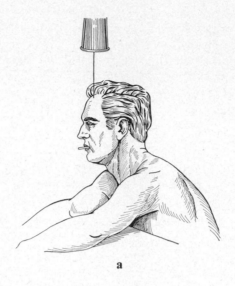

a

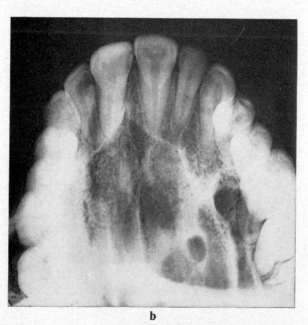

b

FIG. 13–2.   METHOD OF RADIOGRAPHY OF HARD PALATE WITH OCCLUSAL TYPE OF DENTAL FILM: **a**, Positioning of patient; **b**, radiograph.

in these locations, which by direct inspection are difficult to evaluate, since they may be posterior to the visible mucosa, or the patient may be unable to open his mouth.

Soft Tissue Radiography of the Floor of the Mouth with the Aid of the Occlusal Type Dental Film. By placing an occlusal type dental film in the mouth (Fig. 13–1) and directing the x-ray beam perpendicular to it, the soft tissues of the submandibular area are penetrated, as well as the mandible. These soft tissues are not visualized in sufficient detail to distinguish the various anatomic structures such as the salivary glands and ducts, lymph nodes, and tongue—but this method of examination affords a ready means of investigating abnormal calcareous deposits in these structures. Hence an understanding of the normal appearance of this projection is essential.

Soft Tissue Radiography of the Cheek. This can be performed in a similar manner by placing an occlusal film on the inside of the cheek. Care must be exercised in placing the film sufficiently posterior to obtain a visualization of as much of Stenson's duct as possible, since occasionally calcareous deposits in this location may lead to obstructive inflammation and symptoms.

Radiography of the Hard Palate. Apart from the lateral projection previously described, a visualization of the hard palate may be obtained by means of an occlusal film in the mouth as illustrated in Figure 13–2. It will be noted that there are considerable differences in density in the various portions of the hard palate. This is accounted for by the aerated sinuses, the alveolar process, and the bony nasal septum, which overlie the palate. This variation in osseous density is important to consider when one interprets the osseous structure of the hard palate.

The incisive foramen and the major palatine foramen can usually be identified. Frequently, the midline suture as well as the transverse palatine suture can also be noted.

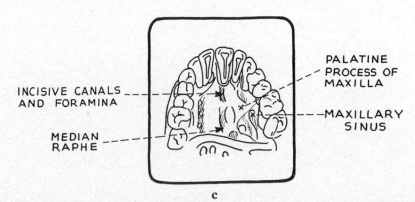

c

FIG. 13–2.   METHOD OF RADIOGRAPHY OF HARD PALATE WITH OCCLUSAL TYPE OF DENTAL FILM: Labeled tracing of **b.**

THE SALIVARY GLANDS

Normal Anatomy. There are three salivary glands, each with a separate duct or ducts opening into the mouth: the parotid, the submaxillary and the sublingual.

The parotid gland is the largest of these and lies on the side of the face, below and in front of the ear, bounded by the zygoma above, the sternomastoid muscle behind, and the ramus of the mandible in front. Approximately one quarter or one third of the gland is usually deep to the posterior margin of the mandible, and extends almost to the pharyngeal wall, being separated from the latter by the branches of the carotid artery, several veins and nerves, and small muscles. Actually, the anterior surface of the gland is wrapped around the posterior margin of the ramus of the mandible. The parotid duct (or Stenson's duct) runs across the masseter muscle superficially, accompanied by branches of the facial nerve. At the anterior margin of the masseter muscle, it turns sharply inward, pierces the buccinator muscle, and opens into the vestibule of the oral cavity on a small papilla opposite the second upper molar tooth. It is approximately 6 cm. in length.

The submaxillary gland lies in the submaxillary triangle on either side of the neck. This gland lies under cover of the body of the mandible for the most part, in its submaxillary fossa. There are a few small lymph nodes embedded in the substance of the gland, and the external maxillary artery runs through its superior and posterior portion. The submaxillary duct (Wharton's duct) runs forward, inward and upward to open into the floor of the mouth, in a papilla on the plica sublingualis close to the frenulum of the tongue. This duct is about 5 cm. in length.

The sublingual gland is the smallest of the salivary glands, and is more deeply situated. It lies under the mucosa of the floor of the mouth, just posterior to the symphysis and in the sublingual fossa of the medial surface of the mandible. It has approximately twelve separate excretory ducts which open on the plica sublingualis, for the most part, but one or two of them may open into the submaxillary duct. This latter point is of importance from the standpoint of sialography, since one of the ducts which opens into the submaxillary duct may be injected by error, and the submaxillary gland visualized instead of the sublingual.

Radiographic Technique of Examination. The salivary glands may be examined by means of plain radiographs, or following the injection of contrast media into the salivary duct. The plain radiographs are of value only when a calculus is suspected. In other instances, the contrast studies are necessary.

With regard to the *plain radiographs*, the following studies may be done:

1. For parotid calculi, a lateral view (in stereoscopic projection preferably) is taken, centering over the gland, with the neck extended and the mouth open.

2. For submaxillary calculi and sublingual calculi, a stereoscopic lateral view is obtained with the mouth closed, and usually it is best to incline the x-ray tube slightly cephalad to prevent superimposition of the two rami of the mandible. Also a view of the floor of the mouth is obtained, with the aid of an occlusal type dental film as previously described.

Sialograms are defined as the radiographic demonstration of the salivary ducts and alveoli, by the injection of contrast media. The technique is as follows:[6]

The duct is dilated with olive-tipped lacrimal probes. A sterile polyethylene

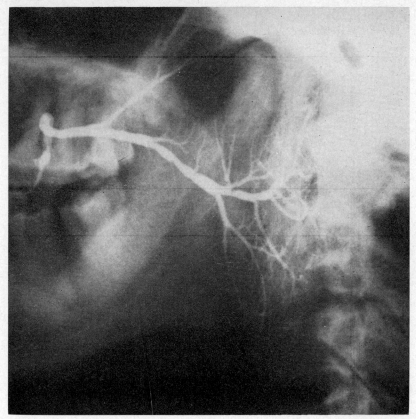

FIG. 13–3.   Normal sialogram of the parotid gland, lateral view. (Courtesy of Dr. L. B. Morettin, Galveston, Texas.)

catheter is thereafter inserted with a wire stylus for rigidity for a distance of 3 to 4 cm. Injection of an iodized oil is thereafter carried out until definite pain occurs. Normally, less than 1 cc. is required. Abnormally, up to 2 cc. may be used. The polyethylene catheter is then plugged and postero-anterior and lateral films are obtained. The patient is then instructed to suck on a lemon for one minute, after which the patient rinses his mouth. Normally, the gland should be empty within five minutes (although a faint "acinar" cloud may persist for up to 24 hours). The latter emptying phase is considered as important as the "filling phase" to be described.

The Normal Filling Phase Sialogram.   The appearance of the normal sialogram simulates the skeletal structure of a leaf (Fig. 13–3).

The parotid duct is somewhat narrower than the submaxillary and angulates sharply as it leaves the masseter muscle and it passes obliquely through the buccinator muscle. There is usually a large forking branch from the parotid duct directed superiorly, called the "socia parotidis," but otherwise the branching ducts tend to join the main duct almost at right angles.

The secondary ductules of the submaxillary duct are less regular than that of the parotid, but otherwise very similar.

The sublingual gland has numerous excretory ducts, and ordinarily only a small segment of the gland is visualized by a single injection. Occasionally, one visualizes a portion of the sublingual gland after injecting the submaxillary duct, since the sublingual excretory duct may empty into the submaxillary duct rather than into the mouth.

THE ESOPHAGUS

Gross Anatomy and Relationships of the Esophagus.   The esophagus extends from the pharynx at the inferior border of the cricoid cartilage to the cardiac orifice of the stomach opposite the eleventh thoracic vertebra. Its course is in the midline anterior to the vertebral column, but it deviates to the left at the base of the neck for a short distance, and at about the level of the seventh thoracic vertebra it passes slowly to the left and anteriorly to reach the esophageal orifice of the diaphragm, and maintains this direction until the stomach is reached.

Its length varies between 25 and 30 cm., and its breadth between 12 mm. and 30 or more mm. in its distended state.

In cross section it usually appears as a flattened tube, or a tube with a stellate lumen.

There are certain anatomic relationships of the esophagus (Fig. 13–4) which are of definite importance:

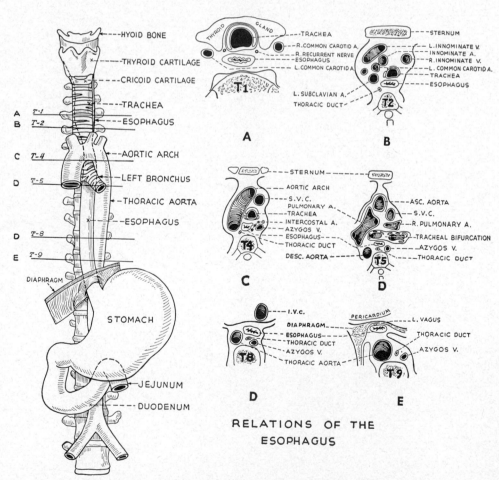

FIG. 13–4.   Relationship of esophagus to contiguous structures at various levels.

In the neck it is loosely connected by areolar tissue with the posterior aspect of the trachea. It is possible, however, for an abnormal structure such as aberrant thyroid tissue to lie between the trachea and esophagus, and hence it is important to obtain a lateral visualization of the base of the neck with barium in the esophagus when studying the thyroid gland.

In the thorax, the trachea lies anterior to the esophagus as far as the fifth thoracic vertebra near which the trachea bifurcates. The arch of the aorta, passing back to reach the vertebral column, crosses to the left side of the esophagus, causing a slight deviation of the esophagus to the right. The thoracic aorta lies first to the left of the esophagus, then posterior to it, and finally, both posterior and to the right of it.

Immediately below the level of the bifurcation of the trachea, the esophagus is crossed by the left bronchus, and in the rest of its thoracic course it lies close to the posterior surface of the pericardium. In this location it is situated in the posterior mediastinum, and is separated from the vertebral column by the azygos vein, thoracic duct and lower thoracic aorta. It is in close proximity with the left atrium, and any enlargement of the latter structure is reflected in displacement of the esophagus posteriorly and to the right (Fig. 11–5).

The two vagus nerves descend to the esophagus after forming the anterior and posterior pulmonary plexuses, and unite with the sympathetic branches to form the anterior and posterior esophageal plexuses. The left vagus then winds anteriorly and the right posteriorly, and the two vagi descend in the esophageal sheath through the diaphragm to reach the stomach.

The esophagus is connected with the esophageal orifice of the diaphragm by strong fibrous tissue throughout its circumference, but any defects in this supportive tissue may cause hiatal protrusion of the stomach.

The abdominal portion of the esophagus is approximately 1 to 3 cm. in length and runs in the esophageal groove on the posterior surface of the liver.

The phrenic ampulla is that portion of the esophagus which lies just above the esophageal orifice of the diaphragm (Fig. 13–5). It is rather bulbous, and variable in dimensions, and radiographically causes confusion with a hiatal hernia of the stomach through the diaphragm. The esophageal ampulla appears as a segmented ovoid structure 3 to 5 cm. in length and 2 to 4 cm. in diameter which is separable from the stomach pattern below. The hiatal herniation of the fundus through the diaphragm is considerably more variable in size, and its rugal pattern can usually be more closely identified with that of the contiguous portion of the stomach.

The cardiac antrum is another name for the intra-abdominal portion of the esophagus. This area has been called the esophageal vestibule also. The vestibule is often situated above the diaphragm, and may be responsible for an appearance which resembles closely a sliding hernia. The inferior esophageal sphincter is situated between the vestibule and the ampulla, but should not be confused with a thick fibrous band occasionally encountered, called a "Schatzki ring" (Fig. 13–5 c).

The diaphragm and its ligamentous esophageal attachments at the esophageal hiatus produce a valve-like action spoken of as "constrictor cardiae."

Normal Points of Narrowness in the Esophagus. There are three definite constrictions in the normal esophagus (Fig. 13–6): one at its cricoid beginning, a second opposite the crossing of the left bronchus, and the third where it passes through the diaphragm. The lumen at the site of the upper two constrictions is smaller than the third, and ordinarily, when a foreign body fails to pass down the esophagus, the site of obstruction occurs at one of the two upper points of narrowness.

The cardiac sphincter is not a true sphincter as is the pyloric sphincter. The sphincteric action is probably secondary to the muscular action of the diaphragm through its esophageal orifice. Thus when the diaphragm contracts as in inspiration, there is a momentary delay of a bolus of food at this level, and during expiration, emptying of the esophagus proceeds normally.

Johnstone[2] has reported that the cardiac sphincter may or may not be at the level of the esophageal hiatus of the diaphragm, and prefers to designate the constrictor action of the diaphragm at the level of the esophageal hiatus as the "constrictor cardiae." The cardiac sphincter, may, on the other hand, produce a slight constriction of the esophagus between the ampulla and the vestibule (inferior esophageal sphincter), and when the vestibule is above the level of the diaphragm, an appearance simulating an hiatal hernia is produced (Fig. 13–6, **d**).

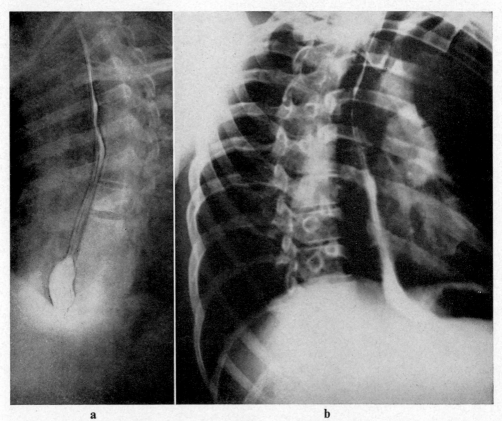

a   b

FIG. 13 5. RADIOGRAPH OF ESOPHAGUS: **a,** Demonstrating the esophageal phrenic ampulla (intensified); **b,** showing rugal pattern of esophagus.

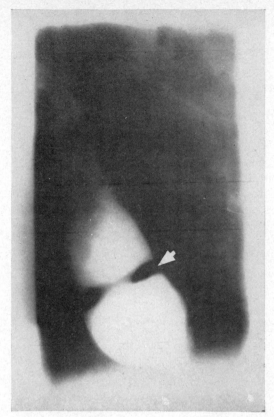

FIG. 13–5. **c,** Radiograph demonstrating Schatzki's ring.7

The Normal Rugal Pattern of the Esophagus. The mucous coat of the esophagus is very loosely connected with the muscular coat by the areolar tissue of the submucous layer. When the esophagus is empty, the mucous coat is thrown into a series of longitudinal folds (Fig. 13–6); otherwise it is very smooth in contrast with the mammillated gastric mucous membrane.

The longitudinal folds of the empty or partially empty esophagus impart to the radiographic picture the typical rugal pattern attributed to this organ. These consist of parallel lines throughout the esophagus which become more closely approximated as the distal funnel end of the esophagus is reached just above the cardia.

Abnormalities in the esophageal wall are reflected to a great extent in alteration of this normal rugal pattern, either by the appearance of abnormal folds, or by the lack of folds.

Venous Drainage of the Lower Esophagus—and Its Importance. The veins of the esophagus form a plexus exteriorly. The venous drainage of the lower esophagus passes to the coronary vein of the stomach, and the latter vein empties into the portal vein. Higher up, the veins of the esophagus empty into the azygos system and thyroid veins. (See Chapter 12.)

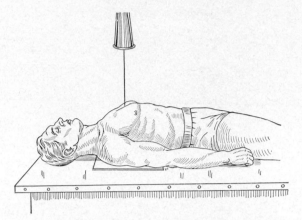

FIG. 13–6. ANTERO-POSTERIOR FILM STUDY OF ESOPHAGUS: **a,** Positioning of Patient.

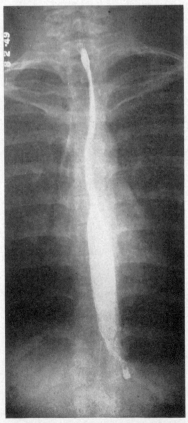

FIG. 13–6. ANTERO-POSTERIOR FILM STUDY OF ESOPHAGUS: **b,** Radiograph.

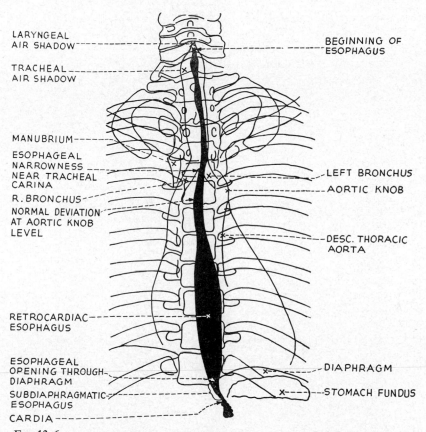

LARYNGEAL
AIR SHADOW

BEGINNING OF
ESOPHAGUS

TRACHEAL
AIR SHADOW

MANUBRIUM

ESOPHAGEAL
NARROWNESS
NEAR TRACHEAL
CARINA

LEFT BRONCHUS

AORTIC KNOB

R. BRONCHUS

NORMAL DEVIATION
AT AORTIC KNOB
LEVEL

DESC. THORACIC
AORTA

RETROCARDIAC
ESOPHAGUS

ESOPHAGEAL
OPENING THROUGH
DIAPHRAGM

DIAPHRAGM

SUBDIAPHRAGMATIC
ESOPHAGUS

STOMACH FUNDUS

CARDIA

FIG. 13–6.   ANTERO-POSTERIOR FILM STUDY OF ESOPHAGUS: **c,** Labeled tracing of **b.**

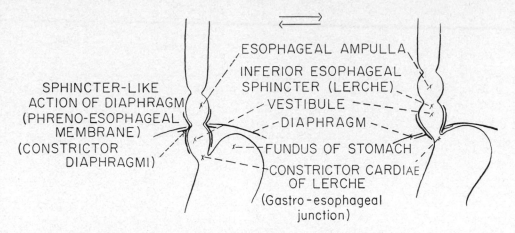

FIG. 13–6. **d,** Diagram illustrating the relationship of the inferior esophageal sphincter, vestibule, ampulla, constrictor diaphragmi and constrictor cardii. (Modified after Johnstone; Lerche; and Poppel, Zaino and Lentino.)

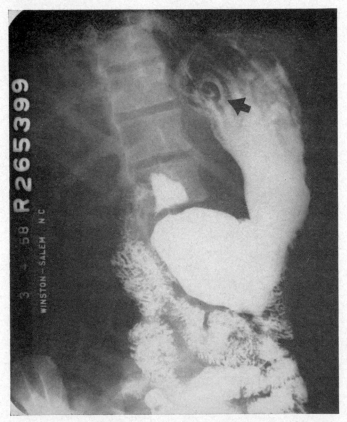

FIG. 13–6. **e,** "Epithelial ring" at the cardio-esophageal junction.

Thus, the esophagus forms a communicating link between the portal circulation on the one hand and the systemic veins on the other, since the azygos vein empties into the superior vena cava.

Obstruction of the portal vein from any cause may, in turn, cause considerable distention of the lower esophageal veins and other tributaries of the coronary vein of the stomach. These irregular distentions are spoken of as "varices," and have the appearance and the same physiologic significance as hemorrhoids in the case of the anal canal. These veins may rupture and cause considerable embarrassment from bleeding. They produce a marked irregularity of the rugal pattern of the lower esophagus, especially when the venous pressure is increased as in the case of forced expiration. Indeed, the relative disappearance of the irregularity in deep inspiration, and reappearance with forced expiration is pathognomonic of esophageal varices.

The Normal Swallowing Function.   The process of deglutition has been very completely described by Barclay[1] and more thoroughly studied by cineradiography in recent times. Indeed the latter expedient has permitted very close analysis. Briefly, the sequence of events is as follows:

1. There is a forward and upward movement of the tongue which displaces the contents of the mouth backward.

2. The larynx rises and the pharyngeal space becomes obliterated for a fraction of a second.

3. With a backward thrust, the base of the tongue forces the bolus downward.

4. Once the bolus has passed the epiglottis, filled the pyriform recesses and entered the esophagus, air begins to enter the nasopharynx, the soft palate relaxes, and the epiglottis and larynx begin to return to their resting position.

5. In frontal projection, the epiglottis produces the appearance of a central ovoid filling defect during the act of swallowing.

6. According to Barclay,[1] the chief function of the epiglottis is to form a trap, along with the vallecula, for saliva running down over the back of the tongue between the acts of deglutition. When food is trapped by the epiglottis, it is forced into the vallecula, thereafter to be swallowed later.

7. Below the level of the upper third of the esophagus, peristaltic action carries the food bolus down into the stomach. The peristalis begins in the posterior pharynx and is shallow in type and not occlusive.

8. The function of the gastro-esophageal segment (Fig. 13–6, **d**) is quite complex, and there is still disagreement in relation to this area. This segment may be divided into a:

(*a*) Phrenic ampulla;

(*b*) Interior esophageal sphincter;

(*c*) Gastro-esophageal vestibule;

(*d*) Constrictor cardiae;

(*e*) Constrictor diaphragmatis, or phreno-esophageal membrane.

The phrenic esophageal ampulla is a physiologic dilatation of the lower esophagus which can be identified particularly when this region is distended by a bolus of food or barium. It may be seen most clearly in full inspiration. The ampulla is accentuated by a contraction or constriction of the esophagus just proximal to it. Just distal to the ampulla there is a contraction in the esophagus at the site of the inferior esophageal sphincter, which coincides in position with the constrictor diaphragmi in deep inspiration.

The anatomic presence of the inferior esophageal sphincter has been demonstrated by Lerche.[3] The narrowing produced in the esophageal appearance in this area is due in part to the contraction of the sphincter and in part to the downward pull of the phreno-esophageal membrane, the upper end of which is attached at this point.

The phreno-esophageal membrane is the anchor ng apparatus for the lower esophagus to the diaphragm. This membrane divid i into an ascending portion which is attached at the level of the inferior esophageal sphincter and into a descending portion which is attached to the muscular coat of the cardia of the stomach in the region of the gastro-esophageal junction. The phreno-esophageal membrane ordinarily serves as a channel for the esophagus, resisting excessive shortening or lengthening of the organ during the act of respiration. On the other hand, in deep inspiration the diaphragm constricts the lower end of the esophagus (constrictor diaphragmatis) and in expiration the area opens up fully. With changes in position, there is a sliding movement of the esophagus in this area so that the relationship of the esophagus to the diaphragm actually changes with respiration.

The gastro-esophageal vestibule corresponds with the abdominal portion of the esophagus. This has been referred to as the gastric antrum or antechamber of the stomach. It extends from the inferior esophageal sphincter to the constrictor cardiae. When the phrenic ampulla is full, the vestibule is ordinarily empty. It is essential that the gastro-esophageal vestibule be recognized so that it may not be mistaken for a sliding hiatal hernia. When the vestibule is empty the longitudinal rugae are thin and parallel and resemble closely the rugal pattern of the esophagus above this level. When the vestibule is full, however, there is an effacement of the rugae and there is a close resemblance to the rugae of the gastric fundus. Hence serial film studies are necessary to differentiate this area accurately.

The constrictor cardiae is at the gastro-esophageal junction and ordinarily is located beneath the diaphragm at the junction of the esophageal and gastric mucosa. There is an abrupt change from the squamous epithelium of the esophagus to the columnar epithelium of the stomach at this site. At times, this epithelial line appears as an epithelial ring and this may be demonstrated radiographically through the gastric air bubble (magenblase) as a ringlike shadow which varies with the degree of contraction or relaxation of the constrictor cardiae.

TECHNIQUE OF EXAMINATION OF THE ESOPHAGUS

The proper examination of the esophagus involves a combination of fluoroscopy and radiography, including spot-film radiography, careful attention to detail being most important.

Fluoroscopy. The patient should, if possible, be first examined in the erect position. The chest is first inspected in the antero-posterior position for any gross abnormality; then, in the right anterior oblique position the region in which the esophagus lies is examined for any opaque abnormality.

Thereafter, the patient is asked to swallow a mouthful of thick barium paste, and his swallowing function and esophageal structure are studied in the postero-anterior and both oblique positions, bearing in mind the physiologic and anatomic features previously described.

The patient may thereafter be asked to swallow a barium capsule or cotton ball soaked in barium sulfate, to visualize any point of obstruction which might not appear by routine examination. Occasionally, a pointed foreign body will catch the cotton ball, and thus become demonstrable. Great caution, however, must be used in the interpretation of interference with the passage of a cotton ball, since this may occur normally. The cotton ball should not exceed 4 mm. in diameter.

Thereafter, the patient is asked to swallow a thin barium sulfate suspension and is once again fluoroscoped in all projections. Forced inspiration and expiration are particularly important from the standpoint of demonstration of possible esophageal varices.

The patient is then placed in the recumbent supine position and asked to swallow another mouthful of thin barium suspension, and the study of the esophagus is repeated. The Trendelenburg position is also employed, particularly when a hiatal hernia is seen or suspected.

Spot-film Radiography. This is of great importance when an abnormality is detected fluoroscopically, since this abnormality may not be demonstrated by routine radiographic procedures.

The following routine films are taken immediately after fluoroscopy.

The Antero-posterior Film Study of the Esophagus (Fig. 13–6). In this projection, the esophagus is tapered superiorly and inferiorly immediately above the diaphragm, and is largely a midline structure, except where it is deviated to the right by the left bronchus impression in the upper part of its course, and below as it courses slightly to the left and anteriorly in the region of the diaphragm. There may be a very slight impression by the left auricular appendage, displacing the esophagus slightly to the right also. If this displacement is more than extremely slight, it is usually indicative of enlargement of the left atrium.

The Right Anterior Oblique Projection (Fig. 13–7). In this projection the esophagus is rather closely applied to the spine in the neck, and to the posterior margin of the pericardium in the thorax. The previously described "aortic" indentation in the region of the left bronchus is also seen to displace the esophagus slightly posteriorly. There is a slight indentation of the esophagus in the region of the left atrium, which is in a posterior position. The clear space behind the esophagus increases above the diaphragm, in view of the gradually increasing anterior course of the esophagus.

The Left Anterior Oblique Projection (Fig. 13–8). In this view, the slight posterior impression produced by the left bronchus is once again seen, but otherwise, the esophagus courses directly down to the diaphragm on the anterior aspect of the thoracic spine.

Iodized Oil Study of the Esophagus. Iodized oil is possibly somewhat less irritating when inhaled into the trachea or bronchial tree than is the barium sulfate suspension. On the other hand, it is more expensive and somewhat more irritating to gastric mucosa.

When a patient gives a history of extreme difficulty in swallowing, followed by considerable coughing, it is usually indicative that the patient inhales the swallowed bolus at least in part. In such instances, it is advisable first to study the patient's swallowing function with iodized oil rather than barium mixture.

This is particularly true in cases of pharyngeal palsies, pseudopharyngeal palsies, and such congenital anomalies as esophageal atresias, where there is usually a communication between the esophagus and the trachea or bronchial tree.

Iodized oil media should not be used for examination beyond the esophagus

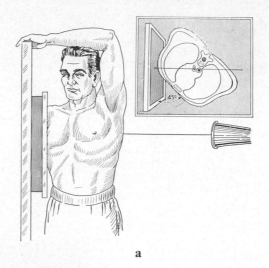

a

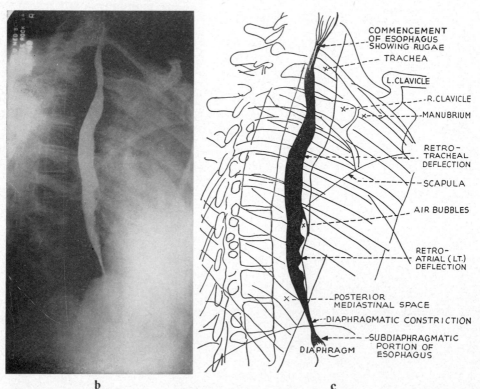

b   c

FIG. 13–7. RIGHT ANTERIOR OBLIQUE VIEW OF ESOPHAGUS (THIS SAME POSITION IS FREQUENTLY TAKEN IN THE RECUMBENT AS WELL): **a,** Positioning of patient; **b,** radiograph; **c,** labeled tracing of **b.**

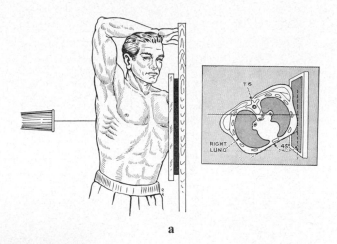

a

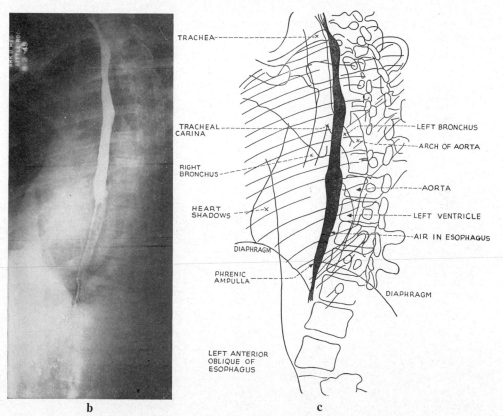

b c

FIG. 13–8. LEFT ANTERIOR OBLIQUE PROJECTION OF ESOPHAGUS: a, Positioning of patient (recumbent may also be used); b, radiograph (intensified); c, labeled tracing of b.

THE STOMACH

Subdivisions of the Stomach.   The stomach is arbitrarily divided into three parts: the fundus, the body and the pyloric portions (Fig. 13–9).

The fundus is that portion of the stomach which lies above a horizontal plane through the junction of the stomach and esophagus (this latter being called the "cardiac orifice" or "cardia"), and the pyloric portion is that part which falls between the incisura angularis and the pylorus. The body is represented by the intervening portion.

The right wall of the cardia merges into the lesser curvature of the stomach, while the left wall is deeply notched by the cardiac incisura.

A pyloric constriction marks the junction between the stomach and duodenum. The pyloric sphincter is sharply demarcated from the duodenum, but blends imperceptibly with the thickened musculature of the pyloric antrum. The pyloric canal traverses the pyloric sphincter and is approximately 5 mm. in length. The gastric mucous membrane is continued into the duodenum without any alteration visible to the naked eye.

The greater curvature corresponds in its greater part with the attachment of the gastrosplenic and gastrocolic ligaments.

Stomach Contour Variations in Accordance with Body Build (Fig. 13–10). Gastric tone and contour normally follow the habitus of the individual very

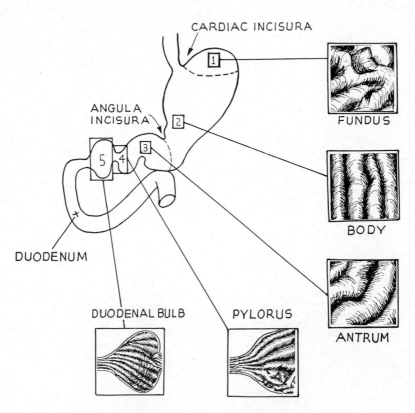

DIFFERENCES IN RUGAL PATTERN

Fig. 13–9.   stomach·   a, Subdivisions and rugal pattern.

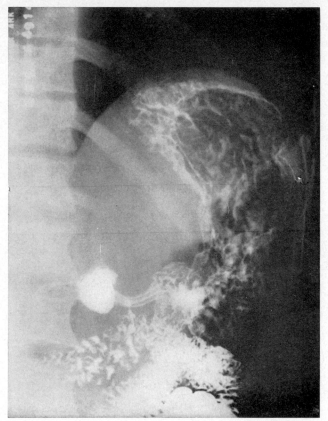

Fig. 13-9. STOMACH: **b,** Radiograph showing rugal pattern. (The distal portion of the pyloric antrum is in a contracted state and its rugal pattern merges imperceptibly with the pattern of the pyloric canal.)

closely. In the individual who is short and stocky, the stomach is usually high in position and "steer-horn" in shape, its lumen being largest above and tapering toward the pylorus. It extends more quickly toward the right. The incisura angularis is difficult to identify, and occasionally the pylorus is the lowermost part of the stomach.

In the sthenic individual, the eutonic stomach is J-shaped, and the body of the stomach tends to be vertical in the frontal projection and uniform in size. The lowermost part of the stomach in the erect position tends to be at the level of the iliac crests.

In asthenic individuals, the stomach tends to be hypotonic, and shaped rather like a fishhook. The greater curvature tends to sag down into the pelvis, with the greatest diameter between the incisura angularis and the adjoining greater curvature.

Each of the stomach types may occur in individuals of any body build, but in general the hypotonic stomach tends to occur more frequently in underweight individuals, whereas the steer-horn type tends to occur more frequently in the overweight. Indeed, according to a recent study which we have conducted,[2] when the hypotonic stomach occurs in an overweight individual, it is almost invariably symptomatic. Likewise, a cascade stomach tends to be symptomatic in an overweight individual, whereas in normal or underweight individuals the cascade stomach is relatively asymptomatic. The symptoms are very vague abdominal distress, sometimes suggestive of peptic ulcer.

The normal relationships of each type of stomach to each type of body build have been carefully worked out and tabulated as shown in Figure 13–11. Measurements can be taken as indicated and should fall within the normal range; if they are outside this normal range, one should be strongly suspicious of displacement of the stomach by some extrinsic lesion (See Table 13–1).

Variations of the Stomach in Different Positions (Fig. 13–10). Gravity will influence the position of the gastric contents and the position and contour of the stomach.

Thus, in the supine recumbent position, there is a tendency for the stomach to move upward. At the same time gastric contents will flow into the fundus, and

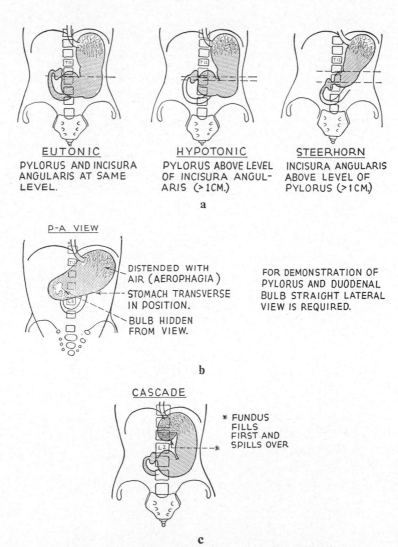

EUTONIC
PYLORUS AND INCISURA ANGULARIS AT SAME LEVEL.

HYPOTONIC
PYLORUS ABOVE LEVEL OF INCISURA ANGULARIS (>1CM.)

STEERHORN
INCISURA ANGULARIS ABOVE LEVEL OF PYLORUS (>1CM.)

a

P-A VIEW

DISTENDED WITH AIR (AEROPHAGIA)
STOMACH TRANSVERSE IN POSITION.
BULB HIDDEN FROM VIEW.

FOR DEMONSTRATION OF PYLORUS AND DUODENAL BULB STRAIGHT LATERAL VIEW IS REQUIRED.

b

CASCADE

* FUNDUS FILLS FIRST AND SPILLS OVER

c

FIG. 13–10. VARIATIONS IN STOMACH CONTOUR. a, In relation to body build and general stomach type. b, The infantile stomach. c, The cascade stomach.

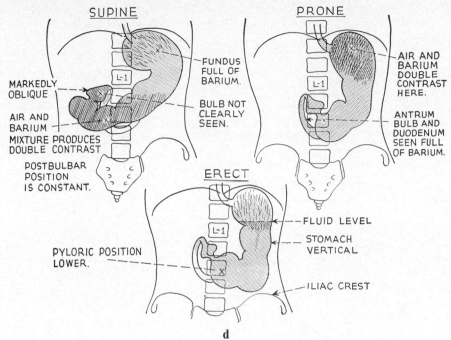

FIG. 13–10. VARIATIONS IN STOMACH CONTOUR. **d,** In relation to body position.

the air in the stomach, which in the erect position is found in the fundus, will move anteriorly and occupy the anterior portion of the body of the stomach. Some of the air is invariably trapped in the pyloric portion also, but if there is sufficient barium suspension in the stomach, the pyloric portion and duodenal bulb will fill with it as well as with entrapped air, producing a double contrast effect.

In the prone recumbent position, the gravity relationship is reversed. The barium mixture usually flows into the pyloric portion while the gas moves into the fundus. At the same time, there is a tendency for the stomach itself to move downward slightly, more closely resembling the appearance in the erect position.

In order to separate the shadows of the pyloric antrum and the duodenal bulb, it is usually necessary to place the patient in a slight right anterior oblique position. Otherwise these structures usually overlie one another.

The lateral projection also finds wide usefulness, in that one can demonstrate positional relationships of the stomach to the pancreas and the omental bursa with greatest accuracy in this projection. The *left* lateral *standing* view is most valuable for this purpose since the relationship of the stomach to retrogastric structures is most accurately depicted thereby. On the other hand, in the *right* lateral *recumbent* position, the stomach swings forward on its two areas of fixation (diaphragm and post-bulbar duodenum), changing its relationship to the retrogastric structures. In this latter view, however, the pyloric antrum and body of the stomach fall anteriorly away from the level of the duodenum, producing a clearer depiction of the pyloro-bulbar area.

When the patient is supine, the stomach does not necessarily fall closely toward the retrogastric structures. This relationship is sometimes altered by the

Table 13–1. Measurements 4, 9, 10, 11, and 13 are defined in Figure 13–11. (From Meschan, I., et al.: South. M.J. 46:878, 1953.)

RELATIONSHIPS OF STOMACH AND DUODENUM TO THE SPINE IN DIFFERENT WEIGHT AND STOMACH TYPE GROUPS
(BOTH ASYMPTOMATIC AND SYMPTOMATIC SUMMATED)

Weight Group	Stomach Type	No. of Cases	4 Rt. Lat. Avg. of Medians	4 Rt. Lat. Range	4 Lt. Lat. Avg. of Medians	4 Lt. Lat. Range	9 Rt. Lat. Avg. of Medians	9 Rt. Lat. Range	10 Rt. Lat. Avg. of Medians	10 Rt. Lat. Range	11 Rt. Lat. Avg. of Medians	11 Rt. Lat. Range	13 Rt. Lat. Avg. of Medians	13 Rt. Lat. Range
NORMAL	J-shape	58	5.5	1—8.5	4	0—8	6.5	4—9.5	3	—1—9	3	0—12.5	4	—0.5—8
NORMAL	Fish-hook	10	4	1.5—6	3	0.5—6.5	6	4—8	3	2.5—4	5.6	3.5—8	4.5	2.5—9
NORMAL	Cascade	13	6	1—13	5.5	1.5—13	6	4.5—6	4.3	2—9.5	6.6	1—11	6	2.5—9
NORMAL	Steer-horn	9	5	0—11	4	1—13	6.5	5.5—8	3.5	—0.5—5	5.5	1.5—9	5	2.5—10
UNDERWT	J-shape	56	4.5	1.5—7	2	0.5—8	5.5	2—11	3	—0.5—7	4	0—9	3	0.5—6.5
UNDERWT	Fish-hook	21	4	0—7.5	2.6	—1.5—4.5	5.5	3.5—8	2.5	0—5	3	1.5—5	2.5	1—4
UNDERWT	Cascade	5	5	2—8	2.6	0—5	6	5.5—6.5	2.5	2—3.5	4.5	4—5	3	2—5
UNDERWT	Steer-horn	3	5	4.5—6	6.5	0.5—7.5	8	6.5—8	4.5	2—6	7	6.5—8	4	1.5—5
OVERWT	J-shape	13	5.5	1.5—10	4	1.5—8.5	6.5	4—9	3.3	2—7	4.5	3.5—9	3.5	1.5—9.5
OVERWT	Fish-hook	5	5	3—	4	0—5.5	5	3—7.5	2.5	0—4	4.5	2—9.5	4.6	3—6.5
OVERWT	Cascade	10	5	2—11	5.5	0—9	7	4—9	4	1—7.5	5	1.5—10	5.6	3—12
OVERWT	Steer-horn	8	6	2.5—9.5	4.6	2.5—8	6	5.5—8	4	3.5—5.5	5	3—7.5	4.5	3—7.5

211

* Asymptomatic cascade is farther from spine than symptomatic

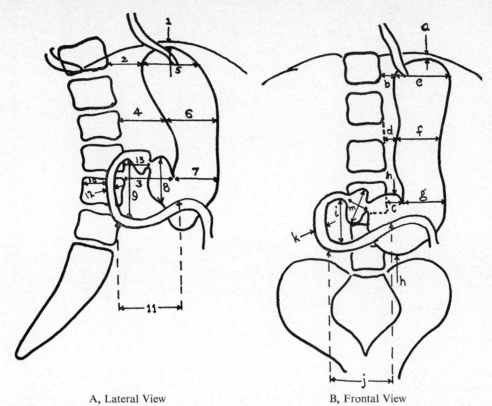

A, Lateral View   B, Frontal View

FIG. 13–11.   Lateral and frontal views of the stomach showing the various measurements which can be taken in an effort to associate the normal stomach with body build. (From Meschan, I., et al.: South. M. J. vol. 46, 1953.)

1, Distance between top of fundus and diaphragm.

2, Cardia of the stomach to the anterior .spine

3, Stomach to anterior spine at the level of the cardia.

4, Stomach to anterior spine midway between cardia and incisura angularis.

5, Horizontal measurement of the fundus at the level of the cardia.

6, Horizontal midway measurement of the body of the stomach at the level of measurement 4.

7, Horizontal measurement of the stomach at the level of the incisura angularis.

8, Maximal vertical measurement of the pyloric antrum.

9, Maximal vertical internal diameter of the duodenal loop.

10, Minimal measurement of the outer margin of the second portion of the duodenum to the posterior margin of the vertebral bodies.

11, Maximal horizontal internal diameter ot the duodenal loop

12, Maximal outer diameter of the second part of the duodenum.

13, Distance between the pylorus and the anterior margin of the spine.

a, Measurement between the diaphragm and top of fundus.

b, Distance between the cardia and lateral margin of spine.

c, Distance between the incisura angularis and lateral margin of the spine.

d, Distance between the stomach and the lateral margin of the spine midway between b and c.

e, Maximal horizontal measurement of the fundus at the level of the cardia.

f, Midway measurement of the body of the stomach at the level of measurement d.

g, Horizontal measurement of the body of the stomach at the level of the incisura angularis.

h, Maximal vertical measurement of the pyloric antrum.

i, Maximal vertical internal diameter of the duodenal loop.

j, Maximal horizontal internal diameter of the duodenal loop.

k, Diameter of the second part of the duodenum.

m, Ratio of the measurement of the base of the bulb over its height from apex to pylorus.

fact that the gas content of the stomach causes it to rise anteriorly. In our experience, therefore, a left lateral study of the stomach, obtained with a horizontal x-ray beam and the patient lying supine, is *less* valuable for study of stomach relationships to retrogastric structures than is the left lateral erect position.

Other Factors Which Influence Gastric Contour (Fig. 13–10).   Vagal stimulation increases gastric tone, whereas sympathetic stimulation decreases it. Thus, when an individual is frightened or otherwise emotionally disturbed, the stomach tends to be hypotonic. These psychic effects are usually temporary. Pathologic processes in the gastrointestinal and biliary tracts will also cause changes in gastric contour, but these are outside the scope of the present text.

Important Anatomic Relationships of the Stomach.   The position of the stomach varies in different individuals, and in the same individual depending upon posture and emotional factors, as well as upon the digestive state (Fig. 13–10). The pylorus may lie as high as the twelfth thoracic vertebra, or as low as the upper sacrum. It may lie in the midline, or to the right or left of it. Associated with these different positions of the pylorus, there is a difference in the position of the first part of the duodenum, and its relation to the head of the pancreas. Likewise, the stomach may be high and the liver low, and vice versa, indicating no definite relation between their relative positions.

Ordinarily, the stomach is obliquely placed in the left upper abdominal cavity (Fig. 13–10), with the fundus somewhat more lateral than the pylorus. In the lateral projection, the fundus is posterior to the liver, in apposition with the diaphragm above and behind. The body of the stomach is anterior, lying immediately under the anterior abdominal wall. The pyloric antrum extends obliquely posteriorly, superiorly, and to the right. Usually the pylorus is situated

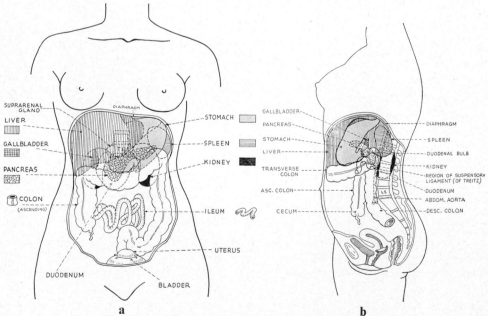

a   b

FIG. 13–12.   IMPORTANT ANATOMIC RELATIONSHIPS OF THE STOMACH: **a,** Antero-posterior view: **b,** lateral view (right, recumbent).

just above the head of the pancreas (Fig. 13–11) in the posterior part of the abdomen, in a plane just anterior (1 to 2 cm.) to the plane of the second part (retroperitoneal portion) of the duodenum.

The hepatogastric and hepatoduodenal ligaments constitute the lesser omentum which is attached to the lesser curvature of the stomach and forms a part of the omental bursa—an anatomic relationship of considerable practical significance.

The spleen lies posterior and somewhat lateral to the body of the stomach, with the gastrosplenic ligament attaching it to the greater curvature of the stomach.

The head of the pancreas lies in the duodenal loop, whereas the body of the pancreas lies posterior to the pyloric portion of the stomach. The tail of the pancreas usually lies just posterior to the body of the stomach, and comes into contact with the medial surface of the spleen. The pancreas forms a large part of the posterior wall of the omental bursa, whereas the posterior wall of the stomach forms the greater part of the anterior wall of this important "sac." Abnormalities of this bursa and the pancreas are therefore frequently reflected in pressure upon the stomach, with alteration of the normal gastric contour.

The transverse colon is loosely connected with the greater curvature of the stomach via the greater omentum, which hangs like an apron over the entire intestinal tract. The splenic flexure of the colon is lateral to the lower greater curvature of the stomach, and closely applied to the undersurface of the spleen.

In most texts dealing with gross anatomy, there is reference to the "stomach chamber" or "bed" in which the stomach is said to lie. Radiographically, the stomach usually extends more inferiorly than is indicated by the dissection of the cadavers.

The Rugal Pattern of Each Subdivision of the Stomach (Fig. 13–9). When the stomach is wholly or partially empty, the muscular layers contract and throw the mucosa into numerous folds or rugae which project into the interior of the stomach. The rugae of the fundus tend to be arranged in a mosaic, which gradually becomes more regular in the body of the stomach. The mosaic appearance is more marked along the greater curvature and this pattern gradually diminishes toward the pylorus.

The rugae tend to remain parallel in a narrow segment on the lesser curvature of the stomach throughout the entire length of the stomach from the cardia to the pylorus.

These longitudinal rugae which begin at the cardia and run the full length of the stomach to the pylorus form the "magenstrasse," which seems to constitute a channel for the usual descent of the food, although not invariably so.

The rugae in the pylorus are thin parallel folds. These parallel folds continue into the duodenal cap or bulb, where they remain parallel, or spiral toward the apex of the duodenal bulb.

Between the rugae, there are minute depressions due to the openings of the small gastric glands, and minute ridges around them, giving the stomach mucosa the so-called mammillated appearance. These minute mammillae are not recognizable radiographically.

The rugal pattern of the stomach must not be thought of as being completely static, in that it can vary in the same individual under different physiologic conditions. Thus, it will vary in accordance with the degree of vascularity of the mucosa and submucosa, and also with the degree of distention of the stomach. Cold tends to make the rugae smaller and more numerous, and certain chemicals such as pilocarpine and physostigmine have the same effect, whereas atropine has the opposite effect.

However, the rugal pattern will change in certain pathologic states such as inflammation, ulceration and neoplastic infiltration, as well as from extrinsic pressure, and the rugae thus become one of the most accurate indices which the radiologic examination of the stomach furnishes. Examination for rugal pattern constitutes one of the most important aspects of the gastrointestinal examination, if not the most important.

MOTOR PHYSIOLOGY OF THE STOMACH

Normal Persistalsis.   Normal peristalsis usually begins high in the body of the stomach, where it is usually quite shallow. As the peristaltic waves descend. they become deeper—being deeper on the greater curvature than on the lesser until the incisura angularis is reached. In the pyloric antrum the waves are usually sufficiently deep to obliterate completely the gastric lumen. Usually, there are two or three simultaneous waves in the stomach at the same time. Ordinarily, it is considered that five or more visible simultaneous peristaltic waves are abnormal, and indicate a state of hyperperistalsis.

Study of Gastric Evacuation.   The stomach will empty its contents when the pressure in the stomach exceeds the pressure in the duodenum, and regurgitation from the duodenum will occur whenever there is a reversal in this pressure relationship. There has been considerable speculation as to the exact function of the pyloric sphincter. Thomas and also Meschan and Quigley have demonstrated the time relationship of contractions of the stomach, pylorus and duodenal bulb (in dogs) and the response of the pylorus to all different types of food stimuli. From these experiments, it would seem that the pylorus does not function to prevent the egress of food *normally*, but rather it serves to prevent the regurgitation of food from the duodenum into the stomach. The contraction and relaxation of the pylorus follow very closely upon identical behavior of the pyloric antrum, whereas the pylorus is closed when the duodenal bulb is contracting, and hence the bolus does not move backward into the stomach, but moves onward down the duodenum. This does not occur at all times, and a certain amount of regurgitation is normal. Regurgitation is to a great extent responsible for the proper neutralization of gastric chyme. These findings are in contradistinction to those advanced by Cannon some years ago, that acid on the stomach side serves to open the pylorus and thus permit gastric evacuation, and acid on the duodenal side causes a closure of the pylorus.

The pyloric antrum, pylorus and duodenal bulb act as a single unit in response to various food stimuli, and it is the pressure gradient which determines which way the food bolus will go. Structurally, the duodenal bulb represents a transition between the duodenum on the one hand and the pyloric antrum on the other. Functionally, a similar relationship exists. Antral and sphincteric contractions occur at the rate of 3 to 5 per minute, and the duodenal bulbar contractions appear as 3 to 5 rhythmic duodenal contractions, superimposed on a basic antral contraction scheme. As one descends into the duodenum, this basic "tonus" rhythm in tune with the antrum tends to disappear, and only the more frequent duodenal contractions persist.

The study of gastric evacuation is not only an index of pyloric contraction as is so often thought, but an indication of the pressure relationships existing between the stomach and entire duodenum, with the pyloric antrum, sphincter and duodenal bulb acting as the fulcrum in this delicate balance. Any factor which can alter the pressure and tone of any part of this unit will alter the rate of gastric evacuation. In some instances, delayed gastric emptying will be due to relative hypotonicity of the stomach, and in others, it will be caused by a hypertonicity of the duodenum.

Factors Influencing Rate of Gastric Evacuation. Of practical importance are the following normal considerations:

The type of meal will alter the rate of gastric evacuation considerably. The presence of any food will depress gastrobulbar peristalsis, and prolong the emptying time by about three times. This may function by means of a reflex, or hormone (enterogastrone) operating from the duodenum. The presence of alkali such as sodium bicarbonate in the stomach will increase the rate of gastric evacuation. Only isotonicity, with no food substances contained in the meal, will not alter the rate of evacuation. Normally, with food-free barium suspension, emptying will begin almost immediately after the introduction of the barium into the stomach, and the main bulk of the meal will have left the stomach in one hour, with no residual trace in two or three hours. Hypoacidity in the stomach will permit the retention of a coating of barium on the gastric mucosa, which in itself is not an indication of abnormality. Six-hour retention of any significant degree is pathologic, and it is customary to obtain a film in six hours for this purpose.

Cascade Stomach (Fig. 13–13). Occasionally, the posterior portion of the fundus of the stomach will fill first, and the remainder of the stomach will fill by overflow from the fundus. This is spoken of as a "cascade" stomach. This may be related to overdistention of the splenic flexure of the colon, or to localized muscular hypertonus. Occasionally it is related to adhesions between the stomach and the diaphragm, but it cannot be properly called a normal variation under these circumstances.

RADIOGRAPHIC METHOD OF STUDY OF THE STOMACH

Ordinarily, the stomach and duodenum are investigated at the same examination, but it is convenient at this time to consider the technique of examination of the stomach.

Fluoroscopy. Fluoroscopy plays an essential part in the examination of the stomach. The examination is begun with the patient in the erect position if at all possible. Prior to the introduction of a contrast medium only the gas bubble or "magenblase" is visible in the fundus. This may contain a fluid level if there is any amount of gastric juice or fluid in the stomach.

The patient is instructed to swallow a mouthful of barium mixture (approximately 100 gm. of barium sulfate suspended in a glassful of water), and

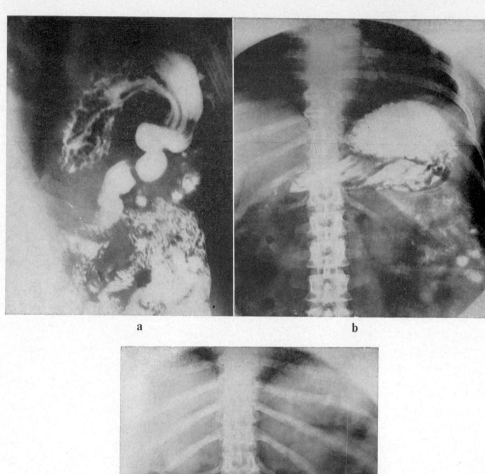

a   b

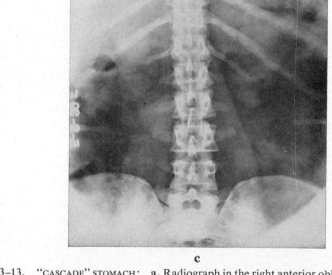

c

FIG. 13–13. "CASCADE" STOMACH: **a,** Radiograph in the right anterior oblique position; **b,** slight cascade stomach in antero-posterior projection; **c,** same as **b** without the barium, showing how the fundus of such a stomach may simulate a mass in the left upper quadrant. (Films **b** and **c** by courtesy of Drs. H. L. Friedell and C. C. Dundon, University Hospitals, Cleveland, Ohio.)

the way in which the barium enters the stomach is carefully studied. It is seen to descend along the lesser curvature at a rate depending on the subject and approaches the lower part of the body and pyloric antrum. In the presence of excessive fluid in the stomach, the barium will drop into the fluid like pellets in a glass of water. The lesser curvature is normally smooth below the cardia and any variation is of definite significance.

This small amount of barium is then massaged into all of the rugal folds of the stomach and duodenal bulb, and the rugal pattern as described above is studied in the frontal as well as the oblique projections. It may at times be necessary to place the patient in the supine or prone positions to accomplish a complete investigation of this pattern at this juncture, but usually the investigator can proceed to examine the stomach when it is full of barium mixture.

When the rugal pattern is satisfactorily studied the patient is then instructed to drink more of the barium mixture, and the swallowing function and esophagus are carefully studied, together with the appearance of the cardiac orifice. Thereafter, the stomach is examined with the aid of compression by the gloved hand in frontal and oblique projections once again, and at this time the contour is examined. The greater curvature has an irregular undulating appearance normally, and abnormal irregularity is difficult to interpret. The splenic flexure of the colon may produce an indentation of the greater curvature also. Both the greater and lesser curvature of the pars pylorica tend to be smoother in outline than the rest of the stomach, but an undulating appearance here is common owing to peristaltic waves. A constant band of contraction or a constant filling defect, however, becomes of definite pathologic significance.

The pyloric canal is ordinarily no greater than 5 mm. in length and 5 to 8 mm. in diameter. The direction of the long axis of the pylorus, like that of the stomach, will depend upon those factors discussed under variation in gastric contour. Tone, body habitus and emotional influences all play a part, as previously indicated. The pylorus is ordinarily centrally placed with respect to the base of the duodenal bulb, and excentricity is likewise of pathologic significance. Its appearance in relation to the duodenal bulb resembles that of a basal stem to its leaf. The rugae of the pyloric canal are quite narrow and parallel, in contrast to the slightly wider rugal pattern of the antrum on the one side, and the bulb on the other.

The rugal pattern of the normal stomach has been discussed above.

Usually, at this point, spot-film compression radiography is carried out and films obtained under fluoroscopic control with compression of any desired parts. The patient is thereafter placed in the supine position, and once again the stomach is studied in the frontal as well as the oblique projections. The competency of the cardiac sphincter is investigated by having the patient strain in suspended respiration against a closed glottis (Valsalva's experiment). To further accentuate this procedure the patient may be placed in the 15-degree Trendelenburg position when it is performed. While the patient is supine, the air in the stomach rises to the antrum and duodenal bulb, and "double contrast" studies of these areas are obtained with "spot-films." Slowly, the patient is turned onto his right side, and the spatial relationships of the stomach and duodenum studied in the lateral projection. Thereafter, with the patient in the prone position, gastric contour and peristalsis are once again carefully scru-

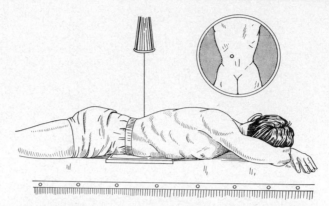

FIG. 13–14.   RECUMBENT POSTERO-ANTERIOR PROJECTION OF STOMACH AND DUODENUM: **a,** Positioning of patient.

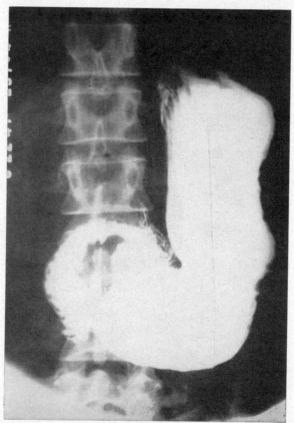

FIG. 13–14.   RECUMBENT POSTERO-ANTERIOR PROJECTION OF STOMACH AND DUODENUM: **b,** Radiograph.

tinized. Spot-film studies of the cardio-esophageal junction are routinely obtained with the Valsalva maneuver while the patient is in the prone position.

Attention is paid throughout this examination to the position, contour, pliability, peristalsis of the stomach, and points of tenderness and masses nearby.

This examination is thereafter followed by certain routine film studies and any special studies as are indicated by the fluoroscopy.

The importance of spot-film compression radiography can hardly be overemphasized in the radiographic study of the gastrointestinal tract. Film visualization of an anatomic part is far more accurate and detailed than is fluoroscopy, and this method of film radiography has the additional advantage of compression, the patient being turned so that the desired anatomy is demonstrated. The permanent recording of a part under fluoroscopic control is possible. It has been repeatedly demonstrated that compression may bring out a defect which otherwise might escape detection.

In addition, the *routine radiographs usually obtained are:* (1) recumbent postero-anterior (prone), straight frontal projection (Fig. 13–14); (2) right anterior oblique prone (Fig. 13–15); (3) right lateral recumbent (Fig. 13–16); (4) postero-anterior full abdominal view in four or six hours for study of the extent of gastric evacuation (Fig. 13–19).

These are demonstrated in the accompanying illustrations, and the various anatomic portions labeled.

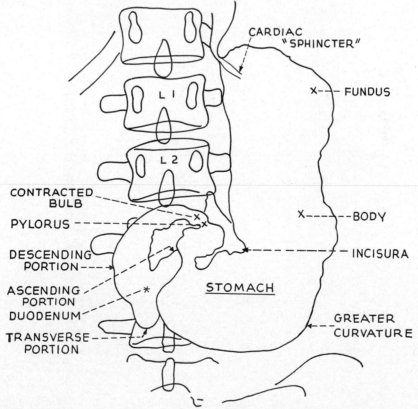

FIG. 13–14. RECUMBENT POSTERO-ANTERIOR PROJECTION OF STOMACH AND DUODENUM: **c,** Labeled tracing of **b.**

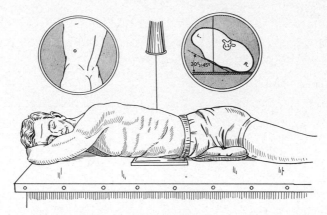

FIG. 13–15.   RIGHT ANTERIOR OBLIQUE PRONE PROJECTION OF STOMACH AND DUODENUM: **a,** Positioning
of patient.

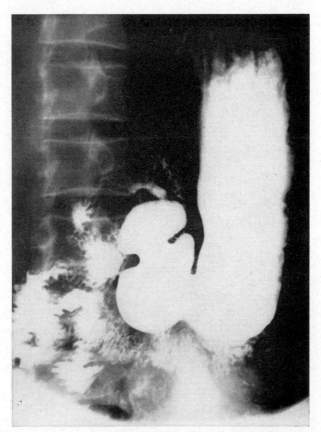

FIG. 13–15.   RIGHT ANTERIOR OBLIQUE PRONE PROJECTION OF STOMACH AND DUODENUM:
b, Radiograph.

Points of Practical Interest With Reference to Figure 13–15:

1. It is often in this position that peristalsis is maximal. Often, when there is an initial delay in gastric evacuation, it is our practice to place the patient in this position for a short while until peristalsis returns and gastric emptying begins.
2. This position is also optimal for passage of a Miller-Abbott or Cantor tube from the stomach into the duodenum, provided the balloon end of the tube is in good relationship with the pyloric antrum. The balloon should not be inflated until this end of the tube reaches the third part of the duodenum.
3. When rigidity of the stomach is suspected, it is well to put the patient in this position and obtain several films in sequence without moving the patient. The films may thereafter be superimposed to study the extent of change over the intervals of time studied. The films obtained should be taken at the rate of two or three per minute.

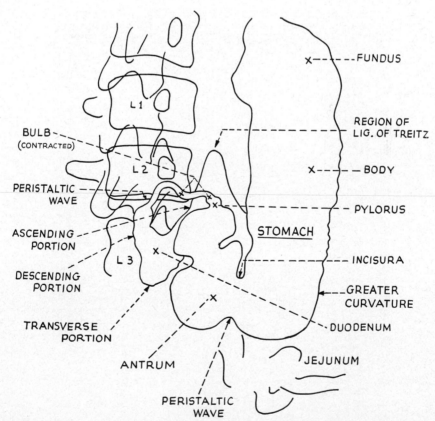

Fig. 13–15.   Right anterior oblique prone projection of stomach and duodenum: **c,** Labeled tracing of **b.**

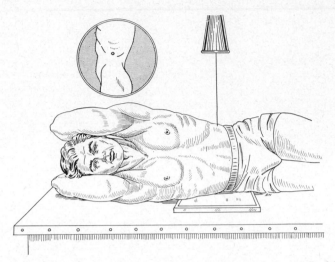

FIG. 13–16.   RIGHT LATERAL RECUMBENT VIEW OF STOMACH AND DUODENUM: **a,** Positioning of patient (both arms may be placed over the head in an alternate position).

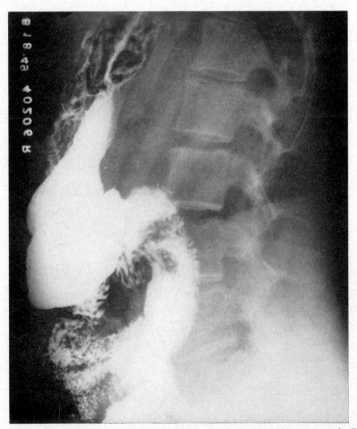

FIG. 13–16.   RIGHT LATERAL RECUMBENT VIEW OF STOMACH AND DUODENUM: **b,** Radiograph.

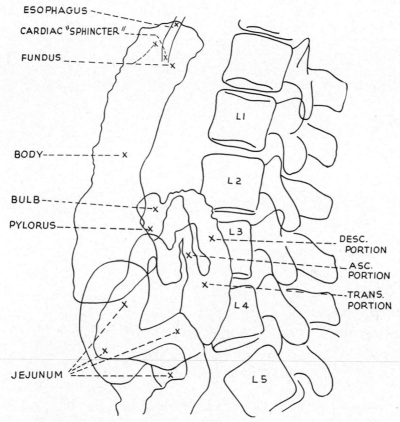

ESOPHAGUS

CARDIAC "SPHINCTER"

FUNDUS

L1

BODY

L2

BULB

PYLORUS

L3

DESC. PORTION

ASC. PORTION

TRANS. PORTION

L4

JEJUNUM

L5

FIG. 13–16.   RIGHT LATERAL RECUMBENT VIEW OF STOMACH AND DUODENUM: **c,** Labeled tracing of

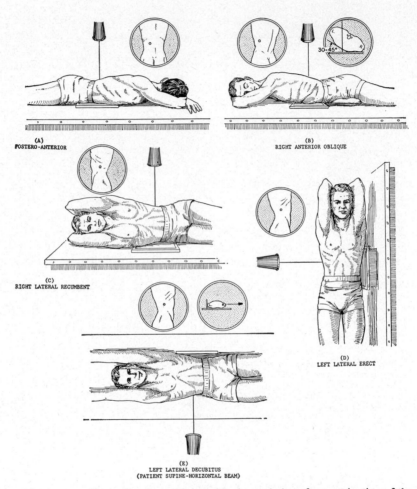

FIG. 13–17. Diagrams illustrating the routine positioning technique for examination of the stomach radiographically, apart from fluoroscopy.

Left Lateral Erect Film of Stomach and Duodenum (Fig. 13–18). The left lateral erect view of the stomach and duodenum is most useful to demonstrate the exact relationship of the stomach to retrogastric structures. Anatomic detail is obscured, and hence this film study is obtained when especially indicated by clinical history suggesting pancreatic or retrogastric disease.

Antero-posterior View of Stomach in Slight Left Posterior Oblique (Fig.13–20). In this position, the air in the stomach rises and when admixed with the barium furnishes a double-contrast visualization of the body, antrum and bulb, and a completely barium-filled fundus. Filling defects and mucosal disturbances are thereby sometimes intensified in these areas.

Air Insufflation of the Stomach. Air may be introduced into the stomach as a special examination either by stomach tube, or indirectly by Seidlitz powders or a carbonated drink. The stomach should be empty for this examination. The direct introduction of air has the advantage of permitting the examination of the dry gastric mucosa, following which the addition of a small amount of barium mixture permits double contrast. The carbonated drink method has the disadvantage of diluting the barium which interferes with its coating property.

In either case the patient is first examined fluoroscopically in all projections, and films in any desired position obtained.

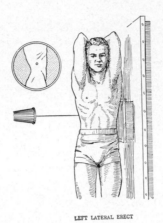

LEFT LATERAL ERECT

FIG. 13–18.   LEFT LATERAL ERECT FILM OF STOMACH: **a,** Position of patient.

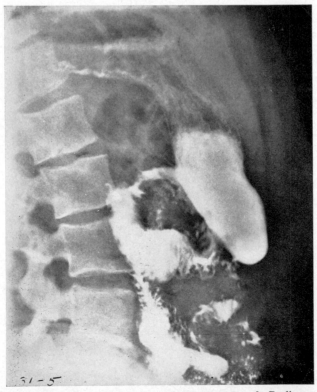

FIG. 13–18.   **LEFT LATERAL ERECT** FILM OF STOMACH: **b,** Radiograph.

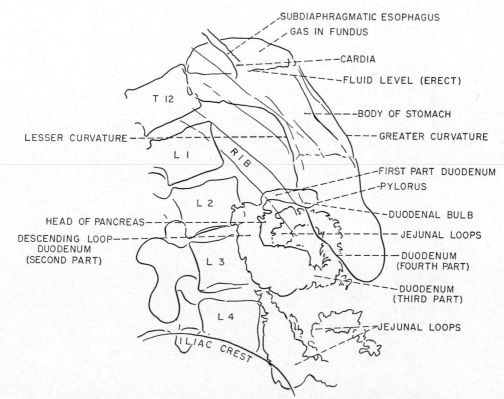

SUBDIAPHRAGMATIC ESOPHAGUS
GAS IN FUNDUS
CARDIA
FLUID LEVEL (ERECT)
BODY OF STOMACH
GREATER CURVATURE
FIRST PART DUODENUM
PYLORUS
DUODENAL BULB
JEJUNAL LOOPS
DUODENUM (FOURTH PART)
DUODENUM (THIRD PART)
JEJUNAL LOOPS

T 12
LESSER CURVATURE
L 1
RIB
L 2
HEAD OF PANCREAS
DESCENDING LOOP DUODENUM (SECOND PART)
L 3
L 4
ILIAC CREST

FIG. 13–18. LEFT LATERAL ERECT FILM OF STOMACH: **c,** Labeled tracing of **b.**

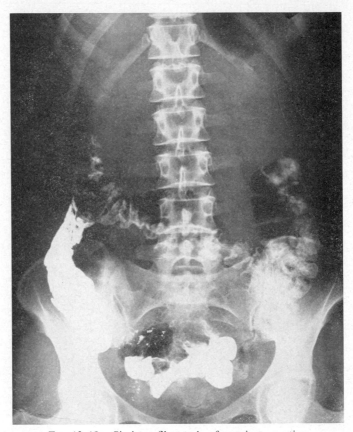

FIG. 13--19.   Six-hour film study of gastric evacuation.

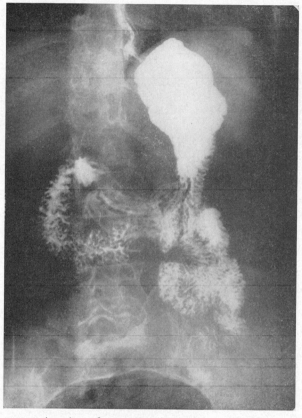

FIG. 13–20. Antero-posterior view of stomach in slight left posterior oblique. Note the excellent double contrast of the distal stomach while the fundus is completely filled with barium.

THE DUODENUM

The duodenum is ordinarily examined simultaneously with the stomach, and its separate consideration here is for the sake of convenience of description only. The first part of the duodenum—the duodenal bulb—is integrated both structurally and functionally with the pyloric antrum. The structure of the remainder of the duodenum resembles that of the small intestine.

The duodenum differs from the rest of the small intestine in several important respects:

1. It has no mesentery, and is fixed to the posterior abdominal wall for the most part.
2. The ducts of the liver, gallbladder and pancreas open into it (at the duodenal papilla, or ampulla of Vater), in the descending part of the duodenum.
3. The duodenum contains some distinctive glands of its own, the duodenal glands of Brunner.
4. It is the shortest, widest, and most fixed portion of the small intestine.

Subdivisions.   The duodenum is variably described as consisting of three or four parts (Figs. 13-14 through 13-16 inclusive):

1. The superior portion, or duodenal bulb, which runs superiorly, backward, and to the right, is in direct continuity with the pylorus of the stomach. This portion has a mesentery of its own for a short distance.
2. The descending portion, which begins at the neck of the gallbladder, and runs down on the posterior abdominal wall, and usually ends opposite about the upper border of the fourth lumbar vertebra on the right of the vertebral column.
3. The inferior part is variably described as one or two separate parts. It consists of a transverse portion (3) which crosses to the left of the midline, across the vena cava, aorta and vertebral column; and ascending portion (4), which ascends on the left of the vertebral column to the inferior surface of the pancreas. There it bends abruptly forward, forming the duodenojejunal flexure.

The duodenum is in the form of a "U," with the superior portion more anterior than the descending part, the transverse portion coming directly forward and to the left, and the ascending portion in the same plane as the superior portion but to the left of the midline.

GROSS ANATOMY AND RELATIONSHIPS OF EACH SUBDIVISION

The Superior Portion, Duodenal Bulb or Cap. Sites of Normal "Fleck" Formation.   This first part of the duodenum is rather conical in shape, approximately 3.5 to 5 cm. in length, and 3 cm. in diameter. It is described as having a base and an apex, the base forming a "stem-and-leaf" relationship with the pyloric canal.

As previously indicated, the rugal pattern of the bulb more closely resembles that of the pyloric antrum than the remainder of the duodenum, tending to be rather parallel, or parallel in spiral fashion from the base to apex. The contraction pattern and motor physiology of the bulb forms a transition between that of the antrum and the distal duodenum.

Radiologically, a "fleck" (from the German meaning "spot") is a loculation of barium of any size from a few millimeters to 2 or more centimeters which strongly suggests a break in the normal mucosal structure and ulceration. In view of the great frequency of ulceration in this area, the detection of a fleck in this location is of extreme importance.

There are certain locations in the duodenal bulb, however, where fleck formation may be a normal variant, and these must be differentiated from the pathologic variety: (1) When the pylorus closes, there may be a dimple of mucosa at the base of the bulb in which the barium may accumulate, giving rise to the appearance of a fleck. (2) The outer periphery of the base of the bulb occasionally acts as a groove, or sinus, in which barium may accumulate, and when seen in profile, gives the appearance of fleck formation at the base of the bulb. (3) The concentration of rugae at the apex of the bulb may simulate fleck formation on occasion also. (4) Flecks of an inconstant variety may be simulated by peristaltic waves passing over the duodenal bulb

The anatomic relationships of the bulb which are of importance are as follows (Fig. 13–12): The duodenal bulb forms the inferior boundary of the foramen epiploicum (foramen of Winslow), and hence a pathologic penetration of the bulb finds ready access into the lesser omental bursa. The hepatic artery is also in contact for a short distance with the superior margin of the bulb. Below, the bulb rests on the head and neck of the pancreas. There are several large blood vessels which come into close contact with this area, and are of considerable importance from the standpoint of possible erosion of an ulcer. On the left side lie the portal vein, gastroduodenal artery (and bile duct); close to the posterior aspect is the right side of the inferior vena cava; and adjoining the inferior margin are the superior pancreaticoduodenal and the right gastro-epiploic vessels.

The common bile duct may occasionally indent the bulb, giving rise to an apparent deformity, and the gallbladder lies in close apposition with the superior and right margins of the first part of the duodenum, occasionally producing an indentation of the duodenum.

The Second, or Descending Part of the Duodenum. Description of Villi and Plicae Circulares. This part of the duodenum is retroperitoneal in position with the root of the transverse mesocolon, crossing it at its middle. The head of the pancreas is in contact with its left margin (Fig. 13–12) and occasionally overlaps it both anteriorly and posteriorly, and along this margin in similar position run the branches of the pancreaticoduodenal arteries. The bile duct, after descending behind the duodenal bulb, passes between the head of the pancreas and this part of the duodenum where it joins with the pancreatic duct. The two together pierce the duodenal wall obliquely, and open by a common orifice on its inner aspect at the apex of the duodenal papilla (ampulla of Vater) medially (Fig. 14–15).

The mucous membrane of this part of the duodenum as well as all parts of the small intestine presents a soft, velvety internal surface which is due to the presence of the minute mucosal processes known as villi. These begin at the edge of the pyloric valve but are quite broad in that location and become narrower as they proceed down the small intestine. The only place they are not found is immediately over the solitary lymph nodules. These villi play an important part in the absorption function of the small intestine.

The mucous membrane of the small intestine is thrown into numerous folds which may to a great extent disappear upon distention, but there are permanent folds known as the plicae circulares (Fig. 13–21) or valvulae conniventes. They are crescentic folds running around the small intestine in circular fashion. They may bifurcate, and they usually project about 8 mm. into the lumen of the small intestine. *They begin in the second part of the duodenum,* and gradually become more prominent, so that in the region of the duodenal papilla, they are very distinct and remain prominent in the rest of the duodenum. The combination of the plicae circulares and the villi imparts a feathery pattern to the duodenum and jejunum when viewed radiographically, in the absence of distention, and this is the typical rugal pattern not only of the duodenum but also of the jejunum. The absence of plicae circulares in the duodenal bulb accounts for its closer resemblance radiographically to the pyloric antrum.

The Horizontal Portion of the Inferior Part of the Duodenum (Third Part). This part is somewhat concave upward, is retroperitoneal, and is crossed by the superior mesenteric vessels and the root of the mesentery near the midline. It crosses the inferior vena cava, and is closely applied to the inferior aspect of the head of the pancreas.

The Ascending Portion of the Inferior Part of the Duodenum (Fourth Part). This part lies on the aorta, the left renal vein, and occasionally also the left renal artery. A previously indicated, it extends obliquely anteriorly and to the left, and its left side lies in contact with some coils of small intestine. In addition to being clothed by peritoneum anteriorly (as is the case of the second and third parts), it is also clothed by peritoneum on its left side.

The duodenojejunal flexure is fixed by the musculus suspensorius (suspensory ligament) of Treitz, opposite the left side of the first or second lumbar vertebrae. This latter suspensory muscle blends with the muscular coat of the duodenum, and passes upward behind the pancreas to blend partially with the celiac artery, and then is attached to the right crus of the diaphragm.

In the neighborhood of the ascending part of the duodenum, there may frequently be present three peritoneal fossae. Two of these, the superior and

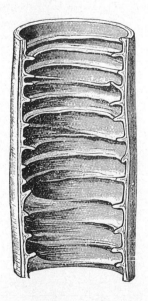

FIG. 13–21. Anatomic presentation of the plicae circulares of the small intestine (jejunum). (From Cunningham's *Text-Book of Anatomy*, edited by Arthur Robinson, published by Oxford University Press.)

inferior duodenal fossae, are formed by slips of fibrous tissue covered by peritoneum extending from the left side of the duodenum to the peritoneal surface adjoining it, and form very small pouches directed caudad and cephalad respectively. The third, however, which is called the paraduodenal fossa, is produced by a fold of peritoneum formed by the inferior mesenteric vein as it courses along the left lateral side of the ascending part of the duodenum. The inferior mesenteric vein is accompanied in part of its course by the left colic artery. This fossa is capable of forming a hernial sac, and therefore may be of some clinical significance.

Importance of a Study of the Duodenal Contour. The duodenum is in a fixed position for the most part, and hence variations from its normal position become of significance in the detection of space-occupying lesions in adjoining structures, such as the pancreas, lesser omental bursa, colon, gallbladder and biliary ducts.

There is, however, a considerable variation in different individuals in the normal contour of the duodenum. To a great extent, this is correlated with body habitus. Thus in pyknic individuals with high steer-horn stomachs (Fig. 13–11) the duodenal loop appears widened; and in asthenic individuals, portions of the duodenal loop will appear to be very close to one another, and overlap one another. Occasionally, there is a redundancy of the first part of the duodenum, with a greater segment peritonealized than is ordinarily seen. In some individuals, the second part of the duodenum may be virtually lacking, and it would appear that the superior part of the duodenum connects almost directly with the horizontal part of the inferior portion of the duodenum.

These normal variations must be constantly borne in mind when radiography of the duodenum is attempted.

RADIOLOGIC METHODS OF STUDY OF DUODENUM

Fluoroscopy. Shortly after the patient swallows his first mouthful of barium, the barium is seen to enter the duodenal bulb under normal conditions. It may be somewhat delayed here, and shortly thereafter it passes on around the duodenum. Although rugal pattern is indicated with this first swallow, the normal bulbar contour cannot be detected until it is filled out completely with the barium mixture. Occasionally there is a tendency for air to become trapped in the duodenal bulb, and this will prevent its complete filling. It will give the erroneous impression that the pyloric canal is excentric. When the bulb is completely filled, compression is applied to observe the rugal pattern when spot compression films are taken as required. In order to visualize the inferior portion of the duodenum it is necessary to place the patient in an oblique position, since otherwise the stomach will obscure the visualization of this part. There is also a tendency for the second part of the duodenum to be overlapped by the duodenal bulb, or the pyloric antrum to overlap this structure, and hence the oblique position is necessary in this instance also.

VARIATIONS IN THE APPEARANCE OF THE DUODENAL BULB (Fig. 13–22). This is by far the most important part of the duodenum from the standpoint of incidence of abnormality. The normal bulb is usually very regular. It tends to be conical, or triangular, in shape, and variations from this configuration are usually of considerable significance. The apex of the bulb is usually surrounded by the feathery mucosa of the duodenum which contains plicae circulares, but

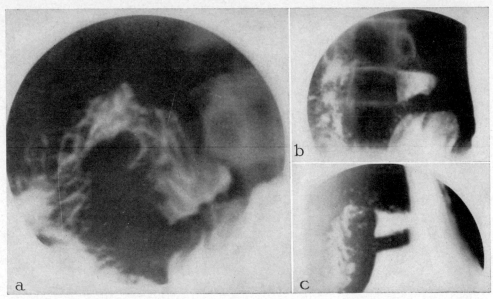

FIG. 13–22.   VARIATIONS IN APPEARANCE OF THE DUODENAL BULB.   **a,** Slight left anterior oblique; **b,** slight right anterior oblique; **c,** almost direct right lateral. In each of these illustrations the descending part of the duodenum is shown on the left also.

the mucosal pattern of the bulb proper usually consists of fairly parallel rugae, or rugae arranged in the form of a spiral.

The body habitus of the individual will to some extent cause some variation in the appearance of the bulb. In the short, squat individual, the bulb tends to be small and posterior, hiding as it were behind the pyloric antrum. Occasionally also, in such individuals, the bulb will extend obliquely downward, especially if the stomach is high and steer-horn in type.

Occasionally, the bulb is large and patulous in type, and tends to remain filled for a considerable period of time.

The normal rugae are ordinarily quite flexible and elastic, and can be quite readily obliterated by pressure, in contrast to the abnormal "fleck" which has already been mentioned.

The posture of the patient will also affect the appearance of the bulb. The duodenal bulb is best seen and most copiously filled with the patient lying obliquely prone on his right side. It is least filled in the supine position.

THE DUODENUM DISTAL TO THE DUODENAL BULB.   The second, third and fourth portions of the duodenum have the normal feathery mucosal pattern already described. They appear as a single loop, with peristaltic waves carrying the barium around this loop.

Occasionally the duodenal papilla in the middle of the descending part of the duodenum will fill with barium, or produce a small filling defect in the contour of the duodenum. This must not be interpreted as abnormal.

There may be a slight hesitation when the barium passes the duodenojejunal junction, and usually an angulation can be detected in this region. This angle tends to be more obtuse in the pyknic individuals.

Film Studies. Radiographs are obtained in accordance with the anatomy visualized with fluoroscopic study, particular emphasis again being placed on spot-film studies.

The positions used to obtain routine films are those described for the stomach.

REFERENCES

1. Barclay, A. E.: The Digestive Tract. London, 1936.
2. Johnstone, A. S.: Observations on the Radiological Anatomy of the Esophago-Gastric Junction. Proc. Radiological Soc. N. America, 1958.
3. Lerche, W.: The Esophagus and Pharynx in Action: A Study of Structure in Relation to Function. Charles C Thomas, Springfield, Ill., 1950.
4. Meschan, I., et al.: The Normal Radiographic Adult Stomach and Duodenum. South. M. J., *46:* 878–887, 1953.
5. Poppel, M. H., Zaino, C., and Lentino, W.: Roentgenographic Study of the Lower Esophagus and the Esophago-Gastric Junction. Radiology, *64:* 690–700, 1955.
6. Rubin, P., and Holt, J. F.: Secretory Sialography in Diseases of the Major Salivary Gland. Am. J. Roentgenol., *77:* 575–598, 1957. (Bibliography.)
7. Schatzki, R., and Gary, J.: Dysphagia Due to a Diaphragm-like Localized Narrowing in the Lower Esophagus. Am. J. Roentgenol., *70:* 911–922, 1953.

CHAPTER 14

The Intestine
beyond the Duodenum;
the Biliary Tract

THE SMALL INTESTINE

Gross Anatomy. The small intestine during life varies considerably in length. It is well known, for example, that the small intestine can be traversed by a Miller-Abbott tube several feet in length, whereas its length at autopsy is usually 20 to 22 feet; probably with good muscle tone during life it varies between 15 and 17 feet. In formalin-hardened bodies, it rarely measures longer than 12 or 13 feet in length. There is a gradual diminution in diameter from the pylorus to the ileocecal valve (valvula coli).

The jejunum and ileum are completely covered with peritoneum and will therefore vary considerably in position, except at the two ends where relative fixation occurs. However, there is usually a fairly regular pattern in the distribution of the small intestine (Fig. 14–1). Thus, the proximal jejunum usually lies in the left half of the abdomen between the level of the pancreas and the intercrestal line. The distal ileum usually lies deep in the pelvis posteriorly, with the terminal ileum arising out of the pelvis to meet the cecum in the right lower quadrant anteriorly. The distal jejunum and proximal ileum are distributed in the right half of the abdomen for the most part.

Major Differences between the Jejunum and Ileum. The main differences between the jejunum and ileum from the radiographic standpoint can be summarized as follows:

1. There is a gradual diminution in diameter as the cecum is approached, and thus the lumen of the ileum is smaller than that of the jejunum.

2. The plicae circulares commence in the second part of the duodenum and the reader is referred to their description in the preceding chapter. The maximum number and size of plicae circulares is found in the midjejunum, and the plicae diminish toward the ileum, and practically cease a little below the middle of this portion. This difference is of major importance in that the mucosal pattern of the ileum differs from that of the proximal jejunum by being considerably smoother and less feathery. Barium tends to have a more clumped

628

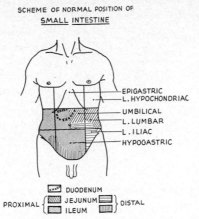

FIG. 14–1.   Approximate distribution of the small intestine within the abdomen.

appearance in the ileum than in the jejunum as a result of this fundamental difference. In the ileocecal region, the rugae tend to be parallel in type and approach the appearance of the rugae in the pylorus.

3. The aggregate lymphatic nodules, or Peyer's patches, are most numerous in the ileum and considerably fewer in number in the jejunum. They are more prominent in young individuals, and tend to atrophy as age advances. They are not ordinarily distinguishable radiographically, and normally do not play a significant role in radiographic diagnosis.

Motility Study of the Small Intestine.   It has been well established that many systemic diseases (such as vitamin deficiency, protein deficiency, certain anemias, allergic states, and so on) are capable of producing considerable change in the motility pattern of the small intestine, and for that reason, a close study of the normal small intestinal motility is imperative.

Cannon[1] was one of the first investigators to demonstrate intestinal motility, both by direct inspection of the exposed intestine in anesthetized animals and also by x-ray studies in the intact animal. He described rhythmic segmentation, pendulum movements and peristaltic waves.

Actually, our present-day concept is not quite so clear-cut as Cannon's description might indicate. Barium usually passes quite rapidly into the jejunum for approximately 30 or 40 cm., and thereafter the movement of the barium column proceeds quite slowly. The lumen of the jejunum is usually sufficiently collapsed to permit a ready and accurate visualization of the rugal pattern. Peristaltic waves are the most common type of motility, but occasionally there is superimposed an over-all movement of a whole segment of small bowel, in a circular motion. The barium column gradually moves on into the ileum, where there is a smoother and less fluffy pattern, and where the barium tends to remain longer in continuous cylinders. Ordinarily, the barium remains clumped in the distal ileum for a considerable period of time, and periodically a peristaltic wave will be seen to carry a small portion of the barium into the terminal ileum which rises out of the pelvis to meet the cecum. Peristaltic waves are intermittent over the terminal ileum. In the distal ileum, there is virtually no rugal pattern

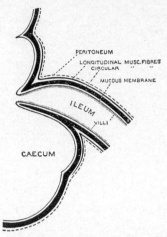

FIG. 14–2. ILEOCECAL JUNCTION: **a,** Diagrammatic section. (From Cunningham's *Text-Book* of *Anatomy,* edited by Arthur Robinson, published by Oxford University Press.)

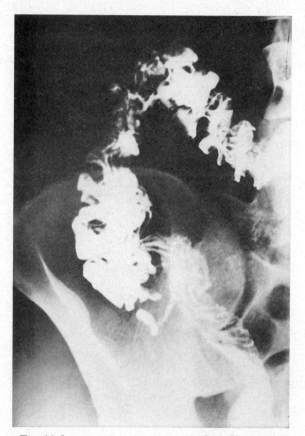

FIG. 14–2. ILEOCECAL JUNCTION: **b,** Spot film study.

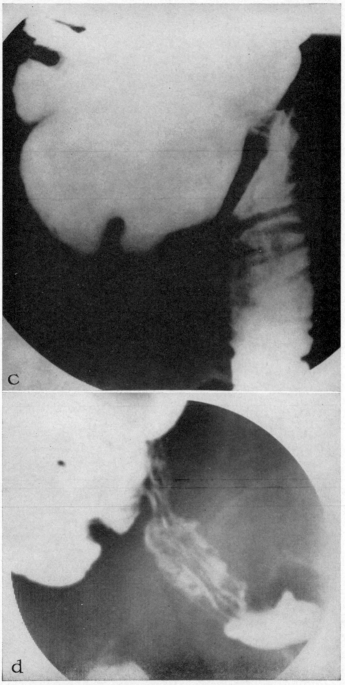

Fig. 14–2. ILEOCECAL JUNCTION: **c** and **d,** Spot film studies.

visible, and all movement is difficult to observe fluoroscopically, since the ileal loops are conglomerated and difficult to palpate in view of their posterior position.

The average time for the head of the barium column to reach the ileocecal region is one and one-half to two hours, but it is not unusual for a period of four hours to elapse before barium appears in the cecum. Abnormality, either primary or secondary, in the emptying of the stomach will of course affect the emptying time of the small intestine, and any abnormality of the terminal ileum may be reflected in a delayed emptying of the stomach.

Special Anatomy of the Ileocecal Valve (Valvula Coli). The terminal ileum projects into the cecum at its termination, producing folds which function as a sphincter. The serosa of the ileum does not participate in this protrusion, and helps to prevent abnormal invagination of the terminal ileum into the ascending colon (called "intussusception"). The filling defect produced by this anatomic structure is readily visualized radiographically (Figs. 14–2, 14–3).

The function of this valve is sphincteric—much like the pyloric valve—but it is unknown if its main function is to prevent regurgitation as is the case with the pyloric sphincter. In performing barium enema examinations, it is possible to force barium from the colon into the terminal ileum in at least half of the cases, and this incompetency is probably of no pathologic significance. Ordinarily, however, in gaseous distention of the colon from any mechanical obstructive cause at a lower level in the colon, the ileocecal valve will prevent passage of the gas back up into the small intestine for a considerable period of time.

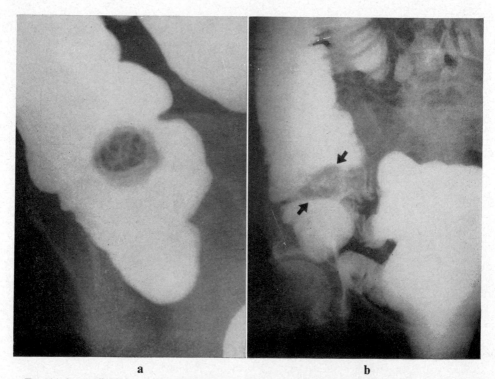

a   b

Fig. 14–3.   Difference between prolapse (a) and prominent ileocecal valves (b). In the former the central slit-like valve orifice is not filled with barium, whereas in the latter it stands out clearly. This is a posteriorly situated valve. (From Hinkel, C. L.: Am. J. Roentgenol., vol. 68, 1952.)

RADIOGRAPHIC METHODS OF STUDY OF THE SMALL INTESTINE

Frequent-interval Film and Fluoroscopy Method (Fig. 14–4). Following a routine examination of the stomach and duodenum, the barium column is fluoroscoped until its movement in the jejunum is very slow. A large postero-anterior film of the abdomen is taken immediately, and at one-half to one hour intervals thereafter until the barium column has reached the ileocecal valve and

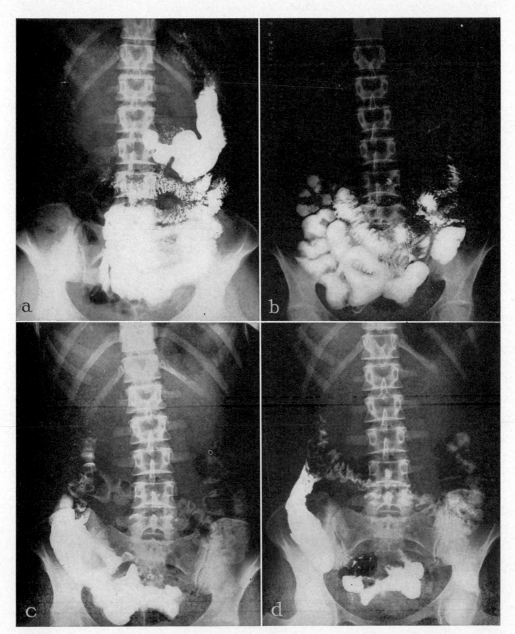

FIG. 14–4. ILLUSTRATIONS TO DEMONSTRATE FREQUENT FILM AND FLUOROSCOPIC METHOD FOR EXAMINATION OF SMALL INTESTINE: **a,** At one hour following administration of the barium; **b,** at two hours; **c,** at three hours; **d,** at six hours.

cecum. The patient is refluoroscoped whenever anything suspicious is seen on one of the interval films. When the barium column has reached the ileocecal region, the patient is refluoroscoped and spot-film compression studies of this region are obtained.

Cold Isotonic Saline Method. Cold isotonic saline has been shown to hasten the motility through the small intestine, and gastric evacuation. Thus, after the administration of the barium sulfate and examination of the stomach and duodenum, the patient is given a glassful of cold isotonic saline to drink. One-half hour later, he is given another glassful of the saline. Under these circumstances, the ileocecal region is reached in one-half to one hour instead of the usual longer intervals. The isotonic saline, however, tends to dilute the barium mixture slightly, and the contrast and detail are not quite so distinct as with the first method. This method has considerable value, since the continuity of the barium column can be more readily followed fluoroscopically, and hence the examination can be performed more efficiently.

Intubation Method. In this method, a Miller-Abbott or Cantor tube is passed into the small intestine as far as desired, and the segment of bowel in question is thereafter examined by the injection of barium mixture locally. The remainder of the small intestine can also be examined by the gradual withdrawal of the tube and the gradual injection of barium mixture at the same time. This method has the advantage of permitting a more exact examination of a desired region of the small bowel, without the interference of overlapping or contiguous loops of bowel. It has the disadvantage of requiring the passage of the tube, which is time-consuming, and quite uncomfortable for the patient. However, it furnishes the most exact method of examining the small bowel.

Small Intestinal Enema Method. This method requires the passage of a tube into the duodenum. Thereafter, the barium is injected as rapidly as desired through the tube and thus forced on its way through the small intestine. As much as 1000 cc. of barium suspension can be injected in a very short interval of time, and the entire small intestine examined fluoroscopically as well as by means of film studies at frequent intervals.

This method has the disadvantage of discomfort to the patient, as well as overlapping of various segments of small intestine, but has the advantage that the examination requires less time.

In each of these examinations scattering of the barium in small clumps or flakes, distention of any segment of the small intestine, or gas in any part of the small intestine in the adult is abnormal. In the child, however, the normal feathery pattern of the small intestine does not appear in the first few weeks or months of life, and there is a lesser tendency for the barium to move as a continuous fine column. Gas in the small intestine of the infant is also normal (in contrast to the adult), and in the infant it is considerably more difficult to distinguish between the normal and abnormal.

It is readily apparent that none of the methods of examining the small intestine is ideal, and all have their disadvantages, as well as advantages. There is still much to be desired in the proper study of the small intestine in the living subject, and our information regarding this examination is only just beginning to accumulate.

THE LARGE INTESTINE

Gross Anatomy.   The large intestine is approximately 5 to 5½ feet in length and varies in diameter from 1½ to 3 inches. Commencing at the cecum, it is further subdivided into ascending colon, transverse colon, descending and iliac colon, sigmoid or pelvic colon, and rectum.

The cecum is found in the right lower quadrant of the abdomen ordinarily, but its position is usually most variable since it is entirely enveloped by peritoneum and lies quite free in the abdominal cavity. It is usually situated anteriorly, with only the omentum and abdominal wall lying over it. The terminal ileum joins the cecum usually on its medial or posterior aspect, and the vermiform appendix springs from the cecum on the same side as the ileocecal junction. The upper end of the cecum is continuous with the ascending colon.

The lower portion of the ascending colon may be on a partial mesentery, and like the cecum be rather anterior in position, but very soon it proceeds posteriorly in most instances, and assumes a partially covered retroperitoneal position. When it reaches the inferior surface of the liver, it turns forward and to the left (forming the hepatic flexure). It lies between the quadratus lumborum laterally, and the psoas major muscle medially. Its posterior surface is ordinarily not peritonealized, thus giving it a relatively fixed position, but it is surprisingly mobile radiographically despite these anatomic limitations.

The hepatic flexure is ordinarily situated lateral and anterior to the descending portion of the duodenum, and posterior to the thin anterior margin of the liver. Its peritoneal relations are similar to those of the ascending colon.

The transverse colon has a long mesentery, and as a result is subject to wide variation in length and position. It usually hangs down in front of the small intestine, a considerable distance from the posterior abdominal wall, with only the greater omentum and anterior abdominal wall lying over it. Its first few centimeters, however, are usually firmly attached to the anterior surface of the second part of the duodenum and the head of the pancreas—a factor of considerable importance when these structures are distended by a space-occupying lesion, since there is in such cases a secondary displacement of this portion of the colon. Toward the left the mesentery shortens, bringing this segment close to the tail of the pancreas, with the stomach lying anterior and to the right. At the inferior surface of the spleen, it passes into the splenic flexure, which is again retroperitoneal but at a higher level than the hepatic flexure.

The splenic flexure is perhaps the most constant part of the colon, being held in position by the phrenicocolic ligament, which is attached laterally to the diaphragm opposite the ninth to the eleventh rib posteriorly.

The descending and iliac portions of the colon are the narrowest parts. The descending colon first lies in contact with the lateral margin of the left kidney, and then in a comparable position with the ascending colon on the right. The posterior surface is not peritonealized and the descending colon is less mobile ordinarily than the ascending.

The iliac colon lies in the iliac fossa and, like the descending colon, is not peritonealized on its posterior surface.

The pelvic or sigmoid colon has a mesentery of its own which accounts for the mobility of this portion of the colon and is somewhat variable in width. It usually lies for the most part in the pelvis minor, but occasionally with marked redundancy it may escape above into the abdominal cavity. In the child at birth, owing to the small size of the pelvis minor, only the terminal part of the pelvic colon lies in this area. In the child, the pelvic colon usually arches over to the right side, and lies in great part in the right iliac fossa. At the termination of the pelvic colon, it arches backward and downward to form the rectosigmoid junction.

The rectosigmoid junction is usually the point of maximum narrowness in the colon, and this narrowness may extend for 1 to 1.5 cm. This narrowness sometimes is difficult to distinguish from an abnormal constriction, and one must familiarize oneself thoroughly with the normal variations of this region (Fig. 14–10, **c**).

The rectum and anal canal are more accurately examined by the proctoscope and sigmoidoscope and by digital palpation than by radiographic methods, and for that reason less radiographic emphasis is placed upon these regions. The rectum has only a partial covering of peritoneum, and has no sacculations; it is very distensible, particularly in its midportion, and this area is therefore called the rectal ampulla. The rectum first follows the hollow of the sacrum and coccyx, and then turns gently forward and finally abruptly downward to join the anal canal. There are three (and sometimes as many as five) crescentic folds, called the plicae transversales (plicae of Houston), which project into the lumen of the rectum. These pass around two thirds of the rectal circumference, and produce indentations on the radiograph of the rectum. They are variable in position and occasionally are poorly developed and virtually absent. It is probable that these are similar in origin to the plicae semilunares of the rest of the colon, but in the absence of the taeniae coli take on a somewhat different appearance. There are creases in addition, however, which involve the entire wall of the rectum in their structure.

Distinguishing Features between the Large and Small Intestine.   Those features which distinguish the large from the small intestine are: (1) the *taeniae coli*, which are longitudinal bands of muscle running along the outer surface of the large intestine, and are symmetrically placed around its circumference; (2) the *appendices epiploicae*, which are small peritoneal processes projecting from the serous coat of the large intestine; and (3) the *haustral sacculations* of the large intestine.

The taeniae coli are the three longitudinal muscle bands into which the longitudinal musculature of the large intestine is principally concentrated; they pass from the cecum to the rectum, where they disappear in a fanning-out process to form a more continuous layer of muscle around the rectum.

The appendices epiploicae usually contain fat and project from the serous coat of the entire large intestine, with the exception of the rectum. Their importance radiologically lies in the fact that occasionally they undergo calcification.

The haustral sacculations are produced by crescentic folds of the entire wall of the large bowel which produce a segmented appearance, each haustral segment measuring 3 to 5 cm. in length. There are creases or folds on the interior of the large intestine which correspond with the external folds, which are called the plicae semilunares of the colon. These plicae differ from those of the small intestine in that: (1) They contain not only the mucosal fold, but the submucosal layer and also a portion of the muscular layer as well; and (2) they are very

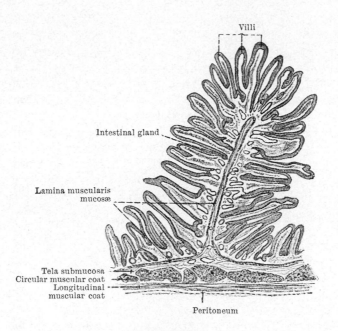

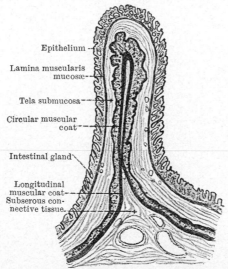

FIG. 14–5. **a,** Diagrammatic presentation of the differences in transverse section between the plicae circulares of the small intestine and plicae semilunares of the large intestine. (From Cunningham's *Text-Book of Anatomy,* edited by Arthur Robinson, published by Oxford University Press.)

SCHEMATIC ILLUSTRATION OF DISTENDED BOWEL

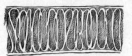

JEJUNUM
(NO INDENTED SEROSA;
COILED SPRING APPEARANCE)

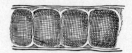

ILEUM
(NO INDENTED SEROSA)

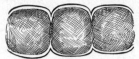

COLON
(NOTE INDENTED SEROSA BY
HAUSTRAE)

FIG. 14–5. **b,** Differences in roentgen appearance of distended small and large intestine.

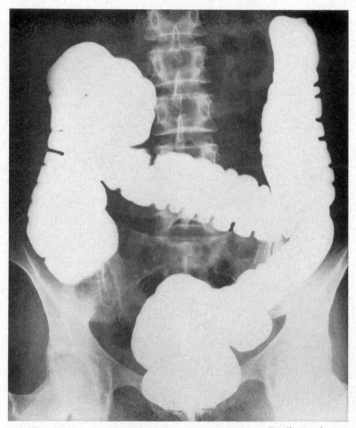

FIG. 14–6. COLON DISTENDED WITH BARIUM: **a,** Radiograph.

much more widely separated—each of these folds extending around one third the circumference of the wall of the large intestine between two taeniae coli.

The radiographic representation of these differences (Fig. 14–5) between the plicae circulares of the small intestine and the plicae semilunares of the colon is of considerable practical significance in attempting to differentiate the gas-distended small and large intestine (Fig. 14–5, **b**). The plicae circulares are very closely placed with respect to one another, and are most conspicuous in the jejunum and least conspicuous in the ileum. Occasionally, they are completely effaced in the ileum. They form a sharp margin with the outer wall of the small bowel, since they are purely mucosal folds, and have no contribution from the outer layers of the wall of the small bowel. The plicae semilunares of the colon, on the other hand, are usually 3 to 5 cm. apart, are most conspicuous in the transverse colon, and have rounded margins, in which there is a contribution from the entire wall of the large intestine.

The widest parts of the colon are the cecum, and the full rectum. There is a gradual diminution in the caliber of the colon from the cecum to the recto-sigmoid junction.

Mucosal Pattern of the Large Intestine. When the colon is full (Fig. 14–6) only the normal haustral pattern of the colon is visible. This is slightly more

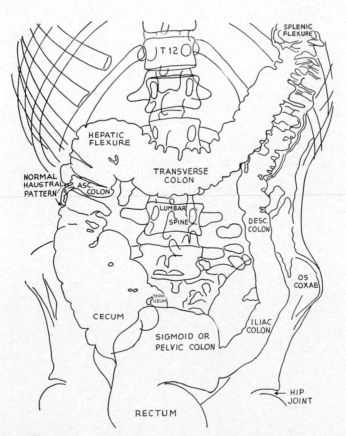

FIG. 14–6. COLON DISTENDED WITH BARIUM: **b**, Tracing.

irregular in the ascending colon than in the transverse, and *may be virtually absent in the descending colon and sigmoid* when the latter portions of the colon are examined radiographically. The haustral appearance of the descending and pelvic colons is therefore variable.

When the colon is empty (Fig. 14–7), its mucosa is thrown into numerous irregular folds. These folds, however, are coarser than those of the small intestine in view of the lack of the plicae circulares and villi. The pattern, however, is an irregular mosaic throughout the colon, except that in the iliac and pelvic colons these folds assume a more regular and parallel appearance. The pattern of the cecum (Fig. 14–8) differs also slightly from that of the rest of the colon, in that there is a greater tendency toward a spiral arrangement of the rugal pattern.

An examination of the rugal pattern of the colon is a very important part of the colonic examination, and for that reason a film after evacuation of a barium enema is never omitted.

Special Anatomy of the Vermiform Appendix. The appendix usually arises from the cecum on its medial or posterior aspects, about 2.5 to 4 cm. from the ileocecal valve. It is extremely variable in size or position. There is a "valve" at its orifice in the cecum which probably does not function in life, although occasionally the appendix even with a patent lumen will not fill immediately at the time of a barium enema, and will be seen to contain barium twenty-four or more hours later.

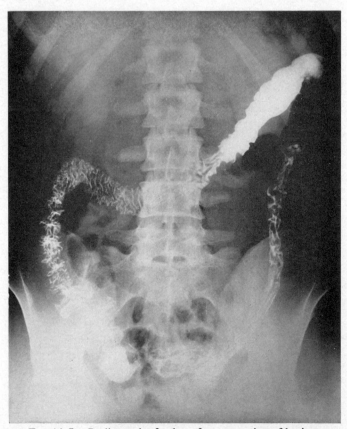

Fig. 14–7. Radiograph of colon after evacuation of barium.

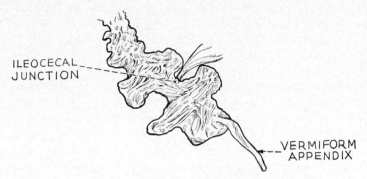

ILEOCECAL
JUNCTION

VERMIFORM
APPENDIX

FIG. 14–8. Representative mucosal pattern of cecum.

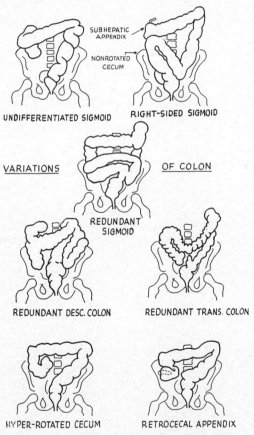

SUBHEPATIC
APPENDIX

NONROTATED
CECUM

UNDIFFERENTIATED SIGMOID RIGHT-SIDED SIGMOID

VARIATIONS OF COLON

REDUNDANT
SIGMOID

REDUNDANT DESC. COLON REDUNDANT TRANS. COLON

HYPER-ROTATED CECUM RETROCECAL APPENDIX

FIG. 14–9. Variations in contour of the colon.

At postmortem examination total occlusion of the lumen of the appendix is found in 3 or 4 per cent of cases, whereas almost total or partial obliteration of the lumen is found in an additional 25 per cent (Cunningham). In individuals past the age of 60, the lumen is obliterated in more than 50 per cent of the cases, and may represent a retrogressive normal change with age.

In disease of the appendix, its lumen is obliterated in practically all (but not all) instances, but since obliteration of the appendix in the adult is such a frequent finding without definite disease, the mere lack of visualization of the appendix radiographically is not indicative of abnormality. However, when the appendix is visualized, it can be taken as good evidence, though not conclusive, of a normal appendix.

Fecal concretions and calculi (called "coproliths") are found in the appendix under many circumstances, and may permit a partial visualization of this structure, despite their presence.

Variation in Size and Position of the Subdivisions of the Colon. The dividing line between anatomic variations and congenital malformations is not a sharp one. Marked redundancies of the sigmoid colon and transverse colon are found so frequently that they can be considered anatomic variants. These various types of redundancies are illustrated in Figure 14–9.

Failures of rotation, however, are congenital aberrations which have considerable practical significance. These are outside the scope of the present text, but the most frequent of these are illustrated (Fig. 14–9). In nonrotation of the cecum, the cecum is seen to lie lateral to the ascending colon, and the appendix ascends toward the liver, giving rise to the so-called subhepatic appendix. In hyper-rotation of the colon, the cecum appears to acquire an extra twist which places it medial to the ascending colon, pointing medially or upward. The appendix is in a variable position in these cases, but is not found in its usual location.

MOTILITY STUDY OF THE LARGE INTESTINE

The passage of a barium mixture as viewed fluoroscopically through the large intestine is very slow, and almost imperceptible. While the contents are still fluid, peristaltic activity and a constant head of pressure from the ileum force the barium column onward. When the barium mixture becomes semisolid or solid, it is a mass movement which forces the passage of the colonic contents. In a matter of seconds, the normal haustral pattern of the colon is seen to disappear, and an entire long segment of the large bowel appears to close down into a ribbon-like structure. This mass movement then gradually passes over the bowel distal to its site of origin and forces the bowel contents toward the rectum. This mass movement may reach the rectum in a matter of fifteen or twenty seconds, and shortly thereafter, the original haustral markings once again make their appearance.

Normally, these mass movements do not occur many times during the day, but during a barium enema examination, especially in an irritable colon, they may be seen repeatedly, eventually forcing the evacuation of the colonic contents.

Some investigators, such as Wright, Cole and others, have described a haustral churning motion, in which the haustra remain in evidence, but change their size. This is a very slow movement, and can be detected ordinarily only in serial radiographic studies.

The rate of movement through the large intestine is very variable, but under ordinary circumstances the cecum is visualized in one and one-half to four hours after the oral administration of barium. The head of the barium column will reach the hepatic flexure in three to six hours and the splenic flexure in six to twelve hours. By twenty-four hours, usually about one-half of the barium has been evacuated, and the remainder scattered in the colon. Ordinarily, the colon is virtually empty of barium in forty-eight hours, except for a few scattered foci. Variations from this sequence are very frequent, and caution must be exercised in the interpretation of abnormal motility of the large intestine.

TECHNIQUE OF RADIOLOGIC EXAMINATION OF THE COLON

The methods of examination are: (1) the plain radiograph of the abdomen; (2) the barium enema, under fluoroscopic visualization, and accompanied by spot-film compression radiography, in addition to certain routine film studies; (3) the barium meal, followed through until the colon is visualized, and thereafter at six hours, twenty-four hours, and further intervals if desired; and (4) the barium-air double-contrast enema.

The Plain Radiograph of the Abdomen. This will be described in greater detail in Chapter 15. In this study, the colon is visualized in accordance with the amount of gas it contains. The caliber of the large bowel can be identified, and haustra can usually be differentiated. A detailed analysis of the bowel is not possible, however, with this negative type of contrast medium, although considerable valuable information, particularly from the standpoint of obstruction, can be gained.

The Barium Enema. Thorough cleansing of the colon prior to the barium enema is essential, since any retained fecal material will obscure the normal anatomy, and give rise to false filling defects and mucosal aberrations. This is usually best accomplished by means of 2 ounces of castor oil given on the night preceding the examination. This aperient has the advantage of not producing an irritation of the large intestine (since its physiologic effect is on small bowel primarily), and it ordinarily cleanses the large bowel quite thoroughly. If desired, other aperients are employed, but we have found them less satisfactory. Approximately two hours prior to the barium enema it is usually desirable to give the patient some cleansing enemas in addition; the two-hour interval is efficacious in permitting adequate time for retained fluid to be reabsorbed in the colon. The cleansing enemas should be given until the returns are clear. Ordinarily the patient is examined without breakfast, since the breakfast meal will introduce gas in the stomach, and occasionally gases in the colon.

The enema tip is introduced while the patient is on the fluoroscopic table. Either an ordinary tip may be employed, or special tips which come equipped with balloons which may be distended with gas or water, so that a rectal plug is provided to prevent involuntary evacuation. Care is employed in the latter technique not to increase the pressure in the bowel excessively, since rupture of a weakened segment may occur. Ordinarily, when the head of the barium column is no more than 3 feet above the table, the pressure will not be excessive.

The barium suspension is made up of U.S.P. barium sulfate mixed with water in a 1:4 up to 1:6 mixture depending upon preference. One teaspoon up to one tablespoon of tannic acid is added. (We have not added the two table-spoonfuls of methylcellulose jell recommended by some.) The barium is introduced slowly with the patient first lying on his left side (supine), and the rectum and pelvic colon are carefully studied fluoroscopically. It is usually advantageous to pause when the pelvic colon is filled to allow the colon to accommodate to the barium mixture, and also to obtain a spot-film study of the pelvic colon in the right anterior oblique position (Fig. 14–10). Sufficient obliquity is employed to demonstrate the entire pelvic colon and the rectosigmoid junction.

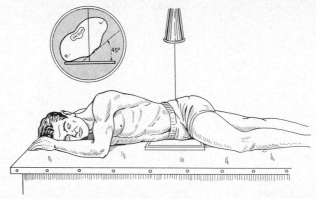

FIG. 14–10.   OBLIQUE STUDY OF PELVIC AND ILIAC COLON: **a,** Position of patient.

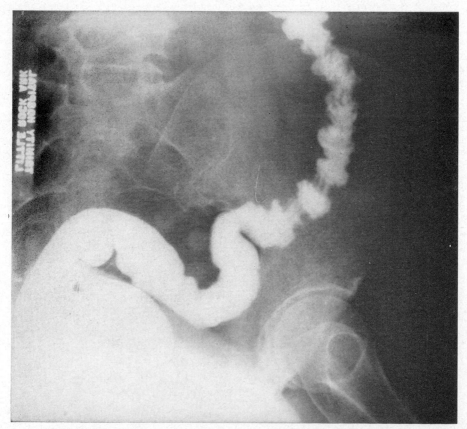

FIG. 14–10.   OBLIQUE STUDY OF PELVIC AND ILIAC COLON: **b,** Radiograph.

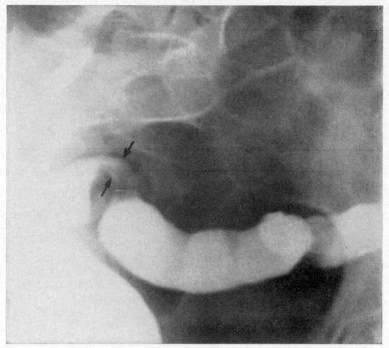

FIG. 14–10.   OBLIQUE STUDY OF PELVIC AND ILIAC COLON: **c,** Film study to demonstrate the narrowness which may occur normally at the rectosigmoid junction.

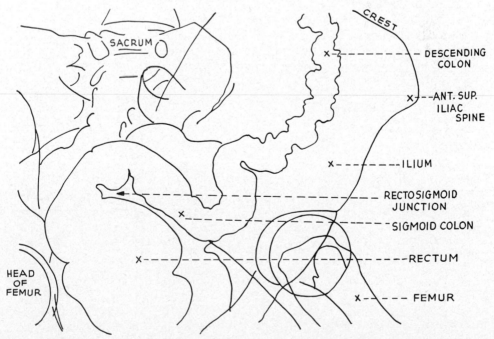

FIG. 14–10.   OBLIQUE STUDY OF PELVIC AND ILIAC COLON: **d,** Labeled tracing of **b.**

The patient is then allowed to turn flat on his back and the descending colon is studied as it is filled. The patient is then turned obliquely on his right side and the splenic flexure is studied completely. Thereafter, the patient is once again placed flat and the transverse colon slowly filled and studied.

The patient is then turned obliquely on his left side once again while the hepatic flexure is filled, and flat on his back thereafter while the ascending colon is filled and studied.

After the cecum is filled, it is studied in both obliquities, and if the terminal ileum and appendix can be filled, they are also examined at this time.

When the fluoroscopic examination is completed (and any spot-film studies desired have been obtained), a postero-anterior film of the full colon (Fig. 14–6) is obtained with the Potter-Bucky diaphragm, employing a rapid exposure technique so that no movement of the colon is detected on the film. A relatively high kilovoltage (90 to 120 KvP) is recommended to make the barium mixture translucent; thus filling defects may be detected in overlapping segments which might otherwise not be seen.[3]

The patient is then allowed to evacuate the barium, and immediately thereafter (so that the barium will not become dehydrated) another postero-anterior film of the empty colon is taken (Fig. 14–7).

We have found it advantageous to introduce about 1 teaspoonful of tannic acid per quart of barium suspension. On the postevacuation film of the colon, it would appear that this mixture permits a better adhesion of the barium to the wall of the large intestine, and thus a better visualization of the mucosal pattern of the colon is obtained. We have found no untoward effects from this adjunct.

Any special studies in obliquity may be obtained otherwise as desired by the examiner.

It is important to emphasize that in the frontal projection of the colon, portions of the hepatic flexure, splenic flexure and pelvic colon will escape observation, since there will be overlapping of parts of the colon. Oblique studies of the flexures and the pelvic colon are essential to reveal them in their entirety. On occasion, when marked redundancy occurs there are certain segments which cannot be seen with accuracy because of overlapping loops of bowel.

The radiographic appearance of the large intestine will vary also with the consistency of the barium suspension employed, and the amount of air introduced with the barium. If the barium has remained in the colon for a considerable period of time it will become dehydrated, and a discontinuous pattern is obtained in which the haustra appear to be separated from one another. Also the colon may appear irregular in caliber. If there is much air in the barium mixture, the barium will appear more radiolucent in some parts than in others, likewise giving rise to an irregular shaded appearance, with a thin barium line around the wall of the colon.

The Barium Meal Method. *This method should never be employed unless it is certain that no colonic obstruction exists.* There is also a tendency for the barium to cake after a time, and a complete and accurate analysis of colonic structure is not possible with this method. As indicated above, this method can be combined with a study of the upper gastrointestinal tract, and films taken at six- and twenty-four-hour intervals after the oral administration of the barium meal. Apart from obtaining a small amount of information regarding the emptying function of the bowel, there is not much accurate information that can be gained from this study. It should certainly not be regarded as a substitute for the barium enema examination. Since it is usually difficult to exclude the possibility of an organic obstruction of the large bowel, we have found it more efficacious to precede the oral barium study by the barium enema. This obviates the necessity for the twenty-four-hour study of the colon following the examination of the upper gastrointestinal tract, and in our laboratory only the two- to six-hour study is obtained thereafter.

The Barium-Air Double-Contrast Enema. There are two types of double-contrast barium enemas: (1) A conventional technique performed after evacuation of a barium enema such as has been described; and (2) a colloidal barium double-contrast enema. Following a complete evacuation of the barium enema, the large intestine may be insufflated with air. It may be necessary for the patient to evacuate more barium at this point to obtain a better mucosal relief pattern. However, after repeating this sequence until only a fine coating of barium remains, air is once again insufflated, and plain or stereoscopic films of the colon are obtained in the postero-anterior, antero-posterior, decubitus, and oblique projections (Fig. 14–11, **a**). These show the colonic walls as thin lines of barium, and these are widely separated by the gaseous distention. Any polypoid masses will be shown in a double relief pattern, being coated by barium. Unless the patient's colon has been thoroughly cleansed beforehand, the interpretation is fraught with hazard, since fecal matter which might be retained would lead to a similar appearance.

The colloidal barium double contrast enema may be performed in one of two ways: (1) the partial filling of the colon with colloidal barium mixture to the splenic flexure or middle of the transverse colon, the aspiration of this, and then the injection of air; or (2) the filling of the colon to the lower descending colon with colloidal barium mixture, followed immediately by the forceful injection of air with rotation of the patient to assist in the proper dispersion of the heavy barium mixture (Fig. 14–11, **b**).

There are various colloidal barium sulfate preparations available,[9, 10] each with specific directions for mixture. Some of these are: Bariloid, which is easy to mix, Barotrast, Baridol and Stabarium. Since the colloidal barium mixture is viscous, pressure is required to force it through the enema tubing. This may be done by elevation of the barium reservoir, "milking" the tube, by "piston" type syringes, or by pumping devices.

In both techniques, after introduction of the barium, the patient is turned under fluoroscopic guidance, even to the complete prone position, so that gravity will assist the air in distributing the barium throughout the colon.

Where suction and controlled drainage are required, various devices are available: (1) The three-way valve box designed by Templeton and Addington[11] which is attached to a sink and works on a Venturi siphon principle; (2) simple Y-tube and clamp devices which permit drainage through one branch of the Y and injection through the other.

Indications for Single- and Double-Contrast Barium Enema. The single-contrast examination has wide usefulness in detection of most abnormalities of the colon including the right half of the colon, ulcerative disease, and terminal ileal disease in many cases. It is less efficient than the double-contrast enema in the detection of small intraluminal tumors. It is unfortunate that both examinations cannot be done on the same day. They are best done one or two days apart as indicated by clinical history. It has been our practice to do the single-contrast study first. In patients with unexplained rectal bleeding (bright red or dark), with a history of polyps, or with polyps found at proctoscopy, the colloidal barium double-contrast enema is scheduled two days later, with a repetition of castor oil preparation the night before the second examination. if any dried barium or feces remains from the previous study, there will be Interference with the accuracy of the double contrast enema.

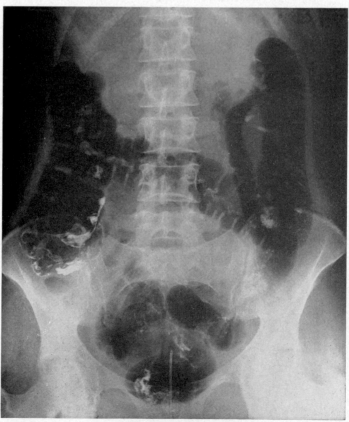

FIG. 14–11. **a,** Barium-air double-contrast enema.

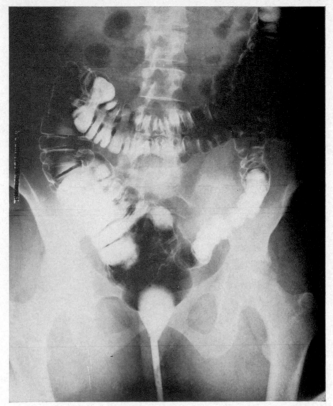

FIG. 14–11. b, Colloidal barium-air double contrast enema.

Special Views of the Rectum and Sigmoid Colon.   There are two additional views of the rectum and sigmoid colon which are useful under special circumstances:

(1) The direct lateral view (Fig. 14–12), which is particularly useful in infants where rectosigmoid constrictions are suspected (as in Hirschsprung's disease).

(2) The Chassard-Lapiné view[7] (also called "sitting," "squat," or "jack-knife" view) (Fig. 14–13, **a, b** and **c**). This view is useful to "separate" the overlapping portions of the rectosigmoid area.

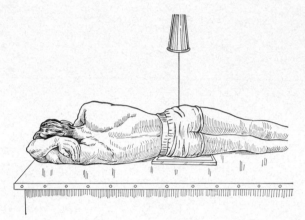

FIG. 14–12.   LATERAL VIEW OF THE RECTOSIGMOID: **a,** Position of patient.

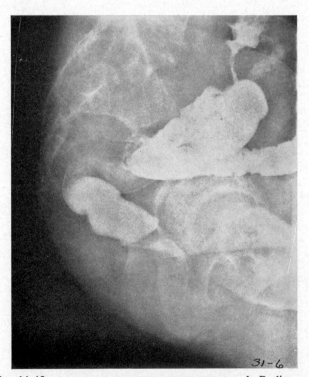

FIG. 14–12.   LATERAL VIEW OF THE RECTOSIGMOID: **b,** Radiograph.

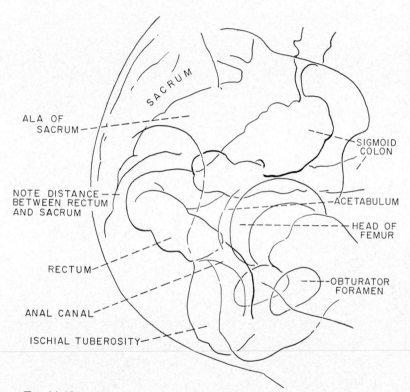

FIG. 14–12.   LATERAL VIEW OF THE RECTOSIGMOID: c, Labeled tracing of b.

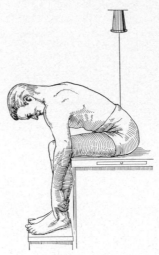

Fig. 14–13.   Chassard-Lapiné view of the rectum and sigmoid colon: **a,** Postion of patient.

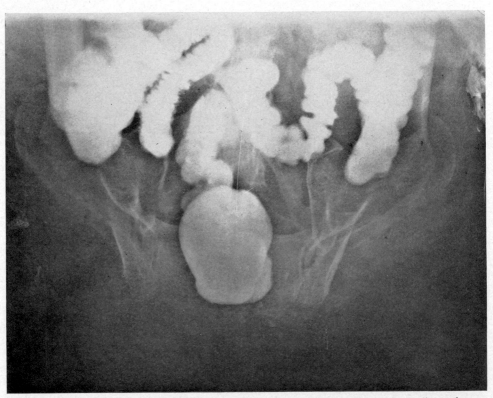

Fig. 14–13.   Chassard-Lapiné view of the rectum and sigmoid colon: **b,** Radiograph.

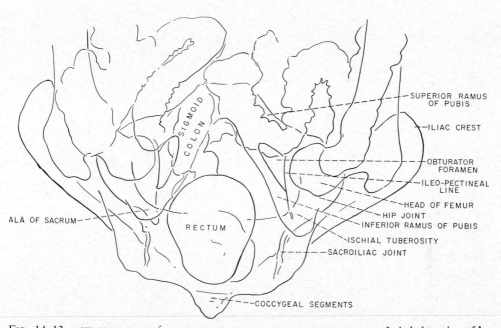

FIG. 14–13.   CHASSARD-LAPINÉ VIEW OF THE RECTUM AND SIGMOID COLON: **c,** Labeled tracing of **b.**

LIMITATIONS OF OUR METHODS OF EXAMINATION OF THE COLON

The limitations in the examination of the colon radiologically as outlined above are as follows:

1. Redundancy and overlapping of portions of the colon may obscure one of the anatomic parts. Hence complete examination of all flexures under fluoroscopic visualization is essential. Occasionally, such complete examination is virtually impossible.

2. Haustral points of narrowness and the rectosigmoid junction may give the impression of abnormal areas of narrowness unless the examiner is thoroughly conversant with the wide variations in the normal appearance of the colon.

3. Although the rectum and anal canal can be visualized, it is impossible to examine these structures as accurately as they can be examined by direct visualization with the sigmoidoscope and proctoscope, and digital examination. *The barium enema is no substitute for the latter two types of examination of these lower regions of the large bowel.*

4. Unless the terminal ileum or appendix has been visualized, it is difficult to be completely certain that the cecum has been seen, and for that reason caution must be observed in assuming that the colon has been completely filled when these latter two structures have not been filled with barium. Unfortunately, it is frequently impossible to fill the terminal ileum and appendix, and experience must dictate when the colon has been entirely distended with barium.

5. Fluoroscopy is not so accurate as the film study for revealing minute mucosal changes such as may be seen in the earliest aberrations of mucosal structure. It is important to become familiar with the normal appearance of both the full and the empty colon in this regard, so that minimal abnormalities can be recognized on the films.

6. When patients are unable to retain the enema and evacuation is forced before complete filling of the colon and cecum, one must not assume that an obstructive abnormality of an organic type must necessarily exist in the colon. A repeat examination, especially with the aid of a rectal balloon, may be more successful.

THE BILIARY TRACT

The radiographic examination of the gallbladder is at the same time both a means of visualization of the anatomic structure of the gallbladder and cystic duct, and a test of hepatobiliary function. One can hardly be considered without the other, and a detailed knowledge of both is essential if we are to carry out the examination with accuracy.

The Microscopic and Gross Anatomy of the Biliary Tract (Figs. 14–14, 14–15). The liver is composed of many hundreds of units called lobules, and each lobule is composed of radial columns of parenchymal cells. Between these columns of cells lie the bile capillaries, the walls of which are the liver cells themselves. On the opposite side of these cells are the stellate cells of the lymph channels and reticuloendothelial system, and the endothelium of the venules leading into the central vein. The bile capillaries empty into interlobular bile ducts, which enter in their turn into larger bile ducts, until finally two chief branches are obtained: a large branch from the right, and a small branch from the left lobe of the liver, called the right and left hepatic ducts respectively (Fig. 14–16). These ultimately unite to form the common hepatic duct.

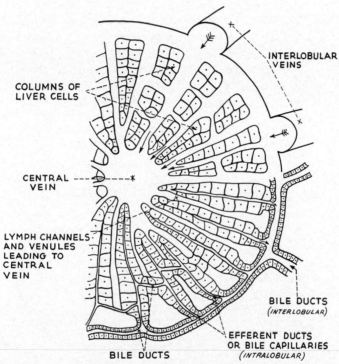

Fig. 14–14. Diagram to illustrate the structure of a liver lobule. (Modified from Cunningham's *Text-Book of Anatomy*, 9th Edition.)

The common hepatic duct passes downward, and just beyond the porta hepatis, it is joined by the cystic duct from the gallbladder to form the common bile duct. The common hepatic duct is about 25 to 30 mm. in length, and about 6 mm. in diameter.

The gallbladder is a pear-shaped enlargement which lies distal to the cystic duct.

The cystic duct is about one half the diameter of the hepatic duct but somewhat longer—about 30 to 37 mm. in length. It pursues a course backward and medially to join the hepatic duct.

The spiral constriction at the neck of the gallbladder (to be described below) is continued into the proximal portion of the cystic duct, called the valvular portion of the cystic duct, in contrast to the nonvalvular portion, or pars glabra.

The common bile duct is about 7.5 cm. in length and about the same diameter as the hepatic duct. It passes downward between the two layers of the hepatoduodenal ligament, with the portal vein behind and the hepatic artery to its left. It then passes behind the superior part of the duodenum, and runs in a groove between the duodenum and head of the pancreas. It then joins with the pancreatic duct (still maintaining a separate lumen) and pierces the

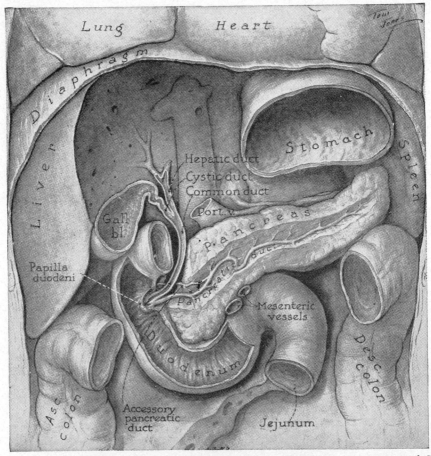

FIG. 14–15. a, The gross anatomy of the biliary system. (From Jones, T.: *Anatomical Studies.* Jackson, Michigan, S. H. Camp and Co., 1943.)

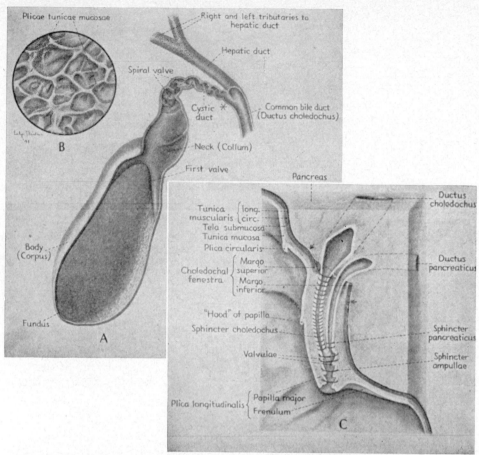

FIG. 14-15. b, GROSS ANATOMY OF BILIARY TRACT: *A*, Interior of the gallbladder and cystic duct; *B*, surface of the mucosa of the gallbladder showing plicae; *C*, diagram of frontal section through duodenum at the inferior duodenal flexure showing the structure and relations of the papilla major (duodenal papilla). (After Boyden in Surgery. From C. M. Jackson and R. F. Blount, in Morris' *Human Anatomy*, Edited by Jackson, The Blakiston Co.)

descending part of the duodenum in its midportion, to open obliquely into the lumen at the duodenal papilla.

The gallbladder is arbitrarily described as consisting of four parts (Fig. 14-15): The distal end or *fundus* usually reaches the anterior border of the liver; the *boay* runs backward, upward, and to the left; the *infunaibulum* is situated between the body and neck, and consists of that portion where the gallbladder begins to taper toward the neck; the *neck* is curved medially toward the porta hepatis, and contains spiral crescentic folds around the interior of its lumen, forming the spiral valve of Heister. The neck of the gallbladder usually curves sharply like the letter "S." This continues into the valvular portion of the cystic duct as previously described. Smooth muscle fibers are found in the fundus and infundibulum, but are almost completely absent in the body; conversely, there is much elastic tissue in the body, and very little in the fundus and infundibulum. The muscle fibers are longitudinal and oblique in the fundus, but circular in the infundibulum, and this circular conformation is continued into the spiral valves. The volume of the gallbladder is about 50 cc.

Usually the gallbladder is not covered with peritoneum on its hepatic side, but occasionally it is suspended from the liver by a short peritoneal ligament. The gallbladder usually rests on the transverse colon in front, and its neck is usually in close proximity with the duodenum.

Variations of the Gallbladder (Fig. 14–17). The major variations of the gallbladder may be classified as follows:

1. VARIATIONS IN SHAPE. The gallbladder may be ovoid, spheroidal or elongated.

2. VARIATIONS IN POSITION. The gallbladder may be deeply embedded in the liver, or it may have a mesentery and lie in the iliac fossa. Its position also varies in relation to the spine. No definite pathologic function has been associated with these unusual locations.

3. CONSTRICTION BY MUCOSAL OR SEROSAL FOLDS. These folds may produce a sacculation of the gallbladder, and the so-called Phrygian cap. This does not have pathologic significance. Also, the gallbladder may be divided longitudinally into separate gallbladders and possess separate cystic ducts.

4. ABSENCE OF THE GALLBLADDER. Rarely, the gallbladder is absent, and in such instances the hepatic ducts have usually been found to be dilated.

5. VARIATIONS IN LENGTH OF DUCTS. Variations in the length of the hepatic ducts, cystic duct and common bile duct may occur.

6. SEPARATE OPENINGS. The common bile duct and pancreatic duct may open separately into the duodenum.

The Function of the Gallbladder. The functions of the gallbladder may be summarized as follows:[12]

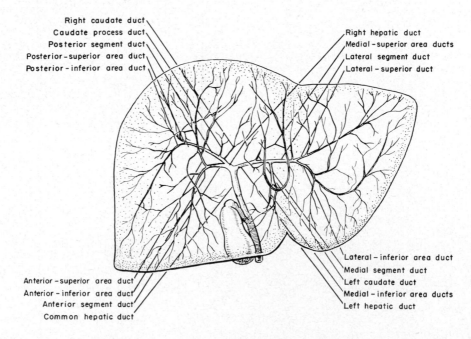

Right caudate duct
Caudate process duct
Posterior segment duct
Posterior-superior area duct
Posterior-inferior area duct

Right hepatic duct
Medial-superior area ducts
Lateral segment duct
Lateral-superior duct

Lateral-inferior area duct
Medial segment duct
Left caudate duct
Medial-inferior area ducts
Left hepatic duct

Anterior-superior area duct
Anterior-inferior area duct
Anterior segment duct
Common hepatic duct

THE ANATOMY OF THE INTRA-HEPATIC BILE FLOW

FIG. 14–16. The anatomy of the intrahepatic bile flow. (Courtesy of Dr. James F. Martin.)

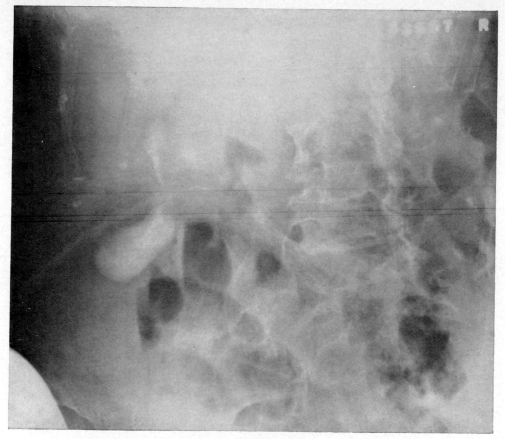

a

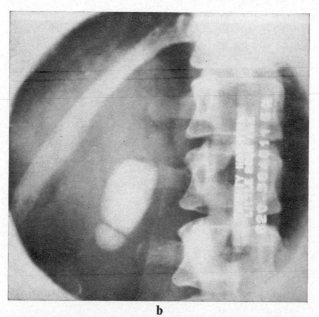

b

FIG 14–17. VARIATIONS IN GALLBLADDER OF RADIOGRAPHIC SIGNIFICANCE: **a,** Ptotic gallbladd lying in the iliac fossa; **b,** mucosal or serosal fold of gallbladder, known as a Phrygian cap.

1. THE RESERVOIR FUNCTION. A part of the bile secreted by the liver is stored in the gallbladder.

2. THE CONCENTRATION FUNCTION. Water and salts are absorbed in the gallbladder whereas the bile pigments are not, and as a result, bilirubin is concentrated about twenty times, cholesterol, bile salts and calcium about five to ten times. In disease of the gallbladder, this concentration function is readily impaired.

3. THE EMPTYING MECHANISM. The exact mechanism involved is not completely understood. It is claimed by some that there is a reciprocal innervation of the gallbladder and sphincter of Oddi, so that vagal stimulation causes contraction of the gallbladder and relaxation of the sphincter. There is also a hormonal influence as follows: When practically any acid or food substance— particularly fats and fatty acids—comes into contact with the duodenal mucosa, cholecystokinin is formed, which is absorbed into the blood stream and causes the gallbladder to empty.

4. THE SECRETORY FUNCTION. The gallbladder apparently secretes constituents of the bile, such as cholesterol and mucin.

Functions of Bile. The main functions of bile can be summarized as follows:

1. It is an important accessory agent in digestion by accelerating the action of pancreatic enzymes.

2. Bile aids materially in the digestion of fats by decreasing surface tension, activating lipase, increasing the solubility of soaps and fatty acids, and materially aiding fatty absorption.

3. It forms a means of eliminating nitrogenous and toxic waste substances.

4. Bile helps to regulate acid-base and calcium balance in the blood stream.

RADIOGRAPHIC EXAMINATION OF THE BILIARY TRACT

Prior to the gallbladder examination, it is well to remove as much gas and fecal material from the gastrointestinal tract as possible. Cascara sagrada or enemas given at least twenty-four hours before the examination may be of considerable assistance. Pitressin may be employed intravenously (0.5 to 1 cc.) in those patients where it would not be contraindicated on the basis of hypertension or arteriosclerosis.

It is also well to obtain a plain film of the entire right side of the abdomen, in the postero-anterior projection, prior to the administration of any dye. The gallbladder itself is not usually delineated with accuracy on such films, but if it should contain calcareous structure, this would immediately be evident from this preliminary study.

A visualization of the gallbladder requires that some form of contrast substance be introduced into it. Tetrachlorphenolphthalein had long been known to be secreted in the bile, and this substance had been used as a test for liver function. Graham and Cole (in 1924) introduced first the bromine radical, and thereafter the heavier iodine radical instead of the chlorine in this compound, and thus obtained a substance which was secreted by the liver in the bile, and concentrated with the bile in the gallbladder. This made it possible to render the bile radiopaque.

In recent years new compounds such as Priodax, Telepaque, Teridax, Monophen, and Cholografin (see Table 14–1) have been introduced which accomplish the same thing without many of the undesirable side effects attributed to the earlier contrast medium. Each of the newer compounds has certain contraindications and some adverse effects which are listed in Table 14–1.

The methods for cholecystography are as follows: (1) *intravenous dye*, such as Cholografin, (2) *oral dye*, such as those enumerated in Table 14–1, and (3) *cholangiograms*.

This latter may be an operative or postoperative procedure and involves the injection of a contrast medium into either the hepatic, cystic or common bile ducts.

The Intravenous Technique.[2, 4]   Cholografin (Biligrafin on the European continent) is an organic iodide administered intravenously in 20 to 40 cc. doses. It is secreted selectively by the liver in sufficient concentration usually to permit a faint concentration of the biliary radicles, common bile duct and gallbladder without dependence upon the concentration function of the gallbladder. Films are taken at ten minute intervals for the first hour and at half hourly intervals thereafter until good visualization is obtained (up to four hours). This method is only moderately satisfactory (Fig. 14–20). It must be used when there is no fistula or tube in the common duct and when the patient continues to have serious symptomatology postoperatively. The examination is contraindicated in the presence of fever (cholangitis or hepatitis) and seldom successful in the presence of jaundice.

The primary indications for intravenous cholangiograms by this technique are:

1. The "postcholecystectomy syndrome": The patient continues to have right upper quadrant discomfort or pain after cholecystectomy.

2. When for any reason stones are suspected in the biliary tree above the level of the cystic duct.

3. When the gallbladder has not been visualized by oral techniques, and its visualization is still desired.

Testing of intravenous sensitivity to Cholografin should never be omitted prior to this study. Indeed, routine administration of anti-histaminics prior to or with the media is advocated by some.

Intravenous cholangiography after cholecystectomy may at times reveal a saclike structure at the site of the amputated cystic duct. This may represent a "reformed gallbladder," and may account for the so-called "postcholecystectomy syndrome" in some patients. This may also represent a false sac created by persistent drainage into a walled-off saccular area at the site of the T-tube insertion in the common duct.

A "scout film" of the gallbladder area is first obtained. Once the gallbladder is found, the patient is rotated in various positions so as to project the gallbladder free from all interfering shadows such as overlying ribs, spine or gas. Ordinarily, the left anterior oblique recumbent projection will project the gallbladder upward toward the ribs, and the straight postero-anterior projection will project the gallbladder closer to the spine. Every effort is made to obtain a clear visualization of the gallbladder.

The spiral valves of Heister must not be misinterpreted as small stones, since they may appear as small negative shadows alternating with positive shadows in the infundibulum and proximal portion of the cystic duct. A typical visualization of the gallbladder and biliary tree by this technique is illustrated in Figure 14–20.

Details of Oral Procedure. On the day before the examination, a fatty meal is given at noon to empty the gallbladder and a light fat-free meal is given at 6:00 p. m Following this, 3 to 5 grams of the oral dye are administered. The drugs presently used are Telepaque, Teridax, Monophen and Priodax. All of the above drugs depend upon their iodine content for visualization and depend upon concentration by the gallbladder. Occasionally the above drugs may produce nausea, diarrhea, or dysuria (Table 14–1).

Nothing is allowed by mouth after the dye is administered until the patient appears for his examination the following morning, fourteen to sixteen hours after taking the dye.

Enemas are administered in the morning if advised by the radiologist. This is done particularly to cleanse the gastrointestinal tract of interfering shadows which may superimpose themselves upon the shadow of the gallbladder and thus obscure detail. On the other hand, some regard a visualization of the media in the colon as a check to note whether or not the dye was actually taken by the patient. When Telepaque is utilized the opaque material can be seen in the gastrointestinal tract. Priodax, on the other hand, is absorbed immediately and is excreted largely by the kidneys and hence is not detected in the gastrointestinal tract.

The first scout film is taken twelve to fourteen hours after the oral administration of the dye. Usually a sufficiently large film is employed to cover the entire area between the costal margin above and the iliac crest below the right lateral abdominal wall and the left lateral aspect of the spine. A scout film (Fig. 14–18) including this entire area should include a gallbladder anomalously placed either over the spine or in the iliac fossa.

Once the gallbladder is found, the patient is rotated in various positions to obtain a clear visualization of this organ on a second film. Every effort is made to obtain this visualization without superposition of rib shadows, calcified cartilages, gas shadows from the colon, or the other bony structures.

Occasionally it is necessary to place the patient on his right side so that the gallbladder drops by gravity and the gas shadows rise; thus, a clear visualization may be obtained employing a lateral decubitus horizontal x-ray beam.

An erect film of the gallbladder region should be routine since this may be an additional expedient for clearing the gallbladder of superimposed shadows. Moreover, if there are stones, very frequently these will either float or settle in the gallbladder and thus become more concentrated and more readily visualized (Fig. 14–19, **c**). This should be a "coned-down" film.

After a satisfactory visualization of the gallbladder is obtained, a fatty meal or stimulant is given and films are taken at fifteen minutes, thirty minutes, one hour, or two hours after the fatty meal until maximal emptying of the gallbladder is seen and until best visualization of the common duct is obtained (Fig. 14–19, **a, b**).

Table 14–1.   Comparison of Some of the Major Compounds Employed for Gallbladder Visualization

	PHARMACOLOGY	CONTRAINDICATIONS	ACCURACY AND ADVERSE EFFECTS
Priodax	Phenylpropionic acid derivative.	1. Acute Nephritis	35% less opacity than Telepaque.
	Insoluble in water but soluble in alkali.	2. Uremia.	60% { nausea, diarrhea, dysuria } vs. 21.4% with Telepaque.
	51.38% Iodine.		More patients require second dose (40%). Fails to visualize 12% of gallbladders—visualized with Telepaque.
	Excreted mostly by kidneys.		
Tele-paque	Ethyl propanoic acid derivative.	1. Acute Nephritis	Fails only in 3% of normal gall-bladders or less with one dose.
	Insoluble in water; soluble in al-kali and 95% alcohol.	2. Uremia	Side reactions less than with Prio-dax as above.
	66.68% Iodine.	3. Gastrointestinal diseases with dis-turbed absorption.	Great opacity may obscure some gallstones.
	Excreted mostly via gastro-intestinal tract.		
Teridax	Tri-iodoethionic acid (ethyl pro-pionic acid derivative).	1. Acute Nephritis	Failure after one examination not always indicative of disease; but after second dose approaches 100% accuracy.
	Insoluble in water; soluble in alkali.	2. Uremia	Not as well worked out as to side reactions as above.
	66.5% Iodine.		Said to produce density intermedi-ate in density between Priodax and Telepaque.
	Excreted mostly by kidneys.		
Mono-phen	Carboxylic acid derivative.	1. Acute Nephritis	60% no adverse signs or symptoms.
	Insoluble in water.	2. Uremia	12% nausea, 1% vomiting, 9% diarrhea, 9% cramps, 3% dysuria
	52.2% Iodine.		
	Excreted mostly by kidneys.		Accuracy stated to be better (?) than Priodax.
Cholo-grafin	Iodipamide (tri-iodobenzoic acid derivative).	*Primary indication:* "Postcholecystec-tomy syndrome"	Sensitivity high. Side effects minimal with slow injection.
	For intravenous use (photosen-sitive).	*Contraindication:* 1. Iodine sensitivity 2. Combined urinary and hepatic disease.	77/85 successful biliary tree vis-ualization.
	64% Iodine.		Visualization faint; usually gall-bladder visualization too faint for significant accuracy.
	With normal liver: 90% ex-creted in feces, 10% in urine. With poor liver function: most-ly excreted by kidneys (hence pyelograms).		

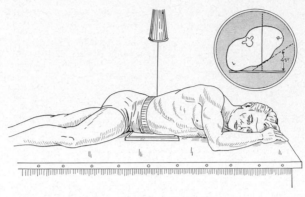

a

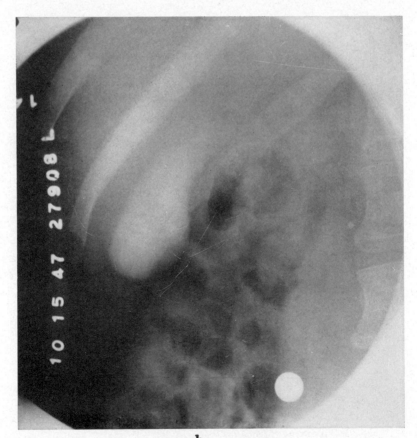

b

Fig. 14–18. RADIOGRAPH OF GALLBLADDER BEFORE FATTY STIMULATION: a, Positioning of patient;
b, radiograph.

Interpretation of Results. When no visualization of the gallbladder is obtained (and assuming adequate absorption of the dye), it may mean any one or more of the following possibilities:

1. Liver function is so poor that bile formation is impeded.
2. There is obstructive disease of the intrahepatic or hepatic bile ducts.
3. There is obstructive disease of the common bile duct.
4. The gallbladder is diseased.

Without further information about the patient, no further interpretation is possible.

When the gallbladder is visualized, the result is interpreted in the light of: (1) anatomic structure and (2) gallbladder function. These two factors are separate entities and not entirely interdependent. Thus, it is not unusual for the gallbladder to concentrate the bile well and respond normally to fatty stimulation, and yet excessive calcium or cholesterol may be deposited as gallstones, indicating that this aspect of its function is abnormal. The size, shape and extent of concentration of the bile are also noted. If the gallbladder is visualized, the size and configuration are noted, and search is made for any abnormal shadows within its lumen. Occasionally, it is also possible to outline the cystic and common bile ducts as well.

Occasionally it is difficult to assess whether adequate absorption of the dye has occurred, but we have found these tests to be very accurate (probably 95 per cent) if the patient took the prescribed dosage and did not vomit the dye.

Cholangiograms. Visualization of the biliary tract is possible at operation by the direct injection of contrast media into the gallbladder, cystic or hepatic duct under direct vision. It is also possible to introduce opaque media into the drainage tube which has been allowed to remain in the biliary tract following operation on the gallbladder. These studies are referred to as cholangiograms. In the latter instance, they can be done while fluoroscoping the patient, and spot-film studies can be obtained during fluoroscopy to supplement the anteroposterior and lateral films which are obtained as a routine.

The opaque media employed are: iodized oil, or water-soluble iodized organic compounds such as Diodrast or Hypaque. Diodrast is used in 35 per cent concentration and Hypaque in 50 per cent, and every care is exercised to avoid air bubbles which may simulate biliary stones.

Films obtained by this type of examination are illustrated in Figure 14–21. If there is no obstruction in the common bile duct, a clear visualization of the duodenum is obtained, along with the delineation of the various biliary ducts already discussed.

Operative cholangiography is an exploratory roentgen diagnostic procedure which is now virtually routine during cholecystectomy.[7] After exposure of the cystic duct, a polyethylene catheter is inserted into the cystic duct and threaded into the hepatic duct. The cystic duct distal to the insertion is clamped. Diodrast, Hypaque or 25 per cent Urokon is injected (about 20 cc.) and a film obtained in the operating room near the end of the injection period with respiration suspended. Experience has shown that this method of exploration will reveal gallstones on many occasions where conventional surgical exploratory techniques will be negative.

Needless to say, T-tube cholangiography under fluoroscopic control with three or four serial injections and spot films in the frontal and oblique projections is far more accurate and should be performed routinely prior to the removal of the T-tube drain.

The most common source of error in either operative or T-tube cholangiography is the introduction of air bubbles with the injection of the contrast media. Air bubbles will resemble negative stones on the radiographs. This error can be avoided by very careful removal of all air from the injection tubing and syringe prior to the injection.

At the completion of either examination as much of the contrast media as possible should be withdrawn to avoid hepatic and pancreatic irritation. Occasionally, mild pancreatitis is experienced subsequent to the above examinations.

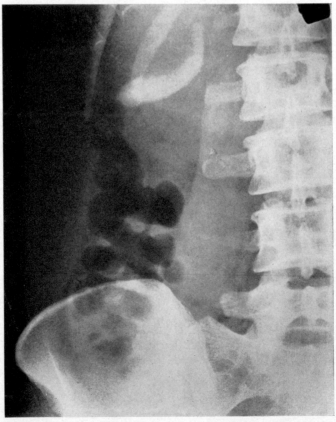

FIG. 14–19.   GALLBLADDER AFTER FATTY STIMULATION: a, Radiograph.

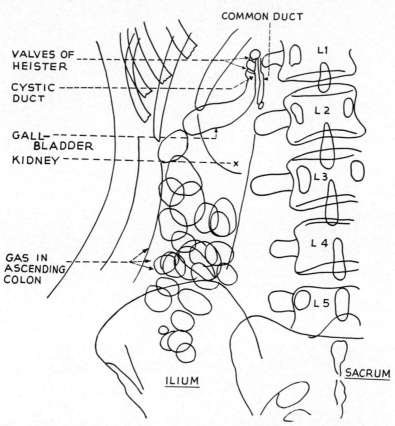

FIG. 14–19.   GALLBLADDER AFTER FATTY STIMULATION: **b,** Labeled tracing of **a.**

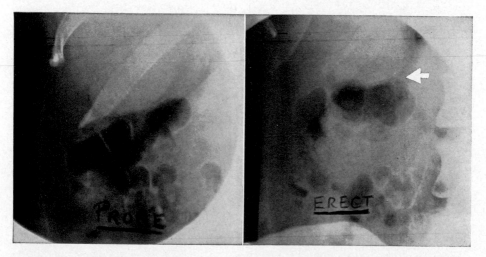

FIG. 14–19.   **c,** An erect film of the gallbladder. Occasionally the contrast medium will gravitate to the bottom of the fundus and form a layer simulating stones. This must be interpreted with caution.

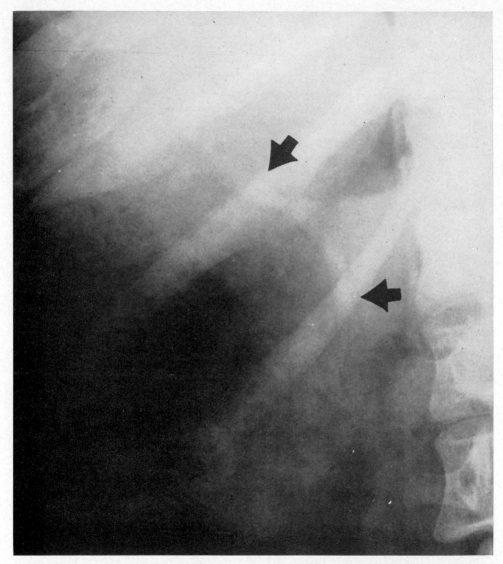

FIG. 14–20.   Faint visualization of the biliary tree by intravenous cholangiography with the aid of intravenous Cholografin. Ordinarily a visualization of this order of density is obtained.

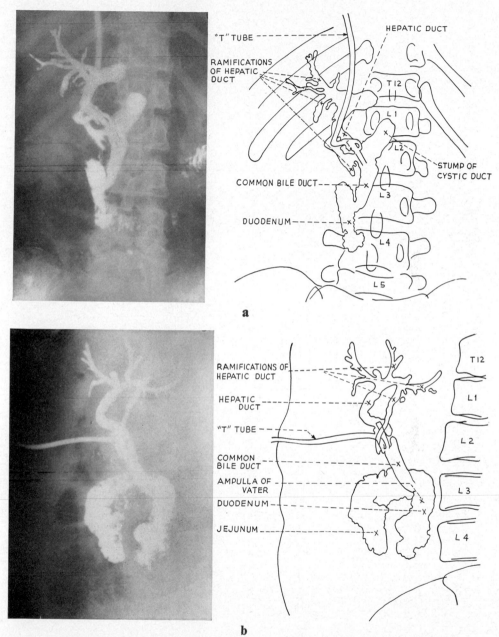

a

b

Fig. 14–21. Representative cholangiograms with iodized oil in **a**, antero-posterior and **b**, lateral projections, with labeled tracings.

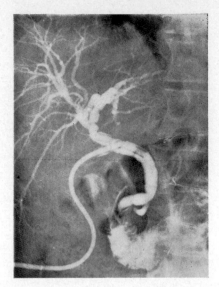

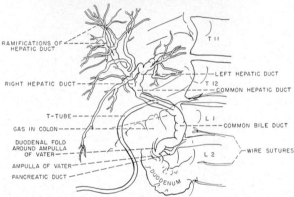

FIG. 14–21. **c,** Thirty-five per cent Diodrast T-tube cholangiogram and its tracing. This contrast medium gives a more complete visualization of all hepatic radicles. This is extremely important since stones may be concealed in the hepatic radicles only to descend later and cause a recurrence of symptoms.

REFERENCES

1. Cannon, W. B.: Am. J. Physiol., *6:* 251, 1901–2.
2. Cohn, E. M., Orloff, T. L., Sclaroff, D. M., and Gershon-Cohen, J.: The Use of Cholografin in the Postcholecystectomy Syndrome. Ann. Int. Med., *42:* 59–68, 1955.
3. Gianturco, C., and Miller, G.: Routine Search for Colonic Polyps by High Voltage Radiography. Radiology, *60:* 496–499, 1953.
4. Hastings-James, R., and Glazebrook, A. J.: Cholographin. Canad. M. A. J., *72:* 561–565, 1955.
5. Hinkel, C. J.: Roentgenologic Examination and Evaluation of the Ileocecal Valve. Am. J. Roentgenol., *68:* 172–182, 1952.
6. Jones, H., Kaplan, H., and Windholz, F.: Air Contrast Colon Examination with Colloidal Barium. Radiology, *56:* 561–566, 1956.
7. Martin, J. F.: Operative Cholangiography. North Carolina M. J., *18:* 537–544, 1957.
8. Moreton, R. D.: Double-Contrast Examination of the Colon with Special Emphasis on Studies of the Sigmoid. Radiology, *60:* 510–517, 1953.
9. Robinson, J. M.: Polyps of the Colon: How to Find Them. Am. J. Roentgenol., *77:* 700–725, 1957.
10. Stevenson, C. A.: The Development of the Colon Examination. Am. J. Roentgenol., *71:* 385–397, 1954.
11. Templeton, F. E., and Addington, E. A.: Roentgenographic Examination of the Colon Using Drainage and Negative Pressure. J.A.M.A., *145:* 702–704, 1951.
12. Wiggers, C. J.: Physiology in Health and Disease. 5th Ed. Lea and Febiger, Philadelphia, 1949.

CHAPTER 15

The Abdomen
and Peritoneal Space

BOUNDARIES, SUBDIVISIONS AND CONTENTS OF THE ABDOMINAL CAVITY

Boundaries and Subdivisions of the Peritoneal Cavity.   The abdominopelvic cavity is that segment of the serous cavity of the trunk which lies below the diaphragm. The anterior wall is composed of the transversalis, internal oblique and external oblique muscles, together with the rectus and pyramidal muscles, the skin and superficial fascia overlying these structures. The posterior wall is composed of the vertebral column, the posterior segment of the pelvis, the inferior portions of the diaphragm, and the quadratus lumborum and psoas muscles. The side walls of the abdomen are formed by the oblique and transverse muscles, and below by the iliacus muscles and the iliac bones.

The abdominal cavity is divisible into the abdominal cavity proper and the true pelvis or pelvis minor. The ribs cover approximately the same area of the abdomen as they do the thorax.

The true pelvis is bounded in front and at the side by as much of the hip bones as lie below the level of the linea terminalis. These are partly clothed by the internal obturator muscle and pelvic fascia. The posterior wall is formed by the anterior aspect of the sacrum and coccyx, covered on each side by the pyriform muscle. The pyriform muscles pass out of the pelvis through the greater sciatic notch, thus closing these potential holes in the cavity. The floor of the pelvis is composed of the levator ani muscles, coccygeal muscles and the endopelvic fascia.

There are certain openings in the abdominal walls which form potentially weak areas through which protrusions (herniations) may occur. These openings occur in the diaphragm to allow passage for the aorta, esophagus and inferior vena cava; in the pelvic floor to allow passage for the urethra, rectum and vagina; in the lower portion of the abdominal wall at the site of the inguinal canals through which the round ligaments and spermatic cords pass, and in the area of weakness formed by the femoral sheath which contains the femoral arteries, veins, lymphatics and femoral canal.

Contents of the Abdomen.   The following structures are found within the abdominopelvic cavity: (1) the peritoneum, mesenteries, omenta and ligaments,

(2) the liver, (3) the spleen, (4) the pancreas, (5) the adrenal glands, (6) the urinary tract, (7) the reproductive organs, (8) the gastrointestinal tract and (9) the blood vessels, lymphatics and nerves.

The gastrointestinal tract, genitourinary tract and cardiovascular system are considered separately.

THE PERITONEUM, MESENTERIES, OMENTA AND LIGAMENTS

The Properitoneal Fat Layer or Tela Subserosa.   Between the transversalis fascia, which covers the inner surfaces of the abdominal muscles, and the peritoneum lies a considerable quantity of extraperitoneal areolar tissue, which contains a variable amount of fat. This is referred to as the "tela subserosa," and its parietal component is called the "properitoneal fat layer," to use a radiologic term (Fig. 15–1).

This layer is of importance radiologically, since it frequently becomes involved in inflammatory processes of the peritoneum, by contiguity, and its demonstration becomes less distinct, thus furnishing a clue to peritoneal involvement.

The tela subserosa continues posteriorly, and is particularly abundant around the kidneys, giving rise to a considerable perirenal fat layer. It is this continuation of the tela subserosa around the kidneys which permits a fairly accurate visualization of these organs without the necessity for contrast media (Fig. 15–1).

The Peritoneum.   The peritoneum is the serous membrane which lines the abdominal cavity and invests most of the abdominal viscera. The peritoneum covering an organ is called "visceral peritoneum"; that lining the abdominal wall, or helping to form mesenteries or omenta, is called "parietal peritoneum." The space between these two layers is actually a potential one and contains a thin layer of fluid under normal conditions. When air is introduced into the peritoneal space, the abdominal organs fall away from the abdominal wall, and this cavity becomes apparent.

The peritoneal space is a completely closed area in the male, but in the female it communicates with the exterior through the uterine tube and uterus, which have openings both to the exterior and into the abdominal cavity.

The Mesenteries.   The mesenteries are folds of peritoneum which unite the abdominal wall with the intestines, and contain the blood vessels and nerves which supply and drain the intestines.

There are separate mesenteries for the small intestine, the transverse colon and the pelvic colon (called "mesentery," "transverse mesocolon," and "pelvic mesocolon" respectively).

The Omenta and Ligaments.   When peritoneal folds are more complex they are termed "omenta" and "ligaments."

The greater omentum is an apron-like fold of peritoneum which is attached to the greater curvature of the stomach, and hangs down in front of the intestines to a variable extent, and then folds back upon itself to attach to the transverse colon. A portion of the anterior layer of the greater omentum continues from the stomach to the spleen, and forms the gastrolienal ligament, and also from the colon to the stomach, where it is called the gastrocolic ligament. Between the anterior and posterior folds is the cavity spoken of as the "omental bursa."

ROUTINE OF EXAMINATION OF KUB FILM

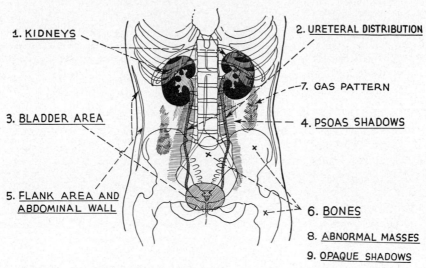

1. KIDNEYS

2. URETERAL DISTRIBUTION

7. GAS PATTERN

3. BLADDER AREA

4. PSOAS SHADOWS

5. FLANK AREA AND ABDOMINAL WALL

6. BONES

8. ABNORMAL MASSES

9. OPAQUE SHADOWS

FIG. 15–1.   **a,** Routine for examination of the recumbent film of the abdomen.

FLANK ANATOMY

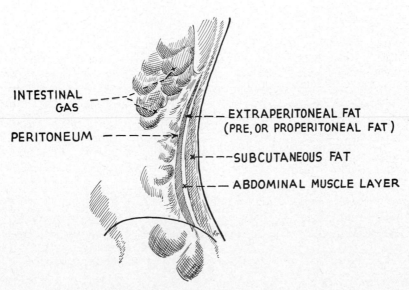

INTESTINAL GAS

EXTRAPERITONEAL FAT (PRE, OR PROPERITONEAL FAT)

PERITONEUM

SUBCUTANEOUS FAT

ABDOMINAL MUSCLE LAYER

FIG. 15–1.   **b,** Diagram demonstrating flank anatomy, showing the relationship of the properitoneal fat layer to the rest of the abdominal wall.

The lesser omentum is a peritoneal fold passing from the inferior surface of the liver to the lesser curvature of the stomach and the first part of the duodenum, and the space posterior to this omentum is the lesser omental bursa which is situated mainly behind the stomach and anterior to the pancreas. The aperture which opens into the lesser omental bursa is called the epiploic foramen, or foramen of Winslow. This has already been described in some detail with respect to the stomach and duodenum (Chap. 13).

RADIOGRAPHIC STUDY OF THE PERITONEAL SPACE AND ABDOMINAL WALL

1. **Antero-posterior Film of the Abdomen, Recumbent.** This is also commonly referred to as a "KUB" film, since it is usually employed in examinations of the urinary tract, and the letters symbolize "kidney, ureter and bladder." The structures delineated in this examination are shown in Figure 15–2. It will be seen that several layers can be identified in the lateral abdominal wall above the iliac crests: the skin and subcutaneous tissues; the muscular layer; the properitoneal fat layer; and finally the abdominal viscera. When inflammatory processes involve the abdominal wall, occasionally abnormal gas shadows may be identified, or the differentiation of these various layers becomes indistinct. Very often in inflammatory disease of the peritoneum, the properitoneal fat layer becomes indistinct, or there may be a diffuse haziness of the structures. It will also be noted that the tela subserosa is continued around the kidney, permitting the outline of that organ to be seen; the psoas muscle shadow and quadratus lumborum muscle shadows are likewise differentiated on both sides. The posterior inferior margin of the layer casts a rather well-defined shadow, beneath both lower poles of the kidneys and under the peritoneum above the iliac crests.

There are variable gas shadows and fecal shadows in the colon and stomach in the adult, and in the small intestine as well in the infant. These tend to obscure soft tissue detail considerably, as well as the detail of the bony structure of the lumbar spine and pelvis. For that reason, if it is desired that such interference be eliminated, and if the patient can be prepared for this examination, it is well to give the patient 2 tablespoonfuls of castor oil the night before the examination, and enemas until returns are clear several hours beforehand. In the event that the examination is an emergency, such preparation is impossible.

2. **Antero-posterior Film of the Abdomen, Erect.** In this study, most of the abdominal viscera tend to descend owing to the action of gravity. Unusual mobility is an indication of abnormality, but the limits of normal in this respect are fairly great. If there is fluid in the gastrointestinal tract as well as gas, fluid levels are obtained. In the small intestine, such fluid levels are frequently an indication of mechanical obstruction. Abnormally, also, there may be air which has escaped into the peritoneal space, in which case it will rise to the highest possible level, and unless there are adhesions which prevent such rise, this gas will usually accumulate under the diaphragm. In obtaining this film, it is important that the diaphragm be absolutely motionless, otherwise a thin stripe of free air will be obscured and may escape detection. A rapid exposure technique should always be employed if free air under the diaphragm is suspected, and in our laboratory we employ a separate chest exposure, or lateral decubitus film of the abdomen (patient lies on his side and a horizontal x-ray

beam is employed to obtain a frontal view of the abdomen), as well as the upright film of the abdomen. The chest film allows for simultaneous examination of that portion of the trunk and helps to exclude referred disease—a very important consideration whenever one is confronted with abdominal complaints.

In the upright film, the soft tissue structures in the anatomic pelvis are less clearly defined, and in general, structural detail is less distinct than in the recumbent film.

3. **Patient Supine; Horizontal X-ray Beam.** In this film study, the patient lies supine, and a horizontal x-ray beam is directed at the abdomen from the patient's side. The main purpose of this examination is to demonstrate free air under the xiphisternum, and also to see any fluid levels which may be present in the small or large intestine. All other detail is generally obscured.

4. **Patient on Side; Horizontal X-ray Beam.** In this examination, the patient lies on one side, and a horizontal x-ray beam is directed at the abdomen from the anterior aspect. Ordinarily, a Potter-Bucky diaphragm is employed, if possible, to obtain better detail. The viscera tend to drop by gravity, but if there are fluid levels present, once again they can be readily demonstrated, and any free air in the peritoneal space rises to the uppermost part of the abdomen where it can be seen. This examination is also helpful when it is desired to eliminate gaseous shadows from one side of the abdomen, since the gas containing loops of bowel will tend to drop away from the side which is uppermost. Kirklin has shown that this can be used efficaciously in gallbladder studies.

Recommended Routine for Study of the Acute Abdomen (Fig. 15–3). The pathologic abdomen is out of the realm of this text, but in this connection it may be pointed out that in the study of a patient for acute abdominal disease, it is well to obtain both a recumbent as well as an erect film of the abdomen, a chest film, and frequently an additional study with the patient on his side, employing a horizontal x-ray beam.

It is also important to note the degree of separation of the gas-containing loops of bowel, since peritoneal disease will often widen the space between adjoining loops of bowel, which is normally about 2 mm. Indeed, this phase of the study is just as important, if not more so, than the examination for the relative clarity of the properitoneal fat line.

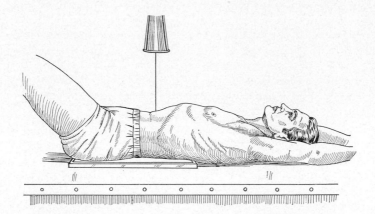

FIG. 15–2.   ANTERO-POSTERIOR VIEW OF ABDOMEN (KUB FILM):   **a,** Positioning of patient.

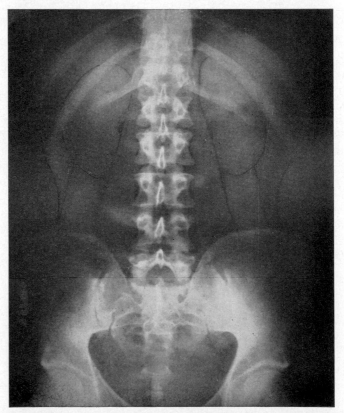

FIG. 15–2.   ANTERO-POSTERIOR VIEW OF ABDOMEN (KUB FILM):   **b,** Radiograph.

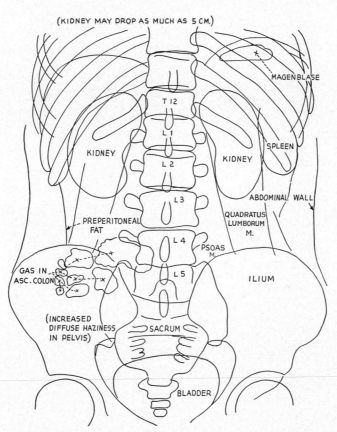

Fig. 15–2. ANTERO-POSTERIOR VIEW OF ABDOMEN (KUB FILM): **c,** Labeled tracing of **b.**

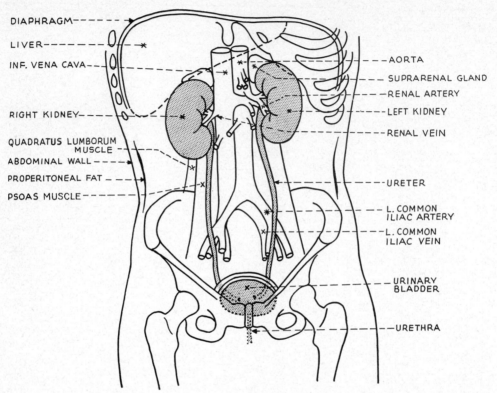

FIG. 15–2. ANTERO-POSTERIOR VIEW OF ABDOMEN (KUB FILM): **d,** Diagram intensifying the urinary
tract and indicating other anatomic relationships.

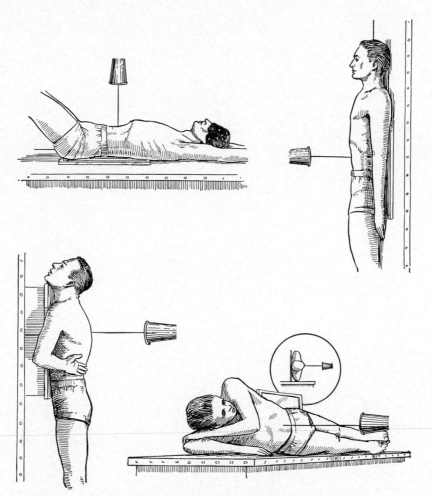

FIG. 15–3. Routine film studies obtained for plain film survey of abdominal disease. Note that a P-A chest film is part of this routine. (Decubitus left lateral may be preferable.)

THE LIVER

Surface Topography; Gross Anatomy. A line connecting the lower border of the fifth rib on the left with the upper border of this rib on the right usually forms the upper border of the superior surface of the liver. This border is ordinarily slightly concave under the xiphisternum. As seen from the front, the lower margin of the liver is found under the costal margin on the right, and passes obliquely upward to the eighth or ninth costal cartilage on the left (Fig. 15–2, **d**).

The liver is maintained in this relationship in the recumbent position, but when erect there is a variable drop of the liver for several centimeters. The position of the liver will also vary with the body habitus and the position of the patient.

The falciform ligament on the anterior and superior surface of the liver divides the liver into a large right lobe and a small left lobe. The quadrate and caudate lobes on the inferior surface of the liver are subdivisions of the right lobe, which are important in that they impart an irregularity to the inferior margin of the liver as it is seen on the plain radiograph of the abdomen.

The left lobe of the liver is contained under the cupola of the left diaphragm and overlies the stomach and the spleen.

Although the liver can be moderately well outlined on the plain radiograph, nevertheless it is rather difficult to detect with certainty even with moderate degrees of enlargement.

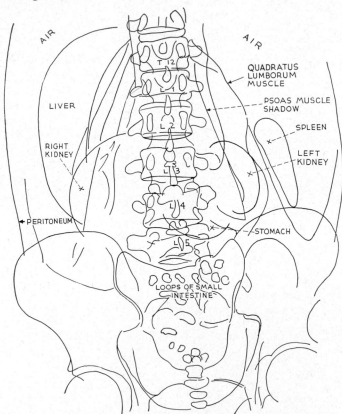

FIG. 15–4. Tracing of a radiograph demonstrating pneumoperitoneum in the erect antero-posterior view of the abdomen.

Areas of calcification as well as bronchovascular markings from the lung may be projected into the liver area from the posterior costophrenic angle of the chest. These must not be misinterpreted as liver abnormalities.

Pneumoperitoneum (Fig. 15–4). The introduction of air into the peritoneal space provides a means of delineating the viscera separately from the abdominal wall. The location, size, mobility, outline and attachments of the various abdominal organs can be detected in this manner.

Normally, there is a fairly wide range of mobility of the liver, spleen and other intra-abdominal organs, and any restriction in motion can be readily detected. Examination of the patient while on his left side allows the air to rise over the right lobe of the liver, and the liver drops into the left abdomen, allowing a clear visualization of the right kidney. When the patient lies on his right side, the left kidney, spleen, splenic flexure and descending colon become visible. When the patient lies prone, with the abdomen suspended between two supports under the thigh and chest, the air rises to the prevertebral space, outlining the structures here.

In the erect position, the liver drops away from the diaphragm and any subphrenic space-occupying lesion becomes readily demonstrable.

Pelvic pneumoperitoneum will be described separately (Chap. 17).

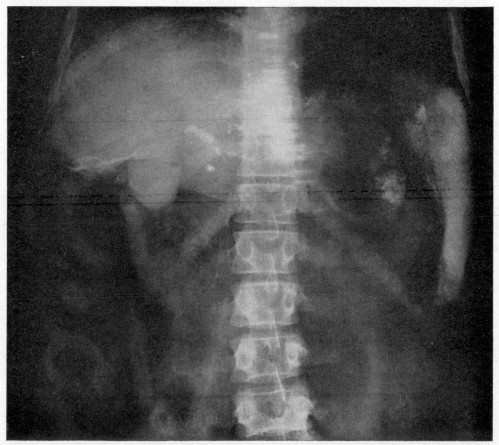

FIG. 15–5. Thorotrast hepatolienography following intravenous injection of 60 cc. of Thorotrast in three days. This film was obtained one week following the last injection.

Pneumoperitoneum is somewhat painful, and there is some question as to whether the information gained is worth the inconvenience of the examination.

SPECIAL RADIOGRAPHIC STUDY OF THE LIVER

Hepatolienography. Thorotrast is a stable suspension of 25 per cent thorium dioxide which when introduced intravenously is stored in the reticuloendothelial system. *In view of the long-lived radioactivity of this compound, it may induce late degenerative, fibrotic, and even malignant changes in the liver and spleen; therefore it must never be used lightly.*

Thorotrast is supplied in 25 cc. ampules, and is freely miscible with water or saline. A total dose of 50 to 75 cc. is necessary over a period of several days, given intravenously. The initial dose should not exceed 10 or 15 cc., but in the absence of symptoms, this may be increased to 25 cc. intravenously in one day. The radiographic examination should be made one or two days after the last dose.

As a result of the fixation of the thorium salts by the reticuloendothelial cells of the liver and spleen, these organs become clearly outlined on the radiograph (Fig. 15–5). Any space-occupying lesions within the liver or spleen are clearly demarcated since they will not become impregnated.

THE SPLEEN

The spleen lies in the left upper quadrant posterior to the stomach, and immediately under the diaphragm. It varies in size considerably, but ordinarily does not project significantly below the horizontal plane at the level of the left costal margin. The diaphragm separates it from the ninth, tenth and eleventh ribs on the left. The medial surface of the spleen is in contact with the tail of the pancreas, and the lower pole of the spleen with the splenic flexure of the colon. The anteromedial portion of the spleen is in contact with the greater curvature of the stomach.

Only the inferior one third or one half of the spleen is visible radiographically on a plain film of the abdomen (Fig. 15–2). It is seen as a tonguelike projection lateral to the stomach, and extending down to the inferior margin of the costal border. It can, however, be detected by means of hepatolienography as previously described (Fig. 15–5).

Ordinarily, the spleen creates a slight impression upon the splenic flexure of the colon, and the greater curvature of the stomach.

Normally, the tiplike projection of the inferior margin of the spleen can be readily identified at the level of the left costal margin, and forms a good basis for measurement of the spleen: the horizontal measurement 2 cm. above the tip of the spleen should not exceed 3.5 cm. (Wyman[2]).

Calcification is very frequent in the region of the spleen, and this may be due to phleboliths, tubercles, calcified infarcts, splenic artery aneurysms and certain cysts (hydatid), but this subject is outside the scope of the present text. Subcapsular calcification may also occur, but this also is most likely a pathologic degenerative change.

THE PANCREAS

Gross Anatomy. The pancreas has already been described to some extent with relation to the stomach and duodenum. It lies transversely and obliquely on the posterior abdominal wall (Fig. 13–11, **a** and **b**), its right end in the concavity of the duodenum and its left end touching the spleen. The greater part of the pancreas lies behind the stomach.

Anatomically it is subdivided into a head, body and tail having the following relationships: The head lies in the concavity of the duodenum with the inferior vena cava and abdominal aorta behind it; the body crosses to the left where it tends to pass upward slightly and posteriorly as it traverses the spine, left kidney and adrenal gland; and the tail touches the inferior part of the spleen.

The body of the pancreas forms the posterior wall of the lesser omental bursa.

These relationships of the pancreas are of considerable importance radiographically, since it is by displacement of contiguous structures that one recognizes its abnormalities. There is no direct means of visualization of this organ without major surgery.

METHODS OF EXAMINATION OF PANCREAS

Plain Postero-anterior Film of the Abdomen. This is useful only if the pancreas contains abnormal calcific deposits, or if there is obvious displacement of the stomach as seen by the gas contained within it.

Barium Meal. The stomach and duodenum are outlined with barium, and displacement of these organs as seen in the postero-anterior and lateral projections is of significance in detecting abnormality in the pancreas.

Passage of Radiopaque Tube into the Stomach and Duodenum. This method basically involves the same principle as the barium meal in that displacements of the tube are interpreted in the light of enlargement of the pancreas or lesser omental bursa. This method has the advantage of not requiring the introduction of an opaque medium, and thus interference with the presence of calcium in the pancreas is not obtained. The stomach and duodenum are not outlined so accurately as they are with an examination with barium, which is a disadvantage.

Introduction of Air into the Stomach. The introduction of air into the stomach outlines the stomach, but not so accurately as does barium. Postero-anterior and lateral views of the abdomen are taken as before, and displacements of the stomach detected in this fashion.

THE ADRENAL GLANDS (SUPRARENALS)

Gross Anatomy. The adrenal glands are two small glands which lie upon the superior poles of each kidney, and are 3 to 5 cm. in height, 3 cm. in width and 1 to 2 cm. in antero-posterior thickness. Each is composed of a thick cortex and a medulla of chromaffin tissue.

The right adrenal is rather pyramidal in shape, having its anterior surface laterally in contact with the liver and with the inferior vena cava, its posterior surface with the diaphragm and its base with the kidney below.

The left gland is more semilunar in shape. Anteriorly it is in contact with the stomach above, with the pancreas below, with the diaphragm posteriorly, and its base with the left kidney below it. The left adrenal lies as much medial to the left kidney as above it, in contrast to the right adrenal which caps the kidney. The amount of peritoneum covering the gland is variable.

The normal adrenal is not clearly visible on the plain radiograph and special contrast studies must be employed to delineate it. This is done by means of perirenal air insufflation (Fig. 15–6) or other gaseous media.

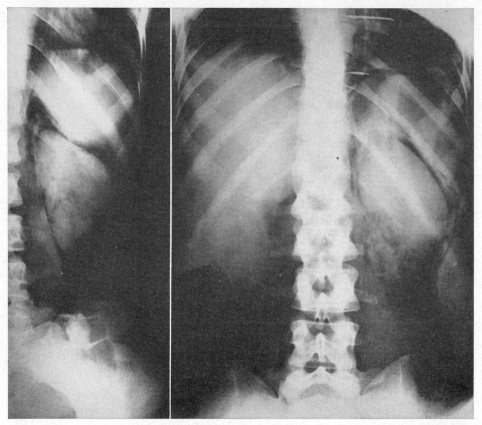

FIG. 15–6.   Perirenal air insufflation around the left kidney and adrenal gland. (Films supplied through the courtesy of Drs. Joelson, Friedell and Dundon, University Hospitals, Cleveland, Ohio.)

Method of Study by Perirenal Air Insufflation (Fig. 15–6). This method involves the introduction of air, oxygen or carbon dioxide directly into the perirenal areolar tissue by needle puncture through the lumbar triangle. Several hundred cubic centimeters are usually necessary and twelve to twenty-four hours must elapse to allow for proper distribution of air around the kidney and adrenal gland. Stereoscopic antero-posterior and lateral films are obtained at 24-hour intervals for approximately three days. Occasionally, the gas diffuses over to the opposite side, and a bilateral visualization is obtained.

When oxygen is used, the examination must be carried out more quickly, since most of this gaseous medium will be absorbed in about six hours. Recently carbon dioxide has been proposed as the safest gaseous medium to employ, since large volumes of this gas can be introduced directly into the blood stream without untoward results. However, the absorption of carbon dioxide is so extremely rapid that diagnostic radiographic detail is impaired. With proper technique, carbon dioxide may well be the best to employ for this purpose.

The presacral route has recently achieved greater popularity for insufflation of gases around the renal and suprarenal areas. In this technique, the needle is inserted through the skin outside the anus into the tela subserosa between the rectum and the sacrum. A finger is placed in the rectum during the needle insertion to help guide its positioning. Approximately 1000 cc. of gas are introduced. During the next two hours, the patient is rotated frequently.

When air is used, an initial film of the suprarenal area is obtained at the two-hour interval and hourly thereafter until maximal visualization is obtained. At this time, it is well to perform intravenous pyelograms, and once again appropriate films of the suprarenal area are obtained. Oblique and stereoscopic films as well as body-section radiographs (5 to 10 cm. from posterior) are now done to aid in the diagnosis.[1]

The adrenal gland on the right is thereafter seen as a pyramidal structure capping the right kidney, and the left adrenal as a semilunar-shaped structure partially capping and medial to the left kidney.

Gas embolism has been described as one of the unfortunate complications of this procedure and, for that reason, it cannot be used indiscriminately as it is never completely without hazard.

REFERENCES

1. Joelson, J. J., Pesky, L., and Rose, F.: The Radiologic Diagnosis of Tumors of Adrenal Gland. Radiology, *62:* 488–495, 1954.
2. Wyman, A. C.: Traumatic Rupture of the Spleen. Am. J. Roentgenol., *72:* 51–63, 1954.

CHAPTER 16

The Urinary Tract

CORRELATED GROSS AND MICROSCOPIC ANATOMY OF THE URINARY TRACTS

THE URINARY TRACT consists of the following major structures: (1) the kidneys—one on either side, (2) the ureters, (3) the urinary bladder and (4) the urethra.

The Kidneys. The kidneys are retroperitoneal bean-shaped organs lying on either side of the vertebral column. The upper poles lie approximately 1 cm. closer to the midline than do the lower, and the right kidney is slightly lower in position than the left. The medial border of the kidney is concave, and contains a slitlike aperture known as the hilus. The average kidney is about 10 to 12 cm. in length, 5 to 6 cm. in width, and about 3 cm. in thickness.

The surface of the kidney is invested by a thin but strong fibrous capsule, and external to this capsule is a considerable quantity of fat tissue known as the adipose capsule. This fatty tissue permits ready identification of the kidney on plain radiographs, since it is considerably more radiolucent than the surrounding muscular structures. This adipose capsule is continuous with the tela subserosa or preperitoneal fat layer. It is the adipose capsule also which is insufflated with air or oxygen in the performance of perirenal air insufflation for diagnosis of adrenal (suprarenal) tumors (Chap. 15).

The kidneys correspond in position with the last thoracic, and upper three lumbar vertebrae, in the recumbent position. A maximum excursion of 5 cm. (or one and one-half vertebral bodies) occurs in the change from the recumbent to the erect positions.

The kidneys are related to other retroperitoneal structures as follows: The medial border of the right kidney is in contact with the descending portion of the duodenum, and most of the lower half of the right kidney is in contact with the ascending colon and hepatic flexure of the colon. The middle one third of the left kidney is in contact with the pancreas; the splenic artery is situated along the upper border of this pancreatic area, and the splenic vein is interposed between the pancreas and the left kidney. A small portion of the lower pole of the left kidney is in contact with the colon, but the rest of the anterior surface of the left kidney is peritonealized. These relations are of considerable importance from the standpoint of displacement by abnormalities of these contiguous organs.

Longitudinal section through the kidney shows it to be composed of the following parts (Fig. 16–1):

686

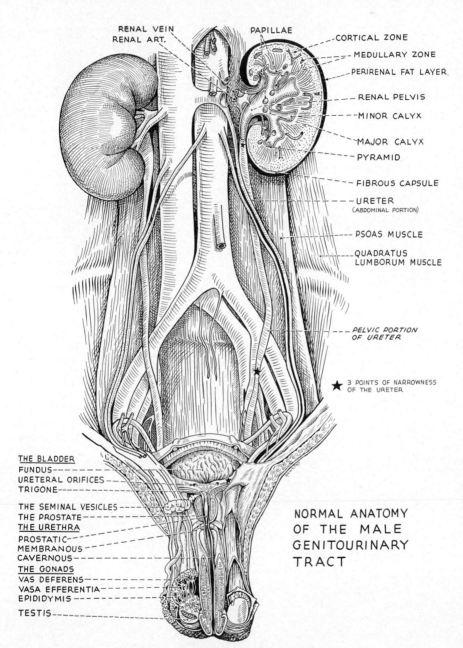

RENAL VEIN
RENAL ART.

PAPILLAE

CORTICAL ZONE

MEDULLARY ZONE

PERIRENAL FAT LAYER

RENAL PELVIS

MINOR CALYX

MAJOR CALYX

PYRAMID

FIBROUS CAPSULE

URETER
(ABDOMINAL PORTION)

PSOAS MUSCLE

QUADRATUS
LUMBORUM MUSCLE

*PELVIC PORTION
OF URETER*

★ 3 POINTS OF NARROWNESS
OF THE URETER

THE BLADDER
FUNDUS
URETERAL ORIFICES
TRIGONE

THE SEMINAL VESICLES
THE PROSTATE
THE URETHRA
PROSTATIC
MEMBRANOUS
CAVERNOUS
THE GONADS
VAS DEFERENS
VASA EFFERENTIA
EPIDIDYMIS

TESTIS

NORMAL ANATOMY
OF THE MALE
GENITOURINARY
TRACT

FIG. 16–1. Gross anatomy of the urinary tract.

1. An *external cortex*, approximately 12 mm. in thickness, containing numerous renal corpuscles, convoluted tubules and minute blood vessels; each renal corpuscle consists of a glomerulus of blood vessels invaginating a spherical glomerular capsule. Each renal unit also contains the first portion of a collecting tubule which is directed radially toward the central portion of the kidney, emptying into larger collecting tubules.

2. An *internal medulla* which contains eight to eighteen pyramidal structures which are called renal pyramids. The bases of the pyramids adjoin the renal cortex, and their apices project into the renal sinus where they constitute the renal papillae. The pyramids are separated from each other by cortex. There are many collecting tubules as well as loops of Henle (which communicate with the convoluted tubules) in each pyramid, and ultimately the collecting tubules empty into the apex of the pyramid (or papilla) through minute openings. The relationship of the calyces and pelvis will be discussed below.

3. *Columns*, which are cortical in origin and lie between the pyramids. These contain the larger arteries after they have entered the kidney (interlobar arteries). These interlobar arteries bend horizontally when they reach the bases of the pyramids and form the arcuate arteries, from which interlobular arteries enter the renal cortex, and *arteriolae rectae* pass into the pyramids.

4. The *renal pelvis* forms the commencement of the duct system leading to the bladder and it is a funnel-shaped expansion of the ureter, partly inside and partly outside the sinus of the kidney. The renal pelvis lies among the larger renal vessels, and is formed as follows:

5. The *minor calyces* are invaginations which surround one or more renal papillae, each being cup-shaped for the reception of urine. These each have a neck or narrow infundibulum and are approximately eight in number.

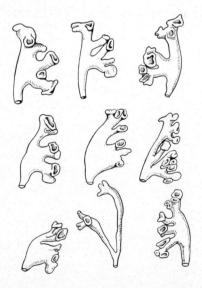

Fig. 16–2.   Variations in configuration of normal renal pelves and calyces.

6. These minor calyces unite into pairs or groups to form two or three *major calyces*, which in turn unite to form the renal pelvis proper.

There are numerous variations in the conformation of the renal pelvis and calyces (these are illustrated in Fig. 16–2). The renal pelvis and calyces are visualized radiographically apart from the renal outline, and a close study of the wide limits of normal is necessary from the standpoint of renal radiographic anatomy.

ANATOMIC VARIATIONS IN THE KIDNEYS. Evidence of superficial lobulation of the kidney, normally present in the infant and child, may be retained to a variable extent in the adult (Fig. 16–9), and this lobulation must be distinguished from the bulbous enlargement of a portion of the kidney which may occur with tumor or cyst formation. There is a variation in size and position of the kidneys which may also be considerable. Other anomalies lie outside the scope of this text.

The Ureter. The ureter is the tubular connection between the kidney and the urinary bladder. It is approximately 25 cm. in length, and is retroperitoneal throughout its course, lying in the subperitoneal fat tissue of the abdomen and pelvis.

The abdominal portion of the ureter lies on the psoas major muscle (Fig. 16–1), and is projected over the tips of the transverse processes of the lumbar vertebrae. The right ureter usually crosses the external iliac artery, and the left ureter the common iliac artery, but this is by no means constant. It crosses the wings of the sacrum just medial to the sacro-iliac joints.

The pelvic portion of the ureter is convex posteriorly and laterally. About the level of the ischial spines, the ureters bend forward and medially to join the lower portion of the urinary bladder in the bladder trigone.

When the right and left ureters reach the bladder they are 4 to 5 cm. apart. They pierce the bladder wall obliquely, and are embedded in its muscular tissue for nearly 2 cm. The openings into the bladder are of a valvular nature, and prevent backflow from the bladder into the ureter.

The lumen of the ureter is variable in size, constantly undergoing peristalsis. There are certain normal areas of constriction (Fig. 16–1) in three locations: (1) at the ureteropelvic junction; (2) where the ureter crosses the external iliac or common iliac artery at the pelvic brim; and (3) where the ureter joins the urinary bladder.

In the female, there is an additional relationship which is of considerable importance. Near the termination of the ureter it lies below the broad ligament of the uterus, and lateral to the cervix and vaginal wall.

The course of the ureter is somewhat variable, and the ureter tends to be redundant in some individuals, particularly following any pregnancy.

The Urinary Bladder (Fig. 16–1). The size and configuration of the urinary bladder vary with the degree of its distention, and to some extent with age. The bladder tends to be extrapelvic in the infant, but in the adult lies in the true pelvis except when distended. It adjoins the pubic symphysis anteriorly, and is separated from the rectum in the male by the ductus deferens and seminal vesicles, and in the female by the uterus and vagina. In the male, the prostate is situated along the inferior aspect of the urinary bladder.

The internal urethral orifice is normally situated at the lowest point of the bladder. It is usually about 2 to 2.5 cm. posterior to the pubic symphysis.

The urinary bladder is peritonealized on its superior aspect only.

For accurate visualization of the bladder a contrast medium is necessary. In view of the globular structure of the distended bladder, it must be studied in several projections to visualize its entire periphery. In the undistended state, it is difficult to be certain of filling defects.

The Urethra (Fig. 16–8). The female urethra is a short channel (Fig. 16–3) from the bladder to the external urethral orifice, which is situated above the opening of the vagina. The male urethra consists of a proximal portion which serves only as a urinary passage and corresponds to the female urethra, and a distal portion which conveys the products of the gonads as well as urine.

The male urethra traverses in turn the prostate gland, the urogenital diaphragm and the entire length of the corpus cavernosum urethrae, to end in the glans penis. The distal portion of the prostatic urethra is slightly wider than the proximal. That portion which is situated between the layers of the urogenital diaphragm is called the membranous portion, and the lumen of this part of the urethra is much narrower than the prostatic portion. That part beyond the membranous portion is slightly dilated again, but narrows as it begins its cavernous portion. Here it maintains a uniform diameter until it reaches the glans, where it dilates once again to form the *fossa navicularis*, beyond which it narrows to a slitlike orifice at the extremity of the glans, which is the narrowest diameter.

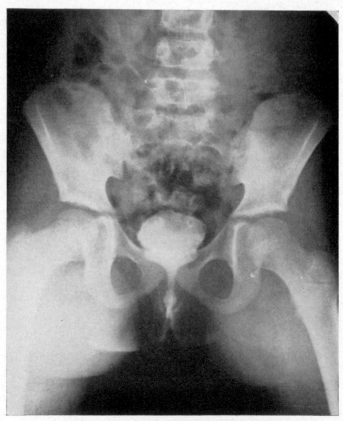

FIG. 16–3.   Normal female urethrogram.

RADIOGRAPHIC EXAMINATION OF THE UROGENITAL TRACT

Preparation of the Patient. Although time may not permit the proper preparation of the patient, and the examination may be successful without it, in a number of cases the examination without preparation is not entirely satisfactory because of the interference by gas and fecal shadows from the gastrointestinal tract. The most satisfactory aperient is usually castor oil taken in a 1 or 2 ounce dose the night preceding the examination, and this is usually followed by two or more enemas on the next morning one-half hour prior to the examination until the enema returns are clear. Aloin, cascara sagrada or phenolphthalein may be utilized in lieu of the castor oil in special cases. One-half to one cubic centimeter of Pitressin approximately one-half hour before the examination may also clear the gastrointestinal tract, but this drug must be used with caution in any individual beyond 40 years of age, or in anyone with a history of cardiovascular disease. It is also probable that it diminishes the concentration of dye by the kidneys, and hence is not desirable.

It is also a good plan to dehydrate the patient as much as possible for a period of at least twelve hours prior to the examination, and hence the patient must have nothing by mouth after the evening meal of the night before except the medication. Dehydration improves the concentration of the dye by the kidneys.

KUB Film. This is an antero-posterior view of the abdomen (Fig. 15–2) with particular emphasis on the urinary tract. This study always forms the initial film prior to either intravenous or retrograde pyelography. The structures visualized and the general technique of this examination have been described in Chapter 15.

This film (as well as the urograms) is usually taken in full expiration, with the patient recumbent. The abdomen is compressed with a taut band or other device so as to diminish the thickness of the part through which the rays must travel. The entire abdomen is included own to the pubic symphysis and if this cannot be done on a single film, two separate exposures (one for the upper abdomen and one for the lower) may be required.

Most films are obtained with the patient supine, although at least one film in the course of an entire urographic study is taken with the patient upright to measure the excursion of the kidneys in the change from the recumbent to the erect position.

Excretory Urography (Fig. 16–4). In the early 1930's, there occurred the gradual introduction of organic iodides that were selectively excreted and concentrated by the kdneys to a great extent, thus permitting a satisfactory radiographic presentation of the urinary tract.[4] Iopax and later Skiodan, followed by Neo-Iopax and Neoskiodan (containing smaller amounts of iodine and less toxicity), were some of the earliest compounds to be employed. At the present time in this country, the most commonly employed organic iodides used for this purpose are 35 per cent Diodrast, 50 per cent Hypaque, 30 per cent Urokon, and 76 per cent Renografin (Table 16–1), in quantities of 20 to 30 cc. in the adult. There are occasional side reactions such as a feeling of warmth, or sensitivity to the iodides such as hives, nausea, vomiting and uvular or laryngeal edema, but these reactions are not ordinarily severe or sufficiently disturbing to impede the utilization of the drugs. *Intravenous* sensitivity tests with 0.5 to 1.0 cc. of the media should be carried out at least several minutes beforehand, and antihistaminic and adrenergic agents should be kept close at hand for use in the event serious sensitivity becomes manifest. (See page 698.)

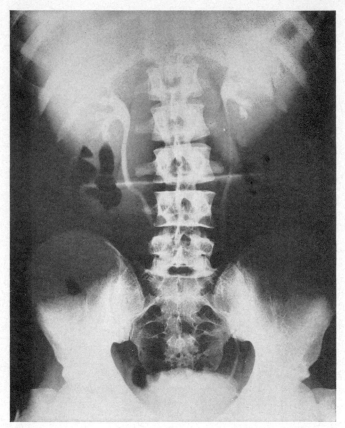

FIG. 16–4. EXCRETORY UROGRAM: **a,** Representative excretory urogram obtained fifteen minutes after the intravenous injection of 30 cc. of 35 per cent Diodrast.

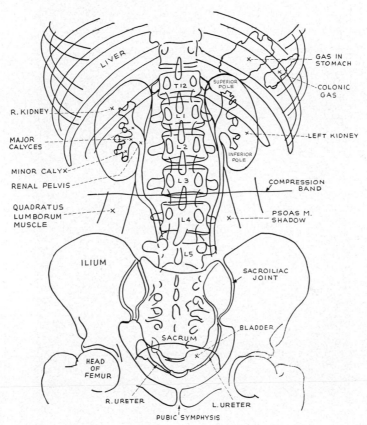

FIG. 16–4.   EXCRETORY UROGRAM: **b,** Tracing of **a.**

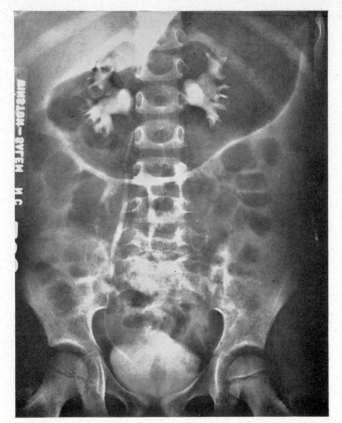

Fig. 16–4. **c,** Intravenous pyelogram on a child with the upper urinary tract demonstrated clearly through a gas-distended stomach.

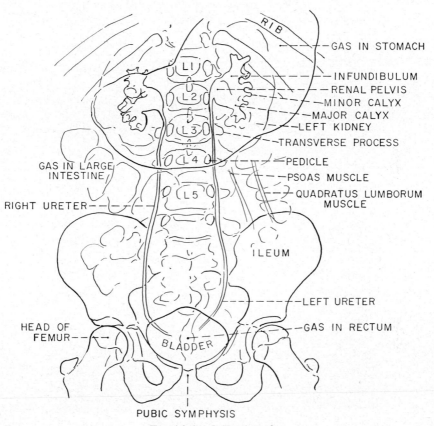

RIB

GAS IN STOMACH

INFUNDIBULUM

RENAL PELVIS

MINOR CALYX

MAJOR CALYX

LEFT KIDNEY

TRANSVERSE PROCESS

PEDICLE

PSOAS MUSCLE

QUADRATUS LUMBORUM MUSCLE

GAS IN LARGE INTESTINE

RIGHT URETER

ILEUM

LEFT URETER

GAS IN RECTUM

HEAD OF FEMUR

BLADDER

PUBIC SYMPHYSIS

L1
L2
L3
L4
L5

FIG. 16–4. **d,** Tracing of c

Table 16–1.   Percentage Comparison of Urological Contrast Media

	% DESCRIPTION OF TRADE PACKAGES	% OF IODINE IN SOLUTION IN TRADE PACKAGES	% IODINE IN DRY CHEMICAL
Renografin	76	36.94	62.1
Urokon	70	46.1	65.8
	50	32.7	65.8
	30	19.8	65.8
Hypaque	50	29.93	59.87
Diodrast	35	17½	50
	70	35	50
Neo-Iopax	50	25.75	51.5
	75	37.8	51.5

Extravasation into the soft tissues or muscles outside a vein is tolerated better with Diodrast than with Neo-Iopax, but it is probably true that side reactions are more common with Diodrast than with the other compounds. It will be recalled that these drugs are employed in double concentration and quantity in angiocardiography.

The purpose of excretory pyelography is to visualize the kidney calyces, pelves, ureters and urinary bladder. The smaller quantity of dye (20 to 30 cc.) is injected rather slowly into an antecubital vein, and films of the abdomen are thereafter obtained at 4 to 5 minutes, 8 to 15 minutes, 25 to 40 minutes, 60 minutes, 90 minutes, 2 hours, and delayed films at hourly intervals if necessary up to 8 hours. Usually only the first three time intervals are adequate. An erect film is usually taken at the 30-minute interval (or when visualization is maximal) as well as one in the recumbent position; oblique films are taken if it is desired to localize a stone or delineate a structure more accurately. Compression of the abdomen has been considered of value by many radiologists, and in some clinics, the feet are elevated above the head in the so-called Trendelenburg position to help concentrate the dye in the upper urinary pathway.

If excretion and concentration are delayed, it is well to obtain films until a good concentration of the dye is seen in the urinary bladder. Otherwise, very frequently the delayed excretion will not permit a visualization of the urinary tracts for several hours.

If in addition a cystogram is desired by this excretory method, oblique studies of the urinary bladder are required. Urethrograms require an oblique study of the urethra while the patient is urinating into a suitable receptacle (voiding cysto-urethrogram). Usually it is more satisfactory to perform urethrograms following the instillation of dye directly into the bladder.

In children similar dyes are used but are injected into the femoral vein if difficulty is encountered with antecubital injection. The amount given is in proportion to the child's age according to the manufacturer's instructions.

If intravenous injection is unsuccessful, gluteal intramuscular injection may be used together with an injection of hyaluronidase to promote absorption. (Diodrast, 35 per cent, is recommended for this purpose.)

In some individuals, particularly infants and children, the clarity of the excretory urogram can be improved by projecting the upper urinary tract through a stomach shadow which is distended with gas. This may be accomplished by giving the patient several swallows of a carbonated drink; or by injecting air into the stomach through a stomach tube (Fig. 16–4, **c** and **d**).

Excretory urography is not only performed to obtain an anatomic evaluation of the urinary tracts, but is also done to determine the functional status of the kidneys. Anatomic detail, however, is usually not so satisfactory as it is with retrograde pyelography, and the latter procedure is usually performed in addition when pathology is suspected, or when it is desired that anatomic minutia be visualized.

Retrograde Pyelography (Fig. 16–5). In contrast to excretory urography, hydration, rather than dehydration, is practiced the night before the examination. A local anesthetic is usually employed for minimizing the discomfort accompanying passage of the cystoscope. After preliminary cystoscopy, the urologist removes the observation telescope and replaces it with the double catheterization element into which the catheters have been placed. After specimens of urine are obtained through each ureteral catheter and a suitable kidney function test performed for each kidney (such as the intravenous phenolsulphonphthalein test), the urologist is then ready to perform the urographic examination with the cooperation of the radiologist.

Fluoroscopic observation of the process of kidney filling is carried out in some clinics, but in most clinics, film studies are the only ones thought necessary. KUB technique is employed with the aid of a special cystoscopic table that has incorporated in it a Potter-Bucky diaphragm.

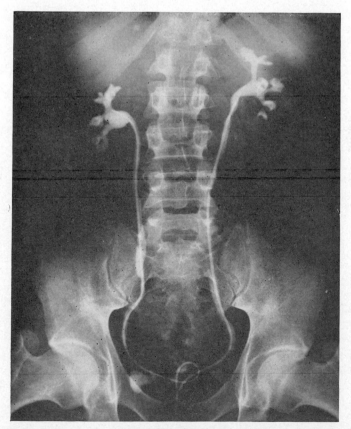

FIG. 16–5. Representative retrograde pyelogram with ureteral catheters in situ.

Various contrast media may be employed, each having special advantages or disadvantages. The intravenous preparations such as Neo-Iopax or Diodrast give the best contrast, but are the most expensive. Twelve to 15 per cent Hippuran gives adequate contrast and is not so costly, but the contrast is not so great as with the latter two drugs. However, in some respects too great a contrast is a disadvantage since it may obscure small stones, although these would be previously seen on a KUB film taken prior to the injection of the dye. Sodium iodide or bromide and thorium nitrate are now seldom employed because of their greater irritative effect.

A plain KUB film is first obtained as with excretory urography, and this is followed after a preliminary injection of 5 to 10 cc. of contrast medium by a film to show the kidney pelves and calyces. Thereafter 10 to 20 cc. of dye is injected while the catheters are withdrawn in order to visualize the ureters in their entirety. The routine film employed is the antero-posterior, but oblique films are taken if there is a calculus in question which may or may not be situated in the ureteral pathway. Stereoscopic films are also made if the occasion demands.

Indications and Contraindications for Excretory Urography and Retrograde Pyelography. The chief advantage of excretory urography is greater comfort to the patient by avoiding the cystoscopic procedure and the avoidance of such secondary symptoms as may arise from this procedure such as pain, colic, fever, and occasionally a retrograde cortical infection of the kidney.

There is usually a somewhat uncomfortable systemic sensation following the intravenous injection of the organic iodides. The patient may feel flushed, and at times he may actually feel nauseated or even vomit. Ordinarily these discomforts are evanescent and disappear quite rapidly. On occasion, sensitivity phenomena of a minor order such as hives and the like are encountered. It is usually desirable to inject a few drops of the organic iodide medium and wait several minutes before injecting the remainder. The intravenous test performed this way is the most accurate sensitivity test. Intra-ocular, subungual or intra-cutaneous tests are not an adequate substitute. Fatalities after intravenous injection have been reported in the literature; the exact cause of such fatalities is not known, but it is estimated that the fatality occurrence is no greater than one in 60,000 examinations.

In certain urologic conditions when catheterization of the ureters is either impossible or possible only with excessive trauma, excretory urography is the method of choice. This is particularly true with large tumors of the urinary bladder obstructing the ureteral orifices, enlargement of the prostate gland, transplantation of the ureters into the bowel, and occasionally in the urologic examination of children.

There are certain advantages in the investigation of anomalies and of trauma to the urinary tract by excretory urography in that it gives one not only structural information but also information in relation to renal function. In trying to assay the latter, however, it must be remembered that this is not an accurate renal function test and that not infrequently there is failure of visualization even in the presence of good function. Sometimes, renal function is only momentarily impaired, as in the case of ureteral calculus when by some reflex phenomenon there is poor excretion from the kidney on the affected side.

As a survey medium for the urologist prior to cystoscopic examination, it permits him to evaluate the kidneys on either side both structurally and to some extent functionally. It allows him, therefore, to concentrate on one side or the other by the retrograde method.

It is probable that renal insufficiency should be regarded as a contraindication to excretory urography. Ordinarily, satisfactory urograms are not obtained when the blood urea nitrogen concentration in the blood is greater than 60 milligrams per cent. When one utilizes the usual dosage (20 to 30 cc. of 35 per cent organic iodide medium), it is probable that no serious or harmful effects are obtained, since ultimately excretion does occur, and while this amount of dye is present within the body no serious sequelae are noted.

Iodine sensitivity is a contraindication to intravenous pyelography.

Intravenous pyelography should not be employed when it is contemplated that the patient will undergo thyroid assay by the iodine uptake technique; the organic iodide medium definitely interferes with an accurate assay of thyroid function for as long as one or two weeks.

The greatest disadvantage of excretory urography is the possibility of relatively poor visualization and detail. When the most accurate detail is required, retrograde pyelography must be employed.

It is often impossible to arrive at a definite diagnosis by intravenous pyelography unless the most accurate detail is obtained regarding kidney calyceal structure. This is particularly true in relation to early renal tuberculosis or affection of the kidneys by renal neoplasms. In such cases it is almost the rule that retrograde pyelography must be performed even after a moderately satisfactory excretory urogram has been obtained. However, a minimal distention of the calyces is produced by this method, compared with intravenous urography, and this must be taken into account in the interpretation.

It is inadvisable to inject contrast medium above a point of obstruction such as an obstructing ureteral calculus, since severe reactions in the patient are often encountered.

While excretory urography is contraindicated in all cases with nitrogenous retention, but may be tolerated by the patient without serious sequelae, retrograde pyelography may prove to be highly dangerous in some medical diseases of the kidney such as pyelonephritis, glomerulonephritis, and arteriolar nephrosclerosis. Anuria may be precipitated.

In general, it should be noted that intravenous and retrograde pyelography are complementary or supplementary procedures and that one does not exclude the utilization of the other.

Pneumopyelograms. Air is injected into the kidney pelvis under manometric control, and pressure is maintained around 20 to 30 mm. of mercury. This procedure has not been used very frequently in this country because of the danger of air embolism, but it has numerous advocates in Europe. It may have particular value when there are abnormalities of the renal pelvis proper, or strictures of the ureter. Carbon dioxide insufflation is safer and hence preferable.

Nephrograms and Nephrotomography[3] (Fig. 16–6). Nephrograms are films of the kidney obtained by intensification of the cortical as well as medullary areas by the concentration of dye.

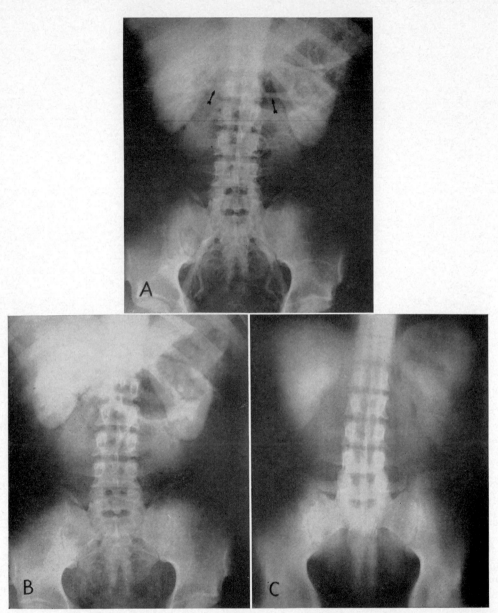

FIG. 16–6. Twenty-five year old normal male subject. *A*, Plain film taken at predetermined circulation time demonstrates arteriogram phase. Good opacification of abdominal aorta, renal arteries (arrows) and other major arterial trunks. Note beginning opacification of the kidneys. *B*, Plain nephrogram. Film taken immediately after arterial phase. *C*, Nephrotomogram demonstrates clearly opacified kidneys without superimposition of extraneous abdominal shadows. (From Evans, J. A., Dubilier, W., Jr., and Monteith, J.: Am. J. Roentgenol., vol. 71, 1954.)

At the present time the two effective methods of producing satisfactory nephrograms are as follows[2]:

1. Transabdominal aortography involving the rapid injection of a small quantity (15 to 20 cc.) of organic iodide directly into the upper abdominal aorta.

2. The rapid intravenous injection of concentrated organic iodine solution by the method developed by Robb and Steinberg for angiocardiography.

However, despite good opacification of functioning renal parenchyma by the intravenous technique, the clarity of the renal mass is sometimes compromised by the superimposition of intestinal contents and gas. Moreover small renal lesions embedded in the substance of the kidney may some times be missed by plain nephrography because of being enveloped by functioning renal parenchyma. However, if body section roentgenography is combined with the intravenous nephrography it is conceivable that confusing superimposed shadows may be eliminated.

The exact technique is as follows:[3]

1. With a patient positioned in the supine position on the radiographic table equipped with body-section apparatus, preliminary plain films and body section radiographs are obtained to be used as control films and to check the roentgenographic technique.

2. A 12 gauge Robb-Steinberg angiocardiographic needle is inserted into an antecubital vein.

3. Arm-to-tongue Decholin circulation time is determined, employing the same injection technique as for contrast substance.

4. With the roentgen tube in mid-position, 50 cc. of 70 per cent Diodrast, or 70 per cent Urokon Sodium, or 90 per cent Hypaque are injected rapidly in one and a half to two seconds into the abducted arm. A film is then exposed at the predetermined circulation time. The first roentgenogram will demonstrate the renal arteries. This is followed as rapidly as possible by a second film which secures the nephrogram. Immediately after the second exposure a body section radiograph is obtained. The elapsed time between the first exposure and the completion of body-section film should not exceed 25 seconds.

If a repeat injection is considered necessary, it is advised that a repeat circulation time be undertaken before the second injection because the circulation time may be delayed after the first injection, presumably due to an increase in the peripheral resistance.

The problem of obscuration by overlying intestinal gas is thereby eliminated and one obtains full advantage of the clear definition of the renal parenchyma. The procedure is of course of greatest value in the differentiation of renal cysts from renal neoplasms.

Cystograms. Cystograms, or radiographs of the urinary bladder (Fig. 16–8), are employed in the following cases: (1) when bladder calculus or other filling defect is suspected; (2) to demonstrate diverticula; (3) when cystoscopy is undesirable or impossible; (4) for demonstration of central or marginal placenta praevia (see Chap. 17).

The most commonly used opaque media employed for this purpose are: 5 to 10 per cent sodium iodide; 12 per cent Hippuran; 12 per cent Diodrast, Hypaque, Urokon, Renografin or Neo-Iopax; air; Lipiodol gum tragacanth mixture; Umbrathor; various mixtures of organic soluble iodides, and sodium iodide. The first two are the most popular for cystograms; the others are not infrequently employed in urethrography.

The usual film studies obtained are (Fig. 16–7, **b, c** and **d**): (1) straight antero-posterior; (2) right posterior oblique (45 degrees); (3) left posterior oblique; (4) Chassard-Lapiné view ("sitting," "squat" or "jackknife view").

Stereoscopic films may be obtained if desired.

If catheterization is not possible, the bladder may be visualized by taking views in similar positions after an intravenous dye has been injected. Care must be taken not to overinterpret filling defects or pressure defects of the undistended urinary bladder.

Urethrograms (Fig. 16–8). This method of examination consists of first obtaining a film of the urethra before the introduction of contrast material into the lumen and thereafter obtaining films of the urethra filled with an opaque medium. Approximately 15 per cent sodium iodide is usually adequate, although any of the media described under cystography may be used. This is injected through a urethral nozzle. A resistance to the injection is encountered when the contrast material has reached the external sphincter of the bladder. After this is overcome, the injection must be continued while the radiographs are obtained, since there is a constant leakage of contrast media into the urinary bladder. Thus not only the anterior urethra but also the membranous and prostatic portions will be visualized.

The patient is placed in an oblique position, with the lower thigh flexed, and the upper thigh extended. The penis is held parallel with the upper thigh. The central ray is directed at the root of the penis.

The film taken prior to the injection of the contrast media is of value in detecting any calculi or foreign bodies which may be present.

A urethrogram in the female is illustrated in Figure 16–3.

Aortography. Aortography has become of particular significance in the investigation of renal lesions. This is more fully considered, however, in Chapter 12.

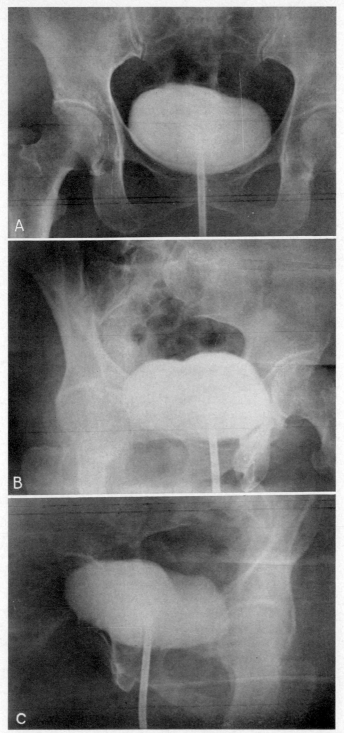

FIG. 16–7.   REPRESENTATIVE NORMAL CYSTOGRAMS: a, Antero-posterior view; b, left posterior oblique
view; c, right posterior oblique view.

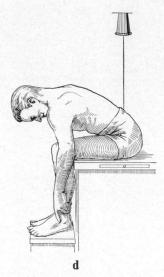

d

FIG. 16–7. CHASSARD-LAPINÉ VIEW OF URINARY BLADDER. (Also called sitting, squat or jackknife view.) **d**, Position of patient.

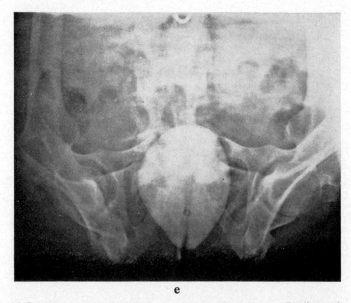

e

FIG. 16–7. CHASSARD-LAPINE VIEW OF URINARY BLADDER: **e**, Radiograph obtained.

Points of Practical Interest With Reference to Figure 16–7:

1. The dynamics activity of the urinary bladder may be studied by obtaining films of the bladder area after voiding. This may show:
   (*a*) Residuum in bladder (bladder retention).
   (*b*) Reflux up the ureters.
2. The thickness of the wall of the bladder is of importance also, and may be gauged readily particularly when the well is hypertrophied in association with cystitis.

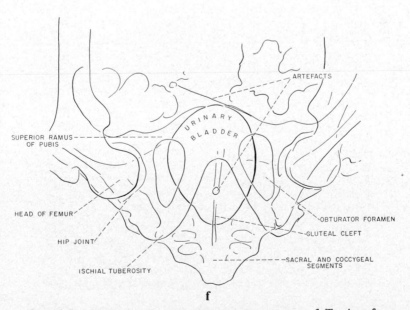

f

Fig. 16–7. Chassard-Lapine view of urinary bladder: f, Tracing of e.

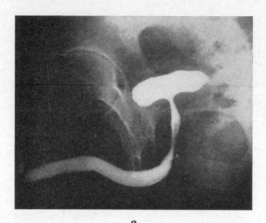

a

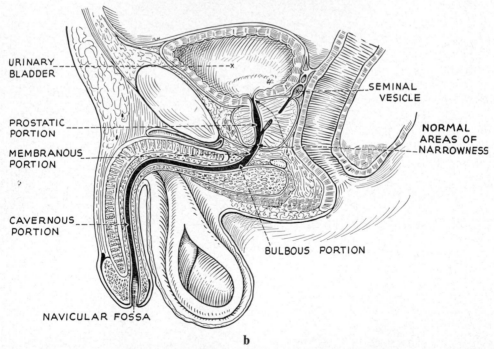

URINARY BLADDER

PROSTATIC PORTION

MEMBRANOUS PORTION

CAVERNOUS PORTION

NAVICULAR FOSSA

SEMINAL VESICLE

NORMAL AREAS OF NARROWNESS

BULBOUS PORTION

b

FIG. 16–8.   Representative normal urethrogram: **a,** Radiograph. (Reproduced with permission of Goodyear, Beard and Weens and publishers of Southern Medical Journal.) **b,** Anatomic sketch of the male urethra and surrounding structures.

THE NORMAL RADIOGRAPHIC APPEARANCE OF THE URINARY TRACT

The Kidney. In addition to the gross anatomic details already described, certain practical considerations deserve our attention.

The radiographic description must concern itself with exact outline, size, position, mobility, general configuration and relationship to contiguous structures. The numerous variations within normal limits as regards these descriptive terms must be recognized.

The outline of the kidney is ordinarily visible on the KUB film because of the surrounding perirenal fat layer. It is usually regularly convex on its outer margin, and concave in its hilus. It tends to be lobulated in the infant, but considerably less so in the adult (Fig. 16–9). One kidney may therefore appear slightly larger than the other. Variations from this become of definite significance in the detection of various abnormalities.

The average level of the kidneys in expiration is as follows: The hilus of the right kidney is usually opposite the second transverse process of the lumbar vertebra, and the left is 1 to 2 cm. higher. The length of the kidney in the male averages 10 to 12 cm., its breadth 5 to 6 cm., and its thickness 3 to 4 cm. The kidneys of the female are slightly smaller.

There is a 1 to 3 cm. excursion of the kidney in respiration, and up to 5 cm. excursion in the change from the recumbent to the erect position (width of one and one-half vertebral bodies).

There is a wide variation in the appearance of the kidney pelves and calyces. A normal kidney pelvis permits an equal drainage from all parts of the kidney, and allows a free flow of urine into the ureter and bladder. Roentgenologically, there is usually a common pelvis, two to three major calyces, and six to fourteen minor calyces. The superior calyces are usually in a direct line with the ureter, whereas the inferior calyces are horizontally placed. On occasion, however, the ureter divides almost immediately into the calyces, with no common renal pelvic basin. The average capacity of a pelvis is 7.5 cc. of fluid, but this may be as high as 20 cc. and still not be considered pathologic.

INFANT   ADULT

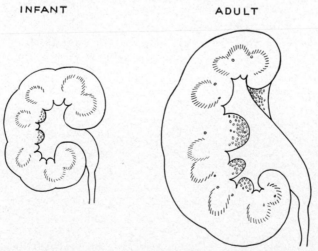

Fig. 16–9.   Infantile renal lobulation and its comparison with the adult renal contour. (After Caffey, with permission of the publishers.)

The major calyces are merely channels, whereas the minor calyces consist of a neck, with an expanded cupped distal end. The cupping is formed by the projection of the minor papillae into the calyces. The edges of the cup must be clean-cut and sharply demarcated. It is important not to mistake the rounded shadow of a calyx seen end on for a clubbed calyx, since the latter appearance is definitely abnormal.

Serial studies show that there are definite changes in the size and contour of the calyces, due to motility, and contraction and relaxation of the pelvis and ureter. These changes must be considered physiologic.

Backflow Phenomena (Figs. 16–10, 16–11).   Occasionally, the dye will enter the collecting tubules, renal veins or lymphatics when introduced in retrograde pyelography. The cause of this phenomenon is not known. Occasionally, it may be due to increased pressure upon introduction of the dye, but this may not be the sole cause. There are five types of backflow: (1) pyelotubular, (2) pyelolymphatic, (3) pyelovenous, (4) pyelosinous and (5) pyelointerstitial.

Pyelotubular backflow is manifest by the dye radiating in straight lines in divergent fashion from a minor calyx.

Pyelolymphatic backflow appears as irregular lines arising from the region of the hilus, and passing inward to the region of the renal glands.

Pyelovenous backflow has the appearance of thick cobwebs or hazy streaking around the major calyx and adjoining neck of the minor calyx. In the living subject, the interlobar, intralobular and arcuate veins are not entered in view of the venous drainage toward the kidney hilus. The veins visualized are the venous plexuses into which the interlobar veins of the kidney drain, since the tissue separating the calyces from the endothelium at these points is extremely thin and easily ruptured. The other types of backflow are also illustrated in Figure 16–10.

Ureters.   The ureter usually leaves the renal pelvis at its most dependent point and passes directly downward into the bladder. Rotation of the kidney will cause some variation in this appearance, and this rotation can be recognized by the appearance of the calyces. The important factor to bear in mind is the presence or absence of interference to drainage from the kidney pelvis, or any potential for such interference.

There is a constant peristalsis over the length of the ureter, and portions of the ureter are not visualized in excretory urography depending upon this factor. For an area of constriction to be abnormal, it must be constant, and be associated with a persistent dilatation of the ureter above this level. Normal areas of narrowness occur at the three locations described above, namely: the ureteropelvic junction, the bifurcation of the iliac vessels, and the point of entrance of the ureter into the urinary bladder.

The average ureteral diameter is 2 to 6 mm.

Slight irregularities in the anatomic course are of no significance if ureteral obstruction is not manifest. A mild degree of tortuosity occurs with deep inspiration also.

The Urinary Bladder.   In the antero-posterior recumbent projection, the neck of the bladder lies just below the upper border of the pubic symphysis, and the fundus rises to a variable distance above the symphysis depending upon the degree of distention. The distended bladder is ellipsoid in shape in

CONFUSING PYELOGRAPHIC APPEARANCES

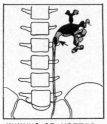

KINKING OF URETER
WITHOUT OBSTRUCTION

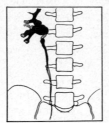

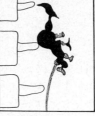

ATYPICAL URETEROPELVIC JUNCTIONS
NORMAL VARIANTS

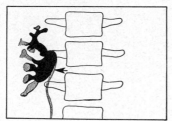

EXTRARENAL PELVIS

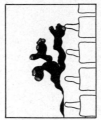

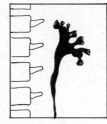

NORMAL VARIANTS OF RENAL CALYCES

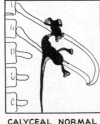

CALYCEAL NORMAL
VARIANTS

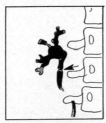

PERISTALSIS IN URETER

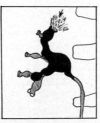

PYELOTUBULAR BACKFLOW

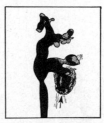

PYELOSINOUS TRANSFLOW

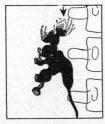

PYELOVENOUS BACKFLOW

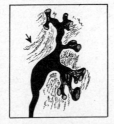

PYELOLYMPHATIC BACKFLOW

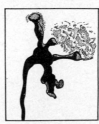

PYELO-INTERSTITAL
BACKFLOW

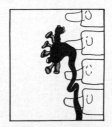

URETERAL KINKING
WITHOUT OBSTRUCTION

FIG. 16–10.

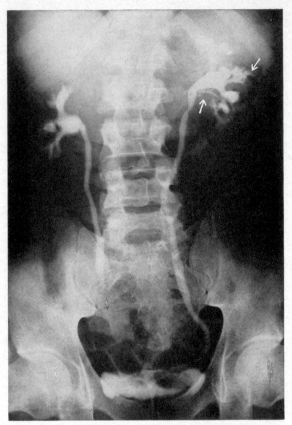

FIG. 16–11.   Intensified radiograph to demonstrate backflow phenomena.

the adult, but in the child tends to be elongated in its long axis. The outline of the bladder is usually smooth when distended, but may be irregular in the partially collapsed state, and one should not regard this appearance as abnormal unless the degree of distention is adequate.

In the male, there may be a minimal rarefaction at the neck of the bladder as a result of the impression of the medial lobe of the prostate. When this impression is more than minimal it is usually but not always an indication of abnormal enlargement of the prostate or seminal vesicles.

In the undistended bladder there are indentations of the dome which likewise may have no significance, since they are usually due to pressure from contiguous organs (such as the pelvic colon) rather than abnormalities.

The Urethra.   The prostatic urethra is slightly spindle-shaped and is 2 to 4 cm. in length. It joins the base of the urinary bladder abruptly. The narrowness of the membranous portion extends for a distance of 1 to 1.5 cm. The outline of the cavernous part of the urethra is fairly uniform throughout.

Occasionally there is a slight reflux into the ejaculatory duct as it opens into the prostatic urethra.

The female urethra is approximately 5 cm. in length and resembles closely the proximal one-third of the male urethra. Normally, its walls are smooth with a minimum lumen of about 3 mm. and a maximum of 8 mm. Irregularities, dilatation or outpouchings are of pathologic significance.

REFERENCES

1. Braasch, W. F., and Emmett, J. L.: *Clinical Urography.* W. B. Saunders Co., Philadelphia, 1951.
2. De Backer, J.: J. belge radiol. *33:* 318–321, 1950 (abst. in Radiol. *58:* 913, 1952).
3. Evans, J. A., Dubilier, W., Jr., and Monteith, M. C.: Nephrotomography. Am. J. Roentgenol., *71:* 213–233, 1954.
4. Wesson, M. B.: *Urologic Roentgenology.* Lea and Febiger, Philadelphia. 1946.

CHAPTER 17

The Genital System

THE MALE GENITAL SYSTEM

Related Gross Anatomy. Each testis (Fig. 17–1) is formed by numerous lobules, each containing coiled tubules called seminiferous tubules. The spermatozoa are formed in these tubules. These lobules and tubules converge posteriorly toward the rete testis, which consists of a network of tubules which empty by coiled ducts into the head of the epididymis. Here the duct of the epididymis is formed and extends in very tortuous fashion to the tail of the epididymis where it becomes the ductus deferens. This latter is a cord-like structure which traverses the posterior aspect of the spermatic cord, and in the vicinity of the trigone of the urinary bladder undergoes slight bulbous dilatation to form the ampulla of the ductus deferens. Near the lower margin of this ampulla, there is a diverticulum-like structure which extends cephalad, and appears racemose in configuration. This is the seminal vesicle. The continuation of the ampulla of the ductus deferens beyond the point of junction with the seminal vesicle is called the ejaculatory duct, and this empties into the lower posterior aspect of the prostatic urethra, one opening on either side of the prostatic utricle. In its course, the ejaculatory duct traverses about two thirds of the length of the prostate.

Technique of Examination. There are only certain portions of the male genital system which can be examined radiographically by presently known methods, and these are not very frequently employed. The examination is confined to a soft tissue study of the prostate, seminal vesicles and scrotal contents, and the direct injection of opaque media into the lumen of the seminal vesicles, vas deferens and ejaculatory duct via the vas deferens.

The usual method employed in the direct injection depends on the exposure of the vas through a small inguinal incision under local anesthesia. This injection is first directed upward to fill the vesicles and then downward to the epididymis to fill the tubules (Fig. 17–2). Either Lipiodol or Diodrast may be used. Urethroscopic catheterization has been employed by a few, but ordinarily this procedure is not very feasible in the normal subject. The latter method also does not permit visualization of the vas deferens, and serves only to outline the ejaculatory ducts and seminal vesicles.

Radiographic Appearances. On a plain radiograph the prostate may be visualized when enlarged as an impression directed upward at the base of the urinary bladder, or calculi may be seen within the prostate, but the outline of the gland cannot be delineated.

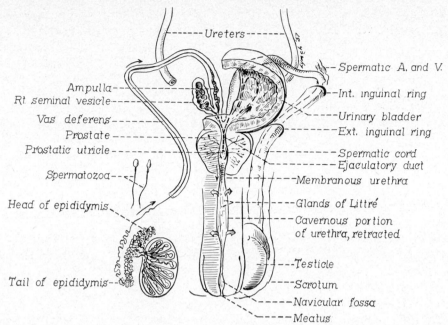

FIG. 17–1. The male reproductive system. (Modified from Dickinson, *Atlas of Human Sex Anatomy*, Williams and Wilkins Co.)

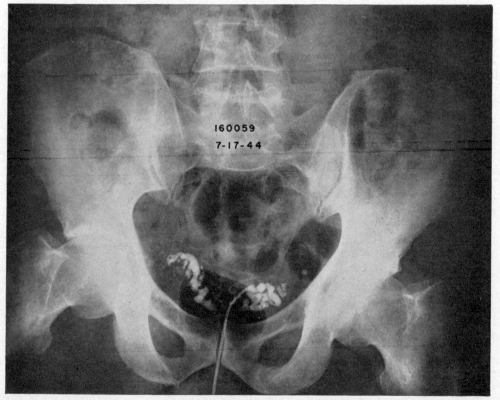

FIG. 17–2 Representative seminal vesiculogram. (Courtesy of Drs. H. Hauser and C. C. Dundon Cleveland, Ohio.)

Using contrast material, the numerous racemose or diverticulum-like tubes of the seminal vesicles are seen as an indefinite mass, and the ductus deferens may be seen as a tubular structure which conforms closely with the anatomic description above. The more distal tubules may be visualized, depending upon the efforts of the investigator, but their examination is very infrequent.

In prostatic carcinoma, the ejaculatory duct may be invaded and occluded, but in the normal subject it may be seen extending beyond the junction of the ductus deferens and the seminal vesicles.

THE FEMALE REPRODUCTIVE SYSTEM

The soft tissue structures of this system will be described first and then a brief account will be given of the bony pelvis and its anatomic variations.

Soft Tissues. The organs of the female genital system consist of two ovaries, two oviducts, the uterus, the vagina and the external genitalia. The suspensory and supplementary structures are the broad ligaments (and mesosalpinx) on either side, the round ligament, the mesovarium and mesometrium (Fig. 17–3).

The broad ligament is the transverse fold of peritoneum which extends across the pelvis minor, dividing it into an anterior and a posterior compartment. This has frequently been compared with a "curtain draped over a clothesline." Projecting into the posterior compartment, and attached a little below the upper margin of the broad ligament, is the mesovarium, with the ovary attached to its free edge. That portion of the broad ligament above this is called the mesosalpinx, and that below, the mesometrium.

The ovaries are two almond-shaped organs—one on either side of the pelvis. Their exact position in nulliparous women is somewhat variable but their long

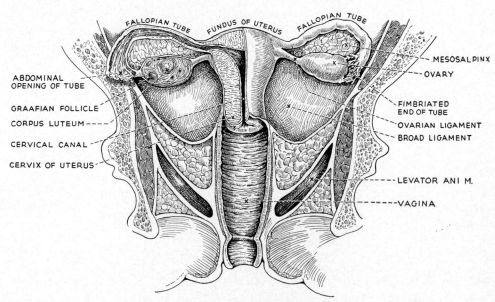

FEMALE REPRODUCTIVE SYSTEM
(FRONTAL SECTION DIAGRAM)

FIG. 17–3.   GROSS ANATOMY OF FEMALE REPRODUCTIVE SYSTEM: **a,** Frontal view.

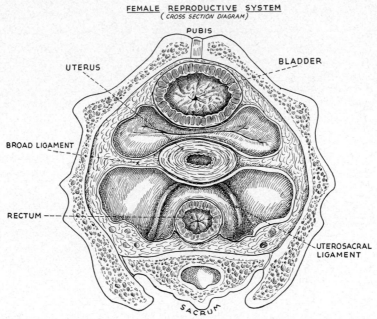

FIG. 17–3. GROSS ANATOMY OF FEMALE REPRODUCTIVE SYSTEM: **b,** Superior cross-sectional diagram

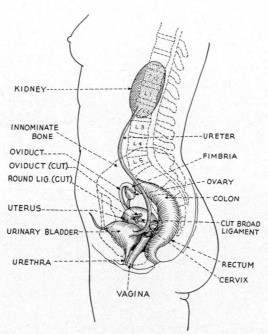

FIG. 17–3. GROSS ANATOMY OF FEMALE REPRODUCTIVE SYSTEM: **c,** Lateral relationships of genitourinary tract.

axis is usually vertical in the erect position. The right ovary is usually slightly larger than the left, and the length varies from 2.5 to 5 cm. The width is ordinarily one half the length and the thickness one half the width.

The oviducts, or uterine tubes, are two trumpet-shaped tubes which run in the superior border of the broad ligament between the uterine horns and the lateral pelvic walls. The dilated end lies over each ovary. Each oviduct is from 7 to 14 cm. in length. Ordinarily, the fimbriated end and mouth of the infundibulum rest upon the medial end of the ovary. The course of the oviducts is rather variable, and may be different on the two sides.

The uterus is a pear-shaped organ with a body or fundus, and a downward extension, the cervix, with supravaginal and vaginal sections. The cavity of the body is flattened transversely and has a triangular shape, being broad above where each cornua communicates with an oviduct and narrow below where it communicates with the canal in the cervix. The direction of the axis of the uterus is quite variable. Ordinarily a moderate degree of anteflexion is considered the normal position, making an angle of 80 to 120 degrees with the horizontal. There may also be a slight list to the right or to the left side.

The vagina extends from the uterus to the external genitalia where it opens to the exterior. Its course roughly parallels the anterior curvature of the sacrum and averages 5 to 7 cm. in length.

Bony Pelvis. In addition to the normal anatomic landmarks of the pelvis described in Chapter 5, certain areas should receive the attention of the radiologist as having an influence on the course of labor. Differences characteristic of male and female types should be borne in mind. These areas are as follows:

1. THE SUBPUBIC ARCH (Fig. 17–4). Note should be made of the bones of the pubic rami, whether they are delicate, average or heavy; whether the pubic angle is wide or curved (female) or narrow and straight (male), and whether the side walls of the forepelvis are divergent, straight or convergent. The configuration of the pelvic arch is a guide to the capacity of the true pelvis.

2. THE ISCHIAL SPINES. These are classified as sharp, average or anthropoid. Sharp spines are definitely a male characteristic and when present, direct the attention to the necessity for a more detailed examination of the pelvis, as they may be associated with converging side walls of the forepelvis. The anthropoid spines are blunt and shallow.

3. THE SACROSCIATIC NOTCH AND SACRUM. The capacity of the posterior pelvic inlet is related to the width of the sacrosciatic notch and the configuration of its apex. The male pelvis shows a long narrow notch with a high rounded apex and the female a wide notch with a blunt apex.

The inclination of the sacrum directly affects the capacity of the birth canal since a forward tilt will offer a barrier to normal delivery. If the forepelvis is wide and divergent, compensation occurs but if convergent, a funnel pelvis will result. The female sacrum is wide and short compared with that of the male.

The curvature of the sacrum on the lateral projection is also important. Normally the sacrum is concave anteriorly. When this curvature is absent owing to any developmental aberration, the midpelvis is diminished and the progress of labor is impeded. The absence of this curvature will be readily apparent from measurements to be described below.

a

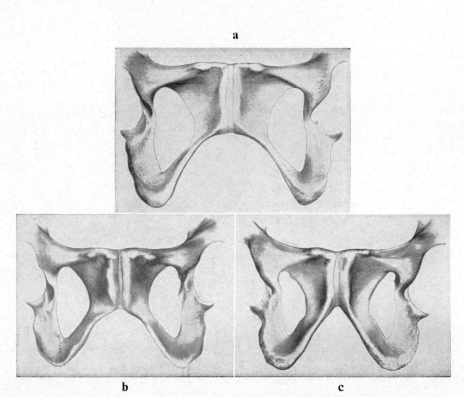

b   c

Fig. 17–4. VARIATIONS IN SIZE AND SHAPE OF THE SUBPUBIC ARCH. **a,** Delicate bones; wide angle; well-curved female type of pubic rami. **b,** Average bones; moderate angle; average curvature of pubic rami. **c,** Heavy bones; narrow angle; straight masculine type of pubic rami. (From Golden. *Diagnostic Roentgenology*, vol. 2, Thomas Nelson and Sons, Publisher.)

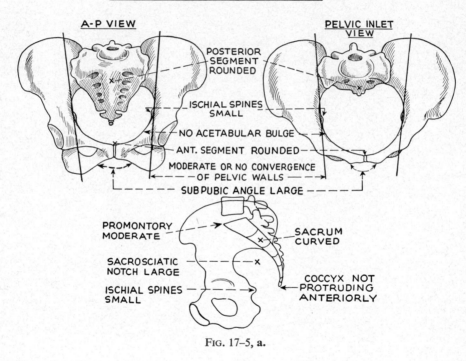

FIG. 17–5, a.

FACTORS STUDIED IN PELVIC ARCHITECTURE

1. PELVIC INLET STUDY *(SEE DIAGRAMS OF DIFFERENT PELVIC TYPES)*

2. PROMINENCE OF ISCHIAL SPINES

3. CONVERGENCE OF LATERAL PELVIC WALLS

4. SUBPUBIC ANGLE

5. CURVATURE OF SACRUM

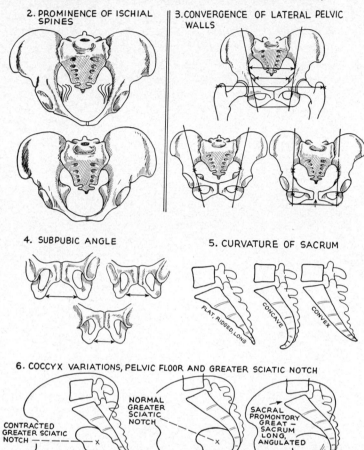

FLAT, RIDGED LONG   CONCAVE   CONVEX

6. COCCYX VARIATIONS, PELVIC FLOOR AND GREATER SCIATIC NOTCH

CONTRACTED GREATER SCIATIC NOTCH -- -- -- X

NORMAL GREATER SCIATIC NOTCH

LARGE, RIGID ANGULATED COCCYX

SACRAL PROMONTORY GREAT -- SACRUM LONG, ANGULATED

MAY BE CALCIFICATION IN SACRO-SCIATIC LIGAMENTS

7. UTERINE AXIS FACTOR IN RELATION TO SACRUM AND SACRAL PROMONTORY

A. AXIS OF UTERUS NEAR SPINE, GOOD FLEXION OF HEAD

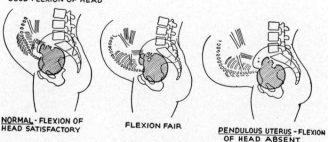

NORMAL - FLEXION OF HEAD SATISFACTORY

FLEXION FAIR

PENDULOUS UTERUS - FLEXION OF HEAD ABSENT

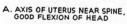

FIG. 17–5, b.

4. THE PELVIC INLET.[3] The pelvic inlet with its variations forms the basis for the classification of all pelves into four major types (Fig. 17–6):

The inlet of the anthropoid pelvis is relatively long in antero-posterior measurements and narrow in transverse diameter. The pelvic arch is usually wider then normal and the sacrosciatic notch is wide and shallow when seen in the lateral view. The anthropoid type is so called because it closely resembles the pelves found in the higher apes.

The gynecoid type pelvis refers to the average type as seen in the human female. The inlet is round or slightly oval, the pubic angle is wide, and the sacrosciatic notch is also wide. The cavity of the pelvis is ample in all directions.

The android pelvis refers to a female pelvis which has marked masculine characteristics. These include what is described as a blunt heart-shaped or wedge-shaped inlet with narrow forepelvis, and the widest diameter is close to the sacral promontory. A narrow masculine type of sciatic notch is present and the sacrum is set forward in the pelvis. The pubic arch is usually narrow.

The platypelloid or flat pelvis is characterized by an inlet with a transversely oval shape. The antero-posterior diameter is short and the greatest transverse diameter of the pelvis is wide—this diameter occurring well in front of the sacrum. The angle of the forepelvis is wide also, but the sacrosciatic notch and subpubic angle will vary in size.

It should be stated that gradations between all types are seen and individual variations should be described as they appear on the radiograph.

The reader is referred to the work of Caldwell and Moloy[3] on this subject.

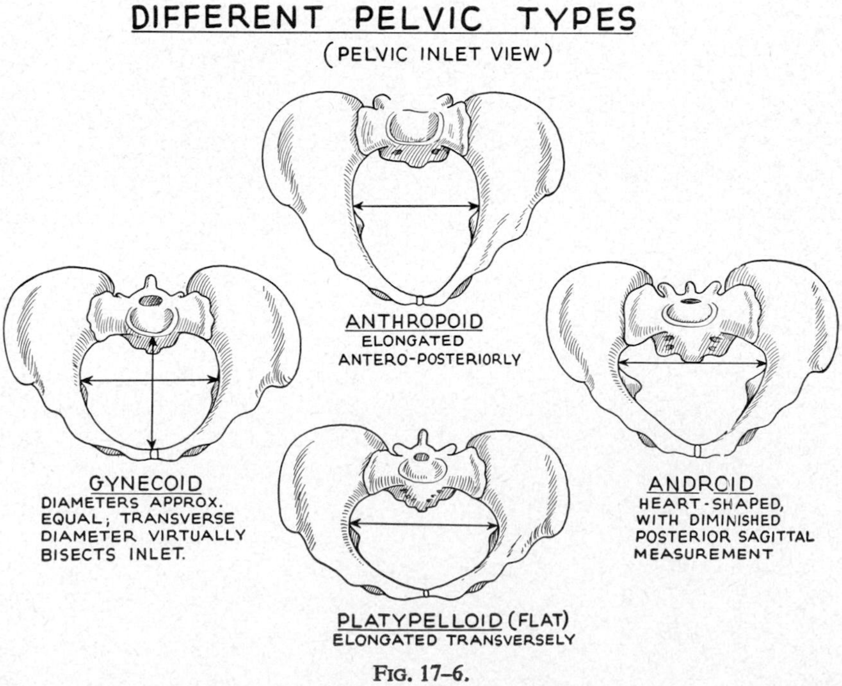

DIFFERENT PELVIC TYPES
(PELVIC INLET VIEW)

ANTHROPOID
ELONGATED
ANTERO-POSTERIORLY

GYNECOID
DIAMETERS APPROX.
EQUAL; TRANSVERSE
DIAMETER VIRTUALLY
BISECTS INLET.

ANDROID
HEART-SHAPED,
WITH DIMINISHED
POSTERIOR SAGITTAL
MEASUREMENT

PLATYPELLOID (FLAT)
ELONGATED TRANSVERSELY

FIG. 17–6.

METHODS OF STUDY OF THE FEMALE GENITAL SYSTEM

In the entire description below of the applications and usefulness of radiographic techniques in investigation of obstetrical and gynecologic problems, the student must bear in mind those aspects of radiologic protection which pertain here (see Chap. 2). The information to be gained must justify the exposure of the patient (and the fetus, if one be present). In any case, radiation exposure of the patient and the fetus in the first trimester of pregnancy is to be avoided unless the problem at hand be a critical one.

Direct Radiography and Its Applications. Antero-posterior, lateral and oblique views of the pelvis are obtained and a considerable amount of information is available from these views (Fig. 17–7):

1. The configuration of the maternal pelvis can be ascertained as judged by the standard bony types described above. It is important to comment on individual bony differences irrespective of the four major pelvic types.

2. An indication of the age of the fetus is obtained or a decision as to the maturity of the fetus can be reached. Perhaps, the best index of the former is the fetal length. Haase has suggested that for clinical purposes the length of the embryo in centimeters may be approximated during the first five months by squaring the number of the month to which the pregnancy has advanced; in the second half of pregnancy by multiplying the month by five as shown in the following table:

At the end of the first month	1 x 1	1 cm. in length
At the end of the second month	2 x 2	4 cm. in length
At the end of the third month	3 x 3	9 cm. in length
At the end of the fourth month	4 x 4	16 cm. in length
At the end of the fifth month	5 x 5	25 cm. in length
At the end of the sixth month	6 x 5	30 cm. in length
At the end of the seventh month	7 x 5	35 cm. in length
At the end of the eighth month	8 x 5	40 cm. in length
At the end of the ninth month	9 x 5	45 cm. in length
At the end of the tenth month	10 x 5	50 cm. in length

There are also several tables and graphs available for computing fetal age from roentgen measurements of the fetal skull (Figs. 17–8, 17–9, 17–10). Thus, from the anthropometric studies of Scammon and Calkins,[5] Paul C. Hodges[4] has prepared graphs from which the age of the fetus is readily determined in terms of weeks, from the occipitofrontal diameter in centimeters (Fig. 17–8) or from the biparietal diameter (Fig. 17–9); a third graph in terms of the average net circumference of a fetal skull obtained from two roentgenograms taken at right angles to one another (Fig. 17–10); and a fourth graph based upon the length of the calcified portion of the femoral shaft, which we consider of less value, roentgenographically, since distortion makes it very difficult to be certain one is obtaining the true length of the femoral diaphysis (graph not reproduced here).

The radiologist may be called upon to offer an opinion as to the maturity of the fetus. Authorities suggest the following as salient criteria:

An ossification center is present in the distal end of the femur in 90 per cent of term fetuses; ossification of the hyoid bone is complete; and five out of six cases will show ossification in the proximal tibial epiphysis.

Less practical standards are the ossification of the essential parts of vertebrae, the first segments of the coccyx, and the metacarpals and phalanges.

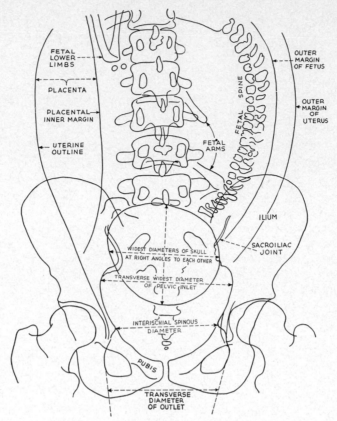

FIG. 17–7. TRACING OF RADIOGRAPH ROUTINELY EMPLOYED IN PELVICEPHALOMETRY: **a,** Antero-posterior (position same as KUB film).

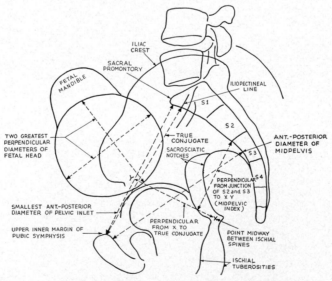

FIG. 17–7. TRACING OF RADIOGRAPH ROUTINELY EMPLOYED IN PELVICEPHALOMETRY: **b,** Lateral (position same as lateral abdomen or lumbar spine).

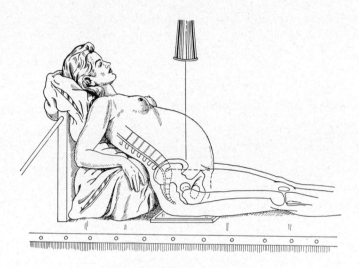

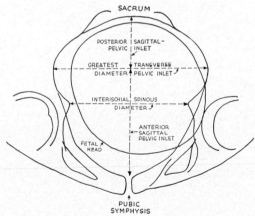

SACRUM

POSTERIOR | SAGITTAL–
PELVIC | INLET

GREATEST _ TRANSVERSE
DIAMETER | PELVIC INLET

INTERISCHIAL SPINOUS
DIAMETER

ANTERIOR
SAGITTAL
PELVIC INLET

FETAL
HEAD

PUBIC
SYMPHYSIS

FIG. 17–7. TRACING OF RADIOGRAPH ROUTINELY EMPLOYED IN PELVICEPHALOMETRY: **c,** Special view of pelvic inlet, showing positioning of patient (note the pelvic inlet is parallel to the table top) and tracing of radiograph so obtained.

It should be remembered that good films are essential to obtain the necessary detail.

3. The presentation and position of the fetus can be determined.

4. The degree of flexion of the fetal head and spine can be noted.

5. The viability of the fetus can be confirmed.

6. The progress of labor can be followed.

7. The diagnosis of multiple pregnancy or fetal abnormality can be made.

8. The detection of the early fetus is possible. Antero-posterior and oblique films of the pelvis are obtained; and the position described under the heading of pelvic pneumoperitoneum is also useful. The oblique films are especially helpful as a small fetus may be obscured by the sacrum in the antero-posterior film. Good films will detect the fetal skeleton as early as three and one-half months.

9. The position of the placenta can be ascertained.

Direct antero-posterior and lateral views of the abdomen are usually sufficient in our experience to delineate the placenta as a crescentic shadow lying

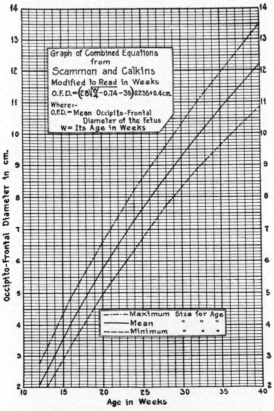

FIG. 17-8. Graph for computation of fetal age in weeks from net occipitofrontal diameter. (From Hodges, in Am. J. Roentgenol., vol. 37.)

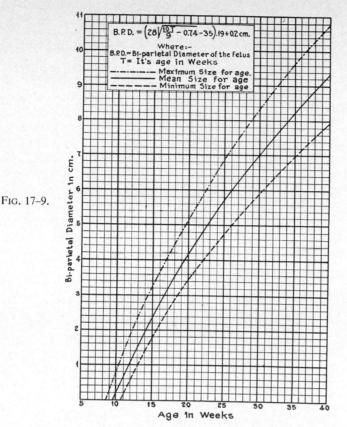

FIG. 17–9.

FIG. 17–9. Graph for computation of fetal age in weeks from biparietal diameter. (From Hodges. in Am. J. Roentgenol., vol. 37.)

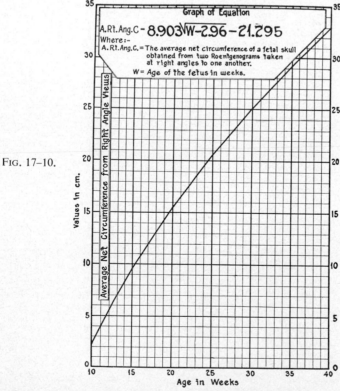

FIG. 17–10.

FIG. 17–10. Graph for computation of fetal age in weeks from average corrected circumference of skull obtained from two radiographs taken at right angles to one another. (From Hodges, in Am. J. Roentgenol., vol. 37.)

between the fetus and boundary of the uterus. A wedge-type barium or plastic filter may be utilized to obtain better detail in placentography.

Combination air rectograms and cystograms are useful in making certain that the placenta is not implanted low in the uterus. When air is injected in the rectum and urinary bladder, and a lateral film of this obtained, a placenta which is implanted low will produce an opacity projected in the air medium (Fig. 17–11) and thus may be recognized.

This method is of value in cephalic presentations, and particularly in a central type of placenta praevia where the placenta intervenes between head and bladder. The erect position must be employed to make sure the fetal head is pressing upon the dome of the urinary bladder, and that gravity and the weight of the fetus are forcing the head downward.

Radiography after the injection of opaque fluid such as Diodrast into the amniotic sac (amniography) has been employed by some, but it frequently induces labor, and has been known to be associated with fetal death of undetermined cause. It is therefore probably seldom, if ever, indicated.

Pelvic Pneumoperitoneum.[2]   A needle is inserted 2 to 3 cm. below and to the left of the umbilicus. Oxygen, carbon dioxide or nitrous oxide is introduced into the peritoneal space with the patient in the Trendelenburg position (hips above the level of the head). Films are thereafter obtained (Fig. 17–12) in the postero-anterior position with the patient tilted head downward approximately 50 degrees and the central x-ray beam centered over the rectum, the beam being directed vertically downward.

Pelvic pneumoperitoneum allows visualization of the ovaries, oviducts and uterine fundus. The uterus appears as (Fig. 17–12) a dome-shaped structure projecting above the pubic symphysis, and measures approximately 3 to 5 cm. on the usual projection. The ovaries are projected on the lateral pelvic walls as ovoid shadows. There is a homogeneous air shadow above.

Hysterosalpingography with Opaque Media (Fig. 17–13). The most common opaque media employed are Lipiodol, Iodochlorol, Lipoiodine, Rayopaque, Skiodan acacia, or Salpix. A suitable cannula, which at the same time obstructs the cervical canal, is inserted into the cervical canal of the uterus. Approximately 6 cc. of the opaque medium is injected and an antero-posterior film is obtained. If there is inadequate filling of any portion another 3 cc. is injected, and stereoscopic films are obtained while injecting an additional 2 to 3 cc. of dye. When iodized oil is used, another film is obtained in twenty-four hours to detect the extent of overflow into the pelvis through the oviducts. Serial films may be obtained if there is an obvious constriction of one of the tubes, and it is desired to detect the constancy of this finding. When Rayopaque or the other absorbable media are employed, serial films at fifteen- to twenty-minute intervals are obtained. Ordinarily, in one to two hours all the dye is reabsorbed and appears in the urinary bladder.

Hysterosalpingography is particularly useful in cases of sterility and to prove or disprove the patency of the tubes. This examination delineates the uterine cavity, shows the length, shape and position of the oviducts, and the patency of one or both tubes. A variable amount of fluid escapes into the pelvis proper.

ROENTGEN STUDY OF THE PLACENTA

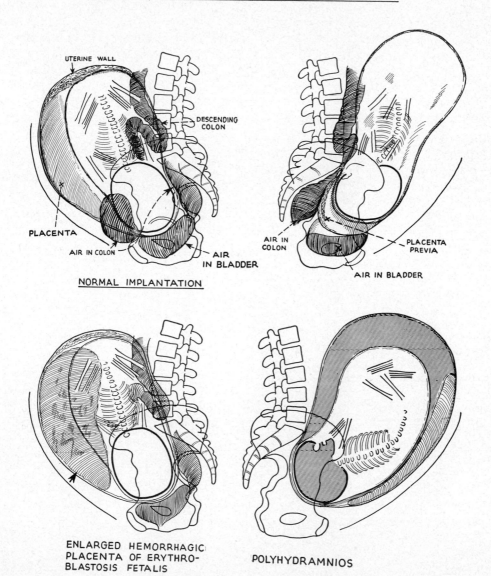

NORMAL IMPLANTATION

ENLARGED HEMORRHAGIC
PLACENTA OF ERYTHRO-
BLASTOSIS FETALIS

POLYHYDRAMNIOS

FIG. 17–11.   Radiographic appearance of normal placental implantation compared with appearances of abnormal implantations. The placenta previa is shown in good contrast by means of air distention of both the bladder and the rectum.

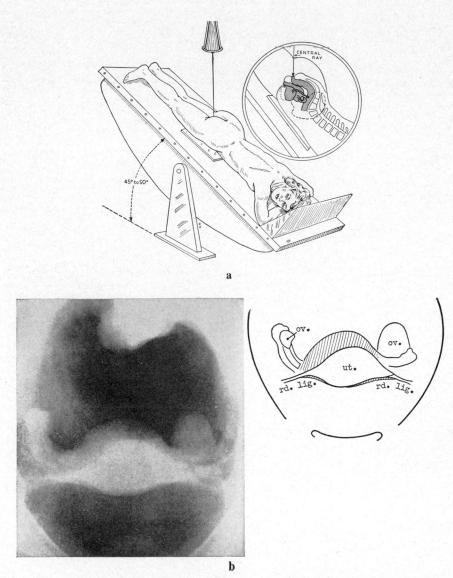

FIG. 17–12.   PELVIC PNEUMOPERITONEUM.   **a,** Position of patient. **b,** Gynecogram with explanatory diagram, showing large left ovary. (**b** from Granjon, A.: Presse med., vol. 61, 1953.)

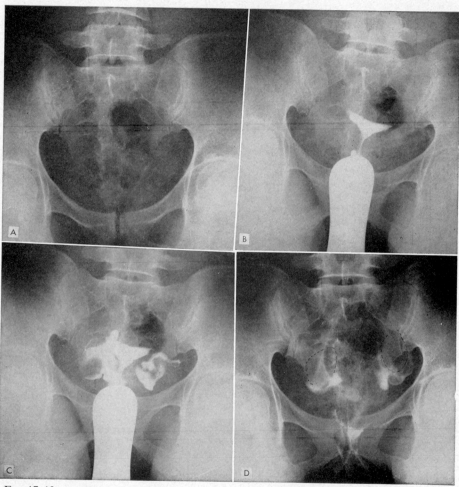

FIG. 17–13. RADIOGRAPHS DEMONSTRATING ROUTINE FILMS OBTAINED BY HYSTEROSALPINGOGRAPHY WITH SOLUBLE, ABSORBABLE MEDIUM. A, Preliminary scout film prior to the injection of the first medium. B, Film obtained after the insertion of the first 2 cc. fraction. C, Radiograph obtained after the fourth insertion of the 2 cc. fraction. This radiograph demonstrates spillage into the pelvic peritoneal space. D, Film obtained 20 minutes after the injection, showing the opaque medium still to be present in the pelvic peritoneal space, but already some of the medium has been absorbed and is appearing in the urinary bladder. Dotted areas indicate the impression of the ovaries upon the contrast medium.

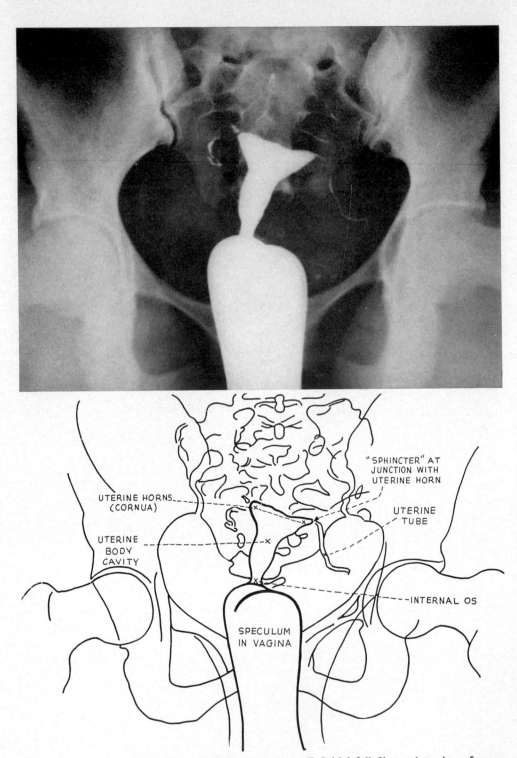

FIG. 17–13. HYSTEROSALPINGOGRAPHY WITH LIPIODOL: *E,* Initial full film and tracing of same.

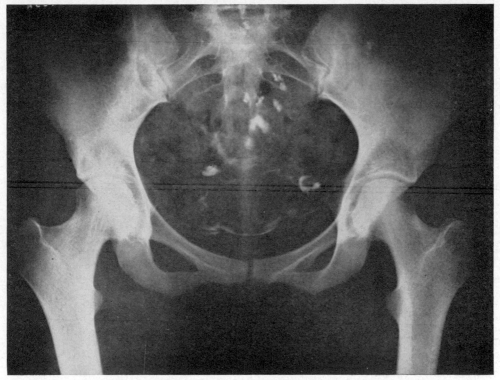

FIG. 17–13. HYSTEROSALPINGOGRAPHY WITH LIPIODOL: *F*, Twenty-four hour film.

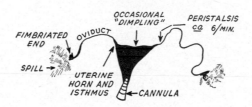

FIG. 17–13. *G*, Diagrams illustrating the normal roentgen findings in hysterosalpingography.

PELVIC MENSURATION AND FETAL CEPHALOMETRY

The purpose of this investigation is to determine by the process of measurements made on radiographs whether or not disproportion exists between the fetal head and maternal pelvis. It should be stated that this examination can only determine the *mathematical* relationship of the fetal head to the maternal pelvis. *No prognostication as to whether or not spontaneous delivery will occur is possible in view of the multitude of other factors which are involved,* such as the extent of molding of the fetal head, or uterine inertia.

These measurements can be made on the routine films described below, but the calculations are complicated by the necessity for correction of the magnification present. This problem is overcome by applying a correction factor for magnification, and different methods of pelvimetry differ primarily in their method of correction.

A teleroentgenographic technique may be employed which minimizes magnification, and the films are usually taken at a distance of 6 feet. This method requires relatively high-powered equipment, but is readily applicable in many hospital laboratories with tall ceilings and floor-to-ceiling tube stands, and we have found it most convenient in our own laboratory. A magnification of approximately 10 per cent is obtained for a part 15 cm. from the film, and this correction is readily applied. A lesser correction is applied for measurement of parts closer to the film. Not only is error in measurement minimized by this method, but one also obtains better detail and an immediate visual impression of the relative size of the fetal head with respect to the pelvis which has proved very valuable.

In cephalic presentations, the same film may be employed for measurement of both the fetal head and the pelvis. In breech presentations, it is advisable to obtain separate films centered over the fetal head, in addition to the films of the pelvis, to obviate distortion caused by divergence of the x-ray beam.

It should be emphasized that the part to be examined should be parallel with the film surface to eliminate distortion, otherwise distortion must also be taken into consideration (see Chap. 1).

In all these examinations, care must be exercised not to alter the position of the patient in the change from the antero-posterior to lateral projection since the one view is utilized to obtain measurements which are utilized in correction for magnification in the other view. Such care is less important in the teleroentgenographic method since small changes in position do not reflect significant changes in magnification; in all other methods, these changes are especially important, particularly in breech presentations, or when the fetal head is not engaged.

Thus, if the patient is supine for the antero-posterior film, the patient should remain so for the lateral view, and a horizontal x-ray beam should be employed.

The erect position has the advantage of simplifying this procedure, but the greater difficulty of obtaining good films in the erect position on a pregnant woman offsets this advantage.

In all methods other than the teleroentgenographic method a considerable inaccuracy will be introduced if the patient does not remain in the same position for both antero-posterior and lateral views; if it is not possible to do this in any installation, a deficiency in accuracy must be recognized and so stated.

The usual views obtained are as follows: (1) antero-posterior view of the pelvis and fetal head (Fig. 17–7, **a**); (2) lateral view of the pelvis and fetal head (Fig. 17–7, **b**); (3) a direct view of the pelvic inlet (Fig. 17–7, **c**). The patient sits on the table top, the back making an angle of about 45 degrees with the table. The patient is adjusted so that the pelvic inlet will be parallel with the table top. The central ray is directed central to the pelvic inlet. If possible, 72-inch film-target distance should be employed to produce a minimum magnification. With short film-target distances, the pelvic inlet will be considerably magnified and somewhat distorted, in view of the relatively great distance of the pelvic inlet from the film. (4) Occasionally a special view of the pelvic outlet is made with the patient sitting and leaning forward, so that the ischial tuberosities are in contact with the table top, and the remainder of the body does not obscure them.

Whatever method of taking these films is employed, it is important to know the film-to-target and film-to-table-top distances accurately to correct for the magnification present.

If a breech presentation is present, additional antero-posterior and lateral views centering over the fetal head are made.

The Customary Measurements Made on the Radiographs (Fig. 17–14). It is important to emphasize that we are comparing the measurements of the particular fetus in question with the maternal pelvis and that the data needed are present on the films and are obtained as described. *No average pelvic or fetal measurements are included, as each case has to be judged on its own merits.*

Having obtained satisfactory films, it is necessary to ascertain the following measurements:

MEASUREMENTS TO GAUGE THE SIZE OF THE INLET. 1. *The greatest transverse diameter of the pelvic inlet* is obtained from the special view of the pelvic inlet and from the antero-posterior view of the pelvis.

2. *The antero-posterior diameter of the pelvic inlet* (true conjugate) is obtained from the lateral projection. The measurement is taken from the posterior margin of the symphysis pubis to the point where the shadow of the iliopectineal line crosses the sacrum, or to the top of the sacral promontory, whichever distance is smaller.

3. *The ratio of the posterior sagittal dimension of the inlet to the total antero-posterior diameter* is obtained. To obtain this measurement, the greatest transverse diameter of the inlet is drawn on the film of the special view of the inlet. Since an accurate measurement for this is available from the antero-posterior view of the pelvis, a magnification correction factor is thus obtained by comparing the latter with the former. On the inlet view a perpendicular is drawn from this greatest dimension to the middle of the sacral promontory and also to the middle of the pubic symphysis. The former measurement is spoken of as the posterior sagittal measurement of the inlet and the latter as the anterior sagittal measurement of the inlet. Accurate correction for these measurements is obtained from the correction factor mentioned above. Ideally, the ratio of the anterior to the posterior sagittal diameters of the inlet should approach unity in a gynecoid pelvis.

Measurements Taken to Gauge the Size of the Midpelvis. 1. *The inter-ischial spinous diameter* is drawn on the antero-posterior view of the pelvis, but may be obtained from the special view of the inlet if a correction factor is known for this view.

2. *The midpelvic index* is obtained by the following proecdure: (*a*) A perpendicular is drawn from the ischial spines to the true conjugate on the lateral projection. (*b*) A second perpendicular is then drawn from the junction of the second and third sacral vertebrae to the perpendicular described in (*a*). This measurement is known as the midpelvic index. The midpelvic index may be considered the radius of a plane surface whose diameter is representative of the plane of the midpelvis. This midpelvic index is doubled and then can be compared with the average diameter of the fetal skull in order to judge the capacity of the midpelvis.

3. *The antero-posterior measurement of the midpelvis* is obtained by measuring the line drawn from the posterior aspect of the pubic symphysis to the middle of the third sacral vertebral body.

Measurements Taken to Gauge the Size of the Pelvic Outlet. 1. A tangent is drawn from the outer margin of the obturator foramen to meet the ischial tuberosity. The distance between these tangents is then measured and is an index of the *transverse diameter of the outlet*.

2. *An antero-posterior diameter of the pelvic outlet* is obtained by drawing a line from the inferior posterior margin of the pubic symphysis to the tip of the sacrum (or coccyx). (It should be specified as to whether or not the sacrum or coccyx was utilized.) Obstetrically the sacral measurement is considered more important.

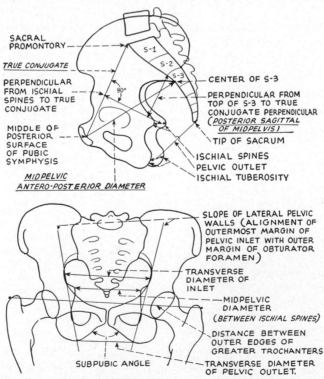

Fig. 17–14. **a,** Diagrams illustrating the various measurements which are obtained from routine antero-posterior and lateral teleroentgenograms of the pelvis for pelvic measurement.

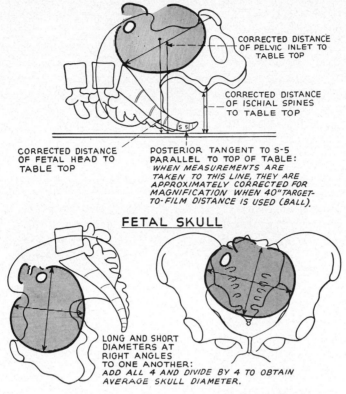

FETAL SKULL

FIG. 17–14. **b,** Diagrams illustrating the various measurements of the fetal head which are obtained and compared with the pelvic measurements.

MEASUREMENTS TO GAUGE THE SIZE OF THE FETAL HEAD. 1. The greatest diameter of the fetal skull is obtained on both the antero-posterior and lateral projections.

2. The greatest diameter perpendicular to (1) is drawn on both the antero-posterior and lateral projections.

3. An average is made of the measurements obtained in (1) and (2). This is spoken of as the *average diameter of the fetal skull.* Two to three millimeters are usually added to this measurement to compensate for the soft tissues of the scalp.

4. The volume of the fetal head may be computed (or obtained readily from nomograms [Fig. 17–15, **a**]), by utilizing the average diameter in (3). The geometric formula volume $= 4/3 \pi r^3$ applies, where r is one-half the diameter.

THE INTERPRETATION OF THE MEASUREMENTS. Having obtained the above measurements of the pelvis and the average diameter of the fetal head, each pelvic measurement is compared with the fetal head diameter. Obviously when the average inlet, midpelvic and outlet diameters exceed the average diameter of the fetal head, no disproportion exists. When the average diameter of the fetal head exceeds the average diameter of any of the above pelvic planes, further computation is necessary as follows:

The average pelvic diameter in question is considered the diameter of a sphere and as such the volume of this sphere is calculated or obtained from nomograms (Fig. 17–15, **a**). This volume is compared with the fetal head volume as previously computed. When the fetal head volume exceeds the volume capacity of the inlet by 70 cc. or less, or the volume capacity of the bispinous diameter by 50 to 220 cc., the incidence of cesarean section would be about 33 per cent. Greater excesses beyond these limits would increase difficult delivery, and cesarean section incidence accordingly,[7] up to 80 to 87 per cent.

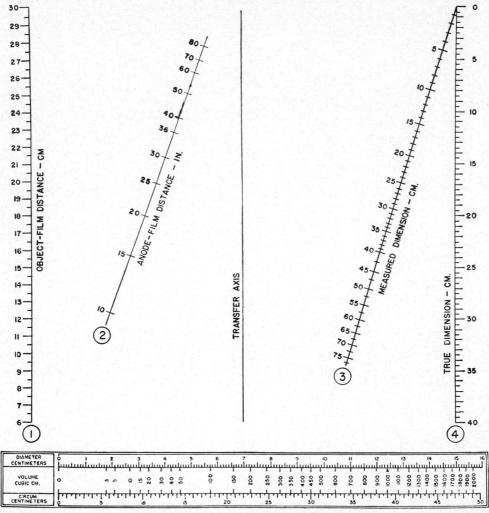

Fig. 17–15. **a,** Nomograms for correction of magnification and for conversion of diameters to volumes. (After Holmquest, from Golden, *Diagnostic Roentgenology,* Thomas Nelson and Sons, Publishers.) With a straight edge, a line is drawn from the object-film distance (*1*) of a certain dimension through the anode-film distance (*2*) used when the film was taken to the transfer axis. From this point on the transfer axis, a line is drawn through the dimension as measured on the film (*3*) which intersects (*4*) at the true, corrected dimension. With the table at the bottom of the nomogram a circumference or a diameter measurement in centimeters can be transposed directly to volume of a similar sphere in terms of cubic centimeters.

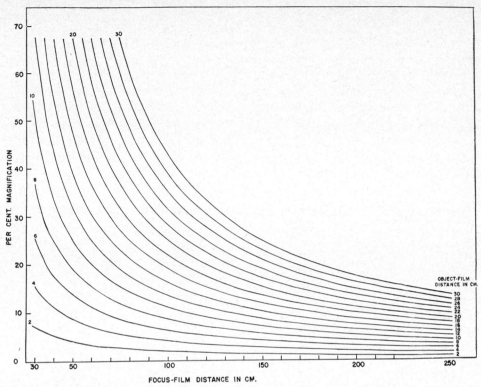

FIG. 17–15. **b,** Graph demonstrating the per cent magnification readily obtained when one knows the focus-film distance in centimeters and the object-film distance in centimeters. (Courtesy of T. H. Oddie, D.Sc.)

It should be emphasized that it is impossible to predict the delivery of the fetus by any mathematical calculation, since there are other variables besides the actual measurements, such as the forcefulness of the contractions, deformities of the pelvis, tumors within the pelvis, uterine inertia, and the like. The main purpose of studying pelvic measurements is to permit a better understanding of the course of labor, and to contribute toward an ultimate decision when all factors have been considered in each individual case. A study of the bony pelvis and the variations described earlier is also important.

Moreover, any consideration of the pelvis without the study of the term fetal head may be considered inadequate. Indeed, probably the greatest contribution of radiology lies in the field of a radiographic study of the progress of the labor.

Method for Correction of Magnification.[6] The degree of magnification will vary in accordance with the distance between the x-ray tube target and the film, and the distance between the diameter (or distance) to be measured and the film. If the dimension in question is parallel with the film surface, distortion is eliminated. If the target-to-film distance is known and also the object-to-film distance, it is possible to calculate accurately the true measurement of the part. This may be accomplished by graphs or nomograms (Fig. 17–15, **a, b**) (Ball, Snow), stereoscopic films (Caldwell and Moloy), metal notched rules placed next to the part being radiographed (Colcher-Sussman), or perforated metal plates superimposed on the radiograph (Thoms).

In those methods that employ calculation, graphs or nomograms to determine the degree of magnification, the basic procedure is as follows:

1. The desired dimension is measured on the one radiograph, whether it be the antero-posterior or lateral view.

2. The distance that this dimension is placed from the film is determined from the other radiograph. Thus, to determine this object-to-film distance for dimensions measured on the antero-posterior view, the lateral radiograph is employed, and vice versa.

3. There will, however, be an error of magnification on this second radiograph also, which must be corrected before it can be applied as the object-to-table-top distance.

4. In order to obtain object-to-film distance, the object-to-table-top distance is first calculated, and to this figure is added the known table-top-to-film distance (usually 5 cm.).

5. Only those dimensions in the central ray can be measured, unless the teleroentgenographic method is employed where beam divergence is negligible.

6. The following triangulation laws are applied (Fig. 17–16):

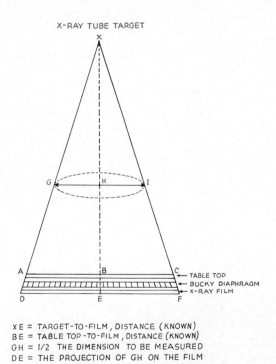

XE = TARGET-TO-FILM, DISTANCE (KNOWN)
BE = TABLE TOP-TO-FILM, DISTANCE (KNOWN)
GH = 1/2 THE DIMENSION TO BE MEASURED
DE = THE PROJECTION OF GH ON THE FILM
     AND HENCE THE MEASUREMENT OBTAIN-
     ED FROM THE FILM (KNOWN)
HB = THE DISTANCE OF DIMENSION GH FROM
     THE TABLE TOP (KNOWN FROM FILM IN
     OPPOSITE VIEW AFTER CORRECTED FOR
     MAGNIFICATION)

FIG. 17–16.   Triangulation method of determining radiographic magnification (see text).

FORMAT FOR REPORTING CEPHALOPELVIC MEASUREMENTS
Measurements

Inlet		Average Normal (cm.)	Volume
(1) A-P		10.5–11.5	
(2) Transverse		11.5–13.5	
Average of A-P and Transverse			*

Midpelvis			Volumes
(1) A-P		11.0–12.0	
(2) Post. Sag. Index		Greater than 5.0	
(3) 2 x P.S.I.		Greater than 10.0	
(4) Interischial spinous		10.0–11.0	
Average (1) + (4)			*
Average (3) + (4)			*

Outlet

Intertub.		9.5–10.5	
Fetal Head		Average Normal	Volumes
A-P view (a) Long			
(b) + to (a)			
Lat. view (c) Long			
(b) + to (c)			
Ave. a, b, c, d.		10.0–11.0	

Relation of Fetal Head Volume to:		Head Greater by:	Pelvis Greater by:
	Pelvic inlet	cc.	cc.
	Midpelvis	cc.	cc.

FIG. 17–17. **a.** (All measurements are recorded after correction for magnification.)

PELVIC ARCHITECTURE
(Encircle)

Inlet:	Gynecoid	Anthropoid	Platypelloid	Android
Inlet Plane:	Near	Horizontal	Oblique	Vertical
Uterine Axis:		Posterior	Oblique ant.	Pendulous
Promontory:		Great	Moderate	Slight
Sacrum:		Concave ant.	Flat	Convex ant.
		Short	Medium	Long
Sacrosciatic Notch:		Acute	Medium	Obtuse
Spines:		Large	Medium	Small
Acetabular Bulge:		None	Slight	Marked
Lateral Wall Converg.:		None	Moderate	Funnel
Subpubic Notch:		Gynecoid	Medium	Android

Position of Fetus:
Engagement of Fetus:
Estimated Age of Fetus:
Position of Placenta:
Amniotic Fluid: Normal—Excess.

FIG. 17–17.   *b*, Format for recording cephalo-pelvic measurements; pelvic architectute. (Modified from Snow, W.: *Roentgenology in Obstetrics and Gynecology.* Springfield, Illinois, Charles C Thomas, 1952.)

$$\frac{GH \text{ (unknown)}}{DE \text{ (known)}} = \frac{XH}{XE} = \frac{XE - (HB + BE) \text{ (known)}}{XE \qquad \text{(known)}}$$

From this equation, it is obvious that all factors are known except GH and hence, simple algebraic solution is possible. Snow's special calculator or Ball's nomograms allow one to obtain this algebraic solution directly.

Method of Reporting.   In reporting, one section is devoted entirely to the various measurements; these are given in tabular fashion (Figure 17–17). The theoretical fetal skull diameter, perimeter and volume are also indicated relative to the dimensions of the pelvic inlet and midpelvis.

The second portion of the report should refer to pelvic architecture and details concerning fetus, placenta and amniotic fluid (Fig. 17–17, **b**).

Radiation Hazard.   Attention is once again drawn to the aspect of radiation hazard, particularly to the fetus, in all roentgen diagnostic studies (see Chapter 2). Certainly, if pregnancy is known, radiation should be avoided in the first trimester of pregnancy at all costs and as much as possible thereafter.

Roentgen studies should be undertaken after carefully weighing the potential risks attendant to radiation exposure as against the information which may be obtained from the study to assist in the management of the clinical problem at hand.

REFERENCES

1. Ball, R. P., and Golden, R.: American Journal of Roentgenology, *49:* 731–741, 1943.
2. Buice, J. W., and Gould, D. M.: Abdominal and Pelvic Pneumography. Radiology, *69:* 704–710, 1957.
3. Caldwell, W. E., and Moloy, H. C.: Anatomical Variations in the Female Pelvis and their Effect in Labor with a Suggested Classification. Am. J. Obst. & Gynec., *26:* 479–503, 1933.
4. Hodges, Paul C.: Roentgen Pelvimetry and Fetometry. Am. J. Roentgenol., *37:* 644–662, 1937.
5. Scammon, R. E., and Calkins, L. A.: *The Development and Growth of the Human Body in the Fetal Period.* University of Minnesota Press, Minneapolis, 1929.
6. Schwarz, G. S.: A Simplified Method of Correcting Roentgenologic Measurements of the Maternal Pelvis and Fetal Skull. Am. J. Roentgenol., *71:* 115–120, 1954.
7. Schwarz, G. S.: Editorial. Radiology, *64:* 874–876, 1955.
8. Schwarz, G. S.: Roentgenometric Classification of Cephalopelvic Disproportion. Radiology, *64:* 742, 1955.
9. Snow, W.: *Roentgenology in Obstetrics and Gynecology.* Charles C Thomas, Springfield, Illinois, 1952.

INDEX